Dentistry: A Multidisciplinary Approach

Dentistry: A Multidisciplinary Approach

Giuseppe Minervini
Stefania Moccia

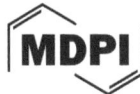

Basel • Beijing • Wuhan • Barcelona • Belgrade • Novi Sad • Cluj • Manchester

Editors

Giuseppe Minervini
Multidisciplinary Department
of Medical-Surgical and
Dental Specialties
University of Campania
"Luigi Vanvitelli"
Naples
Italy

Stefania Moccia
National Research Council
Institute of Food Sciences
Avellino
Italy

Editorial Office
MDPI AG
Grosspeteranlage 5
4052 Basel, Switzerland

This is a reprint of articles from the Special Issue published online in the open access journal *Medicina* (ISSN 1648-9144) (available at: www.mdpi.com/journal/medicina/special_issues/K1P2CLC09A).

For citation purposes, cite each article independently as indicated on the article page online and as indicated below:

Lastname, A.A.; Lastname, B.B. Article Title. *Journal Name* **Year**, *Volume Number*, Page Range.

ISBN 978-3-7258-2178-5 (Hbk)
ISBN 978-3-7258-2177-8 (PDF)
doi.org/10.3390/books978-3-7258-2177-8

© 2024 by the authors. Articles in this book are Open Access and distributed under the Creative Commons Attribution (CC BY) license. The book as a whole is distributed by MDPI under the terms and conditions of the Creative Commons Attribution-NonCommercial-NoDerivs (CC BY-NC-ND) license.

Contents

About the Editors ix

Preface xi

Giuseppe Minervini
Dentistry: A Multidisciplinary Approach
Reprinted from: *Medicina* 2024, 60, 401, doi:10.3390/medicina60030401 1

María-de-Lourdes Chávez-Briones, Gilberto Jaramillo-Rangel, Adriana Ancer-Arellano, Jesús Ancer-Rodríguez and Marta Ortega-Martínez
Identification of the Remains of an Adult Using DNA from Their Deciduous Teeth as a Reference Sample
Reprinted from: *Medicina* 2023, 59, 1702, doi:10.3390/medicina59101702 7

Radu Andrei Moga, Cristian Doru Olteanu, Stefan Marius Buru, Mircea Daniel Botez and Ada Gabriela Delean
Cortical and Trabecular Bone Stress Assessment during Periodontal Breakdown–A Comparative Finite Element Analysis of Multiple Failure Criteria
Reprinted from: *Medicina* 2023, 59, 1462, doi:10.3390/medicina59081462 14

Marcin Mikulewicz, Katarzyna Chojnacka and Zbigniew Raszewski
Comparison of Mechanical Properties of Three Tissue Conditioners: An Evaluation In Vitro Study
Reprinted from: *Medicina* 2023, 59, 1359, doi:10.3390/medicina59081359 32

Yasemin Yavuz, Isa An, Betul Yazmaci, Zeki Akkus and Hatice Ortac
Evaluation of Clinical and Oral Findings in Patients with Epidermolysis bullosa
Reprinted from: *Medicina* 2023, 59, 1185, doi:10.3390/medicina59071185 45

Kelly R. V. Villafuerte, Alyssa Teixeira Obeid and Naiara Araújo de Oliveira
Injectable Resin Technique as a Restorative Alternative in a Cleft Lip and Palate Patient: A Case Report
Reprinted from: *Medicina* 2023, 59, 849, doi:10.3390/medicina59050849 56

Gerardo Guzman-Perez, Carlos Alberto Jurado, Francisco X. Azpiazu-Flores, Humberto Munoz-Luna, Kelvin I. Afrashtehfar and Hamid Nurrohman
Soft Tissue Grafting Procedures before Restorations in the Esthetic Zone: A Minimally Invasive Interdisciplinary Case Report
Reprinted from: *Medicina* 2023, 59, 822, doi:10.3390/medicina59050822 66

Saad Mohammad Alqahtani, Shankar T. Gokhale, Mohamed Fadul A. Elagib, Deepti Shrivastava, Raghavendra Reddy Nagate and Badar Awadh Mohammad Alshmrani et al.
Assessment and Correlation of Salivary Ca, Mg, and pH in Smokers and Non-Smokers with Generalized Chronic Periodontitis
Reprinted from: *Medicina* 2023, 59, 765, doi:10.3390/medicina59040765 77

Giuseppe Minervini, Rocco Franco, Maria Maddalena Marrapodi, Vini Mehta, Luca Fiorillo and Almir Badnjević et al.
Gaucher: A Systematic Review on Oral and Radiological Aspects
Reprinted from: *Medicina* 2023, 59, 670, doi:10.3390/medicina59040670 88

Ali Robaian, Abdullah Alqahtani, Khalid Alanazi, Abdulrhman Alanazi, Meshal Almalki and Anas Aljarad et al.
Different Designs of Deep Marginal Elevation and Its Influence on Fracture Resistance of Teeth with Monolith Zirconia Full-Contour Crowns
Reprinted from: *Medicina* 2023, 59, 661, doi:10.3390/medicina59040661 100

Dila Özyılkan, Özgür Tosun and Aylin İslam
The Impact of Anemia-Related Early Childhood Caries on Parents' and Children's Quality of Life
Reprinted from: *Medicina* 2023, 59, 521, doi:10.3390/medicina59030521 111

Mohammed E. Sayed
The Effect of Dentine Desensitizing Agents on the Retention of Cemented Fixed Dental Prostheses: A Systematic Review
Reprinted from: *Medicina* 2023, 59, 515, doi:10.3390/medicina59030515 128

Amelia Anita Boitor, Elena Bianca Varvară, Corina Mirela Prodan, Sorina Sava, Diana Dudea and Adriana Objelean
The Impact of Simulated Bruxism Forces and Surface Aging Treatments on Two Dental Nano-Biocomposites—A Radiographic and Tomographic Analysis
Reprinted from: *Medicina* 2023, 59, 360, doi:10.3390/medicina59020360 146

Kinga Mária Jánosi, Diana Cerghizan, Florentin Daniel Berneanu, Alpár Kovács, Andrea Szász and Izabella Mureșan et al.
Full-Mouth Rehabilitation of a Patient with Gummy Smile—Multidisciplinary Approach: Case Report
Reprinted from: *Medicina* 2023, 59, 197, doi:10.3390/medicina59020197 161

Alexandru Eugen Petre, Mihaela Pantea, Sergiu Drafta, Marina Imre, Ana Maria Cristina Țâncu and Eduard M. Liciu et al.
Modular Digital and 3D-Printed Dental Models with Applicability in Dental Education
Reprinted from: *Medicina* 2023, 59, 116, doi:10.3390/medicina59010116 172

Anna Kuśka-Kiełbratowska, Rafał Wiench, Anna Mertas, Elżbieta Bobela, Maksymilian Kiełbratowski and Monika Lukomska-Szymanska et al.
Evaluation of the Sensitivity of Selected *Candida* Strains to Ozonated Water—An In Vitro Study
Reprinted from: *Medicina* 2022, 58, 1731, doi:10.3390/medicina58121731 199

Juan Li, Xiaoyan Feng, Yi Lin and Jun Lin
The Stability Guided Multidisciplinary Treatment of Skeletal Class III Malocclusion Involving Impacted Canines and Thin Periodontal Biotype: A Case Report with Eight-Year Follow-Up
Reprinted from: *Medicina* 2022, 58, 1588, doi:10.3390/medicina58111588 209

Carlos A. Jurado, Venkata Parachuru, Jose Villalobos Tinoco, Gerardo Guzman-Perez, Akimasa Tsujimoto and Ramya Javvadi et al.
Diagnostic Mock-Up as a Surgical Reduction Guide for Crown Lengthening: Technique Description and Case Report
Reprinted from: *Medicina* 2022, 58, 1360, doi:10.3390/medicina58101360 221

Hussain D. Alsayed
Misfit of Implant-Supported Zirconia (Y-TZP) CAD-CAM Framework Compared to Non-Zirconia Frameworks: A Systematic Review
Reprinted from: *Medicina* 2022, 58, 1347, doi:10.3390/medicina58101347 231

Jiří Šedý, Mariano Rocabado, Leonardo Enrique Olate, Marek Vlna and Radovan Žižka
Neural Basis of Etiopathogenesis and Treatment of Cervicogenic Orofacial Pain
Reprinted from: *Medicina* **2022**, *58*, 1324, doi:10.3390/medicina58101324 242

Laura Maria Beschiu, Lavinia Cosmina Ardelean, Codruta Victoria Tigmeanu and Laura-Cristina Rusu
Cranial and Odontological Methods for Sex Estimation—A Scoping Review
Reprinted from: *Medicina* **2022**, *58*, 1273, doi:10.3390/medicina58091273 285

Elena-Raluca Baciu, Dana Gabriela Budală, Roxana-Ionela Vasluianu, Costin Iulian Lupu, Alice Murariu and Gabriela Luminița Geleţu et al.
A Comparative Analysis of Dental Measurements in Physical and Digital Orthodontic Case Study Models
Reprinted from: *Medicina* **2022**, *58*, 1230, doi:10.3390/medicina58091230 313

About the Editors

Giuseppe Minervini

Giuseppe Minervini graduated in Dental Medicine in July 2016 with honors. During his undergraduate studies, he participated in an Erasmus project at "Rey Juan Carlos Alcorcon" in Madrid, Spain, from September 2013 to June 2014. He received his Postgraduate Diploma in Orthodontics in December 2020 from the University of Campania, Luigi Vanvitelli, Naples, Italy, and later earned his PhD at the same institution (XXXIV cycle). In 2019, he attended the Tweed Study Course at the Charles H. Tweed International Foundation in Tucson, Arizona. Currently, he serves as an Adjunct Professor at Saveetha Dental College and Hospitals, Saveetha University, Chennai. Dr. Minervini is recognized as one of the top 10 experts worldwide in the field of "Temporomandibular disorders" according to Scopus' rankings. He is a Subject Expert in Dental Materials and a Tutor at the Orthodontics Dentistry School at the University of Campania, Luigi Vanvitelli. His contributions include serving as an Editor for numerous dentistry journals (10 Editorial Boards, 14 Special Issues), and he is an active member of SIDO, EOS, and GSID. With over 188 publications, 70 posters, and an h-index of 32, he is a frequent speaker at national and international conferences. Dr. Minervini has received several awards for his contributions to the field. His research interests include biomedical and biomaterial applications in craniofacial, oral, and temporomandibular districts, as well as orthodontics, orofacial pain, temporomandibular joint disorders, and telemedicine.

Stefania Moccia

Stefania Moccia graduated in Pharmacy (University of Salerno, Italy) in 2013 with 110/110 cum laude. In 2017, she received her PhD in Pharmaceutical Sciences (University of Salerno, Italy) with the project "Novel functional foods from local Italian cultivars for consumers' well-being: from agricultural raw materials to design and development". Since 2014, she has been working at the Institute of Food Sciences (ISA-CNR) as a Contractor, and since 2019, she has worked as a full-time CNR Researcher for the strategic area "Food Production and Nutrition". Her research activity is mainly based on the extraction and characterization of bioactive compounds, in particular polyphenols and carotenoids, from food matrices, on the design and formulation of nutraceuticals, including the development of nanoemulsions, nanoparticles, and delivery systems, and the subsequent evaluation of their biological activity in preclinical models (cell lines and blood samples). In particular, she studies the chemopreventive and antioxidant activity of bioactive compounds (extracts/ purified fractions) from agri-food matrices for their functional characterization to identify the cellular processes involved and the markers of oxidative stress and aging.

Preface

Dear Colleagues,

This Special Issue presents a comprehensive collection of studies showcasing the latest innovations in dentistry, emphasizing the integration of multidisciplinary approaches and technological advancements. With a focus on improving patient outcomes and advancing oral health care, the contributions explore a range of topics, including the development of new biomaterials, minimally invasive techniques, and novel treatment protocols. These innovations have broad applications in restorative dentistry, prosthodontics, oral surgery, implantology, pediatric dentistry, orthodontics, and the management of temporomandibular disorders. The research presented in this reprint reflects the significant progress made in dental science and its application to clinical practice, offering valuable insights for both researchers and clinicians. Special acknowledgment is given to the contributing authors for their valuable insights, as well as to the editors and reviewers for their guidance throughout the process.

Giuseppe Minervini and Stefania Moccia
Editors

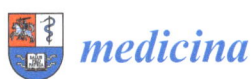

Editorial

Dentistry: A Multidisciplinary Approach

Giuseppe Minervini [1,2]

1. Saveetha Dental College and Hospitals, Saveetha Institute of Medical and Technical Sciences (SIMATS), Saveetha University, Chennai 602105, Tamil Nadu, India; giuseppe.minervini@unicampania.it
2. Multidisciplinary Department of Medical-Surgical and Dental Specialties, University of Campania, Luigi Vanvitelli, 80138 Naples, Italy

In this special issue of Medicina, we delve into the dynamic and ever-evolving world of dentistry, highlighting the remarkable innovations that are shaping the future of oral health and clinical dentistry practice. The articles featured in this issue underscore a critical shift in the dental field: the movement towards a multidisciplinary, technology-driven approach that touches upon various branches, including restorative dentistry, prosthodontics, oral surgery, implantology, pediatric dentistry, orthodontics, and the management of temporomandibular disorders.

The fusion of traditional dental practices with cutting-edge technology is not merely a trend; it is a paradigm shift in how we approach oral health. The advent of new biomaterials, digital modeling, and advanced surgical techniques has revolutionized the way dental professionals diagnose, treat, and manage dental and oral conditions [1]. The articles within this issue also emphasize the growing importance of personalized dental care. Advancements in biomaterials and surgical techniques allow for treatments that are tailored to the unique needs and conditions of each patient. This individualized approach is crucial, especially in complex cases where a standardized treatment may not suffice [2]. Furthermore, the exploration of new frontiers, such as the use of ozonated water for the treatment of Candida infections, represents a significant step towards finding more effective, safer, and less invasive treatment options. This not only enhances patient comfort and recovery but also opens up new avenues for treating a range of dental diseases [3].

Importantly, this issue highlights the critical role of ongoing research and education in the field of dentistry. The advancements we witness today are the results of relentless inquiry and learning [4]. As such, it is imperative for dental professionals to continue engaging in lifelong learning and to remain abreast of the latest developments in their field. This commitment to education and research is what will continue to drive the field forward, ensuring that dental care remains at the forefront of medical science and technology [5,6].

In summary, "Dentistry: A Multidisciplinary Approach" offers a comprehensive overview of the current state and future potential of dental care. It exemplifies how embracing a multidisciplinary, technologically advanced, and patient-centric approach can lead to significant advancements in all branches of dentistry. As we continue to expand the boundaries of what is possible in dental care, it is these principles that will guide us towards a future where oral health is integral to overall health and well-being. These changes have been seen especially in the fields of digital dentistry, tele-dentistry, and TMD treatment [7–10]. In the field of dentistry, recent advancements emphasize a holistic, interdisciplinary approach to treatment, particularly in complex cases. Studies have shown the efficacy of techniques like diagnostic mock-ups for crown lengthening, finite element analysis for bone stress assessment, and innovative approaches for treating malocclusions and cleft lip and palate.

The article "Soft Tissue Grafting Procedures before Restorations in the Esthetic Zone: A Minimally Invasive Interdisciplinary Case Report" presents a case study of a 32-year-old male patient with esthetic concerns regarding his anterior teeth. The patient exhibited generalized clinical attachment loss, gingival recessions, and cervical non-carious lesions. The treatment plan involved plastic mucogingival surgery using tunneling connective tissue grafts and anterior ceramic laminate veneers. The surgical approach focused on improving root coverage and gingival architecture, while the restorative phase aimed to enhance dental esthetics with veneers. The case highlights the importance of an interdisciplinary approach, combining periodontal and restorative treatments, to achieve satisfying esthetic outcomes in complex cases [11]. "The Stability Guided Multidisciplinary Treatment of Skeletal Class III Malocclusion Involving Impacted Canines and Thin Periodontal Biotype" presents a case study of a 16-year-old female patient with dental and skeletal Class III malocclusion, bilaterally impacted maxillary canines, and a thin gingival biotype. The treatment involved orthognathic surgery, subepithelial connective tissue graft surgery, and a segmental arch technique. The study emphasizes the importance of a multidisciplinary approach to addressing complex dental and skeletal issues, highlighting the role of periodontal management in ensuring long-term stability and aesthetic success [12]. The article "Evaluation of the Sensitivity of Selected Candida Strains to Ozonated Water—An In Vitro Study" investigates the sensitivity of Candida strains to ozonated water. The study evaluated the impact of ozonated water at varying concentrations and exposure times on *Candida albicans*, *Candida glabrata*, and *Candida krusei strains*. The findings indicated that all the strains were sensitive to ozonated water, with increased sensitivity correlating with higher concentrations and longer exposure times. The effectiveness of ozonated water against these Candida strains was comparable to 0.2% chlorhexidine gluconate, suggesting its potential as an effective alternative for oral candidiasis treatment [3]. "Diagnostic Mock-Up as a Surgical Reduction Guide for Crown Lengthening: Technique Description and Case Report" discusses a technique using a diagnostic mock-up as a guide for crown-lengthening surgery to improve gingival architecture. This method was applied to a 30-year-old female patient concerned about her "gummy smile" and short clinical crowns. The process involved a diagnostic wax-up, a provisional overlay for surgical guidance, and final restorations with ceramic crowns and veneers. The study highlights the advantages of this technique in achieving desired aesthetic outcomes in complex dental cases [13]. The article "Injectable Resin Technique as a Restorative Alternative in a Cleft Lip and Palate Patient: A Case Report" details the treatment of a 21-year-old female patient with a unilateral left cleft lip and palate. It focuses on the use of an injectable composite resin technique for dental re-anatomization, offering a minimally invasive, efficient, and aesthetically pleasing option. This technique allowed for the successful restoration of the patient's teeth, improving her dental anatomy and aesthetics, with positive results observed after one year [14]. The article "Neural Basis of Etiopathogenesis and Treatment of Cervicogenic Orofacial Pain" discusses the neuroanatomical and neurophysiological basis of cervicogenic pain in cervico-cranial pain syndromes, with a focus on cervico-orofacial syndromes. It covers a wide range of topics, including the clinical anatomy of the cervico-cranial junction, the role of the temporomandibular joint, and the integrative function of the cervico-cranial complex. The article emphasizes the importance of understanding neuroanatomical and neurophysiological neuromuscular relations for effective therapeutic approaches, which are primarily based on orthopedic manual and dental occlusal treatment [15]. The article "Cortical and Trabecular Bone Stress Assessment during Periodontal Breakdown–A Comparative Finite Element Analysis of Multiple Failure Criteria" by Radu Andrei Moga et al. [16] presents a numerical analysis exploring the biomechanical behavior of the mandibular bone under orthodontic forces during periodontal breakdown. It evaluates the appropriateness of various failure criteria (Von Mises, Tresca, maximum/minimum principal stresses, and hydrostatic pressure) for studying bone under these conditions. The study involves 405 simulations across 81 mandibular models with varying levels of bone loss and orthodontic movements (intrusion, extrusion, tipping, rotation, and translation). The results show that Tresca and Von Mises criteria are most suitable for bone stress analysis, displaying a coherent pattern of increasing stress across all movements and levels of periodontal breakdown. The study concludes that Tresca is better suited as a unified criterion for the study of teeth and surrounding periodontium [16]. The article "Modular Digital and

3D-Printed Dental Models with Applicability in Dental Education" explores the impact of digitalization in dental education. It discusses the development and use of modular digital dental models and 3D-printed models in teaching. The study assesses the opinions of dental students regarding these methods, emphasizing their benefits in enhancing practical skills and the understanding of dental procedures. This reflects a significant shift towards integrating advanced technology in dental education, aiming to improve student learning experiences and outcomes [17]. The article "Full-Mouth Rehabilitation of a Patient with Gummy Smile—Multidisciplinary Approach: Case Report" in Medicina describes the comprehensive treatment of a 48-year-old female patient with aesthetic concerns and disturbed masticatory function due to missing posterior teeth and a gummy smile. The treatment plan involved advanced techniques such as diode laser and piezo-surgery, implant installation, and the use of zirconia ceramic for final restorations. This multidisciplinary approach, spanning over two years, significantly improved the patient's dental function and aesthetics. This case underscores the importance of personalized, multifaceted treatment strategies in complex dental cases [18]. The article "Evaluation of Clinical and Oral Findings in Patients with Epidermolysis Bullosa" in Medicina focuses on the oral and dental manifestations in patients with Epidermolysis Bullosa (EB), a genetic skin disorder. The study involves an assessment of clinical and oral findings in 26 EB patients, highlighting various complications like dental caries, enamel hypoplasia, and oral lesions. It underscores the unique dental care requirements of EB patients and suggests the need for specialized treatment approaches [19]. The article "A Comparative Analysis of Dental Measurements in Physical and Digital Orthodontic Case Study Models" by Elena-Raluca Baciu et al. [20] compares manual and digital orthodontic measurements on both physical and digital models. The study aims to determine the reliability of digital models in orthodontic analyses, focusing on the reproducibility of dental arch characteristics. It involves a detailed comparison of different measurement techniques applied to various types of models, including physical models created through traditional pouring and additive manufacturing as well as digital models obtained through scanning. The research concludes that both traditional and digital models are effective for orthodontic teaching, with no significant differences in the measurement results [20]. The article "The Impact of Simulated Bruxism Forces and Surface Aging Treatments on Two Dental Nano-Biocomposites—A Radiographic and Tomographic Analysis" by Amelia Anita Boitor et al. [21] investigates the effects of simulated bruxism forces and aging treatments on two dental nano-biocomposites. It focuses on the radiographic and tomographic analysis of these materials under stress. The study simulates real-life conditions like the consumption of acidic beverages and the use of at-home dental bleaching, aiming to assess the mechanical and functional behavior of these composites under such circumstances. The results provide insights into the suitability of these materials for dental restorations in patients with specific oral conditions, including bruxism [21]. The study "Different Designs of Deep Marginal Elevation and Its Influence on Fracture Resistance of Teeth with Monolith Zirconia Full-Contour Crowns" by Ali Robaian et al. [22] investigates the impact of deep marginal elevation (DME) on the fracture resistance of teeth restored with monolithic zirconia crowns. Forty premolars were divided into four groups, each undergoing different preparation and restoration procedures. The study found that fracture resistance decreased with increasing tooth structure involvement, even with monolithic zirconia crowns. However, DME up to 2 mm below the cemento-enamel junction did not negatively influence fracture resistance, suggesting its viability in clinical scenarios. The study emphasizes the importance of considering tooth preservation and material choice in restorative dentistry [22]. The article "Cranial and Odontological Methods for Sex Estimation—A Scoping Review" by Laura Maria Beschiu et al. [23] provides a comprehensive review of various methods used for sex estimation based on cranial and dental records. The study covers articles published between January 2015 and July 2022, focusing on morphometric, morphologic, and biochemical analyses in living populations, autopsy cases, and archaeological records. The review highlights that cranial and odontological sex estimation methods are highly population-specific and underscores the need for these methods to be applied to and verified in more populations. It also emphasizes the high accuracy of DNA analysis while noting the limitations and challenges of other methods for predicting sex from cranial or odontological records [23]. The article "Comparison of Mechanical Properties of Three Tissue Conditioners: An Evaluation In Vitro Study" by Marcin Mikulewicz et al. [24] compares the mechanical properties of three tissue conditioners (TC) used in dentistry. It focuses on various properties like Shore A hardness, ethanol concentration, sorption, solubility, and adhesion to denture base, evaluated under specific test conditions. The study concludes that materials containing non-phthalate plasticizers showed higher solubility and increased hardness when stored in distilled water compared to those containing phthalates. It emphasizes the importance of understanding the properties of commercial TC for optimal clinical performance and highlights the need for further research to improve these materials, especially considering the use of phthalate-free alternatives [24]. The article "Assessment and Correlation of Salivary Ca, Mg, and pH in Smokers and Non-Smokers with Generalized Chronic Periodontitis" by Saad Mohammad Alqahtani et al. [25] investigates the relationship between salivary calcium, magnesium, pH levels, and periodontitis in smokers and non-smokers. The study, conducted on 210 individuals, reveals significant differences in salivary calcium levels between smokers and non-smokers with periodontitis. It suggests that higher salivary calcium levels in smokers could be a potential marker for periodontitis progression, emphasizing the role of saliva as a diagnostic tool in periodontal diseases [25]. The article "Misfit of Implant-Supported Zirconia (Y-TZP) CAD-CAM Framework Compared to Non-Zirconia Frameworks: A Systematic Review" by Hussain D. Alsayed [26] systematically reviews studies comparing the misfit of yttria-stabilized zirconia (Y-TZP) CAD-CAM implant-supported frameworks with other materials. It includes 11 articles and covers different methods like scanning electron microscopy, one-screw tests, and 3D virtual assessment. The findings suggest that Y-TZP CAD-CAM frameworks have comparable misfits to other materials. However, due to methodological heterogeneity, the numerical misfit values are debatable, highlighting the need for standardized and well-designed in vitro and clinical studies in order to obtain definitive conclusions [26]. The article "Gaucher: A Systematic Review on Oral and Radiological Aspects" by Giuseppe Minervini et al. [27] provides a systematic review of Gaucher disease, particularly focusing on its oral and radiological manifestations. It evaluates the principal findings in the jaw using cone-beam computed tomography and X-ray orthopantomography. The study underlines the importance of dental professionals in the early diagnosis and management of Gaucher disease, emphasizing the role of dental radiographs in detecting jawbone involvement, a common feature in Gaucher patients [27]. The article "Identification of the Remains of an Adult Using DNA from Their Deciduous Teeth as a Reference Sample" by María-de-Lourdes Chávez-Briones et al. [28] presents a unique forensic case. It details the identification of an adult's remains using DNA from their deciduous teeth, kept by the mother. This innovative approach proved crucial in this case, emphasizing the potential of using personal artifacts or saved biological samples as reference DNA in forensic investigations, especially in scenarios where conventional methods are insufficient [28]. The article "The Effect of Dentine Desensitizing Agents on the Retention of Cemented Fixed Dental Prostheses: A Systematic Review" by Mohammed E. Sayed [29] examines the impact of dentine desensitizing agents on the retention of cemented fixed dental prostheses. This systematic review compiles and analyzes data from various studies to determine how these agents affect retention. It evaluates multiple types of desensitizing agents and their interactions with different luting cements. The findings are crucial for clinical decision-making, offering guidance on selecting appropriate desensitizing agents to ensure the optimal retention of dental prostheses [29]. The article "The Impact of Anemia-Related Early Childhood Caries on Parents' and Children's Quality of Life" by Dila Özyılkan et al. [30] explores the relationship between anemia-related dental caries in children and their quality of life, as well as that of their parents. Utilizing the Early Childhood Oral Health Impact Scale (ECOHIS) and the Parental-Caregivers Perceptions Questionnaire (P-CPQ), the study assesses the impact of these dental issues on children and parents. The findings highlight the significant negative impact of anemia-related dental caries on quality of life, underscoring the importance of prioritizing preventive measures and timely dental treatments for affected children [30].

Conflicts of Interest: The author declares no conflicts of interest.

References

1. Vujovic, S.; Desnica, J.; Stevanovic, M.; Mijailovic, S.; Vojinovic, R.; Selakovic, D.; Jovicic, N.; Rosic, G.; Milovanovic, D. Oral Health and Oral Health-Related Quality of Life in Patients with Primary Sjögren's Syndrome. *Medicina* 2023, 59, 473. [CrossRef] [PubMed]
2. Naim, H.; Ahmad, M.; Ageeli, A.A.; Abuarab, R.K.; Sayed, M.E.; Dewan, H.; Chohan, H.; Alshehri, A.H.; Wadei, M.H.D.A.; Alqahtani, S.M.; et al. Radiographic Evaluation of the Gap between Cemented Post and Remaining Gutta-Percha in Endodontically Treated Teeth Performed by Undergraduate Students: A Retrospective Cross-Sectional Study. *Medicina* 2023, 59, 502. [CrossRef] [PubMed]
3. Kuśka-Kiełbratowska, A.; Wiench, R.; Mertas, A.; Bobela, E.; Kiełbratowski, M.; Lukomska-Szymanska, M.; Tanasiewicz, M.; Skaba, D. Evaluation of the Sensitivity of Selected Candida Strains to Ozonated Water—An In Vitro Study. *Medicina* 2022, 58, 1731. [CrossRef] [PubMed]
4. Blasi, A.; Cuozzo, A.; Marcacci, R.; Isola, G.; Iorio-Siciliano, V.; Ramaglia, L. Post-Operative Complications and Risk Predictors Related to the Avulsion of Lower Impacted Third Molars. *Medicina* 2023, 59, 534. [CrossRef]
5. Alssum, L.R.; Alghofaily, M.M.; Aleyiydi, A.S.; Alomar, S.A.; Alsalleeh, F.M. The Incidence of Retrograde Peri-Implantitis in a Single University Dental Hospital Training Center: A Retrospective Analysis. *Medicina* 2023, 59, 560. [CrossRef]
6. Guzman-Perez, G.; Jurado, C.A.; Azpiazu-Flores, F.; Afrashtehfar, K.I.; Tsujimoto, A. Minimally Invasive Laminate Veneer Therapy for Maxillary Central Incisors. *Medicina* 2023, 59, 603. [CrossRef]
7. Minervini, G.; Franco, R.; Marrapodi, M.M.; Ronsivalle, V.; Shapira, I.; Cicciù, M. Prevalence of Temporomandibular Disorders in Subjects Affected by Parkinson Disease: A Systematic Review and Metanalysis. *J. Oral Rehabil.* 2023. [CrossRef]
8. Di Stasio, D.; Lauritano, D.; Gritti, P.; Migliozzi, R.; Maio, C.; Minervini, G.; Petruzzi, M.; Serpico, R.; Candotto, V.; Lucchese, A. Psychiatric Disorders in Oral Lichen Planus: A Preliminary Case Control Study. *J. Biol. Regul. Homeost. Agents* 2018, 32, 97–100.
9. Minervini, G.; Del Mondo, D.; Russo, D.; Cervino, G.; D'Amico, C.; Fiorillo, L. Stem Cells in Temporomandibular Joint Engineering: State of Art and Future Perestives. *J. Craniofacial Surg.* 2022, 33, 2181–2187. [CrossRef]
10. Antonelli, A.; Bennardo, F.; Brancaccio, Y.; Barone, S.; Femiano, F.; Nucci, L.; Minervini, G.; Fortunato, L.; Attanasio, F.; Giudice, A. Can Bone Compaction Improve Primary Implant Stability? An In Vitro Comparative Study with Osseodensification Technique. *Appl. Sci.* 2020, 10, 8623. [CrossRef]
11. Guzman-Perez, G.; Jurado, C.A.; Azpiazu-Flores, F.X.; Munoz-Luna, H.; Afrashtehfar, K.I.; Nurrohman, H. Soft Tissue Grafting Procedures before Restorations in the Esthetic Zone: A Minimally Invasive Interdisciplinary Case Report. *Medicina* 2023, 59, 822. [CrossRef] [PubMed]
12. Li, J.; Feng, X.; Lin, Y.; Lin, J. The Stability Guided Multidisciplinary Treatment of Skeletal Class III Malocclusion Involving Impacted Canines and Thin Periodontal Biotype: A Case Report with Eight-Year Follow-Up. *Medicina* 2022, 58, 1588. [CrossRef] [PubMed]
13. Jurado, C.A.; Parachuru, V.; Villalobos Tinoco, J.; Guzman-Perez, G.; Tsujimoto, A.; Javvadi, R.; Afrashtehfar, K.I. Diagnostic Mock-Up as a Surgical Reduction Guide for Crown Lengthening: Technique Description and Case Report. *Medicina* 2022, 58, 1360. [CrossRef] [PubMed]
14. Villafuerte, K.R.V.; Obeid, A.T.; de Oliveira, N.A. Injectable Resin Technique as a Restorative Alternative in a Cleft Lip and Palate Patient: A Case Report. *Medicina* 2023, 59, 849. [CrossRef] [PubMed]
15. Šedý, J.; Rocabado, M.; Olate, L.E.; Vlna, M.; Žižka, R. Neural Basis of Etiopathogenesis and Treatment of Cervicogenic Orofacial Pain. *Medicina* 2022, 58, 1324. [CrossRef]
16. Moga, R.A.; Olteanu, C.D.; Buru, S.M.; Botez, M.D.; Delean, A.G. Cortical and Trabecular Bone Stress Assessment during Periodontal Breakdown–A Comparative Finite Element Analysis of Multiple Failure Criteria. *Medicina* 2023, 59, 1462. [CrossRef]
17. Petre, A.E.; Pantea, M.; Drafta, S.; Imre, M.; Țâncu, A.M.C.; Liciu, E.M.; Didilescu, A.C.; Pițuru, S.M. Modular Digital and 3D-Printed Dental Models with Applicability in Dental Education. *Medicina* 2023, 59, 116. [CrossRef]
18. Jánosi, K.M.; Cerghizan, D.; Berneanu, F.D.; Kovács, A.; Szász, A.; Mureșan, I.; Hănțoiu, L.G.; Albu, A.I. Full-Mouth Rehabilitation of a Patient with Gummy Smile—Multidisciplinary Approach: Case Report. *Medicina* 2023, 59, 197. [CrossRef]
19. Yavuz, Y.; An, I.; Yazmaci, B.; Akkus, Z.; Ortac, H. Evaluation of Clinical and Oral Findings in Patients with Epidermolysis Bullosa. *Medicina* 2023, 59, 1185. [CrossRef] [PubMed]
20. Baciu, E.-R.; Budală, D.G.; Vasluianu, R.-I.; Lupu, C.I.; Murariu, A.; Geletu, G.L.; Zetu, I.N.; Diaconu-Popa, D.; Tatarciuc, M.; Nichitean, G.; et al. A Comparative Analysis of Dental Measurements in Physical and Digital Orthodontic Case Study Models. *Medicina* 2022, 58, 1230. [CrossRef] [PubMed]
21. Boitor, A.A.; Varvară, E.B.; Prodan, C.M.; Sava, S.; Dudea, D.; Objelean, A. The Impact of Simulated Bruxism Forces and Surface Aging Treatments on Two Dental Nano-Biocomposites—A Radiographic and Tomographic Analysis. *Medicina* 2023, 59, 360. [CrossRef]

22. Robaian, A.; Alqahtani, A.; Alanazi, K.; Alanazi, A.; Almalki, M.; Aljarad, A.; Albaijan, R.; Maawadh, A.; Sufyan, A.; Mirza, M.B. Different Designs of Deep Marginal Elevation and Its Influence on Fracture Resistance of Teeth with Monolith Zirconia Full-Contour Crowns. *Medicina* **2023**, *59*, 661. [CrossRef] [PubMed]
23. Beschiu, L.M.; Ardelean, L.C.; Tigmeanu, C.V.; Rusu, L.-C. Cranial and Odontological Methods for Sex Estimation—A Scoping Review. *Medicina* **2022**, *58*, 1273. [CrossRef] [PubMed]
24. Mikulewicz, M.; Chojnacka, K.; Raszewski, Z. Comparison of Mechanical Properties of Three Tissue Conditioners: An Evaluation In Vitro Study. *Medicina* **2023**, *59*, 1359. [CrossRef] [PubMed]
25. Alqahtani, S.M.; Gokhale, S.T.; Elagib, M.F.A.; Shrivastava, D.; Nagate, R.R.; Alshmrani, B.A.M.; Alburade, A.M.A.; Alqahtani, F.M.A.; Nagarajappa, A.K.; Natoli, V.; et al. Assessment and Correlation of Salivary Ca, Mg, and PH in Smokers and Non-Smokers with Generalized Chronic Periodontitis. *Medicina* **2023**, *59*, 765. [CrossRef]
26. Alsayed, H. Misfit of Implant-Supported Zirconia (Y-TZP) CAD-CAM Framework Compared to Non-Zirconia Frameworks: A Systematic Review. *Medicina* **2022**, *58*, 1347. [CrossRef] [PubMed]
27. Minervini, G.; Franco, R.; Marrapodi, M.M.; Mehta, V.; Fiorillo, L.; Badnjević, A.; Cervino, G.; Cicciù, M. Gaucher: A Systematic Review on Oral and Radiological Aspects. *Medicina* **2023**, *59*, 670. [CrossRef] [PubMed]
28. Chávez-Briones, M.-L.; Jaramillo-Rangel, G.; Ancer-Arellano, A.; Ancer-Rodríguez, J.; Ortega-Martínez, M. Identification of the Remains of an Adult Using DNA from Their Deciduous Teeth as a Reference Sample. *Medicina* **2023**, *59*, 1702. [CrossRef] [PubMed]
29. Sayed, M.E. The Effect of Dentine Desensitizing Agents on the Retention of Cemented Fixed Dental Prostheses: A Systematic Review. *Medicina* **2023**, *59*, 515. [CrossRef]
30. Özyılkan, D.; Tosun, Ö.; İslam, A. The Impact of Anemia-Related Early Childhood Caries on Parents' and Children's Quality of Life. *Medicina* **2023**, *59*, 521. [CrossRef]

Disclaimer/Publisher's Note: The statements, opinions and data contained in all publications are solely those of the individual author(s) and contributor(s) and not of MDPI and/or the editor(s). MDPI and/or the editor(s) disclaim responsibility for any injury to people or property resulting from any ideas, methods, instructions or products referred to in the content.

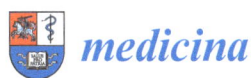

Case Report

Identification of the Remains of an Adult Using DNA from Their Deciduous Teeth as a Reference Sample

María-de-Lourdes Chávez-Briones, Gilberto Jaramillo-Rangel, Adriana Ancer-Arellano, Jesús Ancer-Rodríguez and Marta Ortega-Martínez *

Department of Pathology, School of Medicine, Autonomous University of Nuevo Leon, Monterrey 64460, Mexico; mdlourdes.chavezbrn@uanl.edu.mx (M.-d.-L.C.-B.); gilberto.jaramillorn@uanl.edu.mx (G.J.-R.); adar7035@gmail.com (A.A.-A.); ancerrodriguezj@gmail.com (J.A.-R.)
* Correspondence: marta.ortegamrt@uanl.edu.mx

Abstract: In many forensic cases, the identification of human remains is performed by comparing their genetic profile with profiles from reference samples of relatives, usually the parents. Here, we report, for the first time, the identification of the remains of an adult using DNA from the person's deciduous teeth as a reference sample. Fragments of a skeletonized and burned body were found, and a short tandem repeat (STR) profile was obtained. A woman looking for her missing son went to the authorities. When the DNA profile of the woman was compared to a database, a positive match suggested a first-degree kinship with the person to whom the remains belonged. The woman had kept three deciduous molars from her son for more than thirty years. DNA typing of dental pulp was performed. The genetic profiles obtained from the molars and those from the remains coincided in all alleles. The random match probability was 1 in 2.70×10^{21}. Thus, the remains were fully identified. In the routine identification of human remains, ambiguous STR results may occur due to the presence of null alleles or other mutational events. In addition, erroneous results can be produced by false matches with close family members or even with people who are completely unrelated to the victim, such that, in some cases, a probability of paternity greater than 99.99% does not necessarily indicate biological paternity. Whenever possible, it is preferable to use reference samples from the putative victim as a source of DNA for identification.

Keywords: dental pulp; DNA analysis; human remains; reference sample; teeth; victim identification

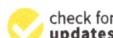

Citation: Chávez-Briones, M.-d.-L.; Jaramillo-Rangel, G.; Ancer-Arellano, A.; Ancer-Rodríguez, J.; Ortega-Martínez, M. Identification of the Remains of an Adult Using DNA from Their Deciduous Teeth as a Reference Sample. *Medicina* **2023**, *59*, 1702. https://doi.org/10.3390/medicina59101702

Academic Editor: Bruno Chrcanovic

Received: 29 July 2023
Revised: 30 August 2023
Accepted: 20 September 2023
Published: 23 September 2023

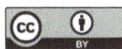

Copyright: © 2023 by the authors. Licensee MDPI, Basel, Switzerland. This article is an open access article distributed under the terms and conditions of the Creative Commons Attribution (CC BY) license (https://creativecommons.org/licenses/by/4.0/).

1. Introduction

One of the main tasks of legal systems in the investigation of criminal cases is the personal identification of unknown human remains. To achieve this purpose, collaboration between forensic anthropologists, pathologists, and odontologists may be crucial. Also, DNA profiling can be used in the identification of skeletonized or highly decomposed human remains. Identification is usually carried out by comparing the genetic profile from the remains with the genotypes of reference samples from relatives, most commonly the parents of the victim. However, in these cases, ambiguous results may occur due to the presence of null alleles or other mutational events, and erroneous results can be produced by false matches with close family members or even with people who are completely unrelated to the victim [1,2].

Thus, in the identification of human remains by DNA typing, it would be ideal to use biological samples of the person from whom the remains are suspected to have come as a reference. However, there are few reports in the literature on the successful use of this strategy. Calacal et al. [3] identified the skeletal remains of two children by directly comparing the genetic profiles derived from the remains with the profiles from children's umbilical tissues, which had been preserved by their mothers. Tanaka et al. [4] identified two corpses in two criminal cases using the toothbrushes of the victims as DNA sources.

Sweet et al. [5] identified a skeleton using a reference sample consisting of cytological smears stained with the Papanicolaou method, obtained from the medical record of the deceased. Other studies have analyzed the feasibility of using objects or samples from the victim, such as cosmetic applicators [6] and archived tumor samples [7], to obtain DNA that can be used to identify human remains; however, these strategies have not been applied in actual criminal cases.

While bloodstains or buccal swabs would be the perfect reference samples from the victim for the identification of unknown remains, they are often not available. Here, we report, for the first time, the use of DNA isolated from deciduous teeth as a reference sample to identify an adult victim in an actual criminal case.

2. Case Presentation

Fragments of a skeletonized and burned body were found on the slopes of a hill. Four of the least damaged bone fragments were selected for DNA extraction. Given the physical condition of the body, we could neither determine to which bones the analyzed fragments belonged nor characteristics such as the sex or the approximate age of the deceased. The outer surfaces of the fragments were cleaned by immersion in 50% commercial bleach for 15 min. Next, they were washed briefly with nuclease-free water (5 washes), then immersed briefly in 100% ethanol and air-dried overnight in a sterile hood. The samples were frozen with liquid nitrogen and pulverized with a pestle and mortar. The bone powder (0.5 g) was decalcified by incubating it with a 0.5 M EDTA solution on a rocking platform at 37 °C for 5 days with three solution changes. Samples were centrifuged, and the pellets were rinsed twice in double-distilled water. DNA extraction was performed using the PrepFiler Express BTA™ Forensic DNA Extraction Kit (Applied Biosystems, Foster City, CA, USA). Lysis buffer from the kit was added to the samples together with 1 M DTT and Proteinase K (2 mg/mL). Samples were incubated overnight in a thermal shaker at 56 °C. Finally, they were centrifuged, and the supernatant was subjected to DNA extraction in the AutoMate™ Instrument (Applied Biosystems) following the manufacturer's instructions. The DNA samples were quantified on the 7500 ABI Real-Time PCR platform using the Quantifiler Trio DNA quantification kit (Applied Biosystems). All samples had DNA concentrations > 0.01 ng/µL and were therefore deemed suitable for DNA typing [8].

DNA typing was carried out using the commercially available multiplex kit AmpFℓSTR® Identifiler Plus (Applied Biosystems), following the protocol provided by the manufacturer. In an attempt to ensure the amplification of as many alleles as possible, the samples were also amplified by the AmpFℓSTR® MiniFiler kit (Applied Biosystems), which has nine loci in common with the previous kit. Capillary electrophoresis was performed in an ABI PRISM® 310 genetic analyzer (Applied Biosystems). Samples were run on a capillary containing POP-4 polymer; allele assignment was determined by comparison with allelic ladders included in the kits, and genotypes were generated using GeneMapper® IDX-v1.4 software (Applied Biosystems).

No alleles from bone fragment number 1 were amplified. Partial consensus profiles (combining the results of both kits) were obtained from fragments 2 and 3. A complete consensus profile was obtained from fragment 4. The genetic profile obtained was stored in a database containing genotypes from unidentified cadavers.

Four years later, a woman looking for her missing son went to the authorities. A saliva sample was obtained according to the usual protocol followed in these cases at our institution. DNA was extracted from the sample using a Chelex protocol [9]. DNA typing was performed as described above for the bone fragments, but only with the Identifiler kit. When the woman's DNA profile was compared to the database, a positive match suggested a first-degree kinship with the person to whom the remains belonged. The woman was asked about the existence of other first-degree relatives of her son, which could allow a complete identification of the remains. She denied the availability of the father and other first-degree relatives of her son. Later in the interview, she recalled that she had kept three deciduous molars from her son in a plastic bag for more than thirty years (Figure 1). She was asked for the molars to see whether they could serve as a reference sample.

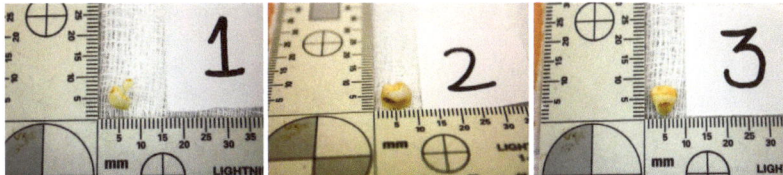

Figure 1. Deciduous molars submitted for DNA typing.

Dental pulp tissue was collected from each molar by sectioning using a carborundum disc. DNA was isolated by Proteinase K digestion and phenol chloroform extraction methods [10] and quantified as described for the bone fragments. DNA typing was performed with the Identifiler and MiniFiler kits as described above. A complete consensus profile was obtained from molar 1. A partial consensus profile was obtained from molar 2. No alleles from molar 3 were amplified.

All the genetic profiles generated are presented in Table 1. The genetic profiles obtained from the bone fragments and the molars coincided in all the alleles. Every locus was sequenced from the bone fragments, and the molars shared at least one allele with the corresponding locus generated from the putative mother. The random match probability and the probability of parentage were calculated using STR allele frequency data from our population and PATPCR software version 2.0.2 [11,12]. The random match probability was 1 in 2.70×10^{21}, and the probability of parentage was 99.9999%. Thus, the remains were fully identified and returned to the victim's biological mother.

Table 1. Comparison of short tandem repeats results of DNA recovered from bone fragments, deciduous molars, and the alleged mother of the victim.

Locus	Bone Fragments	Deciduous Molars	Alleged Mother
Amelogenin	XY	XY	XX
D8S1179	14, 15	14, 15	12, 14
D21S11	32.2, 33.2	32.2, 33.2	29, 33.2
D7S820	10, 10	10, 10	10, 10
CSF1PO	10, 11	10, 11	11, 11
D3S1358	15, 18	15, 18	14, 15
TH01	6, 6	6, 6	6, 6
D13S317	9, 14	9, 14	9, 9
D16S539	11, 12	11, 12	11, 12
D2S1338	18, 25	18, 25	23, 25
D19S433	11.2, 13	11.2, 13	11.2, 15
vWA	16, 17	16, 17	16, 17
TPOX	9, 12	9, 12	8, 9
D18S51	12, 15	12, 15	15, 16
D5S818	11, 12	11, 12	11, 11
FGA	21, 24	21, 24	24, 24

3. Discussion

Dental pulp is a rich source of DNA amenable to genetic analysis; the latter can be used for the positive identification of human remains, especially when soft tissue destruction has occurred. DNA analysis is usually carried out by comparing the genetic profile of the teeth from the remains with the genotypes of reference samples from relatives, most commonly the parents of the victim. For purposes such as crime solving, missing-person cases, and disaster victim identification, this approach has been used for decades [13]. However, to our knowledge, this is the first report of the use of DNA isolated from teeth as a reference sample to identify a victim in a criminal case.

In the case presented here, unambiguous identification was achieved thanks to the matching of DNA profiles generated from the bone fragments with those from the teeth. The DNA profile from the mother served to reinforce the results.

Short tandem repeats (STRs) are the most widely used genetic markers for human identity determination and paternity testing. Their use makes it possible to clarify most legal and forensic cases with a generally very high degree of certainty [14]. As mentioned above, the identification of human remains is generally performed by comparing the genetic profile of the remains with that of first-degree relatives, usually the parents. However, ambiguous STR results may occur due to the presence of null alleles or other mutational events (for specific cases, see [15–28]; for studies in populations, see [29–37]). STRs have mutation rates ranging from 0 to 7×10^{-3}, with an average of 2×10^{-3} [33,34]. The most frequent mechanism causing these mutations is the slippage of the DNA replication complex during DNA synthesis [30]. In the most common mutations, an STR differs only slightly in its size from its presumed predecessor. The gain or loss of tandem repeats could lead to false maternal or paternal exclusions [30,32]. In addition, erroneous results can be produced by false matches with close family members or even with people who are completely unrelated to the victim, such that, in some cases, a probability of paternity greater than 99.99% does not necessarily indicate biological paternity [30,31,38–41]. Poetsch et al. [31] investigated how many wrong paternity inclusions could be detected when comparing 13-15 STRs between 336 children and 348 unrelated men. They found that at least one and up to three "second father(s)" could be found for 23 children. In general, the false inclusion rate ranges between 19% and 23% [40]. These problems are being reported more frequently and are most common in cases where only one putative parent is available [31,40,42]. The inclusion of additional autosomal STR loci may assist in clarifying some ambiguous cases. Sometimes, however, the addition of more loci introduces additional mismatches. Furthermore, it has been observed that the inclusion of more loci does not compensate for the absence of genetic information from the mother or the father [35,40,42–44]. The use of Y-chromosome STRs can help only when the victim is male, and the possibility that a close relative of the putative father is the biological father cannot be ruled out [45]. X-chromosome STRs must be analyzed along with other genetic markers to obtain useful data and can only be used with accuracy when the victim is female, as there are no X-chromosome alleles inherited by descent in a father-son relationship [46]. Other typing systems that may be used to resolve ambiguous cases include the HV1 and HV2 hypervariable regions of mitochondrial DNA, single nucleotide polymorphisms (SNPs), and next-generation sequencing (NGS). However, they are expensive and time-consuming and are not available in most developing countries [47]. Even with these systems, the lack of informative reference samples (first-degree relatives) is the most common problem in identifying unknown corpses [41,48]. Thus, whenever possible, it is preferable to use reference samples from the putative victim as a source of DNA for identification.

In this study, we analyzed three deciduous molars. A complete DNA profile was obtained from only one molar. The efficiency of DNA typing from teeth subjected to various experimental conditions, such as treatment with acids [49] and fire exposure [50,51], has been reported in the literature. In addition, the effect of the duration of the postmortem and postextraction periods in obtaining genetic profiles from the teeth has been analyzed [52,53]. From these and other studies, it can be concluded that the usefulness of teeth to obtain a genetic profile not only depends on the conditions to which they are subjected before analysis but also varies between individuals and even within the same individual. This inter- and intra-individual variation may be due to a wide difference in the number of cells present in each individual tooth, resulting in a different DNA yield. In turn, the different number of cells is due to various factors, including the presence or absence of disease and the age of the subject. Therefore, each identification case must be considered individually [53,54].

It is important to note that the mother's decision to keep some teeth from her son was essential for the resolution of this case. This and similar practices [55] should be promoted, as teeth can be an alternative source of reference DNA for the identification of persons in, for example, mass disasters or criminal cases. Other samples may also be considered for this purpose, such as buccal swabs, hair, and blood spots. Instructions for their collection and preservation, as well as the material required even in a domestic setting, can be easily found on the Internet. However, in this regard, one must be very careful and sensitive and respect the customs and beliefs of a particular society or individual.

Finally, although DNA profiling is an important element for the identification of human remains, several factors can affect the results of this analysis, such as an insufficient amount of extracted DNA or its degradation in cases of poorly preserved samples. In such cases, a multidisciplinary approach may be necessary that considers the use of other disciplines, including forensic anthropology and odontology [56,57].

4. Conclusions

This is the first reported case of the use of DNA isolated from teeth as a reference sample to identify a victim in a criminal case. Whenever possible, it is preferable to use reference samples from the putative victim as a source of DNA for identification.

Author Contributions: Conceptualization, M.O.-M. and M.-d.-L.C.-B.; methodology, M.-d.-L.C.-B., G.J.-R. and M.O.-M.; resources, M.O.-M. and A.A.-A.; literature review, M.-d.-L.C.-B., G.J.-R. and J.A.-R.; writing—original draft preparation, M.-d.-L.C.-B., G.J.-R. and M.O.-M.; writing—review and editing, G.J.-R., A.A.-A. and J.A.-R.; visualization, M.O.-M., M.-d.-L.C.-B. and A.A.-A.; supervision, G.J.-R., A.A.-A. and J.A.-R.; project administration, A.A.-A. and M.O.-M. All authors have read and agreed to the published version of the manuscript.

Funding: This research received no external funding.

Institutional Review Board Statement: The study was conducted in accordance with the Declaration of Helsinki. Ethical approval was not required, as this was a case report.

Informed Consent Statement: Written informed consent was obtained from the mother for the publication of this report.

Data Availability Statement: All data generated or analyzed for this report are included in the published article.

Conflicts of Interest: The authors declare no conflict of interest.

References

1. Ziętkiewicz, E.; Witt, M.; Daca, P.; Zebracka-Gala, J.; Goniewicz, M.; Jarząb, B.; Witt, M. Current genetic methodologies in the identification of disaster victims and in forensic analysis. *J. Appl. Genet.* **2012**, *53*, 41–60. [CrossRef] [PubMed]
2. Watherston, J.; McNevin, D.; Gahan, M.E.; Bruce, D.; Ward, J. Current and emerging tools for the recovery of genetic information from post mortem samples: New directions for disaster victim identification. *Forensic Sci. Int. Genet.* **2018**, *37*, 270–282. [CrossRef] [PubMed]
3. Calacal, G.C.; De Ungria, M.C.; Delfin, F.C.; Lara, M.C.; Magtanong, D.L.; Fortun, R. Identification of two fire victims by comparative nuclear DNA typing of skeletal remains and stored umbilical tissues. *Am. J. Forensic Med. Pathol.* **2003**, *24*, 148–152. [CrossRef] [PubMed]
4. Tanaka, M.; Yoshimoto, T.; Nozawa, H.; Ohtaki, H.; Kato, Y.; Sato, K.; Yamamoto, T.; Tamaki, K.; Katsumata, Y. Usefulness of a toothbrush as a source of evidential DNA for typing. *J. Forensic Sci.* **2000**, *45*, 674–676. [CrossRef] [PubMed]
5. Sweet, D.; Hildebrand, D.; Phillips, D. Identification of a skeleton using DNA from teeth and a PAP smear. *J. Forensic Sci.* **1999**, *44*, 630–633. [CrossRef] [PubMed]
6. Adamowicz, M.S.; Labonte, R.D.; Schienman, J.E. The potential of cosmetic applicators as a source of DNA for forensic analysis. *J. Forensic Sci.* **2015**, *60*, 1001–1011. [CrossRef] [PubMed]
7. Vauhkonen, H.; Hedman, M.; Vauhkonen, M.; Kataja, M.; Sipponen, P.; Sajantila, A. Evaluation of gastrointestinal cancer tissues as a source of genetic information for forensic investigations by using STRs. *Forensic Sci. Int.* **2004**, *139*, 159–167. [CrossRef]
8. Song, L.; Liu, S.; Wu, H.; Fang, S.P.; F, Y.F. Quantification and genotyping of trace samples. *Fa Yi Xue Za Zhi* **2018**, *34*, 656–658.
9. Walsh, P.S.; Metzger, D.A.; Higuchi, R. Chelex 100 as a medium for simple extraction of DNA for PCR-based typing from forensic material. *Biotechniques* **1991**, *10*, 506–513. [CrossRef]
10. Green, M.R.; Sambrook, J. Isolation of high-molecular-weight DNA from mammalian cells using proteinase K and phenol. In *Molecular Cloning. A Laboratory Manual*; Cold Spring Harbor Laboratory Press: New York, NY, USA, 2012; Volume 1, pp. 47–53.

11. Rubi-Castellanos, R.; Anaya-Palafox, M.; Mena-Rojas, E.; Bautista-España, D.; Muñoz-Valle, J.F.; Rangel-Villalobos, H. Genetic data of 15 autosomal STRs (Identifiler kit) of three Mexican Mestizo population samples from the States of Jalisco (West), Puebla (Center), and Yucatan (Southeast). *Forensic Sci. Int. Genet.* **2009**, *3*, e71–e76. [CrossRef]
12. Cerda-Flores, R.M.; Budowle, B.; Jin, L.; Barton, S.A.; Deka, R.; Chakraborty, R. Maximum likelihood estimates of admixture in Northeastern Mexico using 13 short tandem repeat loci. *Am. J. Hum. Biol.* **2002**, *14*, 429–439. [CrossRef] [PubMed]
13. Higgins, D.; Austin, J.J. Teeth as a source of DNA for forensic identification of human remains: A review. *Sci. Justice* **2013**, *53*, 433–441. [CrossRef] [PubMed]
14. Brettell, T.A.; Butler, J.M.; Almirall, J.R. Forensic science. *Anal. Chem.* **2011**, *83*, 4539–4556. [CrossRef] [PubMed]
15. Thangaraj, K.; Reddy, A.G.; Singh, L. Mutation in the STR locus D21S11 of father causing allele mismatch in the child. *J. Forensic Sci.* **2004**, *49*, 99–103. [CrossRef]
16. Turchi, C.; Pesaresi, M.; Alessandrini, F.; Onofri, V.; Arseni, A.; Tagliabracci, A. Unusual association of three rare alleles and a mismatch in a case of paternity testing. *J. Forensic Sci.* **2004**, *49*, 260–262. [CrossRef]
17. Tsuji, A.; Ishiko, A.; Inoue, H.; Kudo, K.; Ikeda, N. Analysis of a paternity case in which the alleged father was deceased: Single locus mismatch. *Fukuoka Igaku Zasshi* **2005**, *96*, 76–80.
18. Singh Negi, D.; Alam, M.; Bhavani, S.A.; Nagaraju, J. Multistep microsatellite mutation in the maternally transmitted locus D13S317: A case of maternal allele mismatch in the child. *Int. J. Legal Med.* **2006**, *120*, 286–292. [CrossRef]
19. Narkuti, V.; Vellanki, R.N.; Gandhi, K.P.; Mangamoori, L.N. Mother-child double incompatibility at vWA and D5S818 loci in paternity testing. *Clin. Chem. Lab. Med.* **2007**, *45*, 1288–1291. [CrossRef]
20. Narkuti, V.; Vellanki, R.N.; Gandhi, K.P.; Doddapaneni, K.K.; Yelavarthi, P.D.; Mangamoori, L.N. Microsatellite mutation in the maternally/paternally transmitted D18S51 locus: Two cases of allele mismatch in the child. *Clin. Chim. Acta* **2007**, *381*, 171–175. [CrossRef]
21. Narkuti, V.; Vellanki, R.N.; Anubrolu, N.; Doddapaneni, K.K.; Gandhi Kaza, P.C.; Mangamoori, L.N. Single and double incompatibility at vWA and D8S1179/D21S11 loci between mother and child: Implications in kinship analysis. *Clin. Chim. Acta* **2008**, *395*, 162–165. [CrossRef]
22. Tsuji, A.; Ishiko, A.; Umehara, T.; Usumoto, Y.; Hikiji, W.; Kudo, K.; Ikeda, N. A silent allele in the locus D19S433 contained within the AmpFlSTR Identifiler PCR Amplification Kit. *Leg. Med.* **2010**, *12*, 94–96. [CrossRef] [PubMed]
23. Lindner, I.; von Wurmb-Schwark, N.; Meier, P.; Fimmers, R.; Büttner, A. Usefulness of SNPs as supplementary markers in a paternity case with 3 genetic incompatibilities at autosomal and Y chromosomal loci. *Transfus. Med. Hemother.* **2014**, *41*, 117–121. [CrossRef] [PubMed]
24. Liu, Y.X.; Zhang, W.Q.; Jia, Y.S.; Zhang, L.; Zhou, F.L.; Mei, K.; Huang, D.X.; Yi, S.H. Multistep microsatellite mutation in a case of non-exclusion parentage. *Forensic Sci. Int. Genet.* **2015**, *16*, 205–207. [CrossRef]
25. Chen, L.; Tai, Y.; Qiu, P.; Du, W.; Liu, C. A silent allele in the locus D5S818 contained within the PowerPlex®21 PCR Amplification Kit. *Leg. Med.* **2015**, *17*, 509–511. [CrossRef] [PubMed]
26. Jia, Y.S.; Zhang, L.; Qi, L.Y.; Mei, K.; Zhou, F.L.; Huang, D.X.; Yi, S.H. Multistep microsatellite mutation leading to father-child mismatch of FGA locus in a case of non-exclusion parentage. *Leg. Med.* **2015**, *17*, 364–365. [CrossRef]
27. Dumache, R.; Puiu, M.; Pusztai, A.M.; Parvanescu, R.; Enache, A. A single step mutation at D3S1358 locus in a DNA paternity testing with 2 alleged fathers. *Clin. Lab.* **2018**, *64*, 1561–1571. [CrossRef]
28. González-Herrera, L.J.; García-Aceves, M.E.; Domínguez-Cruz, M.D.; López-González, P.N.; Sosa-Escalante, J.E.; Rangel-Villalobos, H. A four-step mutation at D22S1045 in one complex paternity case when the brother of the alleged father hypothesis is evaluated. *Int. J. Legal Med.* **2020**, *134*, 1647–1652. [CrossRef]
29. Hering, S.; Müller, E. New alleles and mutational events in D12S391 and D8S1132: Sequence data from an eastern German population. *Forensic Sci. Int.* **2001**, *124*, 187–191. [CrossRef]
30. von Wurmb-Schwark, N.; Mályusz, V.; Simeoni, E.; Lignitz, E.; Poetsch, M. Possible pitfalls in motherless paternity analysis with related putative fathers. *Forensic Sci. Int.* **2006**, *159*, 92–97. [CrossRef]
31. Poetsch, M.; Lüdcke, C.; Repenning, A.; Fischer, L.; Mályusz, V.; Simeoni, E.; Lignitz, E.; Oehmichen, M.; von Wurmb-Schwark, N. The problem of single parent/child paternity analysis—Practical results involving 336 children and 348 unrelated men. *Forensic Sci. Int.* **2006**, *159*, 98–103. [CrossRef]
32. Huel, R.L.; Basić, L.; Madacki-Todorović, K.; Smajlović, L.; Eminović, I.; Berbić, I.; Milos, A.; Parsons, T.J. Variant alleles, triallelic patterns, and point mutations observed in nuclear short tandem repeat typing of populations in Bosnia and Serbia. *Croat. Med. J.* **2007**, *48*, 494–502. [PubMed]
33. Lu, D.; Liu, Q.; Wu, W.; Zhao, H. Mutation analysis of 24 short tandem repeats in Chinese Han population. *Int. J. Legal Med.* **2012**, *126*, 331–335. [CrossRef] [PubMed]
34. Sun, M.; Zhang, X.; Wu, D.; Shen, Q.; Wu, Y.; Fu, S. Mutations of short tandem repeat loci in cases of paternity testing in Chinese. *Int. J. Legal Med.* **2016**, *130*, 1203–1204. [CrossRef]
35. Jin, B.; Su, Q.; Luo, H.; Li, Y.; Wu, J.; Yan, J.; Hou, Y.; Liang, W.; Zhang, L. Mutational analysis of 33 autosomal short tandem repeat (STR) loci in southwest Chinese Han population based on trio parentage testing. *Forensic Sci. Int. Genet.* **2016**, *23*, 86–90. [CrossRef] [PubMed]
36. García-Aceves, M.E.; Romero Rentería, O.; Díaz-Navarro, X.X.; Rangel-Villalobos, H. Paternity tests in Mexico: Results obtained in 3005 cases. *J. Forensic Leg. Med.* **2018**, *55*, 1–7. [CrossRef] [PubMed]

37. Zhang, B.; Li, Z.; Li, K.; Chen, P.; Chen, F. Forensic parameters and mutation analysis of 23 short tandem repeat (PowerPlex® Fusion System) loci in Fujian Han Chinese population. *Leg. Med.* **2019**, *37*, 33–36. [CrossRef]
38. Junge, A.; Brinkmann, B.; Fimmers, R.; Madea, B. Mutations or exclusion: An unusual case in paternity testing. *Int. J. Legal Med.* **2006**, *120*, 360–363. [CrossRef] [PubMed]
39. Narkuti, V.; Vellanki, R.N.; Oraganti, N.M.; Mangamoori, L.N. Paternal exclusion: Allele sharing in microsatellite testing. *Clin. Chem. Lab. Med.* **2008**, *46*, 1586–1588. [CrossRef]
40. Chang, L.; Yu, H.; Miao, X.; Wen, S.; Zhang, B.; Li, S. Evaluation of a custom SNP panel for identifying and rectifying of misjudged paternity in deficiency cases. *Front. Genet.* **2021**, *12*, 602429. [CrossRef]
41. Quiroz-Mercado, J.A.; Ríos-Rivas, R.J.; Martínez-Sevilla, V.M.; Chávez-Marín, G.; Jaimes-Díaz, H.; Santiago-Hernández, J.C.; Maldonado-Rodríguez, R.; Rangel-Villalobos, H. Analysis of fortuitous matches in a STR genotype database from Mexico and its forensic efficiency parameters. *Egypt. J. Forensic. Sci.* **2017**, *7*, 19. [CrossRef]
42. Zhang, M.X.; Gao, H.M.; Han, S.Y.; Liu, Y.; Tian, Y.L.; Sun, S.H.; Xiao, D.J.; Li, C.T.; Wang, Y.S. Risk analysis of duo parentage testing with limited STR loci. *Genet. Mol. Res.* **2014**, *13*, 1179–1186. [CrossRef]
43. Ibarguchi, G.; Gissing, G.J.; Gaston, A.J.; Boag, P.T.; Friesen, V.L. Male-biased mutation rates and the overestimation of extrapair paternity: Problem, solution, and illustration using thick-billed murres (Uria lomvia, Alcidae). *J. Hered.* **2004**, *95*, 209–216. [CrossRef] [PubMed]
44. Børsting, C.; Sanchez, J.J.; Hansen, H.E.; Hansen, A.J.; Bruun, H.Q.; Morling, N. Performance of the SNPforID 52 SNP-plex assay in paternity testing. *Forensic Sci. Int. Genet.* **2008**, *2*, 292–300. [CrossRef] [PubMed]
45. Syndercombe Court, D. The Y chromosome and its use in forensic DNA analysis. *Emerg. Top. Life. Sci.* **2021**, *5*, 427–441. [PubMed]
46. Gomes, I.; Pinto, N.; Antão-Sousa, S.; Gomes, V.; Gusmão, L.; Amorim, A. Twenty years later: A comprehensive review of the X chromosome use in forensic genetics. *Front. Genet.* **2020**, *11*, 926. [CrossRef]
47. Wu, J.; Li, J.L.; Wang, M.L.; Li, J.P.; Zhao, Z.C.; Wang, Q.; Yang, S.D.; Xiong, X.; Yang, J.L.; Deng, Y.J. Evaluation of the MiSeq FGx system for use in forensic casework. *Int. J. Legal Med.* **2019**, *133*, 689–697. [CrossRef]
48. Ge, J.; Budowle, B.; Chakraborty, R. Choosing relatives for DNA identification of missing persons. *J. Forensic Sci.* **2011**, *56* (Suppl. S1), S23–S28. [CrossRef]
49. Robino, C.; Pazzi, M.; Di Vella, G.; Martinelli, D.; Mazzola, L.; Ricci, U.; Testi, R.; Vincenti, M. Evaluation of DNA typing as a positive identification method for soft and hard tissues immersed in strong acids. *Leg. Med.* **2015**, *17*, 569–575. [CrossRef]
50. Garriga, J.A.; Ubelaker, D.H.; Zapico, S.C. Evaluation of macroscopic changes and the efficiency of DNA profiling from burnt teeth. *Sci. Justice* **2016**, *56*, 437–442. [CrossRef]
51. Lozano-Peral, D.; Rubio, L.; Santos, I.; Gaitán, M.J.; Viguera, E.; Martín-de-Las-Heras, S. DNA degradation in human teeth exposed to thermal stress. *Sci. Rep.* **2021**, *11*, 12118. [CrossRef]
52. Raimann, P.E.; Picanço, J.B.; Silva, D.S.; Albuquerque, T.C.; Paludo, F.J.; Alho, C.S. Procedures to recover DNA from pre-molar and molar teeth of decomposed cadavers with different post-mortem intervals. *Arch. Oral Biol.* **2012**, *57*, 1459–1466. [CrossRef] [PubMed]
53. Izawa, H.; Tsutsumi, H.; Maruyama, S.; Komuro, T. DNA analysis of root canal-filled teeth. *Leg. Med.* **2017**, *27*, 10–18. [CrossRef] [PubMed]
54. Higgins, D.; Rohrlach, A.B.; Kaidonis, J.; Townsend, G.; Austin, J.J. Differential nuclear and mitochondrial DNA preservation in post-mortem teeth with implications for forensic and ancient DNA studies. *PLoS ONE* **2015**, *10*, e0126935. [CrossRef] [PubMed]
55. Vij, N.; Kochhar, G.K.; Chachra, S.; Kaur, T. Dentistry to the rescue of missing children: A review. *J. Forensic Dent. Sci.* **2016**, *8*, 7–12. [PubMed]
56. Raffone, C.; Baeta, M.; Lambacher, N.; Granizo-Rodríguez, E.; Etxeberria, F.; de Pancorbo, M.M. Intrinsic and extrinsic factors that may influence DNA preservation in skeletal remains: A review. *Forensic Sci. Int.* **2021**, *325*, 110859. [CrossRef]
57. Baldino, G.; Mondello, C.; Sapienza, D.; Stassi, C.; Asmundo, A.; Gualniera, P.; Vanin, S.; Ventura Spagnolo, E. Multidisciplinary forensic approach in "*complex*" bodies: Systematic review and procedural proposal. *Diagnostics* **2023**, *13*, 310. [CrossRef]

Disclaimer/Publisher's Note: The statements, opinions and data contained in all publications are solely those of the individual author(s) and contributor(s) and not of MDPI and/or the editor(s). MDPI and/or the editor(s) disclaim responsibility for any injury to people or property resulting from any ideas, methods, instructions or products referred to in the content.

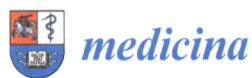

Article

Cortical and Trabecular Bone Stress Assessment during Periodontal Breakdown–A Comparative Finite Element Analysis of Multiple Failure Criteria

Radu Andrei Moga [1,*], Cristian Doru Olteanu [2,*], Stefan Marius Buru [3], Mircea Daniel Botez [3] and Ada Gabriela Delean [1]

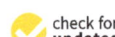

Citation: Moga, R.A.; Olteanu, C.D.; Buru, S.M.; Botez, M.D.; Delean, A.G. Cortical and Trabecular Bone Stress Assessment during Periodontal Breakdown–A Comparative Finite Element Analysis of Multiple Failure Criteria. *Medicina* 2023, 59, 1462. https://doi.org/10.3390/medicina59081462

Academic Editor: João Miguel Marques dos Santos

Received: 20 July 2023
Revised: 6 August 2023
Accepted: 9 August 2023
Published: 15 August 2023

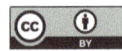

Copyright: © 2023 by the authors. Licensee MDPI, Basel, Switzerland. This article is an open access article distributed under the terms and conditions of the Creative Commons Attribution (CC BY) license (https://creativecommons.org/licenses/by/4.0/).

[1] Department of Cariology, Endodontics and Oral Pathology, School of Dental Medicine, University of Medicine and Pharmacy Iuliu Hatieganu, Str. Motilor 33, 400001 Cluj-Napoca, Romania; ada.delean@umfcluj.ro

[2] Department of Orthodontics, School of Dental Medicine, University of Medicine and Pharmacy Iuliu Hatieganu, Str. Avram Iancu 31, 400083 Cluj-Napoca, Romania

[3] Department of Structural Mechanics, School of Civil Engineering, Technical University of Cluj-Napoca, Str. Memorandumului 28, 400114 Cluj-Napoca, Romania; marius.buru@mecon.utcluj.ro (S.M.B.); mircea.botez@mecon.utcluj.ro (M.D.B.)

* Correspondence: andrei.moga@umfcluj.ro (R.A.M.); olteanu.cristian@umfcluj.ro (C.D.O.)

Abstract: *Background and Objectives:* This numerical analysis investigated the biomechanical behavior of the mandibular bone as a structure subjected to 0.5 N of orthodontic force during periodontal breakdown. Additionally, the suitability of the five most used failure criteria (Von Mises (VM), Tresca (T), maximum principal (S1), minimum principal (S3), and hydrostatic pressure (HP)) for the study of bone was assessed, and a single criterion was identified for the study of teeth and the surrounding periodontium (by performing correlations with other FEA studies). *Materials and Methods:* The finite element analysis (FEA) employed 405 simulations over eighty-one mandibular models with variable levels of bone loss (0–8 mm) and five orthodontic movements (intrusion, extrusion, tipping, rotation, and translation). For the numerical analysis of bone, the ductile failure criteria are suitable (T and VM are adequate for the study of bone), with Tresca being more suited. S1, S3, and HP criteria, due to their distinctive design dedicated to brittle materials and liquids/gas, only occasionally correctly described the bone stress distribution. *Results:* Only T and VM displayed a coherent and correlated gradual stress increase pattern for all five movements and levels of the periodontal breakdown. The quantitative values provided by T and VM were the highest (for each movement and level of bone loss) among all five criteria. The MHP (maximum physiological hydrostatic pressure) was exceeded in all simulations since the mandibular bone is anatomically less vascularized, and the ischemic risks are reduced. Only T and VM displayed a correlated (both qualitative and quantitative) stress increase for all five movements. Both T and VM displayed rotation and translation, closely followed by tipping, as stressful movements, while intrusion and extrusion were less stressful for the mandibular bone. *Conclusions:* Based on correlations with earlier numerical studies on the same models and boundary conditions, T seems better suited as a single unitary failure criterion for the study of teeth and the surrounding periodontium.

Keywords: bone; bone loss; orthodontic force; finite element analysis; orthodontic movement

1. Introduction

The bone structure and periodontal ligament (PDL) are the supporting tissues of the tooth and are subjected to various amounts and forms of stresses during orthodontic treatment [1,2]. Two types of bone can be distinguished: the cortical and the trabecular/cancellous bone, which, biomechanically, should be analyzed as a continuum [1–8]. The trabecular component holds the bone marrow and vascular vessels and has a higher regeneration potential than cortical bone [9]. Both components are anatomically anisotropic materials, with trabecular bone being a highly porous mineralized material while cortical bone is a highly mineralized compact structure [1]. Cortical bone has the function of structural support for surrounding dental tissues and the protection of trabecular/cancellous bone [5].

Bone as a continuum and as a single-stand structure possesses a high adaptation ability to alter its geometry to provide the strongest structure possible with a minimum amount of tissue [7]. The bone structure can also absorb and dissipate energy/stresses and elastically deform, preventing fracture and/or destruction [7]. Its internal structural micro-architecture allows for microcracks/damage (i.e., linear, and diffuse microcracks, and microfractures) and time to heal [7]. Linear microcracks appear as a response to compressive stresses (older age, more brittleness), the diffuse microdamage as a response to tensile stresses (younger age, more ductileness), while microfractures as a response to shear stresses (older age, mixed ductile brittleness, mostly in trabecular bone) [7]. Thus, from a biomechanical engineering perspective, the bone structural behavior depends on the applied loads acting as a ductile material with a certain brittle flow mode [2,7,10–12].

The orthodontic stresses from the tooth are transmitted through the PDL to the bone, while the display areas are also influenced by the tissular anatomy and integrity [8]. Periodontal breakdown is found in orthodontic patients, affecting the biomechanical behavior of the tooth and surrounding support tissues, with higher tissular amounts of stress appearing along with bone loss [2,10–12]. In the bone structure, Burr et al. [7] reported microcracks and microdamage near the resorption and remodeling areas and a decrease in fracture risks in their presence (due to internal micro-architectural changes), which influence the structural stress display. It must be emphasized that the biomechanical behavior in both the intact and reduced periodontium is multifactorial, which depends on the cortical and trabecular structural continuum, material, and structural properties [6].

No studies investigating the mandibular bone stress distribution in a gradual periodontal breakdown under orthodontic loads were found, despite multiple bone-implant FEA (finite element analysis) research studies with a focus on the implant and the surrounding bone [1,5,8,13–18].

Only three reports were found to assess the stress distribution both in the tooth and its intact surrounding support system (0.35–0.5 N of tipping [19,20]; 10 N of intrusion, 3 N of tipping and translation [21]); these showed various qualitative and quantitative results but no correlation with the maximum physiological hydrostatic pressure (MHP) and/or failure criteria type of the analyzed material. These reports employed both ductile (Von Mises) and brittle (maximum principal stress) failure criteria and supplied results that did not entirely match the clinical data.

The orthodontic biomechanical behavior of bone is influenced by the anatomy of tissues, materials, magnitude, and the quantity and quality of the bone [1,14]. There are several tools to analyze the biomechanical behavior of bone and teeth, including in vitro assays (photoelastic stress analysis, static/dynamic mechanical fracture tests) and numerical simulations (finite elements analysis) [1]. FEA is the only method that allows the individual analysis of each component of a structure, providing accurate results if the input data (anatomical accuracy and loading conditions) are correct [1,13]. Only a numerical simulation such as FEA allows for correct biomechanical studies that assess and predict stress distribution in living dental tissues [13,14,17,22].

FEA accuracy also depends on the selection of proper and adequate failure criteria. There are multiple failure criteria, each specially designed to better describe the biomechanical behavior of a certain type of material: brittle-maximum S1 tensile and minimum S3 compressive principal stresses, ductile-Von Mises (VM) overall/equivalent and Tresca (T) shear stress, and liquid/gas-hydrostatic pressure (HP) [2,10–12]. The main difference between these types of materials is related to the way they deform under loads (yielding materials theory) [2,10–12]. The ductile materials suffer from various forms of recoverable deformations, returning to their original form after the force effect has ceased [2,10–12]. The brittle materials, when subjected to various loads, suffer from various degrees of plastic non-recoverable deformations, with modification of their original shape and dimensions (necking and buckling effects) before their fracture and destruction [2,10–12]. Hydrostatic pressure describes a specific physical state where there is no shear stress (which is not adequate for solid materials as ductile and brittle) [2,10–12]. This approach, based on the assessment of material type when performing the FEA analysis, has not been found in other studies (except in our team's earlier studies [2,10–12]) despite its importance for the accuracy of results [22]. Moreover, there are no FEA studies of bone to compare various failure criteria and to select the most adequate one based on the results.

The dental tissues (dentine, cement, dental pulp, neurovascular bundle, PDL, bone, and stainless-steel bracket) are all considered to resemble ductile materials with a certain brittle flow mode [2,10–12]. Only enamel is a brittle material due to its internal micro-architecture [23,24]. Nevertheless, since it represents only an extremely small percentage of the entire volume of dental tissues, and the entire structure behaves as ductile, the adequate and acceptable failure criteria is that of ductile materials [2,10–12,17].

Bone, when subjected to internal stress, undergoes a certain amount of recoverable elastic deformations because of the PDL stress transmitted to the bone, beyond which microfractures appear and bone loss results [14]. According to the engineering composite beam theory, when materials with different elastic modulus (cortical and trabecular bone, PDL and dentine; Table 1) interact and are subjected to a load, the highest stress is located at the first point of contact (i.e., bone cervical third) [14]. Hooke's law states that the deformation of materials depends on their elastic modulus; the higher the modulus, the smaller the deformation [14,22]. In the tooth and surrounding support system, the periodontal ligament, followed by bone, suffers the highest deformation [10–12,14].

Table 1. Elastic properties of materials.

Material	Young's Modulus, E (GPa)	Poisson Ratio, υ	Refs.
Enamel	80	0.33	[2,10–12]
Dentin/Cementum	18.6	0.31	[2,10–12]
Pulp	0.0021	0.45	[2,10–12]
PDL	0.0667	0.49	[2,10–12]
Cortical bone	14.5	0.323	[2,10–12]
Trabecular bone	1.37	0.3	[2,10–12]
Bracket (Stainless Steel)	190	0.265	[2,10–12]

Most bone-implant FEA studies employed the adequate VM failure criteria in intact bone, reporting stress concentrations in the cortical component located in cervical third areas, while in the trabecular component, these occurred in a broader area [1,5,8,13–17,21]; however, they did not address the suitability issues (VM is more suited for homogeneous materials, while bone is non-homogenous). There are biomechanical reports suggesting that the shear stress produced by occlusal loadings contributes to bone resorption around the implants [13]. However, there were no studies found assessing the periodontal breakdown influence over the stress distribution in bone.

For avoiding ischemia, necrosis, and further periodontal loss, the physiological maximum hydrostatic pressure of 16 KPa [2,10–12] should not be exceeded, especially in the well-vascularized dental tissues and dental tissues that are easily deformable under stress (i.e., PDL, dental pulp, and the neuro-vascular bundle (NVB)). However, in the less deformable and vascularized tissues (i.e., dentine, bone), amounts of stress higher than the MHP could appear without significant tissue losses. However, these amounts of stress should not exceed the maximum tensile, shear, and compressive strength of each material (which never occurs in clinical daily practice).

Nevertheless, in orthodontic biomechanics, the PDL is the triggering factor for the orthodontic movements (due to circulatory disturbances) inducing bone remodeling. If these circulatory disturbances are severe and last for a longer period, the inevitable ischemia will lead to necrosis and tissue loss. Usually, in intact periodontium, the orthodontic forces from daily practice are light [25] and up to 1.5 N (approx. 150 gf) [2,10–12]. Nevertheless, there is little information about the orthodontic forces that can be safely applied in the reduced periodontium [10–12]. Earlier studies from our group reported for the PDL, dental pulp, and neurovascular bundle a reduction of applied forces for an 8 mm reduced periodontium to avoid exceeding the MHP. The areas of higher stress were reported to be the cervical third of PDL, with less stress in the apical third, where the NVB is found. Nevertheless, the issues of MHP and correlations with the highly vascularized dental tissues (as PDL, pulp, and NVB) should be approached in a bone study.

In the dental field, the FEA numerical method is well represented in many studies of PDL and implants. The mostly used failure criteria are the Von Mises (VM) overall/equivalent stress [18–22,26–28], Tresca (T) maximum shear stress [2,10–12], maximum principal S1 tensile stress [19,22,29–32], minimum principal S3 compressive stress [22,29,30,32–35], and hydrostatic pressure (HP) [36–40]. However, a recurrent issue in these studies (except in ours [2,10–12]) is the lack of correlations between the inner anatomical micro-structure, the material type resemblance, the criteria suitability, the coherent biomechanical behavior resembling to clinical knowledge, the quantitative results correlated with the physiological maximum hydrostatic pressure (MHP), the orthodontic force dissipation and absorption ability, and the biomechanically correct stress display. Thus, FEA is still approached with care since results are often supplied that contradict clinical knowledge [2,10–12].

In the engineering field, the FEA simulations are extremely accurate since all the above issues related to diverse types of correlations are addressed and the adequate failure criteria and correct input data have been defined. To have the same accuracy of the FEA method in dental studies, it is necessary that a single failure criterion addressing all above correlations is assessed to be scientifically accurate and providing results correlated with clinical and theoretical knowledge [2,10–12]. Previous studies from our group reported the ductile resemblance and showed that only VM and T criteria met all the above expectations, with Tresca proven to be more accurate for the tooth structural components, PDL, and dental pulp with NVB [2,10–12]. Thus, the bone FEA study herein completes the data necessary for assessing the general failure criteria for the tooth and surrounding support periodontium.

The objectives of this FEA analysis are (a) to assess the biomechanical behavior of mandibular bone subjected to light orthodontic forces during a horizontal periodontal breakdown; (b) to assess its suitability for the study in bone of five of the most used failure criteria employed in dental tissue research; (c) to correlate the results with other FEA-related reports of dental tissues to identify a suitable single unitary failure criteria for the study of teeth and the surrounding periodontium.

2. Materials and Methods

The numerical analysis herein is part of a larger stepwise research project (clinical protocol 158/02.04.2018) continuing the investigation of biomechanical behavior of teeth and surrounding periodontal structure during orthodontic movements and various levels of periodontal breakdown.

The earlier analyses of this project, with a focus on the dental pulp, neuro-vascular bundle (NVB), periodontal ligament (PDL), dentine and enamel, were conducted using the same models, boundary conditions, and physical properties as herein [2,10–12].

The 405 FEA numerical simulations were conducted over eighty-one 3D mandibular models holding the second lower premolar obtained from nine patients (4 males/5 females, mean age 29.81 ± 1.45). The selected convenience sample size of nine was acceptable for the accuracy of the results since most of the earlier FEA studies employed a sample size of one (one patient, one 3D model, and few simulations) [1,2,5,8,10–22,26–40]. The research project inclusion criteria were the presence of non-inflamed periodontium and various levels of bone loss, an intact arch and second premolar tooth structure, lack of endodontic treatment and malposition in the region of interest, indication of orthodontic treatment, and regular follow-up. All the situations that were not covered by the above criteria were considered to be exclusion criteria (especially the lack of arch integrity, tooth malposition, more than 8 mm bone-loss cases, and inflamed periodontium).

The lower mandibular region containing the premolars and first molar was examined by CBCT (ProMax 3DS, Planmeca, Helsinki, Finland), obtaining images of various shades of gray, with a voxel size of 0.075 mm.

The radiological Hounsfield gray shade units present on the DICOM slices were examined to identify the dental tissues. The anatomically accurate reconstruction of the tissues was performed through manual segmentation since the automated software algorithm did not accurately identify all the structures. Thus, the enamel, dentine, dental pulp, neurovascular bundle, periodontal ligament, cortical and trabecular bone were reconstructed in 3D (Figure 1). The reconstruction software was Amira 5.4.0 (Visage Imaging Inc., Andover, MA, USA). The base of the bracket, assumed to be of stainless steel, was reconstructed on the vestibular side of the enamel crown. Since the separation of the dentine and the cementum was impossible, and due to similar physical properties, the entire dentine–cementum structure was reconstructed as dentine (Table 1). The PDL had a variable thickness of 0.15–0.225 mm and included the NVB of the dental pulp in the apical third. The 3D models guarded only the second lower premolar, while the other tooth structures were replaced by cortical and trabecular bone. The missing bone and PDL (which were found in the cervical third) were reconstructed as closely as possible to the anatomical reality. Thus, nine models with intact periodontium (one from each patient) were obtained. In each of these models, a gradual horizontal breakdown process (0–8 mm of loss) was simulated by reducing both bone and PDL by 1 mm, obtaining a total of eighty-one models with various levels of bone loss. The 3D intact periodontium models had 5.06–6.05 million C3D4 tetrahedral elements, 0.97–1.07 million nodes, and a global element size of 0.08–0.116 mm.

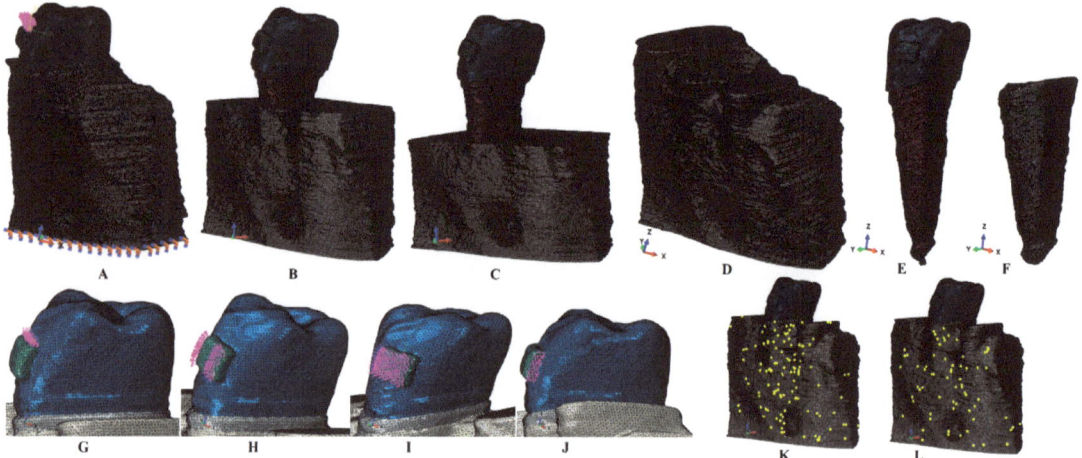

Figure 1. (**A**) 2nd lower right premolar model with intact periodontium, and applied vectors (encastered model base and extrusion loads); (**B**) 4 mm bone loss; (**C**) 8 mm bone loss; (**D**) bone structure (with cortical and trabecular components); (**E**) tooth model with bracket, enamel, dentin and neuro-vascular bundle, (**F**) intact PDL; applied vectors: (**G**) intrusion, (**H**) rotation, (**I**) tipping, (**J**) translation; (**K**) element warnings of the cortical bone component; (**L**) elements warnings of the cortical component.

The surface of the models, due to the manual segmentation technique, displayed a limited number of element warnings and no element errors (Figure 1). Thus, for one of the models shown in Figure 1K,L, the cortical bone mesh displayed 131 element warnings for 3,417,625 elements (i.e., 0.00383%), while for the trabecular mesh, there were only 70 element warnings for 1,699,730 elements (i.e., 0.00411%). The element warnings and surface anomalies were displayed in non-essential areas since the stress areas were quasi-continuous, and both numerical analysis software allowed the passing of the internal checking algorithms.

The numerical analysis was performed using the Abaqus 6.13-1 (Dassault Systèmes Simulia Corp., Maastricht, The Netherlands). Five of the most-used failure criteria were employed: Von Mises maximum overall/equivalent stress (VM), Tresca maximum shear stress (T), maximum S1 tensile principal stress, minimum S3 compressive principal stress, and hydrostatic pressure (HP). Five orthodontic movements were simulated: intrusion, extrusion, rotation, translation, and tipping, under an applied load of 0.5 N (approx. 50 g) on the base of the bracket (Figure 1). This amount of load was selected since it is a light force that is relatively safe to be applied to both the intact and the reduced periodontium; this also enables the results herein to be correlated with earlier studies with a focus on other dental tissues [2,10–12].

The assumed boundary conditions were the homogeneity, linear elasticity, and isotropy, like most of the available numerical analyses [1,2,5,8,10–22,26–40].

The results of the numerical simulations are presented as color-coded projections of the stress display areas (qualitative, Figures 2–6), and quantitative (amounts of stresses, Table 2). The biomechanical behavior displayed by each orthodontic movement and described by each failure criteria were compared and correlated with earlier analysis [2,10–12] to determine if one of the failure criteria is better suited for the study of dental tissues.

Table 2. Maximum stress average values (KPa) produced by 0.5 N of orthodontic forces.

Resorption (mm)			0	1	2	3	4	5	6	7	8
Intrusion	Tresca	a	31.22	36.19	41.17	46.13	51.11	52.35	53.59	54.83	56.08
		m	31.22	31.93	32.64	33.35	34.07	36.06	38.06	40.00	42.06
		c	124.86	127.71	130.56	133.41	136.26	137.26	138.27	139.27	140.28
	VM	a	27.10	31.39	35.68	39.97	44.27	46.03	47.79	49.55	51.31
		m	27.10	27.70	28.31	28.91	29.52	31.76	34.00	36.24	38.48
		c	108.34	110.76	113.19	115.61	118.04	120.59	123.15	125.71	128.27
	P	a	21.94	22.62	23.29	23.96	24.64	25.04	25.45	25.85	26.26
		m	21.94	22.62	23.29	23.96	24.64	25.04	25.45	25.85	26.26
		c	−59.87	−56.71	−53.56	−50.40	−47.25	−44.69	−42.14	−39.58	−37.03
	S1	a	−6.33	−5.51	−4.69	3.87	3.05	3.55	−4.07	−4.57	−5.08
		m	−6.33	−5.51	−4.69	3.87	3.05	5.03	7.01	8.99	10.96
		c	155.22	145.32	135.42	125.52	115.62	121.54	127.47	133.40	139.33
	S3	a	−18.95	−22.68	−26.41	−30.14	−33.88	−33.92	−33.96	−33.96	−34.05
		m	−18.95	−22.68	−26.41	−30.14	−33.88	−33.92	−33.96	−33.96	−34.05
		c	−39.86	−38.36	−36.87	−35.37	−33.88	−33.92	−33.96	−33.96	−34.05
Extrusion	Tresca	a	31.22	36.19	41.17	46.13	51.11	52.35	53.59	54.83	56.08
		m	31.22	31.93	32.64	33.35	34.07	36.06	38.06	40.00	42.06
		c	124.86	127.71	130.56	133.41	136.26	137.26	138.27	139.27	140.28
	VM	a	27.10	31.39	35.68	39.97	44.27	46.03	47.79	49.55	51.31
		m	27.10	27.70	28.31	28.91	29.52	31.76	34.00	36.24	38.48
		c	108.34	110.76	113.19	115.61	118.04	120.59	123.15	125.71	128.27
	P	a	−12.84	−13.38	−13.93	−14.48	−16.65	−19.05	−21.45	−23.85	−26.26
		m	−12.84	−13.38	−13.93	−14.48	−16.65	−19.05	−21.45	−23.85	−26.26
		c	59.87	56.71	53.56	50.40	47.25	44.69	42.14	39.58	37.02
	S1	a	18.90	26.24	33.59	40.93	48.28	49.88	51.49	53.10	54.71
		m	18.90	26.24	33.59	40.93	48.28	49.88	51.49	53.10	54.71
		c	39.87	41.97	44.07	46.18	48.28	49.88	51.49	53.10	54.71
	S3	a	6.33	5.51	4.69	3.87	−3.05	3.55	4.07	4.57	5.08
		m	−9.83	−8.13	−6.44	−4.74	−3.05	−5.03	−7.01	−8.99	−10.97
		c	−155.22	−145.32	−135.42	−125.52	−115.62	−113.52	−111.43	−109.33	−107.24

Table 2. Cont.

Resorption (mm)			0	1	2	3	4	5	6	7	8
Translation	Tresca	a	61.81	71.46	81.11	90.77	100.42	108.97	117.53	126.09	134.64
		m	61.81	71.46	81.11	90.77	100.42	108.97	117.53	126.09	134.64
		c	154.40	159.73	165.07	170.41	175.75	184.09	192.45	200.79	209.14
	VM	a	54.31	62.61	70.92	79.23	87.54	94.94	102.34	109.74	117.14
		m	54.31	62.61	70.92	79.23	87.54	94.94	102.34	109.74	117.14
		c	135.75	140.11	144.48	148.84	153.21	158.85	164.49	170.13	175.78
	P	a	−46.18	−42.14	−38.10	−34.01	−30.02	−26.79	−23.56	−20.33	−17.11
		m	−46.18	−42.14	−38.10	−34.01	−30.02	−26.79	−23.56	−20.33	−17.11
		c	−83.38	−78.39	−73.40	−68.41	−63.42	−59.90	−56.39	−52.88	−49.37
	S1	a	61.60	50.33	39.06	27.79	16.52	27.95	39.39	50.83	62.27
		m	36.62	31.59	26.57	21.54	16.52	27.95	39.39	50.83	62.27
		c	211.59	194.17	176.75	159.33	141.91	136.88	131.86	126.84	121.84
	S3	a	1.13	3.72	6.31	−8.90	−11.50	−10.03	−8.57	7.09	5.62
		m	1.13	3.72	6.31	−8.90	−11.50	−10.03	−8.57	7.09	5.62
		c	−161.14	−140.58	−120.03	−99.48	−78.93	−85.04	−91.16	−97.27	−103.39
Rotation	Tresca	a	63.95	70.54	77.14	83.73	90.33	99.18	108.03	116.88	125.74
		m	63.95	70.54	77.14	83.73	90.33	99.18	108.03	116.88	125.74
		c	255.74	268.98	282.22	295.46	308.71	315.36	322.02	328.68	335.34
	VM	a	55.47	61.21	66.95	72.69	78.43	86.08	91.82	99.47	109.03
		m	55.47	61.21	66.95	72.69	78.43	86.08	91.82	99.47	109.03
		c	221.83	231.67	241.52	251.37	261.22	268.59	275.97	283.34	290.72
	P	a	20.61	21.27	21.94	22.60	23.27	27.44	31.61	35.78	39.95
		m	20.61	21.27	21.94	22.60	23.27	27.44	31.61	35.78	39.95
		c	77.87	82.23	86.59	90.95	95.32	96.17	97.03	97.88	98.74
	S1	a	43.95	53.70	63.45	73.20	82.96	89.68	96.40	103.12	109.84
		m	43.95	46.01	48.07	50.13	52.20	57.90	63.60	69.30	75.00
		c	161.35	134.06	106.78	79.48	52.20	57.90	63.60	69.30	75.00
	S3	a	−5.09	−6.79	−8.49	10.19	11.89	13.71	15.53	−17.35	−19.17
		m	−95.49	−108.74	121.99	−135.24	−148.50	−167.16	−185.83	−204.49	−223.16
		c	−185.93	−208.66	−231.39	−254.12	−276.86	−273.63	−270.41	−267.18	−263.96
Tipping	Tresca	a	61.06	65.40	69.75	74.10	78.45	81.51	84.58	87.64	90.71
		m	61.06	65.40	69.75	74.10	78.45	81.51	84.58	87.64	90.71
		c	122.11	130.81	139.51	148.21	156.91	163.03	169.16	175.29	181.41
	VM	a	53.07	56.78	60.50	64.22	67.94	70.74	73.54	76.34	79.14
		m	53.07	56.78	60.50	64.22	67.94	70.74	73.54	76.34	79.14
		c	106.18	113.58	120.99	128.40	135.81	141.44	147.08	152.72	158.36
	P	a	12.94	14.82	16.70	18.58	20.46	25.31	30.16	35.01	39.87
		m	12.94	14.82	16.70	18.58	20.46	25.31	30.16	35.01	39.87
		c	52.74	62.11	71.49	80.86	90.24	96.93	103.63	110.33	117.03
	S1	a	10.18	16.86	23.54	30.22	36.90	44.14	51.38	58.62	65.86
		m	10.18	16.86	23.54	30.22	36.90	44.14	51.38	58.62	65.86
		c	53.18	49.11	45.04	40.97	36.90	44.14	51.38	58.62	65.86
	S3	a	8.52	10.07	11.63	13.19	14.72	16.01	17.30	18.59	19.89
		m	8.52	9.27	10.03	−10.78	−11.54	−14.43	−17.33	−20.22	−23.12
		c	−171.86	−184.27	−196.69	−209.11	−221.53	−236.44	−251.35	−266.26	−281.18

a—apical third; m—middle third; c—cervical third.

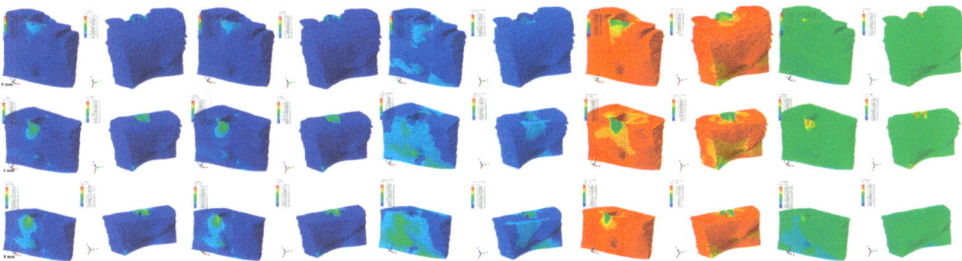

Figure 2. Comparative stress display of the five failure criteria in intact, 4 mm, and 8 mm periodontal breakdown for the extrusion movement under 0.5 N of load—vestibular and lingual views: (**A**) Tresca; (**B**) Von Mises; (**C**) maximum principal S1; (**D**) minimum principal S3; (**E**) pressure.

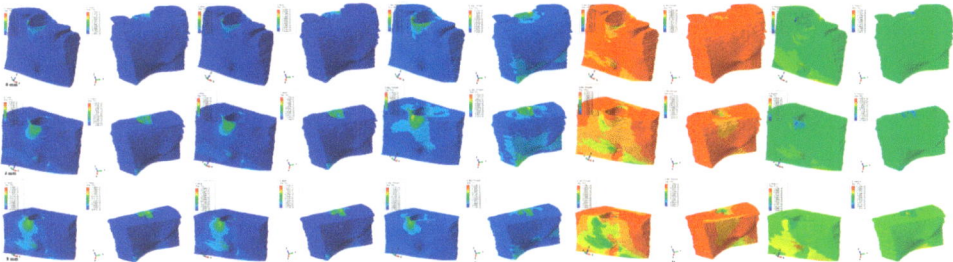

Figure 3. Comparative stress display of the five failure criteria in intact, 4 mm, and 8 mm periodontal breakdown for the intrusion movement under 0.5 N of load—vestibular and lingual views: (**A**) Tresca; (**B**) Von Mises; (**C**) maximum principal S1; (**D**) minimum principal S3; (**E**) pressure.

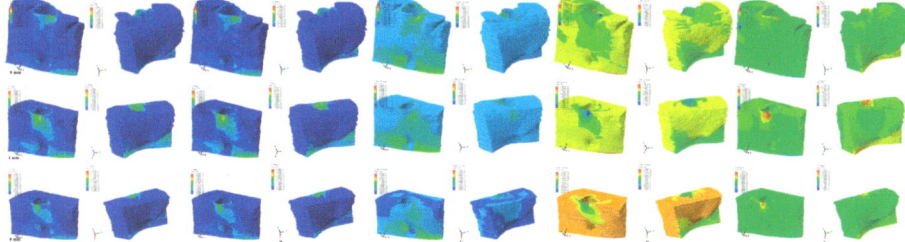

Figure 4. Comparative stress display of the five failure criteria in intact, 4 mm, and 8 mm periodontal breakdown for the rotation movement under 0.5 N of load—vestibular and lingual views: (**A**) Tresca; (**B**) Von Mises; (**C**) maximum principal S1; (**D**) minimum principal S3; (**E**) pressure.

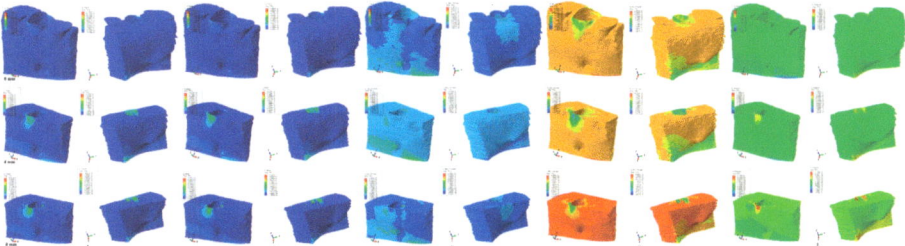

Figure 5. Comparative stress display of the five failure criteria in intact, 4 mm, and 8 mm periodontal breakdown for the tipping movement under 0.5 N of load—vestibular and lingual views: (**A**) Tresca; (**B**) Von Mises; (**C**) maximum principal S1; (**D**) minimum principal S3; (**E**) pressure.

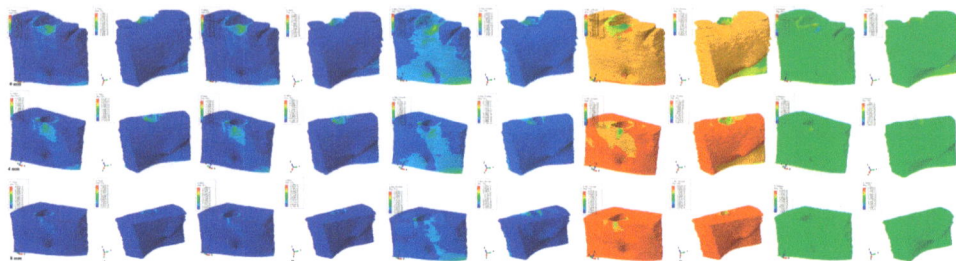

Figure 6. Comparative stress display of the five failure criteria in intact, 4 mm, and 8 mm periodontal breakdown for the translation movement under 0.5 N of load—vestibular and lingual views: (**A**) Tresca; (**B**) Von Mises; (**C**) maximum principal S1; (**D**) minimum principal S3; (**E**) pressure.

3. Results

Our analysis involved eighty-one mandibular models in 405 FEA numerical simulations (Figures 2–6 and Table 2). No influences due to age, sex, or periodontal status were seen.

From the qualitative point of view (i.e., the color-coded stress display from Figures 2–6), both the Tresca and Von Mises failure criteria displayed similar color-coded projections for all five orthodontic movements in both the intact and the reduced periodontium. S1, S3, and HP criteria displayed various color-coded projections of the stress distribution and no visible constant pattern: sometimes resembling T and VM, sometimes showing unusual biomechanical behavior (i.e., different from acknowledged clinical reality). Moreover, the boundary conditions (i.e., encastered base of the model, with zero displacements) significantly influenced the biomechanical behavior of the models when S1, S3, and HP criteria were employed.

From the quantitative point of view (Table 2), the unusual biomechanical behavior was seen in S1 and S3 criteria in the rotation, translation, and tipping movements during the periodontal breakdown with a variable decrease/increase of 0–4 mm and 4–8 mm bone loss. The HP criteria displayed a decrease in the amounts of stress for intrusion, extrusion and translation, and an increase for rotation and tipping. No stress pattern and/or correlations were observed among the S1, S3, and HP criteria despite investigating the same models under the same conditions as T and VM. Only T and VM criteria displayed a constant expected increase pattern during the periodontal breakdown process for all five movements, confirming the acknowledged clinical biomechanical behavior. The rotation movement seemed to be the most bone-stressful of all five criteria. Nevertheless, T and VM displayed rotation and translation, closely followed by tipping, as stressful movements, while intrusion and extrusion were less stressful for the mandibular bone.

All quantitative stresses displayed in the mandibular bone for all five failure criteria exceeded the MHP of 16 KPa in both the intact and the 8 mm reduced periodontium. The highest amount of stress was produced by the rotation at 8 mm of bone loss (335 KPa [0.335 MPa]) under the T criteria. The vestibular cervical third stress was the highest for all criteria, movements, and levels of bone loss. All stresses were lower than the acknowledged physical properties of bone: cortical bone compressive modulus, 16.7 GPa, and compressive strength, 157 MPa; trabecular/cancellous bone compressive modulus, 0.155 GPa, and compressive strength, 6 MPa [1,5,8,13–18].

3.1. Extrusion (Figure 2)

VM (overall stress) and T (shear stress) criteria displayed similar color-coded projections in both the intact and the reduced periodontium. The stressed areas were found in the cervical third of the alveolar wall where the bone is thinner. The cervical third stress location was maintained during the entire periodontal breakdown, with a proportional increase correlated with the bone loss. On the lingual side of the mandibular bone model, due to boundary conditions (base of the model had zero displacements), reduced amounts of stress were displayed. The S1 maximum principal tensile stress displayed from 4 to 8 of bone loss, which was an unusual stress increase both on the vestibular and the lingual surfaces (for such a small extrusion force of 0.5 N). The S3 minimum principal compressive stress displayed an unusual maximum moment of stress increase at 4 mm of loss (on both the vestibular and lingual sides, quantitatively visible in Table 2), despite the cervical third stress having a similar display as T and VM. The HP criteria displayed the same unusual biomechanical stress increase at 4 mm of bone loss, with a further apical third increase on both the vestibular and lingual sides at 8 mm of loss (due to boundary conditions). All quantitative values were higher than MHP.

3.2. Intrusion (Figure 3)

T and VM criteria displayed higher cervical third stress on the vestibular side of the model during the entire periodontal breakdown simulation, with a gradual increase in the apical third from 4–8 mm of loss. The lingual side stress at the base of the model appears to correlate with the progression of bone loss. The quantitative values are like those seen in the extrusion movement. S1 and S3 criteria showed a visible unusual stress display, with higher stresses on both the vestibular and lingual sides, and a decrease in stress from 0–4 mm followed by an increase from 4–8 mm of loss. HP criteria displayed a quantitative cervical stress decrease correlated with bone loss and a light increase in the apical third and base of the model.

3.3. Rotation (Figure 4)

T and VM displayed a cervical third stress increase correlated with the periodontal breakdown on the vestibular side of the bone. Both criteria display stresses found at the base of the models due to the assumption of zero displacements. Rotation produced the highest amounts of stress among all five movements. Both S1 (tensile) and S3 (compressive) criteria displayed unusual extended stress areas for only 0.5 N of rotation and a decrease in quantitative vestibular cervical third stress from 0–4 mm followed by an increase up to 8 mm of loss. HP stress displays mostly vestibular cervical third stress areas (and stress at the base of the model lingual side), and with lower amounts of stress than T and VM.

3.4. Tipping (Figure 5)

Vestibular side cervical third stress was shown during the periodontal breakdown by both T and VM criteria. On the lingual and vestibular sides close to the base of the model, visible stresses were displayed due to assumed boundary conditions. Both criteria displayed a quantitative increase in stresses correlated with the bone loss levels. S1 criteria displayed an unusual stress pattern with less stress in the cervical third and more on the vestibular side close to the base of the model. S3 displayed the highest compressive stress in the cervical third for intact periodontium, while visible stresses (despite the reduced applied force of 0.5 N) were also seen on the lingual side close to the base of the model. Quantitatively, S3 displayed a stress increase correlated with bone loss. S1 criteria displayed an unusual decrease in stress in the cervical third from a 0–4 loss followed by an increase from a 4–8 mm loss. HP criteria displayed a stress increase in both the vestibular cervical third and the lingual side close to the model base.

3.5. Translation (Figure 6)

Both T and VM criteria displayed higher stresses in the vestibular cervical third, with a reduction of the extension correlated with the progress of the periodontal breakdown. Both criteria displayed a correlated quantitative stress increase with the bone loss levels. Both S1 and S3 criteria showed an unusual stress display, and a quantitative decrease from 0–4 mm followed by an increase from 4–8 mm of loss. HP criteria showed almost no stress areas and a constant quantitative stress decrease.

For all five movements and periodontal breakdown levels, the S1, S3 (specific for brittle materials), and HP (specific for liquids/gas) criteria displayed unusually extended and variable stress areas for such a small force (0.5 N/ approx. 50 gf). The quantitative variable stress increase/decrease at the 0–4 and 4–8 mm bone levels and the lack of any biomechanical pattern or correlations seemed to confirm the reduced accuracy of these three criteria. The base of the models was assumed to have no displacements (simulating the stiffness of the mandibular bone); thus, areas of stress found close to the base of the models were expected (similar to other numerical analysis). However, S1, S3 and HP displayed an unusual extension of these stress areas compared with T and VM criteria.

T and VM for all five movements and bone levels displayed a coherent and correlated gradual stress increase pattern (Table 2), the expected biomechanical behavior (Figures 2–6), and a limited stress area at the base of the model. The MHP was exceeded in all simulations (e.g., 6.7–16 times in the vestibular cervical third for T and VM criteria), as expected, since the mandibular bone is anatomically less vascularized, and the ischemic risks are reduced.

The quantitative values provided by T and VM were the highest among all the five criteria. The differences between the T and VM values were approx. 15%, thus falling within the range reported in the literature of 15–30%.

When the qualitative and quantitative results are correlated, T and VM seemed to be more adequate for the study of bone biomechanical behavior than the other three criteria, with T more suited due to its mathematical design for non-homogenous ductile structures with a certain brittle flow mode (dental tissues included [2,10–12]).

4. Discussion

The present study assessed the biomechanical behavior of bone as a single-stand/continuum structure (with both cortical and trabecular/cancellous components) when subjected to stresses projected by 0.5 N of orthodontic force during periodontal breakdown. The experiments were performed through 405 FEA simulations on over eighty-one 3D mandibular models with the second lower premolar included, employing five of the most used failure criteria, with the aim of finding the most suitable criteria for bone analysis. It must be emphasized that this is the only study investigating these issues. Moreover, by correlating the results herein with those from earlier studies [2,10–12], we aimed to identify a single general failure criterion that can be used for the numerical analysis of dental tissues.

During the periodontal breakdown simulations under the five orthodontic movements, only the T (Tresca) and VM (Von Mises) criteria displayed a coherent and correlated pattern, both qualitatively and quantitatively, and a biomechanical behavior resembling that in vivo (Figures 2–6 and Table 2). The other three criteria (S1—maximum tensile, S3—minimum compressive, and HP—hydrostatic pressure) displayed no visible biomechanical behavioral pattern despite investigating the same models and boundary conditions (Figure 1 and Table 1) as T and VM. Between T and VM, due to their mathematical design for different types of internal micro-structures, T seemed to be more suitable than VM (i.e., similar qualitative color-coded projections but with 15% increase in quantitative values, in agreement with other reports [2,10–12]). Both VM and T were designed for ductile materials, the major difference being that T better describes the behavior of non-homogenous materials, while VM is more adequate for homogenous ones [2,10–12]. It must be emphasized that bone has a biomechanical behavior resembling ductile materials (with a certain brittle flow mode), displaying various recoverable elastic deformations when subjected to stresses that totally return to their original form after the forces disappear [1].

The S1 (tensile) and S3 (compressive) failure criteria are adequate for brittle materials (little or no deformations before fracture/destruction), and from the biomechanical point of view, these should display a complementary behavioral pattern and correlation since the tension and compressions are two physical transitional phases of deformation [22]. Nevertheless, no such correlation was seen, suggesting that both S1 and S3 do not meet the necessary accuracy for the study of mandibular bone.

The HP was specially designed for liquids and gas where there are no shear stresses during their behavior [2,10–12]. With HP being suitable for liquids (e.g., circulatory fluids), and since the mandibular bone has a reduced vascularization (being only a percentage of the entire tissue volume), its failure criteria are even less adequate than those of S1 and S3, visible in Figures 2–6.

The FEA analysis of dental tissues needs a single unitary failure criterion that better describes the stress display and provides quantitative results that correlate with clinical data [1]. Both T and VM seem to meet these criteria. In earlier studies [2,10–12] of this issue, both criteria were reported to be suitable for the periodontal ligament, dental pulp, and neuro-vascular bundle, and tooth (dentine/cementum, enamel, and stainless-steel bracket), with T being more adequate than VM.

A failure criterion must also provide results that correlate with the maximum hydrostatic pressure values (about 80% of the systolic pressure) found in the dental tissues, which, if exceeded, would lead to ischemia, necrosis, further periodontal loss, and internal and external orthodontic resorptive processes. Both T and VM criteria were reported to supply quantitative results that met this request, while the other three criteria failed [2,10–12].

There are multiple FEA bone-implant studies on stress distribution [1,5,8,13–18] using uniaxial loading, the VM criteria, and that report concentrations of stress in the cervical third of the bone around the implant, in line with our findings. However, due to the biomechanical behavioral, differences caused by the lack of a PDL and much higher amounts of applied loads than herein (3–10 N [5,18]; 40–800 N [1,8,13–17] vs. 0.5 N), the quantitative results cannot be compared despite the similar boundary conditions and failure criteria. Nonetheless, the qualitative results (the color-coded projection of the VM overall stress) could be correlated with those herein, displaying similar results for the stress distribution areas.

Only three FEA tooth–bone studies of stress distribution were found [19–21], with the same boundary conditions and failure criteria as herein. Merdji et al. [21] (single intact periodontium models, 10 N of intrusion, 3 N of tipping and translation, lower third molar, intact bone, VM criteria, 0.25–1 mm global element size, 142305 elements of the mandibular bone) reported a similar cervical third stress display for all three movements as herein. Nonetheless, some differences are also visible since the Merdji et al. [21] model was of the third molar with a different anatomical geometry (equal thickness of the lingual and vestibular bone, three roots) vs. the second premolar herein (vestibular wall of the alveolar process much thinner than the lingual one especially during periodontal breakdown, two roots). The quantitative amounts of cervical stress were 10.5 MPa for 10 N of intrusion, 11.5 MPa for 3 N of tipping, and 16.83 MPa for 3 N of translation [21] vs. 108.34 KPa (0.108MPa) for 0.5 N of intrusion, 106.18 KPa (0.106 MPa) for 0.5 N of tipping, and 135.75(0.135 MPa) for 0.5 N of translation reported herein. These quantitative differences could be due to the differences between the elements' size and the number of tetrahedral elements of the bone structure (0.25–1 mm/142,305 elements [21] vs. 0.08–0.116 mm/5117355 elements in our analysis).

Using two mandibular models, Field et al. [20] simulated 0.35 N (0.5 N resulting load) of tipping movements (i.e., a single intact periodontium model of 32,812 elements, with incisor, canine, and first premolar, and a single intact periodontium model with canine of 23,565 elements, global element size 1.2 mm, VM, and S1, S3, and HP criteria). The qualitative results (color-coded stress distribution) of Field et al. [20] resembled those herein but with a different color intensity (red high-stress [20] vs. blue-green lower stress in the models herein, which is closer to the clinical biomechanical behavior of a light force). The quantitative results for the bone cervical third stress were 236.3–287.8 KPa VM, 110.1–135.5 KPa S1, and 9.24–(−11.4) KPa S3 [20] vs. 106.18 KPa VM, 53.18 KPa S1, and −171 KPa S3 herein. The differences between Fields et al. [20] and our results come from the modeling issues and the applied forces (e.g., 23565–32812 number of elements and global element size of 1.2 mm vs. 5.06–6.05 million elements, 0.97–1.07 million nodes, and a global element size of 0.08–0.116 mm herein). In additional support of this assumption,

Field et al. [20] reported an HP stress of 32 KPa in the apical third of the PDL and a VM stress of 235.5–324.5 KPa in the PDL, amounts that both exceed the 16 KPa of physiological MHP signaling related to increased risks of ischemia, necrosis, and periodontal loss, which contradicts clinical knowledge [25]. These reports of stress [20] are unusually high (for a light orthodontic force of 0.5 N), signaling potential tissue damage which in reality does not occur [25]; thus, these are in need of an explanation. Nonetheless, no correlation with MHP and clinical biomechanical behavior was found in the Field et al. [20] study.

Field et al. [20] also reported a difference between the single tooth and multiple teeth numerical analyses, with higher amounts of stress and larger extension of the stress areas in the multi-tooth system. However, our herein results are lower than those reported by Field et al. [20], and we expect that that same pattern would be followed by a model with multiple teeth.

Similar correlations have been discussed and shown in earlier studies [10–12] using same models and boundary conditions as herein, but with a focus on the PDL, dental pulp, NVB, and dentine tissues. By using the same failure criteria comparison as herein, both VM and T criteria were proven to be adequate for dental tissues, with T being more accurate. Moreover, 0.5 N of force was proven to be safely applied to PDL, dental pulp, and NVB in both intact and 8 mm periodontal breakdown, with quantitative results lower than the MHP and correlated with the acknowledged clinical biomechanical behavior [10,11]. For the less vascularized tissues, such as dentine, the quantitative amounts of stress were higher than the MHP, as they biomechanically should be (correlating with the amounts of stress in bone herein), with qualitative stress display areas correlated with those present in vascularized ones (PDL, dental pulp, and NVB) [12]. The results herein, both quantitative and qualitative, are in line with the above approach.

Shaw et al. [19] (upper incisor, intact periodontium model of 11,924 elements and 20,852 nodes, VM and S1 criteria) reported, for the same five movements (intrusion, extrusion, tipping, translation, and rotations), lower amounts of cervical stress (1.664 KPa for intrusion/extrusion, 0.6 KPa for translation, 0.54 KPa for tipping, and 0.015 KPa for rotation) and comparable stress display areas. We assume that the differences are due to the anatomical accuracy and geometry of the models (incisive vs. premolar, and 507 times fewer elements than herein).

FEA analysis can supply accurate results as in the engineering field if the same requirements are fulfilled (i.e., proper failure criteria, boundary conditions, and physical properties) [2,10–12]. The selection of the failure criteria is mandatory for the correctness of both qualitative and quantitative results [22]. A single unitary criterion for the FEA analysis of teeth and the surrounding periodontium is needed, and based on the available data, this could be easily identified [2,10–12]. This criterion is scientifically based on the type of internal architecture of the analyzed material (suiting its internal micro-architecture [23,24]) that better describes its biomechanical behavior and provides results that are correlated with the clinical practical data [25] and other numerical analyses [2,10–12]. Bone-implant studies [1,5,8,13–18] exclusively employed, as adequate, the ductile material resemblance VM failure criteria, while bone–tooth studies [19–21] employed multiple criteria: ductile (VM), liquid (HP), and brittle (S1, S3). The PDL studies also employed Von Mises (VM) overall/equivalent stress [18–22,26–28], Tresca (T) maximum shear stress [2,10–12], maximum principal S1 tensile stress [19,22,29–32], minimum principal S3 compressive stress [22,29,30,32–35], and hydrostatic pressure (HP) [36–40]. In all FEA simulations, only the ductile resemblance criteria (VM and T) matched the clinical data [2,10–12].

The dental tissues, despite resembling ductile material, have a certain variable amount of brittleness; thus, when brittle material failure criteria such as S1 and S3 are applied, these can sometimes provide both qualitative and quantitative results matching the adequate ductile criteria as in the above studies [19,22,29–35] and also shown herein in Figures 2–6. However, when conducting a larger survey of multiple movements and various bone loss levels, the non-suitability of S1 and S3 becomes more and more visible (as shown by the herein comparisons in Figures 2–6 and in our earlier studies [2,10–12]). Only one study was found that provided knowledge regarding the differences between the application of various failure criteria and that had similar reports [22] as herein, except for the brittleness of endodontic filing materials. Moreover, this study [22] emphasized the differences that are due to the employment of different brittle failure criteria when analyzing a brittle material and thus the importance of selecting better suited criteria.

The HP criteria (which was also largely employed in the study of PDL based on the rich proportion of fluids contained in the ligament [36–40]) do not describe the shear state since liquids do not go through this physical state (common engineering knowledge). Moreover, when multiple HP studies are compared, the reports are variable and do not match the clinical practical knowledge.

Studies by Wu et al. [38–40] reported various (0.28–3.31 N) optimal forces for the intact PDL subjected to orthodontic movements of the canine, premolar, and lateral incisive. However, despite using the same models and boundary conditions, all three studies reported significant differences for the same movement and tooth (e.g., canine: rotation 1.7–2.1 N [40] and 3.31 N [38]; extrusion 0.38–0.4 N [40] and 2.3–2.6 N [39]; premolar: rotation 2.8–2.9 N [38]), which were all much higher compared with those reported by Proffit et al. [25] (0.1–1 N), Moga et al. [10,11] (0.5 N), and Hemanth et al. [31,32] (0.3–1 N). Hofmann et al. [36,37], in two studies using the same HP failure criteria for the PDL, reported unusual qualitative and quantitative results for 0.5–1 N of intrusion, which contradicted his earlier study and the existing clinical knowledge. Maravic et al. [26], despite using a single FEA model, supplemented the numerical analysis with an in vivo–in vitro study, reporting numerical results that did not accurately match the experimental ones.

The common issue found for all the FEA studies [19–21,26,28,29,31–34,36–40] was the small sample size of only one (one patient, a single 3D model, subjected to few orthodontic movements, generally in intact periodontium, and aleatory, using one or two failure criteria). This study and our earlier [2,10–12] studies tried to address these issues by increasing the sample size to nine, using multiple various bone loss levels, and rationally selecting the failure criteria (nine patients, eighty-one models and 405 numerical simulations), thus obtaining different and more accurate results.

There are few studies (i.e., limited to PDL investigations) that approach the study of biomechanical behavior of dental tissues during the periodontal breakdown, while all numerical FEA examinations are of the intact periodontium. Moreover, there is no standardization (due to the lack of biomechanical engineering knowledge) for conducting finite element studies in the dentistry field [1]. Thus, there is a need for studies to supply data that address this issue, since numerical simulations are the only possible method to study living tissues.

The boundary conditions assumed in the FEA studies for dental tissues were homogeneity, isotropy, and linear elasticity [1,2,5,8,10–22,26–40], despite the acknowledged anisotropy, non-homogeneity, and nonlinear elasticity of dental tissues. However, in order for all the above assumptions to supply accurate results, some issues must be addressed. If the applied loads are around 1 N, small movements and displacements are produced, and all tissues display biomechanical linear–elastic isotropic behavior despite their nonlinear anisotropic behavior under higher loads [2,10–12]. Few studies have addressed the differences between linear and non-linear behavior (and limited only to PDL behavior). Hemanth et al. [31,32] investigated these differences under light forces up to 1 N (intrusion and tipping of an upper incisor) and reported up to 20–50% less quantitative applied force needed for non-linearity vs. linearity. However, these two studies [31,32] did not address the essential issue of the adequate material-type failure criteria for PDL, since they used for comparison the S1 tensile and S3 compressive brittle criteria for the analysis of a ductile behavior resemblance material such as PDL. Another potential issue that could influence the results seems to be the accuracy of the analyzed 3D model (i.e., only 148,097 elements and 239,666 nodes and idealized anatomy) when extremely fine, small, and sensitive interactions occur both within and between anatomical elements.

The issues of assuming non-homogeneity in dental tissues demand an extremely complicated mathematical equations approach, internal micro-architecture tissue 3D modeling, and high computing resources, which simply are not possible to be performed manually since this type of modeling software is not available. However, in the engineering field, this problem has been approached and addressed by mathematically designing failure criteria for both ductile non-homogenous materials (T) and homogenous (VM) materials, thus supplying the only practical solution currently possible.

The anatomical accuracy of the models influences the correctness of the results, especially if small tissues under small displacements are investigated. Due to difficulties related to the creation of anatomically accurate 3D models (possible through a manual segmentation technique), and since the automated software detection algorithm encounters difficulties in identifying the differences of various shades of gray on the CBTC slices, most numerical analyses have a reduced sample size that is limited to only one model or use idealized models that do not accurately follow the anatomical accuracy. However, the downside of manual segmentation is the presence of a limited number of surface anomalies and irregularities (as in the models herein) that usually do not influence the accuracy of the results since these are in non-essential areas and the internal software mesh-testing algorithm allowed the simulations.

Due to all these limitative issues, and since FEA analysis (here included) cannot entirely reproduce the clinical situation and biomechanical behavior, correlations with clinical behavioral biomechanics and physiological constants (such as MHP) are mandatory for confirming the numerical results. Thus, there is a need to have a multidisciplinary engineering and medical/dental knowledge approach that discusses all the above-mentioned issues, our team's work herein and in earlier [2,10–12] studies being the first in this direction. Nevertheless, despite all the above limitative issues, FEA is still the only available method to study the stress and strain distribution in the tissue components of an anatomical tissue.

5. Practical/Clinical Implications

Periodontal breakdown is found in orthodontic patients, with little available information about the stress distribution under light orthodontic forces (0.5 N). The clinician needs to know not only the areas most affected by orthodontic stresses but also the amount of stress that could appear during the most stressful orthodontic movements to be able to individualize the treatment and correlate it with bone loss levels. Another practical issue is related to the fact that, based on the results herein, a single unitary suitable failure criterion for the study of teeth and the surrounding periodontium can be seen, which is strictly correlated with the physical properties and ductile resemblance of dental tissues. The researcher benefits from the biomechanical correlations herein, which supply important data for further studies that are needed for a better understanding of the biomechanical behavior of periodontal breakdown and for minimalizing the risks of further tissue loss.

6. Conclusions

For the numerical analysis of bone, the ductile failure criteria are suitable (both T and VM are adequate for the study of bone), with Tresca being more adequate than VM.

The S1, S3, and HP failure criteria, due to their distinctive design dedicated to brittle materials and liquids/gas, only occasionally correctly described the distribution of stresses in the bone.

For all five orthodontic movements and bone levels, only T and VM displayed a coherent and correlated gradual stress increase pattern along with the periodontal breakdown.

The quantitative values provided by T and VM were the highest among all five criteria (for each movement and level of bone loss).

The MHP (maximum physiological hydrostatic pressure) was exceeded in all simulations, since the mandibular bone is anatomically less vascularized, and the ischemic risks are reduced.

T and VM displayed rotation and translation, closely followed by tipping, as stressful movements, while intrusion and extrusion were less stressful for the mandibular bone.

Based on correlations with other earlier numerical studies on the same models and boundary conditions, T can be seen as a suitable single unitary failure criterion for the study of teeth and the surrounding periodontium.

Author Contributions: Conceptualization: R.A.M.; Methodology: R.A.M.; Software: R.A.M., S.M.B. and M.D.B.; Validation: R.A.M., A.G.D., S.M.B., M.D.B. and C.D.O.; Formal analysis: R.A.M., M.D.B. and S.M.B.; Investigation: R.A.M. and S.M.B.; Resources: R.A.M.; Data Curation: R.A.M.; Writing—original draft preparation: R.A.M.; Writing—review and editing: R.A.M., A.G.D. and C.D.O.; Visualization, Supervision, and Project administration: R.A.M., A.G.D. and C.D.O.; Funding acquisition: R.A.M., A.G.D. and C.D.O. All authors have read and agreed to the published version of the manuscript.

Funding: The authors were the funders of this research project.

Institutional Review Board Statement: The research protocol has been approved by the Ethical Committee of the University of Medicine (code 158 on 2 April 2018).

Informed Consent Statement: Informed oral consent was obtained from all subjects involved in the study.

Data Availability Statement: Not applicable.

Conflicts of Interest: The authors declare that they have no conflict of interest.

References

1. Prados-Privado, M.; Martínez-Martínez, C.; Gehrke, S.A.; Prados-Frutos, J.C. Influence of Bone Definition and Finite Element Parameters in Bone and Dental Implants Stress: A Literature Review. *Biology* **2020**, *9*, 224. [PubMed]
2. Moga, R.A.; Olteanu, C.D.; Botez, M.D.; Buru, S.M. Assessment of the Orthodontic External Resorption in Periodontal Breakdown-A Finite Elements Analysis (Part I). *Healthcare* **2023**, *11*, 1447.
3. Osterhoff, G.; Morgan, E.F.; Shefelbine, S.J.; Karim, L.; McNamara, L.M.; Augat, P. Bone mechanical properties and changes with osteoporosis. *Injury* **2016**, *47* (Suppl. S2), S11–S20.
4. Wang, L.; You, X.; Zhang, L.; Zhang, C.; Zou, W. Mechanical regulation of bone remodeling. *Bone Res.* **2022**, *10*, 16. [CrossRef] [PubMed]
5. Tawara, D.; Nagura, K. Predicting changes in mechanical properties of trabecular bone by adaptive remodeling. *Comput. Methods Biomech. Biomed. Eng.* **2017**, *20*, 415–425.
6. Hart, N.H.; Nimphius, S.; Rantalainen, T.; Ireland, A.; Siafarikas, A.; Newton, R.U. Mechanical basis of bone strength: Influence of bone material, bone structure and muscle action. *J. Musculoskelet. Neuronal Interact.* **2017**, *17*, 114–139.
7. Burr, D.B. Why bones bend but don't break. *J. Musculoskelet. Neuronal Interact.* **2011**, *11*, 270–285.
8. Cicciù, M.; Cervino, G.; Milone, D.; Risitano, G. FEM Investigation of the Stress Distribution over Mandibular Bone Due to Screwed Overdenture Positioned on Dental Implants. *Materials* **2018**, *11*, 1512. [CrossRef]
9. Wu, V.; Schulten, E.; Helder, M.N.; Ten Bruggenkate, C.M.; Bravenboer, N.; Klein-Nulend, J. Bone vitality and vascularization of mandibular and maxillary bone grafts in maxillary sinus floor elevation: A retrospective cohort study. *Clin. Implant. Dent. Relat. Res.* **2023**, *25*, 141–151. [CrossRef]
10. Moga, R.A.; Buru, S.M.; Olteanu, C.D. Assessment of the Best FEA Failure Criteria (Part II): Investigation of the Biomechanical Behavior of Dental Pulp and Apical-Neuro-Vascular Bundle in Intact and Reduced Periodontium. *Int. J. Env. Res. Public. Health* **2022**, *19*, 15635. [CrossRef]
11. Moga, R.A.; Buru, S.M.; Olteanu, C.D. Assessment of the Best FEA Failure Criteria (Part I): Investigation of the Biomechanical Behavior of PDL in Intact and Reduced Periodontium. *Int. J. Env. Res. Public. Health* **2022**, *19*, 12424. [CrossRef] [PubMed]
12. Moga, R.A.; Olteanu, C.D.; Daniel, B.M.; Buru, S.M. Finite Elements Analysis of Tooth-A Comparative Analysis of Multiple Failure Criteria. *Int. J. Env. Res. Public. Health* **2023**, *20*, 4133. [CrossRef] [PubMed]
13. Yamanishi, Y.; Yamaguchi, S.; Imazato, S.; Nakano, T.; Yatani, H. Effects of the implant design on peri-implant bone stress and abutment micromovement: Three-dimensional finite element analysis of original computer-aided design models. *J. Periodontol.* **2014**, *85*, e333–e338. [CrossRef]
14. Pérez-Pevida, E.; Brizuela-Velasco, A.; Chávarri-Prado, D.; Jiménez-Garrudo, A.; Sánchez-Lasheras, F.; Solaberrieta-Méndez, E.; Diéguez-Pereira, M.; Fernández-González, F.J.; Dehesa-Ibarra, B.; Monticelli, F. Biomechanical Consequences of the Elastic Properties of Dental Implant Alloys on the Supporting Bone: Finite Element Analysis. *BioMed Res. Int.* **2016**, *2016*, 1850401. [CrossRef] [PubMed]

15. Shash, Y.H.; El-Wakad, M.T.; Eldosoky, M.A.A.; Dohiem, M.M. Evaluation of stress and strain on mandible caused using "All-on-Four" system from PEEK in hybrid prosthesis: Finite-element analysis. *Odontology* **2023**, *111*, 618–629. [PubMed]
16. Park, J.M.; Kim, H.J.; Park, E.J.; Kim, M.R.; Kim, S.J. Three dimensional finite element analysis of the stress distribution around the mandibular posterior implant during non-working movement according to the amount of cantilever. *J. Adv. Prosthodont.* **2014**, *6*, 361–371. [CrossRef]
17. Aunmeungtong, W.; Khongkhunthian, P.; Rungsiyakull, P. Stress and strain distribution in three different mini dental implant designs using in implant retained overdenture: A finite element analysis study. *ORAL Implantol.* **2016**, *9*, 202–212.
18. Merdji, A.; Bachir Bouiadjra, B.; Achour, T.; Serier, B.; Ould Chikh, B.; Feng, Z.O. Stress analysis in dental prosthesis. *Comput. Mater. Sci.* **2010**, *49*, 126–133. [CrossRef]
19. Shaw, A.M.; Sameshima, G.T.; Vu, H.V. Mechanical stress generated by orthodontic forces on apical root cementum: A finite element model. *Orthod. Craniofacial Res.* **2004**, *7*, 98–107. [CrossRef]
20. Field, C.; Ichim, I.; Swain, M.V.; Chan, E.; Darendeliler, M.A.; Li, W.; Li, Q. Mechanical responses to orthodontic loading: A 3-dimensional finite element multi-tooth model. *Am. J. Orthod. Dentofac.* **2009**, *135*, 174–181. [CrossRef]
21. Merdji, A.; Mootanah, R.; Bachir Bouiadjra, B.A.; Benaissa, A.; Aminallah, L.; Ould Chikh el, B.; Mukdadi, S. Stress analysis in single molar tooth. *Mater. Sci. Eng. C Mater. Biol. Appl.* **2013**, *33*, 691–698.
22. Perez-Gonzalez, A.; Iserte-Vilar, J.L.; Gonzalez-Lluch, C. Interpreting finite element results for brittle materials in endodontic restorations. *Biomed. Eng. Online* **2011**, *10*, 44.
23. Giannini, M.; Soares, C.J.; de Carvalho, R.M. Ultimate tensile strength of tooth structures. *Dent. Mater. Off. Publ. Acad. Dent. Mater.* **2004**, *20*, 322–329.
24. Chun, K.; Choi, H.; Lee, J. Comparison of mechanical property and role between enamel and dentin in the human teeth. *J. Dent. Biomech.* **2014**, *5*, 1758736014520809. [CrossRef] [PubMed]
25. Proffit, W.R.; Fields, H.; Sarver, D.M.; Ackerman, J.L. *Contemporary Orthodontics*, 5th ed.; Elsevier: St. Louis, MO, USA, 2012.
26. Maravić, T.; Comba, A.; Mazzitelli, C.; Bartoletti, L.; Balla, I.; di Pietro, E.; Josić, U.; Generali, L.; Vasiljević, D.; Blažić, L.; et al. Finite element and in vitro study on biomechanical behavior of endodontically treated premolars restored with direct or indirect composite restorations. *Sci. Rep.* **2022**, *12*, 12671. [CrossRef]
27. Gupta, M.; Madhok, K.; Kulshrestha, R.; Chain, S.; Kaur, H.; Yadav, A. Determination of stress distribution on periodontal ligament and alveolar bone by various tooth movements—A 3D FEM study. *J. Oral. Biol. Craniofacial Res.* **2020**, *10*, 758–763. [CrossRef]
28. Huang, L.; Nemoto, R.; Okada, D.; Shin, C.; Saleh, O.; Oishi, Y.; Takita, M.; Nozaki, K.; Komada, W.; Miura, H. Investigation of stress distribution within an endodontically treated tooth restored with different restorations. *J. Dent. Sci.* **2022**, *17*, 1115–1124. [CrossRef]
29. Vikram, N.R.; Senthil Kumar, K.S.; Nagachandran, K.S.; Hashir, Y.M. Apical stress distribution on maxillary central incisor during various orthodontic tooth movements by varying cemental and two different periodontal ligament thicknesses: A FEM study. *Indian. J. Dent. Res. Off. Publ. Indian. Soc. Dent. Res.* **2012**, *23*, 213–220.
30. McCormack, S.W.; Witzel, U.; Watson, P.J.; Fagan, M.J.; Groning, F. Inclusion of periodontal ligament fibres in mandibular finite element models leads to an increase in alveolar bone strains. *PLoS ONE* **2017**, *12*, e0188707.
31. Hemanth, M.; Deoli, S.; Raghuveer, H.P.; Rani, M.S.; Hegde, C.; Vedavathi, B. Stress Induced in the Periodontal Ligament under Orthodontic Loading (Part I): A Finite Element Method Study Using Linear Analysis. *J. Int. Oral. Health* **2015**, *7*, 129–133. [PubMed]
32. Hemanth, M.; Deoli, S.; Raghuveer, H.P.; Rani, M.S.; Hegde, C.; Vedavathi, B. Stress Induced in Periodontal Ligament under Orthodontic Loading (Part II): A Comparison of Linear Versus Non-Linear Fem Study. *J. Int. Oral. Health* **2015**, *7*, 114–118. [PubMed]
33. Reddy, R.T.; Vandana, K.L. Effect of hyperfunctional occlusal loads on periodontium: A three-dimensional finite element analysis. *J. Indian. Soc. Periodontol.* **2018**, *22*, 395–400. [PubMed]
34. Jeon, P.D.; Turley, P.K.; Moon, H.B.; Ting, K. Analysis of stress in the periodontium of the maxillary first molar with a three-dimensional finite element model. *Am. J. Orthod. Dentofac.* **1999**, *115*, 267–274. [CrossRef]
35. Jeon, P.D.; Turley, P.K.; Ting, K. Three-dimensional finite element analysis of stress in the periodontal ligament of the maxillary first molar with simulated bone loss. *Am. J. Orthod. Dentofac. Orthop.* **2001**, *119*, 498–504.
36. Hohmann, A.; Wolfram, U.; Geiger, M.; Boryor, A.; Kober, C.; Sander, C.; Sander, F.G. Correspondences of hydrostatic pressure in periodontal ligament with regions of root resorption: A clinical and a finite element study of the same human teeth. *Comput. Methods Programs Biomed.* **2009**, *93*, 155–161.
37. Hohmann, A.; Wolfram, U.; Geiger, M.; Boryor, A.; Sander, C.; Faltin, R.; Faltin, K.; Sander, F.G. Periodontal ligament hydrostatic pressure with areas of root resorption after application of a continuous torque moment. *Angle Orthod.* **2007**, *77*, 653–659. [CrossRef] [PubMed]
38. Wu, J.; Liu, Y.; Li, B.; Wang, D.; Dong, X.; Sun, Q.; Chen, G. Numerical simulation of optimal range of rotational moment for the mandibular lateral incisor, canine and first premolar based on biomechanical responses of periodontal ligaments: A case study. *Clin. Oral. Investig.* **2021**, *25*, 1569–1577.

39. Wu, J.; Liu, Y.; Wang, D.; Zhang, J.; Dong, X.; Jiang, X.; Xu, X. Investigation of effective intrusion and extrusion force for maxillary canine using finite element analysis. *Comput. Methods Biomech. Biomed. Eng.* **2019**, *22*, 1294–1302.
40. Wu, J.L.; Liu, Y.F.; Peng, W.; Dong, H.Y.; Zhang, J.X. A biomechanical case study on the optimal orthodontic force on the maxillary canine tooth based on finite element analysis. *J. Zhejiang Univ. Sci. B.* **2018**, *7*, 535–546. [CrossRef]

Disclaimer/Publisher's Note: The statements, opinions and data contained in all publications are solely those of the individual author(s) and contributor(s) and not of MDPI and/or the editor(s). MDPI and/or the editor(s) disclaim responsibility for any injury to people or property resulting from any ideas, methods, instructions or products referred to in the content.

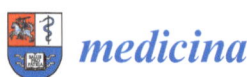

Article

Comparison of Mechanical Properties of Three Tissue Conditioners: An Evaluation In Vitro Study

Marcin Mikulewicz [1], Katarzyna Chojnacka [2] and Zbigniew Raszewski [3,*]

[1] Department of Dentofacial Orthopaedics and Orthodontics, Division of Facial Abnormalities, Medical University of Wroclaw, Krakowska 26, 50-425 Wroclaw, Poland; marcin.mikulewicz@umw.edu.pl
[2] Department of Advanced Material Technologies, Faculty of Chemistry, Wroclaw University of Science and Technology, Smoluchowskiego 25, 50-372 Wroclaw, Poland; katarzyna.chojnacka@pwr.edu.pl
[3] SpofaDental, Markova 238, 506-01 Jicin, Czech Republic
* Correspondence: zbigniew.raszewski@envistaco.com; Tel.: +420-70220800

Abstract: *Introduction:* Tissue conditioners have been widely used in various clinical applications in dentistry, such as treating inflamed alveolar ridges, temporarily relining partial and complete dentures, and the acquisition of functional impressions for denture fabrication. This study aimed to investigate the mechanical properties of the most prevalent tissue conditioner materials on the market, including Tissue Conditioners (TC), Visco Gel (VG), and FITT (F). *Materials and Methods:* The three tissue conditioners, TC, VG, and F, were assessed based on the parameters mentioned above. The following tests were performed based on the ISO 10139-1 and ISO 10139-2 requirements: Shore A hardness, denture plate adhesion, sorption, water solubility, and contraction after 1 and 3 days in water. Additional tests are described in the literature, such as ethanol content and gelling time. The tests were carried out by storing the materials in water at 37 °C for 7 days. *Results:* The gel times of all tested materials exceeded 5 min (TC = 300 [s], VG = 350 [s]). In vitro, phthalate-free materials exhibited higher dissolution in water after 14 days (VG = -260.78 ± 11.31 μg/mm^2) compared to F (-76.12 ± 7.11 μg/mm^2) and experienced faster hardening when stored in distilled water ($F = 33.4 \pm 0.30$ Sh. A, VG = 59.2 ± 0.60 Sh. A). They also showed greater contractions. The connection of all materials to the prosthesis plate was consistent at 0.11 MPa. The highest counterbalance after 3 days was observed in TC = 3.53 ± 1.12%. *Conclusions:* Materials containing plasticizers that are not phthalates have worse mechanical properties than products containing these substances. Since phthalates are not allowed to be used indefinitely in medical devices, additional research is necessary, especially in vivo, to develop safe materials with superior functional properties to newer-generation alternatives. In vitro results often do not agree fully with those of in vivo outcomes.

Keywords: tissue conditioners; phthalate-free alternatives; gelling time; adhesion; solubility; GC; Visco Gel; FITT; denture fabrication; biocompatibility

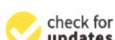

Citation: Mikulewicz, M.; Chojnacka, K.; Raszewski, Z. Comparison of Mechanical Properties of Three Tissue Conditioners: An Evaluation In Vitro Study. *Medicina* 2023, 59, 1359. https://doi.org/10.3390/medicina59081359

Academic Editors: Giuseppe Minervini and Stefania Moccia

Received: 9 June 2023
Revised: 14 July 2023
Accepted: 20 July 2023
Published: 25 July 2023

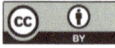

Copyright: © 2023 by the authors. Licensee MDPI, Basel, Switzerland. This article is an open access article distributed under the terms and conditions of the Creative Commons Attribution (CC BY) license (https://creativecommons.org/licenses/by/4.0/).

1. Introduction

Tissue conditioners (TC) are dental materials used to address inflammation or pressure points on the alveolar ridge, temporary relining of partial and complete dentures, and the creation of functional impressions for denture fabrication or restoration. These soft relining materials can be divided into temporary and long-term solutions. Some requirements for both types of materials overlap [1] [Nowakowska-Toporowska et al., 2018]. An ideal material of this type should have the following characteristics: resistance to fungal and bacterial growth, low water absorption, increased color stability, stain resistance, tear resistance, strong bonding with the denture base, dimensional stability, low glass transition temperature, easy processing, long shelf life, biocompatibility, high energy dissipation, and good elasticity [2–4]. One of the main problems with TC is their susceptibility to colonization of microorganisms due to water solubility and degradation, which can exacerbate denture stomatitis [5].

Currently, TC are being enhanced with various types of additives that possess antibacterial properties. These additives include nature-based raw materials such as terpinene-4-ol and cinnamaldehyde [6], Cocos nucifera oil [7,8], lemongrass [9], as well as special fillers such as surface prereacted glass ionomer [10], zinc oxide nanoparticles [10], ZnOAg nanoparticles [11], and substances with drug properties such as cetylpyridinium chloride [12], poly(acryloyloxyethyltrimethyl ammonium chloride)-grafted chitosan [13], and bioactive glass [14].

However, it is important to note that these studies conducted in the laboratory phase have not resulted in commercially available products with such enhanced properties. Therefore, it is important to compare the existing materials so that the dentist can choose the best material for a particular clinical situation.

Typically, these materials consist of a mixture of powder and liquid that combine to form a soft gel [15,16]. The powder component is composed of finely ground poly (ethyl methacrylate polymer) with a granule size ranging between 30 and 40 microns. On the other hand, the liquid component is a mixture of ethanol and plasticizer. A physical reaction occurs when the plasticizer is absorbed into the polymer, and the presence of ethanol accelerates this process, significantly reducing the required time from several hours to mere minutes [2].

However, it is important to be aware that certain TC may contain harmful plasticizers, such as phthalates, which have been linked to adverse effects on the human endocrine system. Recent studies have indicated that prenatal exposure to phthalates is associated with adverse effects on neurodevelopment, including lower IQ, attention and hyperactivity problems, and poorer social communication. The effects of these substances on the adult body can damage the liver, kidneys, lungs, and reproductive system. To address these concerns, the Consumer Product Safety Improvement Act and its final rule in 2018 have banned eight phthalates in children's products under federal legislation [17,18].

In response to safety concerns regarding phthalates, alternative plasticizers have been developed for use in TC. Citrate or sebacate-based plasticizers are among the new generation of materials that are currently available on the market. However, further research is still necessary to evaluate the safety and efficacy of these alternative materials [19,20].

The clinical shelf life of TC is relatively short, typically lasting from a few days to a week. Factors such as chewing forces, fluid consumption, and food intake contribute to the rapid leaching of plasticizers from the material. This process results in the hardening and degradation of TC over time. Additionally, the high sorption capacity of these materials leads to color changes and facilitates the quick colonization of various microorganisms, making it challenging to maintain proper hygiene when using soft relining materials. Routine cleaning with a toothbrush and toothpaste can easily remove or tear these materials [21,22].

The hypothesis of this study posits that phthalate-free alternatives for TC will exhibit physical properties that are comparable to or even superior to those containing phthalates.

2. Materials and Methods

The tests were conducted using the following materials: Visco Gel (Dentsply), Charlotte, NC, USA) which consists of 120 g of powder (transparent poly (ethyl methacrylate)), 90 mL of liquid (a mixture of ethanol and citrate-based plasticizer), and 15 mL of separator based on Vaseline oil. GC Tissue Conditioner includes 90 g of white PEMA powder, 90 g of liquid (composed of dibutyl sebacate and ethanol), and a 12 g coating agent (consisting of ethyl acetate and dissolved polymer). Kerr FITT from Kerr (Brea, CA, USA) contains liquid (ethanol, butyl phthalate, and butyl glycolate plasticizer), and 100 g of white powder based on poly (ethyl methacrylate). These materials were subjected to various mechanical tests, as shown in Figure 1, and tested materials are presented in Table 1.

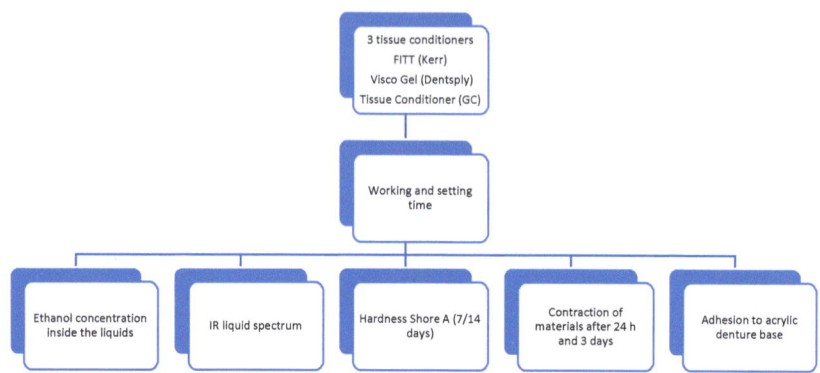

Figure 1. Graphical scheme of the tests carried out.

Table 1. Materials and instruments used for testing.

Material	Producer	LOT
Tissue conditioner	GC (Tokyo, Japan)	1801121
FITT	Kerr (Scafati, Italy)	9529105
Visco Gel	Dentsply (Constance, Germany)	1805000667

Several mechanical tests were conducted for each material, following the standard ISO 10139-1:2018 Dentistry, Soft lining materials for removable dentures, with the number of samples specified by the standard [23].

The gelling time was determined by measuring the time it took for the mixture of powder and liquid to form a soft gel (which indicates the ease of use). Shore A hardness, which measures the material's resistance to indentation, was evaluated for samples stored in water at 37 °C for 7 and 14 days. This test provides insights into the material's ability to absorb masticatory forces and its long-term shelf life. Adhesion to the denture plate was tested by measuring the force required to separate the material from the denture plate, with higher ethanol content indicating more washing out and a shorter lifespan on the denture surface. Ethanol content was measured by drying the samples. Sorption and solubility in water were determined by measuring the change in mass of the samples when immersed in water. Contraction after 1 and 3 days of water immersion was measured by comparing the dimensions of the samples before and after immersion, providing information on the dimensional stability of the materials. The presence of plasticizers in the materials was performed using infrared spectrophotometry. An overview of all the test methods is presented in Figure 1.

2.1. Working a Gelling Time

The materials were mixed according to the manufacturer's instructions. For example, in the case of Kerr FITT, 1.5 g of powder was mixed with 1 g of liquid in a plastic jar using a spatula. The container was then tilted to check if the material was flowing, and the working time of the material was considered to have ended at this point. The surface of the material was touched with a clean PE stick until it adhered to the stick's surface, indicating the gelation time of the material. Time measurements were carried out using a calibrated stopwatch. All tests were conducted under laboratory conditions at a temperature of 23 °C. A total of 20 tests were performed for each measurement, resulting in a total of 60 samples. A description of this study can be found in Saeed et al. [24], Murata et al. [25].

2.2. Shore A Measurements

Samples for Shore A hardness were prepared using a 40 × 6 mm high metal cylinder form. The mold was covered with polyester foil and flat metal slabs on both sides. After a

30-min interval, the form was disassembled and the samples were removed. The initial measurement was conducted using a Shore A HD3000 durometer (Hildebrand, Oberboihingen, Germany) after 1 h. A total of 10 samples were prepared for each material, and each sample was measured four times from both sides (a total of 30 samples and 120 measurements).

Subsequently, the samples were placed in distilled water at 37 °C. After the designated period, the samples were dried, and new hardness tests were performed. Following the testing procedure, the samples were immersed in fresh distilled water and stored for an additional 7 days to simulate long-term use, as required by the ISO 10139-1:2018 Dentistry, Soft lining materials for removable dentures, Part 1: Materials for short-term use [23], and in accordance with previous studies by Saeed et al. [24] and Nowakowska-Toporowska et al. [1].

2.3. Ethanol Concentration

Samples weighing 2 g of liquid were stored at 37 °C until a constant mass was achieved. The determination of a constant mass was based on consecutive weight measurements using an analytical balance. If two successive measurements did not differ by more than 0.001 g, the concentration of ethanol was determined as the difference in mass before and after drying. A total of 10 samples were utilized for each material, resulting in a total of 30 samples. The Denver 300 balance (Denver Instruments, Paris, OH, USA), calibrated for accuracy, was employed for the testing process. For a detailed description of the test procedure, please refer to Murata et al. [25].

2.4. Sorption and Solubility

Following the mixing instructions, the materials were poured into a metal form with a diameter of 20 mm and a thickness of 2 mm. The form was then covered with polyester foil and metal slabs on both sides. After a 30-min interval, the form was opened, and the gel-shaped materials were extracted. For each solubility and sorption test, a total of 20 samples were prepared, resulting in a total of 60 samples.

One hour after removing the samples from the form, they were weighed (M1) and placed in covered plastic jars filled with distilled water. The first group of samples was stored for 7 days at 37 °C, while the second group was stored for 14 days under the same conditions. This was completed to simulate the clinical short-term or long-term use of the material.

After the storage period, the tissue conditioner was removed from the water, dried using paper, and weighed again (M2). Subsequently, the materials were transferred to a desiccator for drying until a constant mass was achieved (M3). For the testing process, a calibrated Denver 300 balance (Denver Instruments, Paris, OH, USA) was used.

Sorption was calculated using Equation (1), recommended by ISO 10139-1:2018 [23]:

$$\text{Sorption} = \frac{(M2 - M1)}{M1} \quad (1)$$

Solubility was obtained from the differences, recommended by ISO 10139-1:2018 [21]:

$$\text{Solubility} = \frac{(M1 - M3)}{M1} \quad (2)$$

For a detailed description of the test, see Saeed et al. [24].

2.5. Adhesion between Two Materials

To measure the adhesion force between the denture base material and the soft relining, a tensile test was performed. Samples of hot curing resins, specifically Superacryl Plus (Spofa Dental, Jicin, Czech Republic), were polymerized in metal forms with dimensions of 25 × 25 × 3.2 mm. After the curing process, the surface of the acrylic plate was coated with TC in a 10 × 10 mm area. A second acrylic plate was then placed on top to create a joint. The soft material was allowed to cure at room temperature for 24 h.

The following day, the samples were placed onto a tearing strength instrument, specifically the Shimadzu KN 50 (Shimadzu, Kyoto, Japan). The elongation speed of the breaking head was 5 mm/min. The samples were elongated at the connection point made with the soft material. The test concluded when the sample split into two pieces.

A total of 20 samples were prepared for each test, resulting in a total of 60 samples used. A detailed description of the test can be found in ISO 10139-2:2018 and Chladek et al. [26]. The scheme is shown in Figure 2.

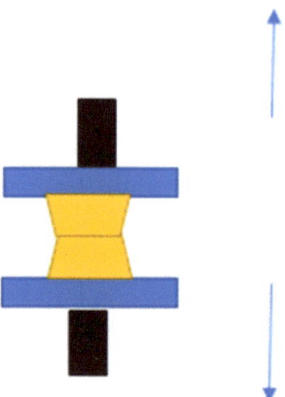

Figure 2. The samples and the breaking method (black attachment to the elongation machine, blue: acrylic plates, yellow: tissue conditioner).

2.6. Contraction

TC are clinically used for functional impressions; for this reason, they must be time stable. To measure the shrinkage of materials over specific time intervals, we used a method commonly used to measure changes in elastomeric impression materials. A specially calibrated metal block was used, featuring lines spaced 24.805 mm apart, each line measuring 50 µm. The samples were in the form of cylinders with a diameter of 30 mm and a thickness of 2 mm. The TC were mixed in accordance with the manufacturer's recommendations and applied onto the metal block, which complied with ISO 10139-2:2016 Dentistry—Soft lining materials for removable dentures—Part 2: Materials for long-term use [23].

After 20 min, the materials were removed from the mold and placed in distilled water at 37 °C. Following 24 h, the distance between the lines on the samples was measured using a Karl Zeiss microscope (Zeiss, Jena, Germany) equipped with a measuring device capable of capturing the distance between the two reference lines (M2). The contraction of the material was determined using the following formula. The water was replaced with a fresh portion, and the process was repeated after 3 days. Each day, the water was replaced with new water.

A total of 20 samples were prepared for each material, resulting in a total of 60 samples. The contraction was calculated based on Equation (3), which is recommended by the ISO 10139-1:2018 standard [23] and described in Chladek et al. [26].

$$\text{Contraction} = \frac{24.805 - M2}{24.805} * 100\% \tag{3}$$

2.7. Infrared Spectroscopy

The monomer samples were analyzed using the Nicolet ID7 apparatus (Thermo Scientific, Waltham, MA, USA). Each sample underwent 64 scans [27]. The test involved placing one drop of liquid onto the measurement window of the instrument and pressing it with a specialized glass to prevent the evaporation of volatile components. After the measurement, the slide was cleaned using enatol (Sigma Aldrich, Prague, Czech Republic).

Each material sample was measured three times, resulting in a total of nine measurements. The identification of plasticizers was performed using a data library.

2.8. Statistical Analysis

Statistical analysis was performed with nine repetitions for each parameter, providing a robust dataset for the study. The data were expressed as mean ± standard error of the mean. A one-way analysis of variance (ANOVA) was performed to test for significant differences between the different tissue conditioner materials, including GC, Visco Gel, and FITT. A p-value < 0.05 was considered statistically significant. Posthoc tests were performed following the ANOVA analysis. GraphPad Software Inc., located in San Diego, CA, USA, was used for the statistical analysis. The use of ANOVA enables reliable determination of differences between the tested materials and ensures the statistical significance of the results.

3. Results

3.1. Working and Gelling Time

Table 2 shows the results of the working and gelling times for commercial products.

Table 2. Working and gelling time of tissue conditioner materials.

Tissue Conditioner Material	Mixing Ratio (g)	Work Time (s)	Gel Time (s)
GC Tissue Conditioner	1.2:1	162 ± 2 *	302 ± 5 *
FITT	1.5:1	92 ± 3 *	231 ± 9 *
FITT	1.2:1	121 ± 4 *	300 ± 6 *
Visco Gel	1.5:1	149 ± 4 *	350 ± 8 *

* p value < 0.01.

The results show that the GC Tissue Conditioner has the longest working time (162 ± 2 [s]), while FITT (mixing ratio 1.3:1) has the shortest working time and gel time (92 ± 3 [s]). The Visco Gel material has the longest gelling time (350 ± 8 [s]).

3.2. Hardness Shore A

Table 3 presents the changes in Shore A hardness after 7 and 14 days in distilled water at 37 °C.

Table 3. Changes in Shore A hardness after 7 and 14 days in distilled water at 37 °C of different tissue conditioner materials.

Composition	Initial Shore A Hardness (°)	Shore A Hardness after 7 Days (°)	Shore A Hardness after 14 Days (°)
GC Tissue Conditioner 1.2/1 *	19.1 ± 0.3 p = 0.01	28.6 ± 0.2 p = 0.04	51.3 ± 0.4 p = 0.01
FITT 1.5/1 *	12.7 ± 0.1	39.1 ± 0.3 p = 0.035	38.1 ± 0.2 p = 0.035
FITT 1.2/1 *	11.0 ± 0.1	13.3 ± 0.2 p = 0.048	33.4 ± 0.3 p = 0.047
Visco Gel 1.5/1 *	17.0 ± 0.1 p = 0.0087	40.0 ± 0.1 p = 0.0088	59.2 ± 0.6 p = 0.009

* Mixing ratio between powder and liquid [g].

Initially, the Shore A hardness of the tested materials was below 20 degrees (F = 11.0 ± 0.10 Sh. A, TC = 0.19.1 ± 0.30 Sh. A). After storage in distilled water, the hardness of all materials increased significantly (F = 38.1 ± 0.20 Sh. A, VG = 59.2 ± 0.60 Sh. A).

3.3. Ethanol Concentration

Table 4 shows the concentration of ethanol in the different products.

Table 4. Ethanol concentration for different products.

Material	Ethanol (%)
GC Tissue Conditioner	12
Visco Gel	11
FITT	19.5

The highest concentration of ethanol was measured for the FITT [19.5%] and the lowest concentration was measured for the Visco-gel [11%]. However, it is important to note that the difference between these results was not statistically significant.

3.4. Adhesion between Materials

Table 5 presents the adhesion between the soft material and the denture base.

Table 5. Adhesion between soft material and denture base, by the tensile test of two acrylic pieces joined by a tissue conditioner.

Material	Adhesion (MPa)
GC Tissue Conditioner 1.2/1 *	0.110 ± 0.013
FITT 1.2/1 *	0.117 ± 0.009
FITT 1.5/1 *	0.105 ± 0.006
Visco-gel 1.5/1 *	0.110 ± 0.007

* Mixing ratio between powder and liquid [g].

The study results indicate that no significant difference was observed in the connection between the various TC and the denture base. In all cases (100%), the separation of the sample occurred in an adhesive manner at the border between the soft material and the acrylic material. Figure 3 illustrates the surface of the acrylic plate after the tissue conditioner material was torn off.

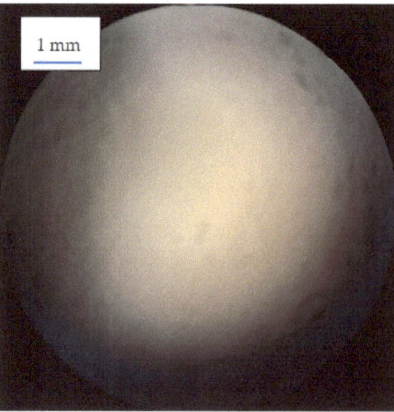

Figure 3. Acrylic disc after tearing off the tissue conditioners from their surface. The lack of traces of soft material proves the type of adhesive connection (magnification 25×).

3.5. Sorption and Solubility

Table 6 provides an overview of the sorption and solubility results for the tissue conditioners.

Table 6. Results from the sorption and solubility of commercial products.

Material	Sorption after 7 Days (μg/mm^2)	Solubility after 7 Days (μg/mm^2)	Sorption after 14 Days (μg/mm^2)	Solubility after 14 Days (μg/mm^2)
GC Tissue Conditioner 1.2/1 *	30.18 ± 3.45	−23.31 ± 4.15	−102.11 ± 2.5	−142.19 ± 3.00
GC Tissue Conditioner 1.2/1 * with lacquer	26.66 ± 5.55	−23.06 ± 2.88	−102.51 ± 2.27	−132.73 ± 3.12
FITT 1.5/1 *	39.36 ± 4.39	−10.27± 2.71	−23.37 ± 2.36 p = 0.029	−76.12 ± 7.11 p = 0.0096
FITT 1.5/1 *	43.55 ± 5.11	−13.78± 3.82	−44.68 ± 3.06 p = 0.048	−106.52 ± 3.27 p = 0.099
Visco Gel 1.5/1 *	33.15 ± 2.32	−27.45 ± 4.32	−1980.59 ± 9.88 p = 0.0001	−260.78 ± 11.31 p = 0.001

* Mixing ratio between powder and liquid [g].

The sorption and solubility values obtained are expressed as negative values because, instead of absorbing water and increasing in mass, the materials dissolve rapidly. Consequently, the measured mass (M2) is smaller than the initial mass (M1).

Among the materials tested, FITT demonstrated the smallest changes in sorption and solubility, with a value of −76.12 ± 7.11 μg/mm^2. In contrast, Visco Gel exhibited significant changes over time, with a value of −260.78 ± 11.31 μg/mm^2.

3.6. Contraction

Table 7 presents the results of the contraction of the materials after 1 and 3 days of immersion in distilled water.

Table 7. Contraction of materials [%] stored in distilled water for a period of 1 and 3 days.

Material	24-h Contraction (%)	3 Days of Contraction (%)
FITT 1.2/1 *	99.11 ± 1.2	97.39 ± 1.05
FITT 1.5/1 *	98.96 ± 1.14	97.36 ± 1.26
GC Tissue Conditioner 1.2/1 *	97.63 ± 1.33	96.47 ± 1.12
Visco-gel 1.5/1	There is no possibility of seeing the lines.	There is no possibility of seeing the lines.

* Mixing ratio between powder and liquid [g].

Immediately after gelling, a 50-micron line was visible in all tested materials. However, after 24 h, such lines were not detectable in Visco-gel. The surface of the material appeared to be overdried.

The smallest shrinkage was observed in the FITT material (mixing ratio 1.2:1) after 24 h (99.11 ± 1.2 [%]). The largest shrinkage occurred in the Tissue Conditioner after 3 days (96.47 ± 1.12 [%]). However, it is important to note that the difference between these results was not statistically significant.

3.7. Infrared Spectroscopy

The infrared scans and SDS analysis reveal the composition of the materials. The FITT material (Kerr) contains butyl phthalate and butyl glycolate, the Visco Gel material (Dentsply) contains acetyl tributyl citrate, and the Tissue Conditioner material (GC) contains dibutyl sebacate. The spectrum is shown in Figure 4.

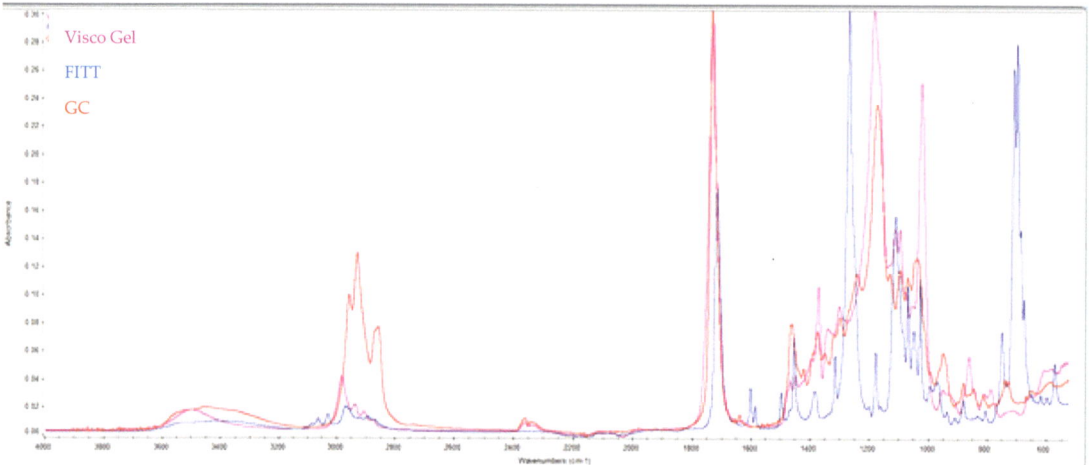

Figure 4. Infrared spectrum of the liquids of TC test materials.

For the FITT there are characteristic FT-IR peaks in the spectrum (cm^{-1}): 1724.9 (carbonyl ester), 1280.9 and 1074.4 (–C–O–stretching), 742.46 (ortho disubstitution) (Blue color). Acetyl tributyl citrate exhibits characteristic peaks, such as the C=O absorption at 1738 cm^{-1}, which is observed at slightly higher wavenumbers than the phthalate. Additionally, the strong asymmetric C–O stretching at 1182 cm^{-1} is typical of citrates (Pink color). The material from GC contains peaks at 2927–2852 cm^{-1}, attributed to alkene (–CH$_2$) groups, while intense peaks at 1159 and 1735 cm^{-1} are indicative of C–O and C=O formation, respectively.

4. Discussion

This study aimed to investigate the mechanical properties of three commercially available TC. However, the initial hypothesis was not confirmed as the materials containing nonphthalate plasticizers did not exhibit superior properties compared to the FITT material.

A very important feature of soft relining materials is their ability to absorb chewing forces in the oral mucosa following surgical treatment. Shore A hardness is a measurable parameter that indicates the material's ability to cushion and relieve pressure in sensitive regions. An excessive increase in hardness compromises the material's primary function. During storage in water, the materials experience an increase in hardness due to the leaching of ethanol and plasticizers. Similar findings of gradual hardness increase have been reported by other authors [2,22,28].

For soft and extra-soft materials, Shore A hardness values should be below 25 °C after 24 h of aging in distilled water at 37 °C. After 28 days of aging, Shore A hardness values should be below 55 °C [26]. The current study's results align with previous studies demonstrating an increase in hardness over time for TC [29,30]. However, it is important to note that the magnitude of hardness increase varied among the tested materials. For instance, GC Tissue Conditioner exhibited an increase in hardness from 19.0 to 50 Shore A after 14 days, while FITT 1.2/1 increased from 11.1 to 33.4 Shore A during the same period. These findings emphasize the importance of material selection based on the desired hardness, which may vary depending on the specific clinical situation [31].

Ethanol is an important component in TC as it accelerates the gelling process of the material. However, it is known to be washed out in the oral environment within the first 24 h. In the conducted tests, the content of evaporated alcohol ranged from 11% for the Visco Gel material to 19.5% for the FITT material. Excessive alcohol content can lead to a positive reaction in a breathalyzer test shortly after denture relining [32].

The choice of gelling agent in TC is also crucial as it affects their overall performance. Researchers are exploring alternative gelling agents to improve long-term stability and performance [9,21,33,34]. Some attempts have been made to prepare materials without ethanol as a gelling agent.

GC Tissue Conditioner, for example, incorporates a special lacquer to reduce solubility and enhance the adhesion between the denture base and the relining material [35]. However, the results of the current study did not support these claims. The adhesion of soft lining materials to acrylic was found to be the same for all tested products (0.11 MPa), consistent with findings from other authors [36,37]. Wang et al. suggested that the adhesive strength between the denture plate and tissue conditioner may depend on the specific plasticizer used, as demonstrated in their study on various citrates [38].

Phthalates, which are known to have adverse effects on the human body, are a concern when in prolonged contact with materials like TC. They can lead to reproductive system changes, and their decomposition products can negatively affect the kidneys and lungs. Currently, FITT material contains phthalates, while Tissue Conditioner and Visco Gel utilize alternative plasticizers [18].

The results of the conducted tests clearly demonstrate that TC exhibit sorption (water uptake) and solubility after a relatively short period (7 days). However, after 2 weeks, these materials start to dissolve, and the amount of water absorbed becomes lower than the eluted plasticizer, resulting in negative sorption values. Among the tested materials, Visco Gel from Dentsply showed the highest degradation after 14 days (-260.78 ± 11.31 µg/mm^2), compared to FITT (-76.12 ± 7.11 µg/mm^2), which contains tributyl citrate according to the IR analysis. The citrate plasticizer with a straight chain structure is more easily eluted compared to the aromatic structure found in the Kerr material. A higher powder/liquid mixing ratio (lower plasticizer concentration) leads to less sorption and leaching for FITT. These findings are consistent with previous studies [2,9,24,26,38–41].

Another important application of TC is for making functional impressions. During this process, the material is applied under the denture base for a short period, typically ranging from 2 to 24 h. It gradually adapts to the oral cavity, undergoing deformation to ensure proper function. It is crucial for the material to maintain its dimensions during this period. The tested materials in this study exhibited low shrinkage, with less than 1% after 24 h and less than 2% after 3 days (FITT 1.5/1: $98.96 \pm 1.14\%$ after 1 day, $97.36 \pm 1.26\%$ after 3 days). However, the Visco Gel material showed significant dimensional changes after 24 h, and its surface appeared dry, making it difficult to observe the 50-micron lines. These results align with previous studies on materials such as Coe Super Soft and older formulas of Visco Gel containing phthalates [41].

The test results for tissue conditioner materials (GC, Visco Gel, and FITT) demonstrate differences in various properties, including working and gelling times, hardness, ethanol content, adhesion, sorption, solubility, and contraction. These differences can significantly impact the performance and properties of the materials, affecting factors such as gelling rate, solubility, and adhesion to the denture base [42]. It is crucial for dental professionals to understand these properties in order to choose the most appropriate tissue conditioner material for their patients. Furthermore, TC have the potential to serve as drug delivery systems and research efforts have been made to develop TC with antimicrobial properties [43–48].

4.1. Future Perspectives

This study provides valuable information on the mechanical properties of commercially available TC. However, further research is required to improve these materials and enhance their clinical performance. It is important to consider the biocompatibility of TC, particularly with the increasing use of phthalate-free alternatives. Researchers should incorporate findings on cytotoxicity and potential adverse effects of alternative plasticizers on oral mucosal cells into the evaluation and comparison of TC to ensure their safety and performance standards for clinical use [16]. Addressing the susceptibility of TC to microbial colonization is also important. The evaluation of alternative gelling agents is necessary since ethanol has drawbacks such as rapid evaporation and potential interference with breath analyzers. Optimizing material properties for patient-specific needs is essential, as different TC exhibit varying mechanical properties, which can be advantageous depending on the clinical situation. Pursuing these research directions has the potential to significantly enhance the clinical utility of TC, leading to better patient outcomes and overall satisfaction.

4.2. Clinical Significance

The clinical significance of phthalates in medical devices is an important issue that needs attention. The emergence of newer generation materials intended as phthalate alternatives could potentially display inferior functional properties when compared to traditional materials. Therefore, it is essential to conduct comprehensive research aimed at optimizing the properties and clinical performance of these novel materials [49,50]. For instance, a comparison can be made between acrylic and silicone materials, such as GC Reline II Soft, to determine their suitability.

5. Conclusions

➢ The concentration of ethanol has a significant impact on the gelling time of TC, whereby higher concentrations result in shorter working and gelling times.
➢ TC with a higher alcohol content exhibit increased solubility.
➢ Straight-chain plasticizers, such as citrate, can be easily washed out of TC, leading to higher sorption and solubility of the materials.
➢ Lacquer presents an intriguing alternative for GC products, as it reduces the sorption of TC.
➢ Materials containing nonphthalate plasticizers demonstrate higher solubility and increased hardness in in vitro tests when stored in distilled water.
➢ Understanding the properties of commercial TC is essential for their optimal clinical performance.

Author Contributions: Conceptualization: Z.R.; Data curation: Z.R., K.C. and M.M.; Formal analysis: K.C. and M.M.; Investigation: Z.R.; Methodology: Z.R.; Resources: Z.R.; Supervision: M.M.; Visualization: Z.R., K.C. and M.M.; Writing—original draft: K.C. and M.M.; Writing—review & editing: Z.R., K.C. and M.M. All authors have read and agreed to the published version of the manuscript.

Funding: This research received no external funding.

Institutional Review Board Statement: Not applicable.

Informed Consent Statement: Not applicable.

Data Availability Statement: Data sharing is not applicable to this article.

Conflicts of Interest: The authors declare no conflict of interest.

References

1. Nowakowska-Toporowska, A.; Malecka, K.; Raszewski, Z.; Wieckiewicz, W. Changes in hardness of addition-polymerizing silicone-resilient denture liners after storage in artificial saliva. *J. Prosthet. Dent.* **2019**, *121*, 317–321. [CrossRef] [PubMed]
2. Parker, S.; Braden, M. Effect of composition on the gelation of tissue conditioners. *Biomaterials* **1996**, *17*, 1827–1832. [CrossRef]
3. Prasad, D.; Anupama Prasad, B.; Rajendra Shetty, V.; Shashidhara Krishna, D. Tissue Conditioners: A Review. *Nitte Univ. J. Health Sci.* **2014**, *4*, 156–161. [CrossRef]
4. Hong, G.; Wang, W.Q.; Sun, L.; Han, J.M.; Sasaki, K. The Dynamic Viscoelasticity of Dental Soft Polymer Material Containing Citrate Ester-Based Plasticizers. *Materials* **2020**, *13*, 5078. [CrossRef] [PubMed]
5. Hejazi, M.; Zareshahrabadi, Z.; Ashayeri, S.; Saharkhiz, M.J.; Iraji, A.; Alishahi, M.; Zomorodian, K. Characterization and Physical and Biological Properties of Tissue Conditioner Incorporated with *Carum copticum* L. *Biomed. Res. Int.* **2021**, *2021*, 5577760. [CrossRef] [PubMed]
6. de Fátima Souto Maior, L.; Maciel, P.P.; Ferreira, V.Y.N.; de Lima Gouveia Dantas, C.; de Lima, J.M.; Castellano, L.R.C.; Batista, A.U.D.; Bonan, P.R.F. Antifungal activity and Shore A hardness of a tissue conditioner incorporated with terpinen-4-ol and cinnamaldehyde. *Clin. Oral. Investig.* **2019**, *23*, 2837–2848. [CrossRef]

7. Krishnamoorthy, G.; Narayana, A.I.; Peralam, P.Y.; Balkrishanan, D. To study the effect of Cocos nucifera oil when incorporated into tissue conditioner on its tensile strength and antifungal activity: An in vitro study. *J. Indian Prosthodont. Soc.* **2019**, *19*, 225–232. [CrossRef]
8. Choonharuangdej, S.; Srithavaj, T.; Chantanawilas, P. Lemongrass-Incorporated Tissue Conditioner with Adjustable Inhibitory Effect Against Candida albicans: An In Vitro Study. *Int. J. Prosthodont.* **2022**, *35*, 338–342. [CrossRef]
9. Tonprasong, W.; Inokoshi, M.; Tamura, N.; Uo, M.; Wada, T.; Takahashi, R.; Hatano, K.; Shimizubata, M.; Minakuchi, S. Tissue Conditioner Incorporating a Nano-Sized Surface Pre-Reacted Glass-Ionomer (S-PRG) Filler. *Materials* **2021**, *14*, 6648. [CrossRef]
10. Homsiang, W.; Kamonkhantikul, K.; Arksornnukit, M.; Takahashi, H. Effect of zinc oxide nanoparticles incorporated into tissue conditioner on antifungal, physical, and mechanical properties. *Dent. Mater. J.* **2021**, *40*, 481–486. [CrossRef]
11. Mousavi, S.A.; Ghotaslou, R.; Akbarzadeh, A.; Azima, N.; Aeinfar, A.; Khorramdel, A. Evaluation of antibacterial and antifungal properties of a tissue conditioner used in complete dentures after incorporation of ZnO–Ag nanoparticles. *J. Dent. Res. Dent. Clin. Dent. Prospect.* **2019**, *13*, 11–18. [CrossRef]
12. Asahara, E.; Abe, Y.; Nakamori, K.; Okazaki, Y.; Makita, Y.; Hasebe, A.; Tsuga, K.; Yokoyama, A. Controlled release, antimicrobial activity, and oral mucosa irritation of cetylpyridinium chloride-montmorillonite incorporated in a tissue conditioner. *Dent. Mater. J.* **2022**, *41*, 142–149. [CrossRef] [PubMed]
13. Lee, H.L.; Wang, R.S.; Hsu, Y.C.; Chuang, C.C.; Chan, H.R.; Chiu, H.C.; Wang, Y.B.; Chen, K.Y.; Fu, E. Antifungal effect of tissue conditioners containing poly (acryloyloxyethyltrimethyl ammonium chloride)-grafted chitosan on Candida albicans growth in vitro. *J. Dent. Sci.* **2018**, *13*, 160–166. [CrossRef] [PubMed]
14. Raszewski, Z.; Nowakowska, D.; Wieckiewicz, W.; Nowakowska-Toporowska, A. Release and Recharge of Fluoride Ions from Acrylic Resin Modified with Bioactive Glass. *Polymers* **2021**, *13*, 1054. [CrossRef]
15. Jones, D.W.; Sutow, E.J.; Graham, B.S.; Milne, E.L.; Johnston, D.E. Influence of Plasticizer on Soft Polymer Gelation. *J. Dent. Res.* **1986**, *65*, 634–637. [CrossRef] [PubMed]
16. Hashimoto, Y.; Tanaka, J.; Suzuki, K.; Nakamura, M. Cytocompatibility of a Tissue Conditioner Containing Vinyl Ester as a Plasticizer. *Dent. Mater. J.* **2007**, *26*, 785–791. [CrossRef]
17. Jafari, A.; Shadman, N. Tissue conditioners in prosthodontics: A literature review. *J. Dent.* **2014**, *15*, 1–9.
18. Rokaya, D.; Srimaneepong, V.; Sapkota, J.; Qin, J.; Siraleartmukul, K.; Siriwongrungson, V. Polymeric materials and films in dentistry: An overview. *J. Adv. Res.* **2018**, *14*, 25–34. [CrossRef]
19. Miettinen, H.; Kivilahti, J. Biocompatibility of dental materials. In *Handbook of Oral Biomaterials*; Narhi, T.O., Ed.; CRC Press: Boca Raton, FL, USA, 1991; pp. 31–55. ISBN 9780849369086.
20. Shillingburg, H.T., Jr.; Hobo, S.; Whitsett, L.D.; Jacobi, R.; Brackett, S.E. *Fundamentals of Fixed Prosthodontics*, 3rd ed.; Quintessence Publishing: Chicago, IL, USA, 1997; ISBN 0867151735.
21. Tonpraatt, J.G.; Varghese, N.M.; Correya, B.A.; Saheer, M.K. Tissue Conditioners: A Review. *J. Dent. Med. Sci. (IOSR-JDMS)* **2015**, *14*, 54–57.
22. Ntounis, A.; Kamposiora, P.; Papavasiliou, G.; Divaris, K.; Zinelis, S. Hardness Changes of Tissue Conditioners in Various Storage Media: An in Vitro Study. *Eur. J. Prosthodont. Restor. Dent.* **2015**, *23*, 9–15.
23. ISO 10139-1:2018; Dentistry, Soft Lining Materials for Removable Dentures, Part 1: Materials for Short-Term Use. ISO: Geneva, Switzerland, 2018.
24. Saeed, A.; Zahid, S.; Sajid, M.; Ud Din, S.; Alam, M.K.; Chaudhary, F.A.; Kaleem, M.; Alswairki, H.J.; Abutayyem, H. Physico-Mechanical Properties of Commercially Available Tissue Conditioner Modified with Synthesized Chitosan Oligosaccharide. *Polymers* **2022**, *14*, 1233. [CrossRef]
25. Murata, H.; Kawamura, M.; Hamada, T.; Saleh, S.; Kresnoadi, U.; Toki, K. Dimensional stability and weight changes of tissue conditioners. *J. Oral. Rehabil.* **2001**, *28*, 918–923. [CrossRef] [PubMed]
26. Tonsdek, G.; Żmudzki, J.; Kasperski, J. Long-Term Soft Denture Lining Materials. *Materials* **2014**, *7*, 5816–5842. [CrossRef]
27. Bosch-Reig, F.; Gimeno-Adelantado, J.V.; Bosch-Mossi, F.; Doménech-Carbó, A. Quantification of minerals from ATR-FTIR spectra with spectral interferences using the MRC method. *Spectrochim. Acta Part. A Mol. Biomol. Spectrosc.* **2017**, *181*, 7–12. [CrossRef] [PubMed]
28. van Vliet, E.M.; Reitano, J.S.; Bergen, G.P.; Whyatt, R.M. A review of alternatives to di (2-ethylhexyl) phthalate-containing medical devices in the neonatal intensive care unit. *J. Perinatol.* **2011**, *31*, 551–560. [CrossRef]
29. Wyszyńska, M.; Białożyt-Bujak, E.; Chladek, G.; Czelakowska, A.; Rój, R.; Białożyt, A.; Gruca, O.; Nitsze-Wierzba, M.; Kasperski, J.; Skucha-Nowak, M. Analysis of Changes in the Tensile Bond Strenght of Soft Relining Material with Acrylic Denture Material. *Materials* **2021**, *14*, 6868. [CrossRef]
30. Pinto, L.; Zanatta, R.F.; Lima, G.S.; Ogliari, F.A.; Moraes, R.R. Effect of the plasticizer's concentration on mechanical and thermal properties of PMMA used in dentistry. *J. Appl. Polym. Sci.* **2017**, *134*, 45234. [CrossRef]
31. Kitagawa, Y.; Yoshida, K.; Takase, K.; Valanezhad, A.; Watanabe, I.; Kojio, K.; Murata, H. Evaluation of viscoelastic properties, hardness, and glass transition temperature of soft denture liners and tissue conditioner. *Odontology* **2020**, *108*, 366–375. [CrossRef]
32. Wilson, J. Alcohol levels in tissue conditioners: High enough to fail the breathalyser? *Eur. J. Prosthodont. Restor. Dent.* **1994**, *2*, 137–140.

33. Vankadara, S.K.; Hallikerimath, R.B.; Patil, V.; Bhat, K.; Doddamani, M.H. Effect of Melaleuca alternifolia Mixed with Tissue Conditioners in Varying Doses on Colonization and Inhibition of *Candida albicans*: An In Vitro Study. *Contemp. Clin. Dent.* **2017**, *8*, 446–450. [CrossRef] [PubMed]
34. Mori, T.; Takaset, K.; Yoshida, K.; Okazaki, H.; Murata, H. Influence of monomer type, plasticizer content, and powder/liquid ratio on setting characteristics of acrylic permanent soft denture liners based on poly(ethyl methacrylate/butyl methacrylate) and acetyl tributyl citrate. *Dent. Mater. J.* **2021**, *40*, 918–927. [CrossRef]
35. Sampaio, F.N.; Pinto, J.R.; Turssi, C.P.; Basting, R.T. Effect of sealant application and thermal cycling on bond strength of tissue conditioners to acrylic resin. *Braz. Dent. J.* **2013**, *24*, 247–252. [CrossRef]
36. Monzavi, A.; Siadat, H.; Atai, M.; Alikhasi, M.; Nazari, V.; Sheikhzadeh, S. Comparative evaluation of physical properties of four tissue conditioners relined to modeling plastic material. *J. Dent. (Tehran)* **2013**, *10*, 506–515.
37. Dorocka-Bobkowska, B.; Medyński, D.; Pryliński, M. Recent advances in tissue conditioners for prosthetic treatment: A review. *Adv. Clin. Exp. Med.* **2017**, *26*, 723–728. [CrossRef] [PubMed]
38. Wang, W.T.; Yang, T.C.; Wang, T.M.; Lin, L.D. Evaluation of the Bond Strength of New Tissue Conditioner with Addition of PMMA Resin. *J. Indian. Prosthodont. Soc.* **2018**, *18* (Suppl. S1), S21. [CrossRef] [PubMed]
39. Murata, H.; Chimori, H.; Hong, G.; Hamada, T.; Nikawa, H. Compatibility of tissue conditioners and denture cleansers: Influence on surface conditions. *Dent. Mater. J.* **2010**, *29*, 446–453. [CrossRef]
40. Murata, H.; Narasaki, Y.; Hamada, T.; Mc Cabe, J.F. An alcohol-free tissue conditioner--a laboratory evaluation. *J. Dent.* **2006**, *34*, 307–315. [CrossRef]
41. Murata, H.; Hamada, T.; Harshini Toki, K.; Nikawa, H. Effect of addition of ethyl alcohol on gelation and viscoelasticity of tissue conditioners. *J. Oral. Rehabil.* **2001**, *28*, 48–54. [CrossRef]
42. Hashimoto, Y.; Kawaguchi, M.; Miyazaki, K.; Nakamura, M. Estrogenic activity of tissue conditioners in vitro. *Dent. Mater.* **2003**, *19*, 341–346. [CrossRef]
43. Chow, C.K.; Matear, D.W.; Lawrence, H.P. Efficacy of antifungal agents in tissue conditioners in treating candidiasis. *Gerodontology* **1999**, *16*, 110–118. [CrossRef]
44. Abe, Y.; Ueshige, M.; Takeuchi, M.; Ishii, M.; Akagawa, Y. Cytotoxicity of antimicrobial tissue conditioners containing silver-zeolite. *Int. J. Prosthodont.* **2003**, *16*, 141–144.
45. Catalán, A.; Pacheco, J.G.; Martínez, A.; Mondaca, M.A. In vitro and in vivo activity of Melaleuca alternifolia mixed with tissue conditioner on Candida albicans. *Oral. Surg. Oral. Med. Oral. Pathol. Oral. Radiol. Endod.* **2008**, *105*, 327–332. [CrossRef] [PubMed]
46. Kolawole, O.M.; Cook, M.T. In situ gelling drug delivery systems for topical drug delivery. *Eur. J. Pharm. Biopharm.* **2023**, *184*, 36–49. [CrossRef]
47. Urban, A.M.; Morikava, F.S.; Schoeffel, A.C.; Novatski, A.; Moraes, G.S.; Cachoeira, V.S.; Matioli, G.; Sanches Ito, C.A.; Ferrari, P.C.; Neppelenbroek, K.H.; et al. Characterization, antifungal evaluation against *Candida* spp. strains, and application of nystatin:β-cyclodextrin inclusion complexes. *Curr. Drug Deliv.* **2022**, *20*, 1533–1546. [CrossRef] [PubMed]
48. Zahid, I.; Zafar, M.S. Role of antifungal medicaments added to tissue conditioners: A systematic review. *J. Prosthodont. Res.* **2016**, *60*, 231–239.
49. Sivakumar, I.; Aras, M.A.; Madhavan, R.; Karthigeyan, S. Use of tissue conditioners in prosthodontics. *Int. J. Biol. Med. Res.* **2015**, *5*, 4564–4567.
50. Maciel, J.G.; Sugio, C.Y.C.; de Campos Chaves, G.; Procópio, A.L.F.; Urban, V.M.; Neppelenbroek, K.H. Determining acceptable limits for water sorption and solubility of interim denture resilient liners. *J. Prosthet. Dent.* **2019**, *121*, 311–316. [CrossRef]

Disclaimer/Publisher's Note: The statements, opinions and data contained in all publications are solely those of the individual author(s) and contributor(s) and not of MDPI and/or the editor(s). MDPI and/or the editor(s) disclaim responsibility for any injury to people or property resulting from any ideas, methods, instructions or products referred to in the content.

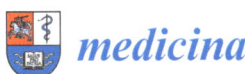

Article

Evaluation of Clinical and Oral Findings in Patients with Epidermolysis bullosa

Yasemin Yavuz [1,*], Isa An [2], Betul Yazmaci [3], Zeki Akkus [4] and Hatice Ortac [5]

1. Restoratif Dentistry, Faculty of Dentistry, Harran University, Şanlıurfa 63000, Turkey
2. Şanlıurfa Training and Research Hospital, Şanlıurfa 63000, Turkey
3. Pediatric Dentistry, Faculty of Dentistry, Harran University, Şanlıurfa 63000, Turkey
4. Faculty of Medicina, Department of Statistic, Dicle University, Diyarbakır 21000, Turkey
5. Uludag University, Bursa 16000, Turkey
* Correspondence: yyavuz-21@hotmail.com

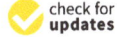

Citation: Yavuz, Y.; An, I.; Yazmaci, B.; Akkus, Z.; Ortac, H. Evaluation of Clinical and Oral Findings in Patients with Epidermolysis bullosa. *Medicina* 2023, *59*, 1185. https://doi.org/10.3390/medicina59071185

Academic Editors: Giuseppe Minervini and Stefania Moccia

Received: 15 May 2023
Revised: 9 June 2023
Accepted: 14 June 2023
Published: 21 June 2023

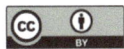

Copyright: © 2023 by the authors. Licensee MDPI, Basel, Switzerland. This article is an open access article distributed under the terms and conditions of the Creative Commons Attribution (CC BY) license (https://creativecommons.org/licenses/by/4.0/).

Abstract: *Introduction:* Epidermolysis bullosa (EB) is a genetically inherited disease characterized by recurrent bullae and erosions on the skin with numerous signs of dental caries and poor oral hygiene. The aim of this study was to investigate the general clinical and oral findings of patients with EB. *Materials and Methods:* In this prospective study, the clinical and oral findings and family history of 26 cases with EB were evaluated. The type of EB, gender, age, parental consanguinity, dental caries, oral findings, distribution of lesions and presence of associated anomalies, clinical and oral findings correlated with gender were recorded. *Results:* All 26 patients with EB had a history of consanguinity and siblings with EB to varying degrees. In our study, malnutrition, anemia and growth retardation, gastrointestinal system complications, hair thinning, hand and nail deformity, ocular problems and renal disease (in one case) were observed with variable frequencies. When the intraoral findings of the patients were investigated, extensive dental caries in all EB types, enamel hypoplasia in junctional EB (JEB) and the presence of tooth-root to be extracted in dystrophic EB (DEB), intraoral bullae and lesions, ankyloglossia, vestibular sulcus insufficiency, microstomia and maxillary atrophy were observed. Three cases had restorative treatment and one case had prosthetic rehabilitation. *Conclusions:* Oral involvement can be seen with varying frequencies depending on the type of EB and the severity of the disease. It may result from delayed oral and dental rehabilitation due to physical disabilities, limitations and more pressing medical problems. Microstomy, pain from mucosal lesions, and restricted access to the mouth can be caused by poor oral hygiene. Oral complications and caloric needs of individuals with EB should be determined, and individual prophylaxis should be applied to prevent caries formation and protect teeth.

Keywords: epidermolysis bullosa; bullae; oral hygiene; dental caries

1. Introduction

Epidermolysis bullosa (EB) is an inherited disease with 30 different phenotypes and genotypes characterized by mechanical fragility of the skin. The presence of recurrent bullae and erosions on the skin and abnormal wound healing are characteristic features of all types of EB [1]. Problems may be observed on epithelial tissue surfaces, such as gastrointestinal, cardiovascular, genitourinary-system, eye, oral-cavity and dental tissues [2]. EB is caused by mutations in at least 20 different genes encoding various structural and signaling proteins within the epidermis and at the dermis–epidermis junction. These mutations lead to a decrease in the level of proteins that ensure epidermis–dermis integrity and to the development of bullae by the separation of skin layers [3].

EB is classified into four main hereditary types according to the ultrastructural level of bullae within the skin [4]. EB simplex (EBS), junctional EB (JEB), dystrophic EB (DEB) and Kindler EB [1,5]. Subclassification is determined according to clinical phenotypic features, extracutaneous tissue involvement, genetic transmission route and the specific gene affected [5]. Symptoms first appear at birth, but in some patients they may appear in adolescence and later. This may delay making the correct diagnosis until adulthood [6]. There is no approved treatment for EB. The goals in treatment are the prevention of bulla formation, wound care, reduction of pain, early recognition and management of extracutaneous complications [6].

EB is a disease that has multiple oral cavity findings and requires a special treatment approach in terms of oral and dental health.

Although individuals with EB with type VII collagen mutations have a developmentally normal tooth, oral mucosal tissues can be severely affected because they are exposed to oral functions from an early age [7]. Oral lesions are characterized by erythema, blistering and their consequences (e.g., erosion, ulceration, crusting, and atrophic scarring). The number, frequency and severity of lesions depend on the type of disease [7]. Functional sequelae, such as ankyloglossia, microstomy and vestibular sulcus insufficiency, extensive caries, enamel defects and inadequate oral hygiene, require special attention in individuals with EB [7].

EB is a disease that has many oral cavity findings and requires a special treatment approach in terms of oral and dental health. Although individuals with EB with type VII collagen mutations have developmentally normal teeth, their oral mucosal tissues may be severely affected [6]. Dentists are involved in oral treatment planning as part of a multidisciplinary team. Examination of oral soft and hard tissue manifestations of each type of hereditary EB will help in planning long-term treatment approaches [5].

The aim of this study is to investigate the general clinical and oral findings (mucous and dental tissue) of patients with EB and to offer suggestions to help dental health management.

2. Materials and Methods

In this prospective study, 26 patients who were clinically, histopathologically and genetically diagnosed with EB, followed up in the dermatology and venereology clinic and consulted to our restorative dentistry and pedodontics clinics between August 2022 and January 2023 were included. Patients' clinical and oral findings and family history were evaluated. The type of EB, gender, age, parental consanguinity, dental caries, oral findings, lesions and presence of accompanying anomalies were determined and recorded in the detailed anamnesis form.

Ethical approval for this study was obtained from the ethics committee of Harran University Faculty of Medicine (Number: HRU/22.13.08). Informed consent was obtained from all participants and their families. The study was conducted in accordance with the Declaration of Helsinki and Good Clinical Practice guidelines.

In statistical analyses, continuous data were calculated as a mean ± standard deviation (SD) and categorical data were calculated as a frequency (%). Pearson Chi-square test and Fisher's Exact Test were used to investigate the relationship between general clinical and oral findings and gender. $p < 0.05$ was considered to be statistically relevant. SPSS 25.0 SPSS Inc., PASW Statistics for Windows, Version, 25.0 (Chicago, IL, USA) was used for statistical analysis.

3. Results

Of the 26 patients diagnosed with EB, 11 were female and 15 were male. Of the 26 patients clinically diagnosed with EB, 2 were EBS, 1 was JEB and 23 were DEB (Figure 1). When the relationship between the parents was analyzed, it was found that 100% of the cases had a history of consanguinity to different degrees and 50% of the cases had a sibling with EB.

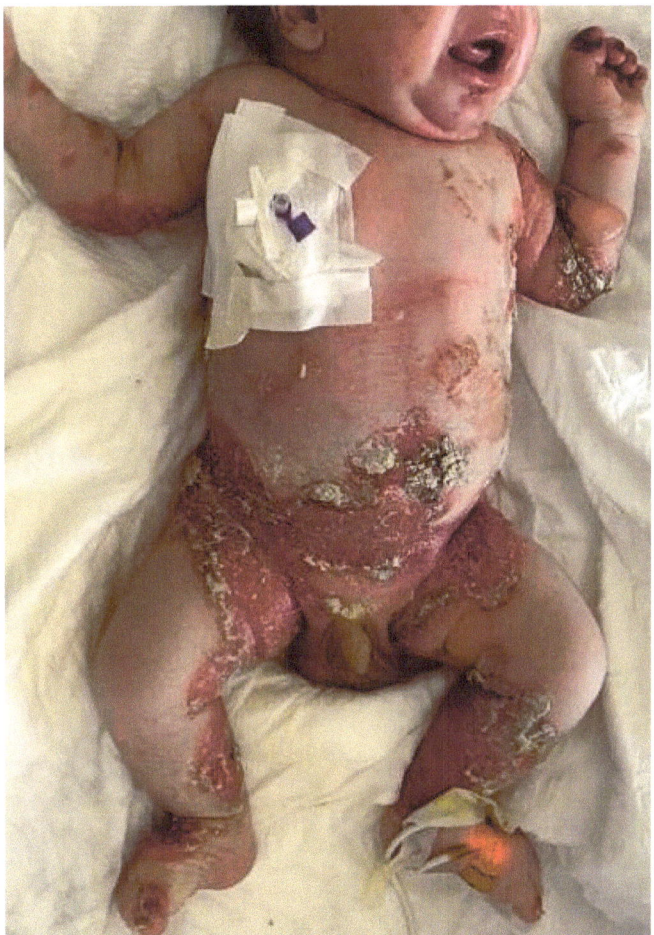

Figure 1. Diffuse bullae and erosion are seen in a patient with a diagnosis of dystrophic epidermolysis bullosa.

In our study, malnutrition was observed in 80.7%, anemia in 46%, growth retardation in 61.5%, ocular problems in 42%, various gastrointestinal system complications in 76.9%, hair thinning in 38%, hand and nail deformities in 88% and renal problems in one case. In 26 cases, no hearing problems were observed.

When the intraoral findings of the patients were investigated, extensive dental caries, enamel hypoplasia in JEB and presence of tooth-root to be extracted in DEB, intraoral bullae and lesions in 92%, ankyloglossia and vestibular sulcus insufficiency in 73%, and microstomia and maxillary atrophy in 69% were observed in all EB types (Figures 2–4). In three cases, treated tooth restorations were seen, and in one case, fixed prosthetic zirconium restoration was seen. General clinical findings reported according to EB type are shown in Table 1, and oral findings are shown in Table 2.

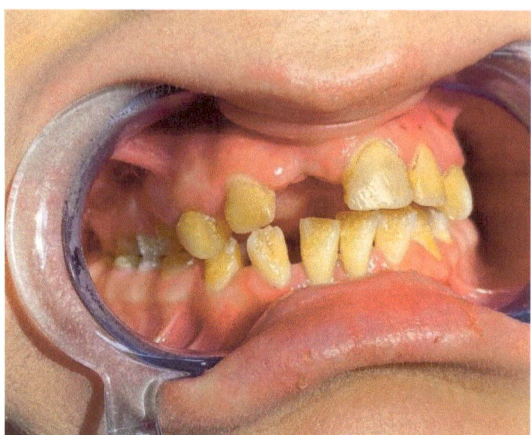

Figure 2. Enamel hypoplasia.

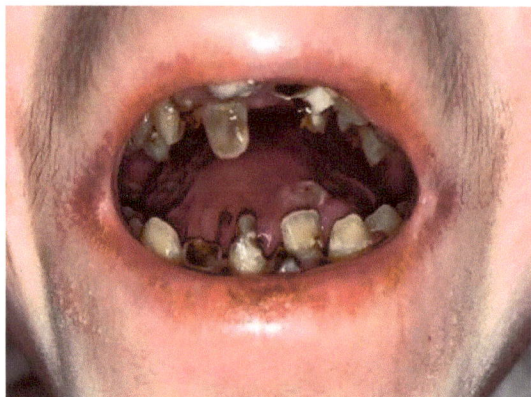

Figure 3. Common dental caries and tooth to be extracted.

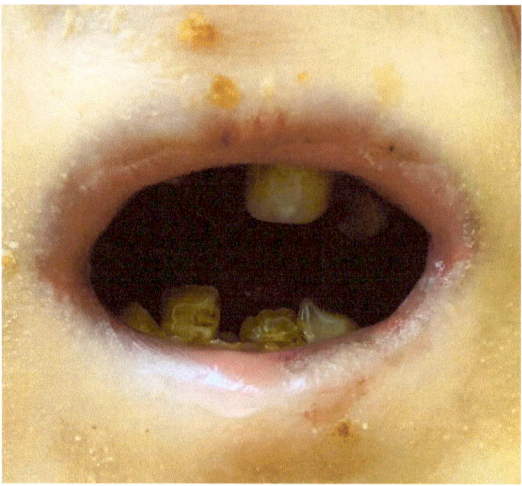

Figure 4. Microstomy.

Table 1. Clinical and demographic characteristics of epidermolysis bullosa patients.

		Epidermolysis bullosa Simplex (n:2)	Junctional Epidermolysis bullosa (n:1)	Dystrophic Epidermolysis bullosa (n:23)	Number of Cases (n)
Gender	Male	1		14	15
	Female	1	1	9	11
Age (year)		2 and 5	21	0.2–30	26
Parental consanguinity		2	1	23	26
Number of affected siblings		0	0	13	26
Malnutrition		0	0	21	26
Anemia		0	0	12	26
Growth retardation		0	0	16	26
Ocular involvement		0	0	11	26
Auricular involvement		0	0	0	26
Renal involvement		0	0	1	26
Gastrointestinal system involvement		1	1	20	26
Hair involvement		0	1	9	26
Hand and nail deformity		0	1	22	26

Table 2. Oral findings in patients with epidermolysis bullosa.

Oral Findings		Epidermolysis bullosa Simplex	Junctional Epidermolysis bullosa	Dystrophic Epidermolysis bullosa	Number of Cases (n)
Gender	Male	1		14	15
	Female	1	1	9	11
Age (year)			21	0.2–30	26
Tooth decay		12	10	280	26
Enamel hypoplasia		0	1	0	26
Extracted tooth		0	1	17	26
Tooth to be extracted		0	0	141	26
Periodontal disease		0	1	17	26
Intraoral bulla and erosion		1	1	23	26
Ankyglossia		0	0	19	26
Microstomy		0	0	18	26
Maxillary atrophy		0	0	18	26
Vestibular sulcus insufficiency		0	0	19	26
Restorative treatment history		0	1	2	26
History of prosthetic rehabilitation		0	1	0	26

4. Discussion

EB is a disease caused by genetic defects transmitted in an autosomal dominant or autosomal recessive manner. It has been classified into four main categories according to the topographic location of the bulge within the cutaneous basement membrane [8].

In our study, 88% of individuals with EB had dystrophic variant DEB, one of its four subtypes. DEB is an inherited skin disorder characterized by bullae, erosions and chronic ulcers in the sublamina densa. It has been identified as the COL7A1 gene encoding type VII collagen. In the study conducted by Vahidnezhad et al., COL7A1 mutations in closely related families were compatible with autosomal recessive inheritance [9].

In our study, it was observed that all cases with EB had a history of consanguinity between parents to varying degrees. It was determined that 46% of individuals with EB were siblings. When the gender differences of the affected individuals were examined, no statistically significant difference was observed ($p > 0.05$). The kinship findings we obtained in our study were in parallel with many previous studies that reported that the likelihood of inherited genetic defects in future generations would be higher in societies where consanguineous marriages are common [9,10].

Particular cases of EBS with mild forms of clinical symptoms of EB may not attract the attention of family members or may lead parents to hide such genetic disorders for fear of being ostracized. However, in severe cases of EB, affected individuals are easily included in hospital records [11].

In our study, 88% of EB patients had DEB. DEB patients with mutations in the COL7A1 gene, which encodes type VII collagen, were enrolled in hospital records for their needs.

Nutrition in the first years of an individual's life is very important for growth and development. Any factor that causes an inadequate nutrient intake during this period predisposes to growth and developmental retardation [12,13].

Manjunath et al. found that dietary modification significantly improved the nutritional status in children with recessive dystrophic epidermolysis bullosa (RDEB) and dominant dystrophic epidermolysis bullosa (DDEB) subtypes. They found that moderate and severe malnutrition in children with EB was significantly associated with the severity of the disease [12].

In our study, all of the developmental delay belonged to the DEB type. Esophageal dilatation was performed in four patients with dysphagia. Growth retardation in individuals with EB can be attributed to various gastrointestinal complications and malnutrition. Dysphagia, esophageal stricture and constipation are the most common gastrointestinal (GI) complications described in DEB [14].

In our study, GI system problems were seen in 76.9% of patients with different severities. It has been reported in previous studies that trauma-induced swelling of the squamous layer of the esophagus following solid food intake and scar tissue formation after healing may cause esophageal strictures [14].

Inadequate nutrient absorption due to bleeding in the GI tract mucosa and cicatrization has been reported to be among the factors causing anemia [15,16].

In our study, growth retardation was observed in 61.5%, malnutrition in 80.7% and anemia in 46% of EB cases. No statistically significant difference was found between EB cases when compared according to the gender variable ($p > 0.05$).

EB is a devastating connective tissue disease that can cause blistering of the ocular surface, including the cornea, conjunctiva and eyelids, poor wound healing and even blindness. Ophthalmic symptoms have been reported to be more common in RDEB caused by VII collagen function and JEB caused by the absence of laminin 5 [17,18].

Chen et al. found that patients with EB showed significant stromal thickening compared to the control group, and visual loss was associated with increased stromal thickness [18].

In our study, various ocular problems were seen in 42% of patients. No statistically significant difference was found when these findings were compared according to the gender variable among cases with EB ($p > 0.05$) (Figure 5).

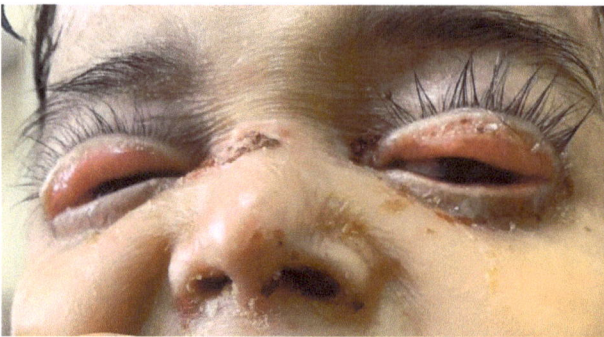

Figure 5. Cicatricial ectropion.

Most patients with DEB have deformities of the fingers and toes of the extremities, and all tissue structures may be affected. Dermal fibrosis, pseudosyndactyly, contractures, atrophic fingers and atrophic thumb tips, nail loss and the entire hand may be covered with an epithelial cocoon [19].

Similar findings were observed in our cases. Although the anatomy of the nail differs from that of the skin, the antigenic expression of components of the nail bed, proximal nail fold and basement membrane region of the nail bed is similar to that of normal skin. Although the presence or absence of nail changes is not used as an absolute criterion for a differential diagnosis between the different subtypes of EB, nail dystrophy and loss are seen, especially in JEB and RDEB. Toenails of the big toe are more severely affected due to trauma [20]. In our cases, nail and hand deformities were not seen in EBS, whereas nail dystrophy and absence were present in JEB. Hand and nail deformities were present in all cases of DEB (Figure 6).

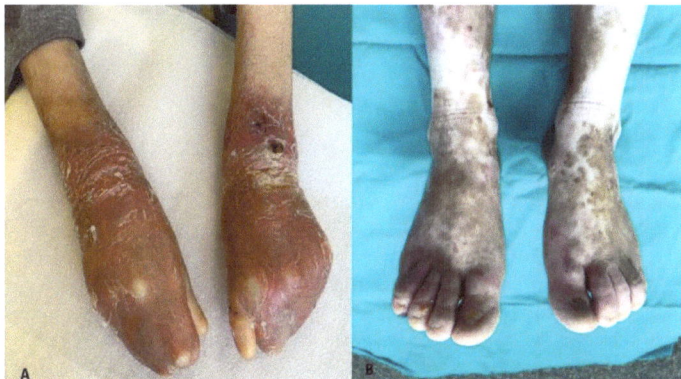

Figure 6. Finger adhesions (**A**) and nail dystrophy (**B**).

No statistically significant difference was found in terms of hand and nail dystrophy when compared according to the gender variable ($p > 0.05$).

Advances in dermal–epidermal-based molecular biology have shown that clinical trials of gene therapy have the potential to make positive changes in the lives of patients with EB [21].

Increased donor cells were found in the skin of children with recessive dystrophic epidermolysis bullosa who underwent allogeneic bone marrow transplantation. Stem cell research may be promising for patients with the most severe forms of EB [22,23].

Oral findings and dental involvement of EB vary according to subtypes. Oral clinical features, such as perioral tissue involvement, microstomia, as well as intraoral soft tissue involvement, such as mouth ulcers, peeled tongue, ankyloglossia, vestibular obliteration, periodontal disease and oral cancer, can be seen. Hard tissue involvement may be accompanied by extensive caries, enamel hypoplasia (local or general), delayed eruption and occlusal anomalies [5,24–26].

In our study, intraoral bullae and lesion, ankyloglossia, microstomy, vestibular sulcus insufficiency and maxillary atrophy were observed in all individuals with DEB. In de Azevedo et al.'s study of clinical signs of EB and salivary changes, the RDEB group showed all the features of ankyloglossia in relation to the oral mucosa, and the JEB group showed deformity in the skin and nails. In saliva analysis, the authors observed no difference between the control and EB groups [27].

In terms of dental caries development, all individuals with EB should be managed as high caries risk patients. The high prevalence of caries in individuals with DEB is due to the frequent consumption of high-sugar drinks and soft carbohydrate foods to increase caloric intake in the diet. This means that teeth are in contact with foods with a high cariogenicity for a longer period of time [28,29].

The absence of collagen VII during embryonic development may impair glandular formation. Individuals with EB may have changes in the salivary glands, mammary glands, and skin sebaceous glands [27].

The salivary flow rate, pH and buffering capacity were not found to be different in individuals with EB compared to normal individuals [27,30,31].

In the Prevalence study, it was reported that although the values of all salivary parameters (salivary flow rate, pH and buffering capacity) obtained from individuals with EB were slightly lower than those without EB, there was no significant difference when these parameters were compared with healthy individuals [30].

This suggests that the extensive dental caries seen in EB is most likely attributable to non-salivary factors, such as enamel involvement, soft tissue changes, inadequate oral hygiene and a soft high carbohydrate diet [29,31].

Enamel structural defects (hypoplasia) have been described in EB patients and are associated with EB genetic mutations that also affect ameloblastic differentiation [7]. Individuals with EB caused by mutations in laminin-332 (Lama3, Lamb3, Lamc2), α6β4-integrin (TGB4, ITGA6) gene and type XVII collagen (Col17A1) are associated with enamel hypoplasia. These proteins are involved in the formation of tooth enamel during amelogenesis [5,6,8].

In our study, developmental enamel defects were seen only in JEB. Although the teeth are structurally normal, inadequate oral hygiene due to microstomia and restricted access to the mouth, pain from mucosal blisters, and a high carbohydrate soft diet may increase the rate of dental caries. No statistically significant difference was found when comparing patients according to the gender variable in terms of dental caries ($p > 0.05$). Wright et al.'s study confirms that the development of caries is not a specific manifestation of EB but rather a consequence of the disruption of oral health-related habits [32].

In their study, Harris et al. reported significantly higher rates of dental caries in children with DEB compared to control groups. Due to difficulty swallowing food, cases with EB tend to eat small amounts of pureed high-carbohydrate foods and drinks throughout the day. This is one of the factors that may explain the high caries experience [29].

In our study, tooth loss was low in all individuals with DEB, but the excess of tooth-root and caries to be extracted was remarkable.

These findings may be explained by the fact that patients primarily focus on vital systemic complications and postpone oral and dental health problems. There are studies reporting that this may be a reflection of the dental treatment needs of dentists and the difficulties in performing restorative treatment [29].

In addition, it has been reported that loss of grasping ability of the fingers due to pseudosyndactyly, difficulty in tooth-brushing, and easy blistering of the oral mucosa in the slightest trauma may negatively affect oral hygiene [29].

In these patients, topical fluoride applications and chlorhexidine mouthwashes may be useful in reducing the burden of cariogenic microorganisms [32].

The oral mucosa originates from ectoderm invagination during the embryologic period. In disorders primarily associated with the skin, mucosal tissues may also be affected. Patients with EB have bullae and ulceration of the oral mucosa. In cases of EBS, bullae tend to be few, to be small in size (<1 cm) and to heal without scarring. Mucosal lesions, which are more common in JEB cases, may heal without obvious scarring, but in severe JEB cases, perioral lesions exhibit granulation tissue. DEB cases often have extremely fragile mucous membranes characterized by tissue fragility. It has been reported that scar-healing ulcerations may have a much higher risk of ankyloglossia, loss of palatal rugae and lingual papillae, vestibule obliteration and microstomia [33].

In our study, no intraoral bullae were observed in EBS cases. The JEB case had intraoral bullae and enamel hypoplasia. Patients with DEB had extensive intraoral soft tissue involvement, including bullae, microstomia, ankyloglossia and obliteration of the oral vestibule. Microstomia, ankyloglossia and vestibular obliteration were not seen in other EB types. When all EB cases were evaluated in terms of microstomia, ankyloglossia and vestibular obliteration according to gender, no statistically significant difference was found ($p > 0.05$).

Mild cases of EB do not need special treatment, but all EB cases should be managed carefully because of their susceptibility to mucosal fragility. Severe forms of EB require special precautions to minimize soft tissue trauma during dental treatments. It has been reported that due to difficulties in oral health care, all EB cases should be encouraged to use fluoride toothpaste, chlorhexidine mouthwash or a spray [29,34–39].

5. Conclusions

In conclusion, oral involvement can be seen with varying frequencies depending on the type of EB and the severity of the disease:

(1) The presence of extensive caries in individuals with DEB may result from delayed oral and dental rehabilitation due to physical disabilities, limitations and more pressing medical problems.
(2) Microstomy, pain from mucosal lesions, and restricted access to the mouth can be caused by poor oral hygiene.

Nutrition is an important factor for healthy growth and development; therefore, dental treatment needs should be provided without being neglected in the early period. The oral complications and caloric needs of individuals with EB should be determined, and individual prophylaxis should be applied to prevent caries formation and protect teeth.

Author Contributions: Conceptualization, software, resources, writing-original draft, Y.Y.; methodology, I.A.; investigation, B.Y.; formal analysis, Z.A. and H.O. All authors have read and agreed to the published version of the manuscript.

Funding: This research received no external funding.

Institutional Review Board Statement: The study was conducted in accordance with the Declaration of Helsinki, and Human right.

Informed Consent Statement: Informed consent was obtained from all subjects involved in the study.

Conflicts of Interest: The authors declare no conflict of interest.

References

1. Fine, J.D. Inherited epidermolysis bullosa. *Orphanet J. Rare Dis.* **2010**, *5*, 12. [CrossRef] [PubMed]
2. Bruckner, A.L.; Bedocs, L.A.; Keiser, E.; Tang, J.Y.; Doernbrack, C.; Arbuckle, H.A.; Berman, S.; Kent, K.; Bachrach, L.K. Correlates of low bone mass in children with generalized forms of epidermolysis bullosa. *J. Am. Acad. Dermatol.* **2011**, *65*, 1001–1009. [CrossRef]
3. Kulali, F.; Özbakir, H.; Kundak, S.; Kalkanli, O.H.; Dilem, E.R.İ.Ş.; Çolak, R.; Çalkavur, Ş. Epidermolizis bülloza: Olgu serisi. *Jinekoloji-Obstet. Ve Neonatoloji Tıp Derg.* **2019**, *16*, 69–73.
4. Bardhan, A.; Bruckner-Tuderman, L.; Chapple, I.L.; Fine, J.D.; Harper, N.; Has, C.; Heagerty, A.H. Epidermolysis bullosa. *Nat. Rev. Dis. Primers.* **2020**, *6*, 78. [CrossRef] [PubMed]
5. Krämer, S.; Lucas, J.; Gamboa, F.; Diago, M.P.; Oltra, D.P.; Guzmán-Leteiler, M.; Paul, S.; Molina, G.; Sepúlveda, L.; Araya, I.; et al. Clinical practice guidelines: Oral health care for children and adults living with epidermolysis bullosa. *Spéc. Care Dent.* **2020**, *40*, 3–81. [CrossRef]
6. Bruckner, A.L.; Losow, M.; Wisk, J.; Patel, N.; Reha, A.; Lagast, H.; Gault, J.; Gershkowitz, J.; Kopelan, B.; Hund, M.; et al. The challenges of living with and managing epidermolysis bullosa: Insights from patients and caregivers. *Orphanet J. Rare Dis.* **2020**, *15*, 1. [CrossRef]
7. Joseph, C.; Marty, M.; Dridi, S.M.; Verhaeghe, V.; Bailleul-Forestier, I.; Chiaverini, C.; Kémoun, P. Oral health status in patients with inherited epidermolysis bullosa: A comparative multicenter study. *Quintessence Int.* **2023**, *54*, 34–43.
8. Wright, J.T. Oral Manifestations in the epidermolysis bullosa spectrum. *Dermatol. Clin.* **2010**, *28*, 159–164. [CrossRef]
9. Simmer, J.P.; Hu, J.C.-C.; Hu, Y.; Zhang, S.; Liang, T.; Wang, S.-K.; Kim, J.-W.; Yamakoshi, Y.; Chun, Y.-H.; Bartlett, J.D.; et al. A genetic model for the secretory stage of dental enamel formation. *J. Struct. Biol.* **2021**, *213*, 107805. [CrossRef]
10. Vahidnezhad, H.; Youssefian, L.; Zeinali, S.; Saeidian, A.H.; Sotoudeh, S.; Mozafari, N.; Abiri, M.; Kajbafzadeh, A.-M.; Barzegar, M.; Ertel, A.; et al. Dystrophic Epidermolysis Bullosa: COL7A1 Mutation Landscape in a Multi-Ethnic Cohort of 152 Extended Families with High Degree of Customary Consanguineous Marriages. *J. Investig. Dermatol.* **2017**, *137*, 660–669. [CrossRef]

11. Gülşen, E.; Yavuz, İ. Epidermolizis Bülloza. *HRU IJDOR* **2021**, *1*, 19–30.
12. Horn, H.; Tidman, M. The clinical spectrum of dystrophic epidermolysis bullosa. *Br. J. Dermatol.* **2002**, *146*, 267–274. [CrossRef] [PubMed]
13. Manjunath, S.; Mahajan, R.; De, D.; Handa, S.; Attri, S.; Behera, B.N.; Bhasin, S.L.; Bolia, R. The severity of malnutrition in children with epidermolysis bullosa correlates with disease severity. *Sci. Rep.* **2021**, *11*, 16827. [CrossRef]
14. Colomb, V.; Bourdon-Lannoy, E.; Lambe, C.; Sauvat, F.; Rabia, S.H.; Teillac, D.; De Prost, Y.; Bodemer, C. Nutritional outcome in children with severe generalized recessive dystrophic epidermolysis bullosa: A short- and long-term evaluation of gastrostomy and enteral feeding. *Br. J. Dermatol.* **2012**, *166*, 354–361. [CrossRef] [PubMed]
15. Freeman, E.; Köglmeier, J.; Martinez, A.; Mellerio, J.; Haynes, L.; Sebire, N.; Lindley, K.; Shah, N. Gastrointestinal complications of epidermolysis bullosa in children. *Br. J. Dermatol.* **2008**, *158*, 1308–1314. [CrossRef]
16. Liy-Wong, C.; Tarango, C.; Pope, E.; Coates, T.; Bruckner, A.L.; Feinstein, J.A.; Schwieger-Briel, A.; Hubbard, L.D.; Jane, C.; Torres-Pradilla, M.; et al. Consensus guidelines for diagnosis and management of anemia in epidermolysis bullosa. *Orphanet J. Rare Dis.* **2023**, *18*, 38. [CrossRef]
17. Laimer, M.; Prodinger, C.; Bauer, J.W. Hereditary epidermolysis bullosa. *J. Dtsch. Dermatol. Ges.* **2015**, *13*, 1125–1133. [CrossRef]
18. Chen, V.M.; Mehta, N.; Robbins, C.C.; Noh, E.; Pramil, V.; Duker, J.S.; Waheed, N.K. Anterior-segment spectral domain optical coherence tomography in epidermolysis bullosa. *Ocul. Surf.* **2020**, *18*, 912–919. [CrossRef]
19. Figueira, E.C.; Murrell, D.F.; Coroneo, M.T. Ophthalmic Involvement in Inherited Epidermolysis Bullosa. *Dermatol. Clin.* **2010**, *28*, 143–152. [CrossRef]
20. Bernardis, C.; Box, R. Surgery of the Hand in Recessive Dystrophic Epidermolysis Bullosa. *Dermatol. Clin.* **2010**, *28*, 335–341. [CrossRef]
21. Tosti, A.; de Farias, D.C.; Murrell, D.F. Nail Involvement in Epidermolysis Bullosa. *Dermatol. Clin.* **2010**, *28*, 153–157. [CrossRef] [PubMed]
22. Marinkovich, M.P.; Tang, J.Y. Gene Therapy for Epidermolysis Bullosa. *J. Investig. Dermatol.* **2019**, *139*, 1221–1226. [CrossRef]
23. Niti, A.; Koliakos, G.; Michopoulou, A. Stem Cell Therapies for Epidermolysis Bullosa Treatment. *Bioengineering* **2023**, *10*, 422. [CrossRef]
24. Arpag, O.F.; Arslanoglu, Z.; Altan, H.; Kale, E.; Bilgic, F. Epidermolysis bullosa in dentistry: Report of three cases and review of the literature. *J. Int. Dent. Med. Res.* **2015**, *8*, 133–139.
25. Volovikov, O.; Velichko, E.; Razumova, S.; Said, O.B. The First Case Report about Noninvasive Impression Taking in Orthodontic Patient with Epidermolysis Bullosa. *J. Int. Dent. Med. Res.* **2021**, *14*, 1587–1591.
26. Filho, G.A.N.; Caputo, B.V.; de Carvalheira, A.A.; Costa, C.; Giovani, E.M. Dentistry approach of epidermolysis bullosa: Two case reports. *J. Int. Dent. Med. Res.* **2013**, *6*, 109–112.
27. De Azevedo, B.L.R.; Roni, G.M.; Dettogni, R.S.; Torrelio, R.M.F.; Leal, L.F.; da Gama-de-Souza, L.N. Epidermolysis bullosa in oral health: Clinical manifestations and salivary alterations. *Clin. Oral Investig.* **2023**, *27*, 3117–3124. [CrossRef] [PubMed]
28. Wright, J.T.; Fine, J.D.; Johnson, L. Dental caries risk in hereditary epidermolysis bullosa. *Pediatr. Dent.* **1994**, *16*, 427.
29. Wagner, J.E.; Ishida-Yamamoto, A.; McGrath, J.A.; Hordinsky, M.; Keene, D.R.; Woodley, D.T.; Chen, M.; Riddle, M.J.; Osborn, M.J.; Lund, T.; et al. Bone marrow transplantation for recessive dystrophic epidermolysis bullosa. *N. Engl. J. Med.* **2010**, *363*, 629–639. [CrossRef]
30. Harris, J.A.; Bryan, R.; Lucas, V.S.; Roberts, G.J. Dental disease and caries related microflora in children with dystrophic epidermolysis bullosa. *Pediatr. Dent.* **2001**, *23*, 438.
31. Prevalence, H.D.C. Higher Dental Caries Prevalence and Its Association with Dietary Habits and Physical Limitation in Epidermolysis Bullosa Patients: A Case Control Study. *J. Contemp. Dent. Pract.* **2016**, *17*, 211–216.
32. Wright, J.; Childens, N.K.; Evans, K.L.; Johnson, L.B.; Fine, J.-D. Salivary function of persons with hereditary epidermolysis bullosa. *Oral Surg. Oral Med. Oral Pathol.* **1991**, *71*, 553–559. [CrossRef] [PubMed]
33. Polizzi, A.; Santonocito, S.; Patini, R.; Quinzi, V.; Mummolo, S.; Leonardi, R.; Bianchi, A.; Isola, G. Oral Alterations in Heritable Epidermolysis Bullosa: A Clinical Study and Literature Review. *BioMed Res. Int.* **2022**, *2022*, 6493156. [CrossRef] [PubMed]
34. Merlya, R.; Darmawan, S.; Taufan, B. The Precede-proceed Model Implementation in Preventive Oral Health Programs for School-aged Children: A Scoping Review. *J. Int. Dent. Med. Res.* **2023**, *16*, 423–428.
35. Hendiani, I.; Prasetyo, B.C.; Evangelina, I.A.; Rizqita, P.A. The Effects of Using Conventional and Self-Ligating Brackets on Oral Hygiene and Periodontal Health Status: A Rapid Review. *J. Int. Dent. Med. Res.* **2023**, *16*, 384–393.
36. Komara, I.; Sopiatin, S.; Hafizh, F.R.; Miranda, A.; Metta, P. Oral Health Management through Plaque Control in Gingivitis with Autism Spectrum Disorder (ASD): A Rapid Review. *J. Int. Dent. Med. Res.* **2023**, *16*, 340–347.
37. Hernawati, S.; Sulistiyani, S. Management of Varicella Zoster and Ulcer Manifestation in the Oral Cavity of a 5-years-old Patient. *J. Int. Dent. Med. Res.* **2019**, *12*, 1610–1612.

38. Reza, M.; Subita, G.P.; Pradono, S.A. Oral Health Status and Subjective Complaint of Oral Dryness of Methadone User at Jakarta Drug Dependence Hospital—Indonesia. *J. Int. Dent. Med. Res.* **2019**, *12*, 1577–1584.
39. Jafar, Z.J. Oral Health and Nutritional Status in Relation to Intelligence Quotient (IQ) of Children in Baghdad. *J. Int. Dent. Med. Res.* **2019**, *12*, 1487–1491.

Disclaimer/Publisher's Note: The statements, opinions and data contained in all publications are solely those of the individual author(s) and contributor(s) and not of MDPI and/or the editor(s). MDPI and/or the editor(s) disclaim responsibility for any injury to people or property resulting from any ideas, methods, instructions or products referred to in the content.

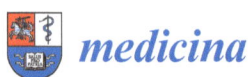

Case Report

Injectable Resin Technique as a Restorative Alternative in a Cleft Lip and Palate Patient: A Case Report

Kelly R. V. Villafuerte [1,2,*], Alyssa Teixeira Obeid [3] and Naiara Araújo de Oliveira [2]

[1] South America Center for Education and Research in Public Health, Universidad Privada Norbert Wiener, Lima 15046, Peru
[2] Dental Division, Restorative Dentistry of the Craniofacial Anomalies Rehabilitation Hospital—HRAC, University of São Paulo, Bauru 17012-230, Brazil
[3] Department of Dentistry, Endodontics and Dental Materials, University of São Paulo, Bauru 17012-901, Brazil
* Correspondence: kelly.vargas@uwiener.edu.pe

Abstract: *Objective*: The objective of this study is to present a case report in which the injectable composite resin technique was used as a restorative alternative for dental re-anatomization in a patient with cleft lip and palate and aesthetic complaints. *Materials and Methods*: The treatment plan included the re-anatomization of the maxillary premolars and canines using a flowable composite resin. This resin was injected and cured through a transparent matrix, which was a copy of the diagnostic wax-up model. Some parameters such as application time and marginal adaptation were also observed when performing the restorations. Additionally, old composite resin restorations on the upper lateral incisors were replaced using the incremental technique with conventional resins, which helped to assess color stability and fracture/wear deterioration for both restorative techniques. *Results*: The clinical case report shows that the injectable technique was a simple and quick method for restoring the anatomy of teeth (shape and contour) in one session, since the injectable resin can be easily applied in interproximal areas without the need to manually sculpt the resin. In this case, no clinical, visual, or photographic differences were found in marginal discoloration, color stability, and fracture/wear deterioration for the two restorative techniques after one year of follow-up. *Conclusions*: The professional may have another clinical option for restorative treatment in the case of small re-anatomizations. In addition, the injectable technique seems to require less operator skill and chair time and better marginal adaptation in cases of small anatomical changes.

Keywords: composite resin; cleft lip; cleft palate; operative dentistry

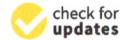

Citation: Villafuerte, K.R.V.; Obeid, A.T.; de Oliveira, N.A. Injectable Resin Technique as a Restorative Alternative in a Cleft Lip and Palate Patient: A Case Report. *Medicina* **2023**, *59*, 849. https://doi.org/10.3390/medicina59050849

Academic Editor: Bruno Chrcanovic

Received: 6 March 2023
Revised: 14 April 2023
Accepted: 21 April 2023
Published: 28 April 2023

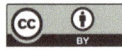

Copyright: © 2023 by the authors. Licensee MDPI, Basel, Switzerland. This article is an open access article distributed under the terms and conditions of the Creative Commons Attribution (CC BY) license (https://creativecommons.org/licenses/by/4.0/).

1. Introduction

Through nanotechnology, it has become possible to improve dental restorative materials such as composite resins, especially fluid resins [1–3]. By providing nanoscale filler particles, it is possible to add a greater volume of filler to the resin matrix, favoring physical–mechanical characteristics [2,4] and improving optical properties [5]. In addition, due to the volumetric increase in filler content, the resin presents better handling, viscosity, and flow characteristics [6], offering good adaptation to the internal wall of the cavity, thus allowing its use in anterior and posterior restorative procedures [7].

Studies [8,9] indicate that high-volume fluid resins offer better polishing and shine than conventional resins. Thus, the use of this type of resin (or universal injectable) has become common among professionals, leading to the use of various techniques, such as the injectable fluid resin technique. Because it has a simple protocol [1], requires less skill from the operator and less working time, and offers lower cost to patients [10,11], some clinicians opt for indirect treatments due to a lack of skill in using direct resins or in cases of extensive aesthetic restorations [12].

Patients with cleft lip and palate require extensive restorative treatments due to a series of dental anomalies [13]. The cleft lip and palate are caused by the interruption of normal development during the early embryonic period of pregnancy, having a complex phenotype [14]. In addition, the existence of the sub-phenotype was emphasized based on the coexistence of dental anomalies alongside the main phenotypes of cleft, such as unilateral and bilateral cleft lip and palate, isolated palate cleft, or lip cleft [14–16]. Facial appearance is central to the psychosocial development of individuals with cleft lip, alveolus, and palate, who often exhibit characteristics of social introversion [17,18]. One of the main reasons may be dental anomalies, which have been shown to be higher in individuals with cleft compared to the normal population [19], including dental agenesis, supernumerary teeth, microdontic upper lateral incisors, the ectopic eruption of teeth, delayed tooth eruption, and enamel hypoplasia, which are frequent in these patients [13,14,20,21]. Additionally, the presence of soft tissue bands connecting the cleft to the base of the nostril or the alveolar margin, known as Simonart's bands, is common [22,23]. These bands may contribute to a higher prevalence of distal upper lateral incisors to the cleft compared to patients without this condition [23]. Simonart's band could assist in the relationship in the upper arch, with a better prognosis in treatment; however, it is not the only factor that will guarantee good resolution [23]. Therefore, these conditions result in long treatments carried out in hospitals and specialized places. Although dental treatments in most patients are usually completed between the ages of sixteen to eighteen years old, some require additional aesthetic or functional treatment during adulthood [24].

The injectable fluid resin technique is classified as a minimally invasive direct/indirect technique that preserves tooth structure [2]. In some cases, it does not require prior or dental preparation and can be performed in one or several teeth in the same session [1,2], through analog or digital diagnosis, to optimize aesthetic (shape and contour) and functional (occlusal) parameters [25]. The anatomical shape of the patient's natural dentition can also be used to create the initial model, which will depend on the type of restorative approach to be selected [1,2]. In addition, this technique can be used in both deciduous teeth [2,26] and permanent teeth [1,2,25,27–29], offering various applicability, including applications related to direct veneers [4,25], re-anatomization, and diastema closure [12,27]. However, the search for information in the literature about this technique returns scarce results due to its relative newness in restorative dentistry and the limitation of clinical studies. This is the first case report of the injectable resin technique presented step by step in a patient with cleft lip and palate.

This clinical report aims to describe the use of the injectable fluid resin technique, with some modifications to the technique, for the re-anatomization of canines in a young patient with cleft lip and palate. Some parameters were observed during the execution of the technique, such as application time and marginal adaptation. In addition, restorations were performed on adjacent teeth (lateral incisors) using an incremental technique with conventional resins, which aided in the assessment of visual and photographic color stability and wear resistance between the two restorative approaches after one year of follow-up.

2. Case Presentation

A female patient, 21 years old with unilateral left cleft lip and palate, presented at the Dentistry Department of the Hospital for Rehabilitation of Craniofacial Anomalies at the University of São Paulo (HRAC/USP) with aesthetic complaints in the anterior upper region. After anamnesis and clinical examination, it was noted that teeth 13 and 23 had been re-anatomized into 12 and 22 after orthodontic treatment was completed when the patient was 16 years old (Figure 1). The patient received a bone graft in the region of the cleft with recombinant human Bone Morphogenetic Protein-2 (rh-BMP2) when she was 12 years old. The patient had agenesis of tooth 22 and tooth 12 had a short root. After the bone graft and during orthodontic treatment for correction, the patient had the option of having an implant in the region of teeth 12 and 22, but she and her parents wished to simplify the treatment by extracting tooth 12, undergoing mesialization of their teeth with orthodontic treatment, and maintaining group occlusion instead of canine guidance. It was observed that after 5 years of completed orthodontic treatment, the patient maintained a stable occlusion without recessions in the premolars. The resin on the "lateral" teeth was opaque with recurrence (small diastemas between 12 and 11 and on the distal of 22). Thus, the patient was dissatisfied with the color of her teeth and did not want to repeat orthodontic treatment. Therefore, treatment options were presented after initial case planning with photos and aesthetic evaluation. Restorative techniques were recommended and explained, but dental bleaching and a combination of restorative techniques were chosen, including the injectable composite resin technique to re-anatomize teeth 14 and 24 into 13 and 23 and replacement of the restorations of teeth 12 and 22 using the direct composite resin technique (Filtek XT Z350 B2B and B2E, 3M, Two Harbors, MN, USA) and closing diastemas.

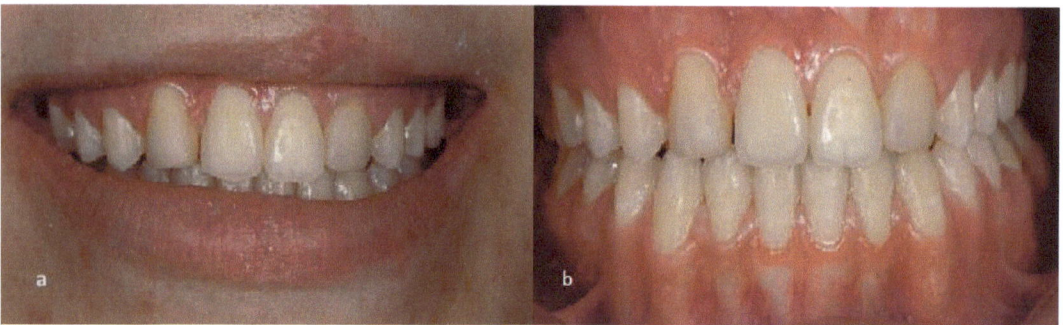

Figure 1. Initial photos of the 21-year-old patient. (**a**) Smile; (**b**) intraoral view of the teeth.

First, an initial impression of the upper and lower arches was taken with alginate to make trays for at-home bleaching with 10% carbamide peroxide (Whiteness Perfect 10%, FGM, São Paulo, SP, Brazil) for 3 h a day for 30 days. With this step, the patient went from the initial color A3 on the Vita Classical scale to B1 (Figure 2). After the completion of bleaching, a new impression was made with condensation silicone to wax the teeth to be re-anatomized (Figure 3). Based on the case planning and wax-up, the patient chose not to undergo periodontal surgery and instead opted to improve the proportion of the gingival contour. Thus, it was decided to re-anatomize teeth 14 and 24 into 13 and 23 using the transparent matrix technique with injectable composite resin (Tetric N-Flow BL L, Ivoclar Vivadent, SP, Brazil).

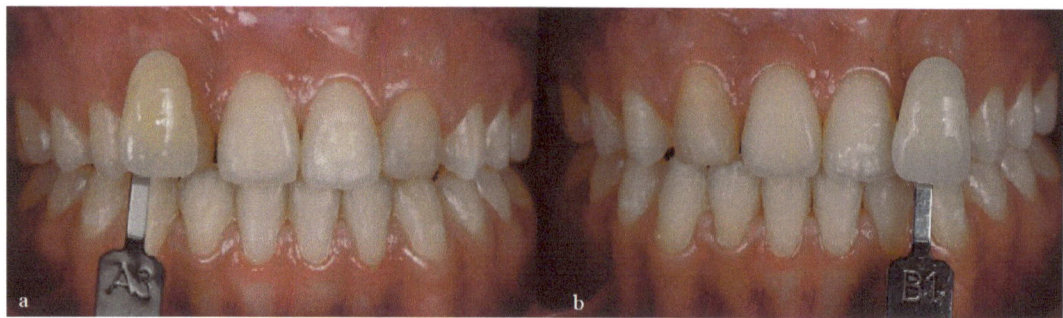

Figure 2. Photos of the bleaching treatment: (**a**) initial color (A3 on the Vita Classical scale); (**b**) final color (B1 on the Vita Classical scale).

For the injectable technique, the waxing model was replicated by molding the wax-up. Subsequently, a transparent plate made of ethylene/vinyl acetate copolymer (EVA) was used, which is a modification of the original protocol that uses a silicone matrix. However, no damage was observed from this adaptation. Therefore, the plate was taken to a vacuum laminator to obtain the transparent matrix. Later, small holes were made in the transparent matrix with high-speed diamond tips in the region of the buccal cusps of the premolars that would be re-anatomized to give access to the tip of the fluid resin to be injected as a transfer vehicle between the tooth and the resin (Figure 4).

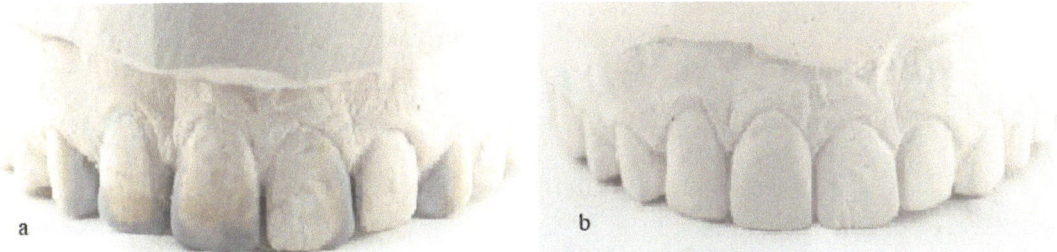

Figure 3. (a) Analog waxing; (b) copy of the wax-up for making the transparent matrix for treatment with the injectable composite resin technique.

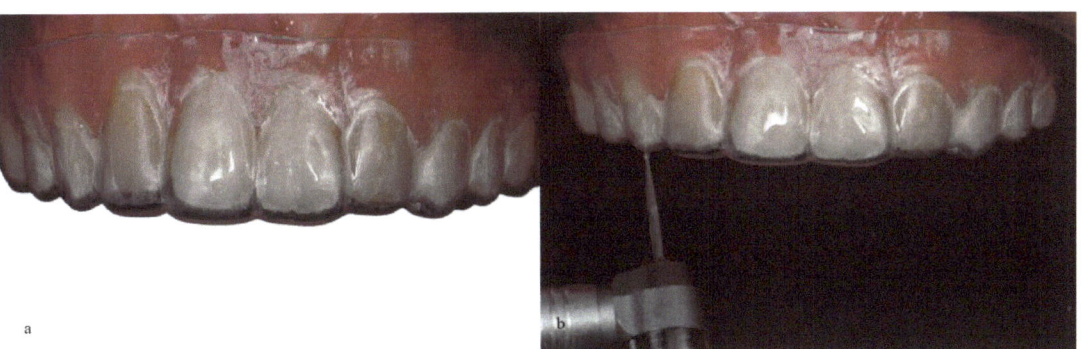

Figure 4. (a) Transparent matrix positioned over the patient's teeth. (b) Drilling with diamond burs to open small holes in the transparent matrix.

Before the matrix was inserted into the oral cavity, a proper fit on the teeth was verified so that the fluid resin could be injected adequately. Prior to this, prophylaxis was performed using pumice stone paste to remove the biofilm and leave the dental surface clean. Subsequently, adjacent teeth were covered with polytetrafluoroethylene (PTFE) tape to prevent material adhesion to undesired dental surfaces and to allow optimal integration in the interproximal region during composite resin infiltration. Teeth 14 and 24 were etched with 37% phosphoric acid for 30 s, followed by a 30 s rinse, gentle drying with air jets to remove excess moisture, the application of the adhesive system (Prime & Bond 2.1; Denstiply, Sirona, SP, Brazil) (Figure 5), and 30 s of light curing (Radi Call SDI, Trevose, PA, USA). When the transparent matrix was positioned, fluid resin was injected to fill the space in tooth 14 between the tooth and the silicone matrix (Figure 6). When the space was filled with the material, light curing was performed for 60 s. The same procedure was repeated for tooth 24 (Figure 6). After the restorations were completed, the matrix was removed, the excess material was removed with a No. 12 surgical blade, and additional light curing was performed for 20 s.

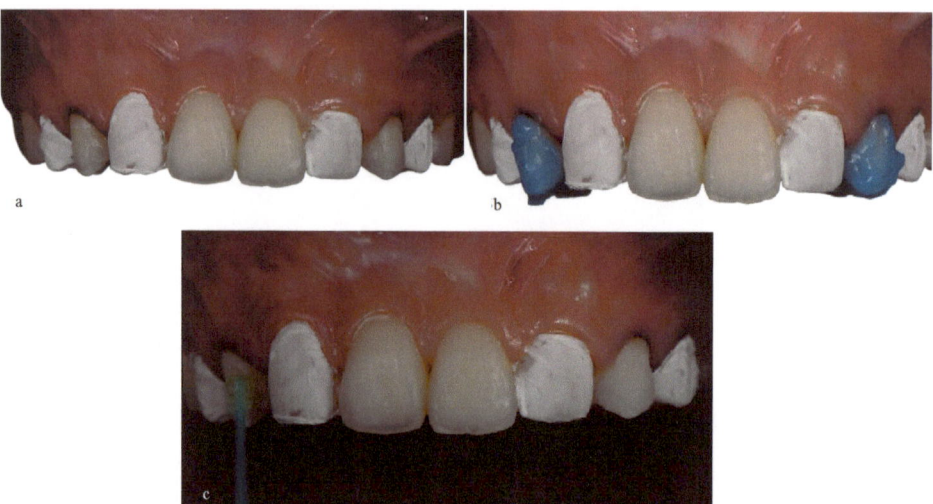

Figure 5. (a) Isolation of adjacent teeth with polytetrafluoroethylene tape and the placement of gingival retraction cords. (b) Phosphoric acid attack. (c) Application of the adhesive system.

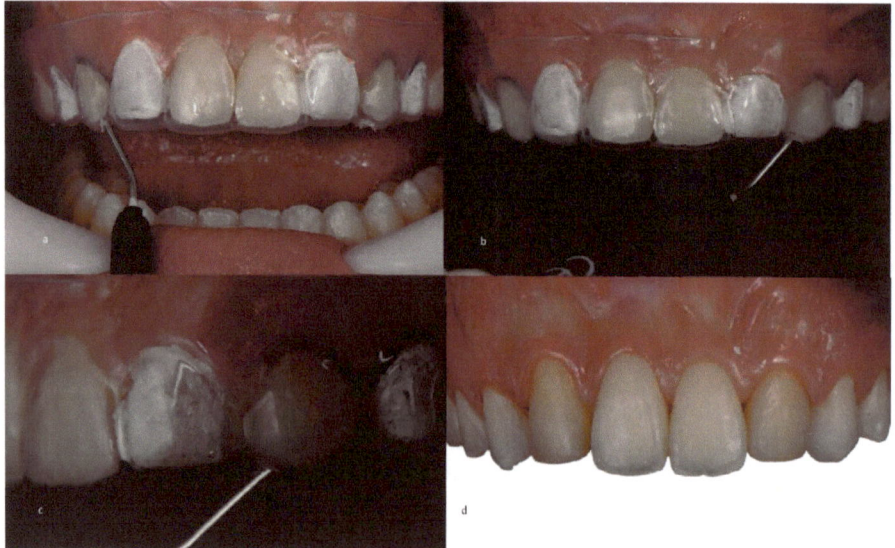

Figure 6. (a) Placement of the matrix on the teeth. (b) The tip of flowable composite resin inserted into holes. (c) Injection of the fluid composite into the transparent matrix, which was light-cured afterward. (d) Completed restorations after removal of the transparent matrix, Teflon tape, and gingival retractor cord.

A glycerin gel was also applied during restoration for final photopolymerization that inhibited the oxygen layer, thus preventing discoloration of the restoration. Occlusion was checked with 12 and 8 μm articulating paper (AccuFilm, Parkell, Long Island, NY, USA), verifying the absence of premature contacts and correct occlusal guidance (anterior and group guide). The composite resin colors to be used on teeth 13 and 23 were selected prior to the resin infiltration procedures on teeth 14 and 24. Teeth 13 and 23, which had already been re-anatomized into "12 and 22," had the old composite resins carefully removed and replaced using the direct composite resin technique (Filtek XT Z350 B2B and B2E, 3M ESPE) (Figure 7).

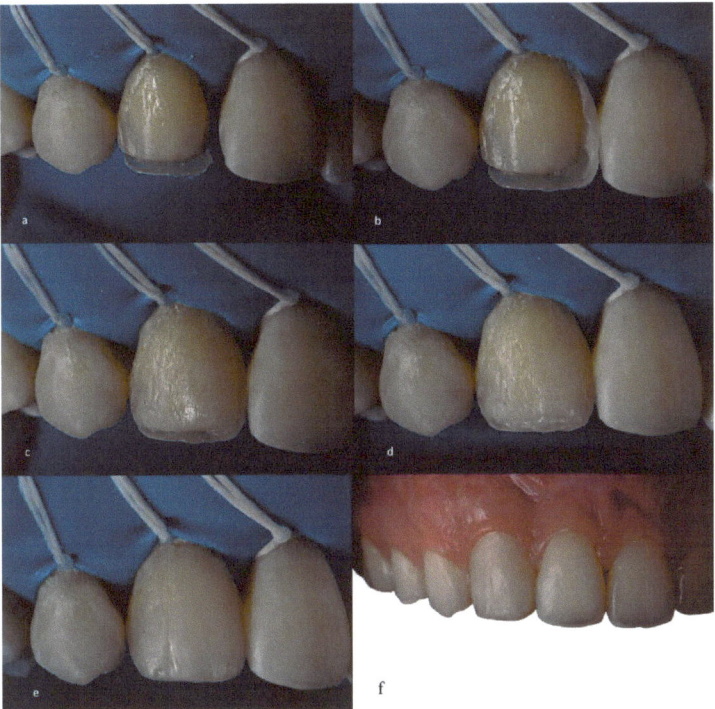

Figure 7. (**a–f**). Direct restoration sequence using the incremental technique with a conventional composite resin.

The patient was satisfied with the restorative treatment, exhibiting a more harmonious and age-appropriate smile. They chose not to alter the shape or add resin to teeth 11 and 21, as their desired outcome had already been achieved (Figure 8).

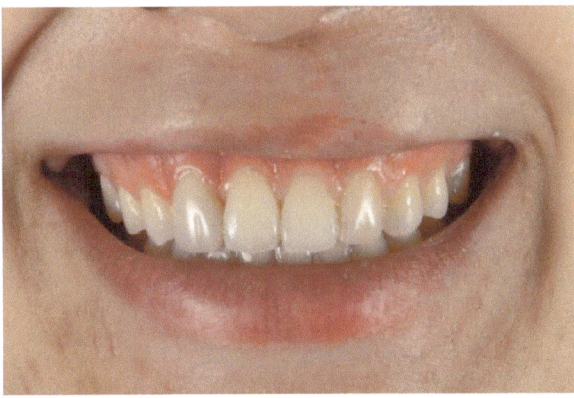

Figure 8. Natural smile. The final result of the restorations after finishing and polishing.

After 1 year, the patient was called for a check-up, and new photos were taken after prophylaxis. The restorations made with the injectable resin technique did not show marginal discoloration or fracture, presenting similar results to the incremental composite resin technique, which also did not change (Figure 9). Therefore, no finishing or polishing was performed.

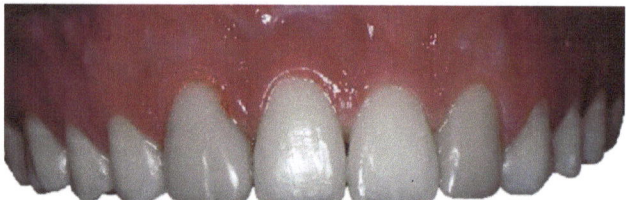

Figure 9. Photo after 1 year of restorations. Intraoral view after performing prophylaxis.

3. Discussion

In the literature, different restorative approaches have been proposed to perform aesthetic restorations. The present case describes the use of the injectable fluid resin technique with some modifications, which allowed for the re-anatomization of the upper premolars in canines in a young patient with cleft lip and palate, as well as a direct restorative approach with composite resin for teeth 12 and 22.

The use of the injectable fluid resin technique was chosen for the premolars as there is evidence in the literature that new fluid composite resins with higher load values (61 to 71% by weight) offer better material adaptation to the cavity walls as well as to the posterior walls, with fewer failures compared to conventional resins. In addition, recent studies [8,9,30,31] show that higher-load fluid resins offer higher mechanical properties (flexural strength and flexural modulus), higher resilience, a high modulus of elasticity [30,31], wear resistance, and better polishing and shine than conventional universal resins [8,9]. Another advantage of this technique is the low cost and good aesthetic results, since the silicone matrix is a replica of the diagnostic wax-up. Thus, the position, shape, and contour are more faithful compared to other incremental techniques [10]. In addition, this technique provides the possibility of restoring one or more teeth, even in cases involving posterior teeth [32]. However, reports in the literature indicate that some care must be taken to avoid periodontal biological complications [10,25,29]. One study [10] indicated that to avoid invasion of the biological distance, the retraction cord should be placed in the gingival sulcus to prevent the fluid resin from flowing more than 0.5 mm; other authors [25,29] indicated that the transparent matrix can be cut following the gingival margin and at the sulcular level, thus obtaining better control of excess material and facilitating its removal. In this clinical case, the placement of a retraction cord in the gingival sulcus was chosen, thus avoiding infiltration of the fluid resin into the gingival sulcus.

The treatment of a patient with cleft lip and palate should be guided by rehabilitation principles, such as physiology, stability, aesthetics, hygiene conditions, and individual expectations [33], which are important to the guidance and initiation of dental treatment. Anomalies of number and form in the teeth behind the cleft lip are common in patients with cleft lip and palate [13,14,20], and when trying to rehabilitate this area, it is common to re-anatomize teeth and sometimes not follow the principals of gold proportions in aesthetic rehabilitation. In this case report, the canines that were re-anatomized in the lateral incisors presented an unfavorable dental proportion in relation to the golden ratio. They ended up with a width close to the central teeth, which required the application of anatomical principles of illusion to create the appearance of narrower teeth. This technique involves altering the position of the vertical edges, favoring the principles of the golden ratio, which is considered one of the options to assist us in aesthetics. The injectable technique seems to be an interesting alternative in the restorative treatment of these patients considering situations where aesthetic treatment should be optimized in a specialized location, such as HRAC/USP. The hospital from this study is a world-class reference in the treatment of cleft lip and palate and hearing loss, was founded in the 1960s, and offers multidisciplinary treatment to numerous patients during the year. Thus, patients who come for dental treatment stay at HRAC for a few days depending on their needs. Analyzing the case report of this article, the technique used facilitated the dental session and promoted the result expected by the patient, without additional appointments.

The injectable technique is generally a simple treatment option for patients looking to improve aesthetics, especially in cases of small re-anatomizations. Therefore, randomized controlled clinical studies are required to demonstrate the long-term effectiveness of the technique. A recent study [34] related to the longevity of restorations, as well as the selection and use of restorative materials alone, indicates that the success of restorations will depend on a series of patient-related risk factors, such as age, the individual's associated risks, parafunctional habits, and the size of the restoration, since the greater the amount of dental structure replaced by a polymeric composite, the greater the mechanical challenges imposed on the restoration.

Thus, the authors indicate that the impact of photopolymerization on the longevity of restorations has been widely discussed in the literature [34,35], and there is enough evidence that the differences between resins from different manufacturers are not an important factor that influences the longevity of composite restorations [34,36,37]. Therefore, this study indicates that professionals are free to select materials based on handling preferences, color availability, technical aspects, and ease of polishing [34,36,37].

In this clinical case report, no differentiations were found between restorative techniques in relation to marginal discoloration and fracture resistance. Therefore, the clinic may have another clinical option for restorative treatment in the case of small re-anatomizations in young patients. However, the clinic should always consider patient-related risk factors such as age, lifestyle, and parafunctional habits, which play an important role in the success of restorations [34].

In addition, one of the limitations of case reports, although they can be useful to present interesting or unusual clinical findings, is that they should not be used as definitive evidence to support the effectiveness of treatment. However, they can be useful to suggest new research hypotheses that can be investigated in more rigorous clinical studies.

4. Conclusions

Smile rehabilitation in patients with cleft lip and palate should be associated with aesthetic and conservative techniques. Among the restorative treatment options, the use of the injectable fluid resin technique seems to be an interesting option for cases involving small re-anatomizations and requiring less chair time and good marginal adaptation. Furthermore, no color change or fracture was observed after one year of follow-up.

Author Contributions: K.R.V.V. contributed toward conceptualization, the treatment plan, execution of the treatment, and writing—original draft preparation; A.T.O. contributed to the methodology and critical review of the manuscript; N.a.d.O. contributed to the treatment plan, clinical case photos, and critical review of the manuscript. All authors have read and agreed to the published version of the manuscript.

Funding: The APC was funded by Universidad Privada Norbert Wiener S.A.

Institutional Review Board Statement: Ethical review and approval were waived for this study due to the nature of the article (case report).

Informed Consent Statement: Informed consent was obtained from the person involved in the study.

Data Availability Statement: Data can be obtained from the corresponding author, Kelly R. V. Villafuerte, PhD., upon reasonable request. Furthermore, the authors report that there is no financial interest in companies whose materials were included in this case report.

Acknowledgments: The authors would like to thank the Hospital for the Rehabilitation of Craniofacial Anomalies for all the structure and materials provided to support this case report.

Conflicts of Interest: The authors declare no conflict of interest.

References

1. Terry, D.A.; Powers, J.M. A predictable resin composite injection technique, Part I. *Dent. Today* **2014**, *33*, 96–101. [PubMed]
2. Terry, D.; Powers, J. Using injectable resin composite: Part two. *Int. Dent. Afr.* **2014**, *5*, 64–72.
3. Bayne, S.C.; Thompson, J.Y.; Swift, E.J., Jr.; Stamatiades, P.; Wilkerson, M. A characterization of first-generation flowable composites. *J. Am. Dent. Assoc.* **1998**, *129*, 567–577. [CrossRef] [PubMed]
4. Baroudi, K.; Rodrigues, J.C. Flowable Resin Composites: A Systematic Review and Clinical Considerations. *J. Clin. Diagn. Res.* **2015**, *9*, Ze18–Ze24. [CrossRef]
5. Terry, D.A.; Powers, J.M.; Blatz, M.B. The Inverse Injection Layering TECHNIQUE. *J. Cosmetic Dent.* **2018**, *34*, 48–62.
6. Tangutoori, T.; Devendra, C.; Ravi, N.; Atul, B.; Sharma, Y.; Eliezer, R. Flowable Resin Composites—A Systematic Review and Clinical Considerations. *World J. Adv. Sci. Res.* **1982**, *1*, 186–191.
7. Lai, W.L.; Saeedipour, H.; Goh, K.L. Dataset on mechanical properties of damaged fiber composite laminates with drilled vent-holes for the resin-injection repair procedure. *Data Brief* **2019**, *24*, 103912. [CrossRef]
8. Imai, A.; Takamizawa, T.; Sugimura, R.; Tsujimoto, A.; Ishii, R.; Kawazu, M.; Saito, T.; Miyazaki, M. Interrelation among the handling, mechanical, and wear properties of the newly developed flowable resin composites. *J. Mech. Behav. Biomed. Mater.* **2019**, *89*, 72–80. [CrossRef]
9. Ujiie, M.; Tsujimoto, A.; Barkmeier, W.W.; Jurado, C.A.; Villalobos-Tinoco, J.; Takamizawa, T.; Latta, M.A.; Miyazaki, M. Comparison of occlusal wear between bulk-fill and conventional flowable resin composites. *Am. J. Dent.* **2020**, *33*, 74–78.
10. Geštakovski, D. The injectable composite resin technique: Minimally invasive reconstruction of esthetics and function. Clinical case report with 2-year follow-up. *Quintessence Int.* **2019**, *50*, 712–719. [CrossRef]
11. Geštakovski, D. The injectable composite resin technique: Biocopy of a natural tooth-advantages of digital planning. *Int. J. Esthet. Dent.* **2021**, *16*, 280–299. [PubMed]
12. Ypei Gia, N.R.; Sampaio, C.S.; Higashi, C.; Sakamoto, A., Jr.; Hirata, R. The injectable resin composite restorative technique: A case report. *J. Esthet. Restor. Dent.* **2021**, *33*, 404–414. [CrossRef]
13. Camporesi, M.; Baccetti, T.; Marinelli, A.; Defraia, E.; Franchi, L. Maxillary dental anomalies in children with cleft lip and palate: A controlled study. *Int. J. Paediatr. Dent.* **2010**, *20*, 442–450. [CrossRef] [PubMed]
14. De Lima Pedro, R.; Faria, M.D.; de Castro Costa, M.; Vieira, A.R. Dental anomalies in children born with clefts: A case-control study. *Cleft Palate Craniofac J.* **2012**, *49*, e64–e68. [CrossRef] [PubMed]
15. Letra, A.; Menezes, R.; Granjeiro, J.M.; Vieira, A.R. Defining subphenotypes for oral clefts based on dental development. *J. Dent. Res.* **2007**, *86*, 986–991. [CrossRef]
16. Sá, J.; Mariano, L.C.; Canguçu, D.; Coutinho, T.S.; Hoshi, R.; Medrado, A.P.; Martelli-Junior, H.; Coletta, R.D.; Reis, S.R. Dental Anomalies in a Brazilian Cleft Population. *Cleft Palate Craniofac. J.* **2016**, *53*, 714–719. [CrossRef]
17. Peter, J.P.; Chinsky, R.R.; Fisher, M.J. Sociological aspects of cleft palate adults: IV. Social integration. *Cleft Palate J.* **1975**, *12*, 304–310.
18. Kapp-Simon, K.A.; McGuire, D.E. Observed social interaction patterns in adolescents with and without craniofacial conditions. *Cleft Palate Craniofac J.* **1997**, *34*, 380–384. [CrossRef]
19. Tannure, P.N.; Oliveira, C.A.; Maia, L.C.; Vieira, A.R.; Granjeiro, J.M.; Costa Mde, C. Prevalence of dental anomalies in nonsyndromic individuals with cleft lip and palate: A systematic review and meta-analysis. *Cleft Palate Craniofac. J.* **2012**, *49*, 194–200. [CrossRef]
20. Lourenço Ribeiro, L.; Teixeira Das Neves, L.; Costa, B.; Ribeiro Gomide, M. Dental anomalies of the permanent lateral incisors and prevalence of hypodontia outside the cleft area in complete unilateral cleft lip and palate. *Cleft Palate Craniofac. J.* **2003**, *40*, 172–175. [CrossRef]
21. Paradowska-Stolarz, A.; Mikulewicz, M.; Duś-Ilnicka, I. Current Concepts and Challenges in the Treatment of Cleft Lip and Palate Patients—A Comprehensive Review. *J. Pers. Med.* **2022**, *12*, 2089. [CrossRef] [PubMed]
22. Ariawan, D.; Vitria, E.E.; Sulistyani, L.D.; Anindya, C.S.; Adrin, N.S.R.; Aini, N.; Hak, M.S. Prevalence of Simonart's band in cleft children at a cleft center in Indonesia: A nine-year retrospective study. *Dent. Med. Probl.* **2022**, *59*, 509–515. [CrossRef] [PubMed]
23. Yatabe, M.S.; Garib, D.G.; Janson, G.; Poletto, R.S.; Ozawa, T.O. Is the presence of Simonart's band in patients with complete unilateral cleft lip and palate associated with the prevalence of missing maxillary lateral incisors? *Am. J. Orthod. Dentofacial Orthop.* **2013**, *144*, 649–653. [CrossRef]
24. Stock, N.M.; Feragen, K.B.; Rumsey, N. "It Doesn't All Just Stop at 18": Psychological Adjustment and Support Needs of Adults Born With Cleft Lip and/or Palate. *Cleft Palate Craniofac J.* **2015**, *52*, 543–554. [CrossRef] [PubMed]
25. Brinkmann, J.C.-B.; Albanchez-González, M.I.; Peña, D.M.L.; Gil, I.G.; García, M.J.S.; Rico, J. Improvement of aesthetics in a patient with tetracycline stains using the injectable composite resin technique: Case report with 24-month follow-up. *Br. Dent. J.* **2020**, *229*, 774–778. [CrossRef]
26. Maroulakos, G.; Maroulakos, M.P.; Tsoukala, E.; Angelopoulou, M.V. Dental Reshaping Using the Composite Resin Injection Technique After Dental Trauma and Orthodontic Treatment. *J. Dent. Child.* **2021**, *88*, 144–147.

27. Coachman, C.; De Arbeloa, L.; Mahn, G.; Sulaiman, T.A.; Mahn, E. An Improved Direct Injection Technique With Flowable Composites. A Digital Workflow Case Report. *Oper. Dent.* **2020**, *45*, 235–242. [CrossRef]
28. Surendar, S.; Abraham, A. Diastema closure using a predictable flowable resin composite injection technique–A case report. *Indian. Assoc. Conserv. Dent. Endod.* **2017**.
29. Hosaka, K.; Tichy, A.; Motoyama, Y.; Mizutani, K.; Lai, W.J.; Kanno, Z.; Tagami, J.; Nakajima, M. Post-orthodontic recontouring of anterior teeth using composite injection technique with a digital workflow. *J. Esthet. Restor. Dent.* **2020**, *32*, 638–644. [CrossRef]
30. Sumino, N.; Tsubota, K.; Takamizawa, T.; Shiratsuchi, K.; Miyazaki, M.; Latta, M.A. Comparison of the wear and flexural characteristics of flowable resin composites for posterior lesions. *Acta Odontol. Scand.* **2013**, *71*, 820–827. [CrossRef]
31. Prabhakar, A.R.; Madan, M.; Raju, O.S. The marginal seal of a flowable composite, an injectable resin modified glass ionomer and a compomer in primary molars–an in vitro study. *J. Indian. Soc. Pedod. Prev. Dent.* **2003**, *21*, 45–48. [PubMed]
32. Kitasako, Y.; Sadr, A.; Burrow, M.F.; Tagami, J. Thirty-six month clinical evaluation of a highly filled flowable composite for direct posterior restorations. *Aust. Dent. J.* **2016**, *61*, 366–373. [CrossRef] [PubMed]
33. Freitas, J.A.; Almeida, A.L.; Soares, S.; Neves, L.T.; Garib, D.G.; Trindade-Suedam, I.K.; Yaedú, R.Y.; Lauris Rde, C.; Oliveira, T.M.; Pinto, J.H. Rehabilitative treatment of cleft lip and palate: Experience of the Hospital for Rehabilitation of Craniofacial Anomalies/USP (HRAC/USP)—Part 4: Oral rehabilitation. *J. Appl. Oral. Sci.* **2013**, *21*, 284–292. [CrossRef] [PubMed]
34. Demarco, F.F.; Cenci, M.S.; Montagner, A.F.; de Lima, V.P.; Correa, M.B.; Moraes, R.R.; Opdam, N.J.M. Longevity of composite restorations is definitely not only about materials. *Dent. Mater.* **2022**, *39*, 1–12. [CrossRef]
35. Balagopal, S.; Geethapriya, N.; Anisha, S.; Hemasathya, B.A.; Vandana, J.; Dhatshayani, C. Comparative evaluation of the degree of conversion of four different composites polymerized using ultrafast photopolymerization technique: An in vitro study. *J. Conserv. Dent.* **2021**, *24*, 77–82. [CrossRef]
36. Moraes, R.R.; Cenci, M.S.; Moura, J.R.; Demarco, F.F.; Loomans, B.; Opdam, N.J.C.O.H.R. Clinical performance of resin composite restorations. *Curr. Oral. Health Rep.* **2022**, *9*, 22–31. [CrossRef]
37. Da Rosa Rodolpho, P.A.; Rodolfo, B.; Collares, K.; Correa, M.B.; Demarco, F.F.; Opdam, N.J.M.; Cenci, M.S.; Moraes, R.R. Clinical performance of posterior resin composite restorations after up to 33 years. *Dent. Mater.* **2022**, *38*, 680–688. [CrossRef]

Disclaimer/Publisher's Note: The statements, opinions and data contained in all publications are solely those of the individual author(s) and contributor(s) and not of MDPI and/or the editor(s). MDPI and/or the editor(s) disclaim responsibility for any injury to people or property resulting from any ideas, methods, instructions or products referred to in the content.

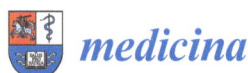

Case Report

Soft Tissue Grafting Procedures before Restorations in the Esthetic Zone: A Minimally Invasive Interdisciplinary Case Report

Gerardo Guzman-Perez [1], Carlos Alberto Jurado [2], Francisco X. Azpiazu-Flores [3], Humberto Munoz-Luna [4], Kelvin I. Afrashtehfar [5,6,*] and Hamid Nurrohman [7,*]

1. Department of Graduate Periodontics, Multidisciplinary Educational Center in Oral Rehabilitation (CEMRO), Tarímbaro 58893, Mexico
2. Department of Prosthodontics, The University of Iowa College of Dentistry and Dental Clinics, Iowa City, IA 52242, USA
3. Department of Restorative Dentistry, Gerald Niznick College of Dentistry, University of Manitoba, Winnipeg, MB R3E 3N4, Canada
4. Private Dental Technician, Irapuato 36643, Mexico
5. Division of Restorative Dental Sciences, Clinical Sciences Department, Ajman College of Dentistry, Ajman City P.O. Box 346, United Arab Emirates
6. Department of Reconstructive Dentistry and Gerodontology, School of Dental Medicine, University of Bern, 3010 Bern, Switzerland
7. Missouri School of Dentistry & Oral Health, A.T. Still University, Kirksville, MO 63501, USA
* Correspondence: kelvin.afrashtehfar@unibe.ch (K.I.A.); h.nurrohman@gmail.com (H.N.)

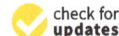

Citation: Guzman-Perez, G.; Jurado, C.A.; Azpiazu-Flores, F.X.; Munoz-Luna, H.; Afrashtehfar, K.I.; Nurrohman, H. Soft Tissue Grafting Procedures before Restorations in the Esthetic Zone: A Minimally Invasive Interdisciplinary Case Report. *Medicina* **2023**, *59*, 822. https://doi.org/10.3390/medicina59050822

Academic Editor: Rafael Delgado-Ruiz

Received: 28 February 2023
Revised: 12 April 2023
Accepted: 19 April 2023
Published: 23 April 2023

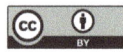

Copyright: © 2023 by the authors. Licensee MDPI, Basel, Switzerland. This article is an open access article distributed under the terms and conditions of the Creative Commons Attribution (CC BY) license (https://creativecommons.org/licenses/by/4.0/).

Abstract: An esthetically pleasing smile is a valuable aspect of physical appearance and plays a significant role in social interaction. Achieving the perfect balance between extraoral and intraoral tissues is essential for a harmonious and attractive smile. However, certain intraoral deficiencies, such as non-carious cervical lesions and gingival recession, can severely compromise the overall aesthetics, particularly in the anterior zone. Addressing such conditions requires careful planning and meticulous execution of both surgical and restorative procedures. This interdisciplinary clinical report presents a complex case of a patient with esthetic complaints related to asymmetric anterior gingival architecture and severely discolored and eroded maxillary anterior teeth. The patient was treated using a combination of minimally invasive ceramic veneers and plastic mucogingival surgery, resulting in a successful outcome. The report emphasizes the potential of this approach in achieving optimal esthetic results in challenging cases, highlighting the importance of an interdisciplinary team approach in achieving a harmonious balance between dental and soft tissue aesthetics.

Keywords: dental esthetics; restorative dentistry; permanent dental restoration; dental ceramics; treatment outcome; patient care team; soft tissue surgical procedures; periodontal plastic surgery

1. Introduction

Dental esthetics play a crucial role in modern society, as an esthetic smile is associated with kindness, popularity, intelligence, and high social status [1]. Achieving an aesthetically pleasing smile requires a harmonious balance between various intraoral and extraoral elements, including the lips, teeth, and gingival tissues [2–6]. Gingival esthetics, also known as "pink esthetics", is a critical determinant of overall dental esthetics, as they frame any esthetic restorative work performed on the teeth [1]. Therefore, conditions such as gingival recession can significantly compromise the esthetic outcome, especially when multiple anterior maxillary teeth are involved [7,8]. Over the years, several surgical procedures have been proposed to manage these complex cases, including coronally repositioned flaps, lateral sliding flaps, free gingival grafts, and subepithelial connective tissue grafts using tunneling and envelope flap techniques [7–12]. These procedures aim to establish a harmonious gingival architecture, increase the amount of keratinized gingiva, and reduce hypersensitivity related to denuded root surfaces [13]. However, to achieve satisfactory results, precise surgical techniques must be employed and attention to detail is necessary to prevent the formation of post-surgical defects, such as scarring, keloid-like defects, and loss of the interdental papilla [7,9]. Data have shown that the outcomes of the surgical treatment of gingival recession are positive. A recent Cochrane systematic review evaluating root coverage procedures for single and multiple recession has reviewed 48 randomized controlled trials in which gingival recessions were addressed with subepithelial connective tissue grafts plus coronally advanced flap and tissue guided regeneration with resorbable membranes plus connective tissue grafts and it concluded that all procedures can be successfully provided for treating single or multiple gingival recessions [14].

Ceramic dental laminate veneers are a well-documented and predictable treatment for modifying the shade of whitening-resistant teeth, improving the shape of teeth with acquired malformations and loss of facial enamel, correcting minor rotations, and closing moderate diastemas [15–18]. Contemporary dental ceramic systems have improved mechanical and optical properties [19–21]. When ceramic restorations are conditioned and combined with resin-based cement, a strong and long-lasting chemical, the micromechanical bond can be created between the ceramic and the underlying tooth substrate [22,23]. Despite significant advances in adhesive dentistry, the success of treatment with dental veneers depends on several factors, including thorough planning, adequate preparation and conditioning of the tooth structure, satisfactory design and conditioning of the restorations, and preparation of the receptor dental and gingival tissues to ensure the harmonious integration of the restorations with the rest of the mouth [24,25]. This clinical report presents the interdisciplinary management of a patient with esthetic complaints related to asymmetric anterior gingival architecture and severely discolored and eroded maxillary anterior teeth. The patient was treated with a combination of minimally invasive ceramic laminate veneers and plastic mucogingival surgery.

2. Materials and Methods

A 32-year-old male patient presented to the clinic indicating that he did not like the esthetics of his anterior teeth (Figure 1A,B).

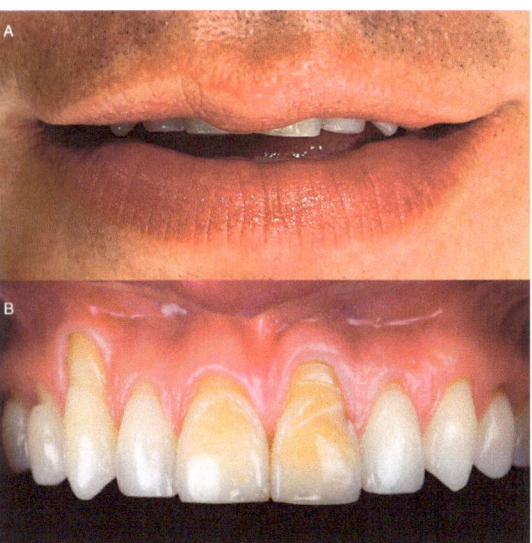

Figure 1. Initial situation. (**A**) Smile. (**B**) Intra-oral frontal.

After a medical questionary, the patient was classified as an ASA type 1 patient systematically healthy with no medical conditions to be concerned about prior to dental care. Additionally, he expressed suffering from severe root sensitivity when drinking or eating. At the initial consultation, the patient expressed that he used to chew on citrus fruits with his anterior teeth and that lemon juice was a big part of his diet until he noticed defects in his anterior teeth. Intraorally, generalized loss of clinical attachment and Miller type 1 gingival recession was observed in the maxillary right first premolar, right canine, and both maxillary central teeth. Additionally, cervical non-carious lesions were noticed on teeth maxillary right first premolar, right canine, right lateral, right central, and maxillary left central, and significant loss of facial enamel was noticed on both maxillary central teeth, giving the teeth a lower color value than the adjacent anterior teeth (Figure 2A,B).

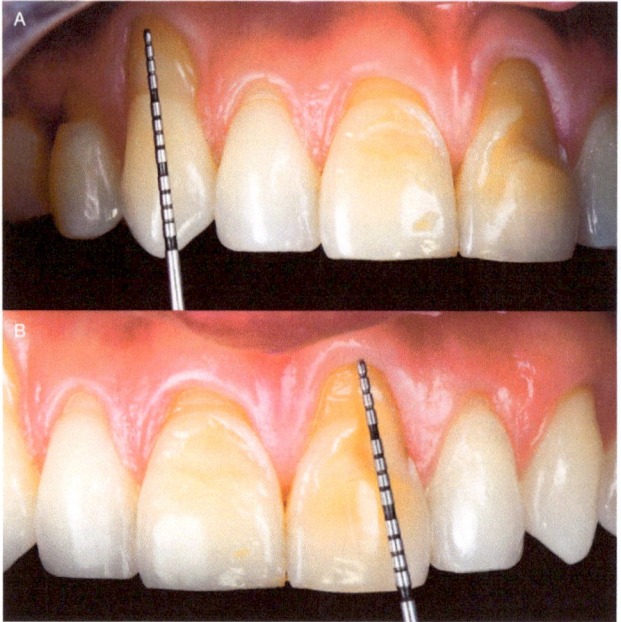

Figure 2. Initial intra-oral situation. (**A**) Measurement of Miller Class 1 recession on the maxillary right canine. (**B**) Measurement of Miller Class 1 recession on a maxillary left central incisor.

When the endodontic condition of the anterior teeth was assessed, all the teeth responded positively to electrical and thermal tests. Additionally, no signs of parafunction or occlusal interferences were noticed during the examination. Subsequently, the clinical findings were presented to the patient and three treatment options were offered: (1) no treatment provided with only monitoring of the gingival conditions and address whenever patient decides; (2) only restorative prosthesis such as veneers from canine to canine to improve the shade and shape of the anterior dentition; and (3) soft tissue grafting procedure to treat the gingival recession following with veneers from canine to canine.

The patient was more interested in the third option and it was further explained that it would consist of plastic mucogingival surgery involving tunneling connective tissue grafts, and anterior ceramic veneers were presented. The treatment's limitations, possible complications, length, and financial aspects were discussed; after considering all these factors, the patient decided to proceed with the proposed treatment.

On the day of the surgery, bilateral anterior superior alveolar, nasopalatine, and left greater palatine blocks were performed with Lidocaine 2% with 100,000 units of epinephrine (Lignospan Standard; Septodont, Saint-Maurdes-Fosses, France). Subsequently, the tunneling procedure was performed from maxillary right first premolar to maxillary left lateral tooth; a partial thickness dissection was performed using periodontal microsurgical instrumentation. Additionally, the root surfaces were mechanically debrided and the smear layer was chemically removed using 24% ethylenediaminetetraacetic acid (EDTA) gel (Straumann PrefGel; Straumann, Basel, Switzerland) for 2 min, followed by abundant irrigation with saline solution (Figure 3A,B).

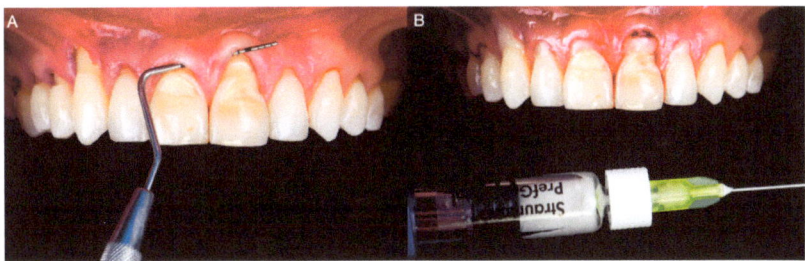

Figure 3. (**A**) Tunneling procedure. (**B**) 24% ethylenediaminetetraacetic acid gel application to prepare the denudated root surfaces.

Subsequently, a partial thickness flap was reflected approximately 4–5 mm from the lingual marginal gingiva of the maxillary right second molar, extending to the lateral tooth in the same quadrant. A 55 × 5 mm band of connective tissue was obtained from the glandular and adipose regions of the palate. During the harvesting procedure, absolute care was taken to preserve the periosteum of the donor site. Subsequently, the connective tissue graft was trimmed to fit the receptor sites (Figure 4A,B) and was inserted and secured below the partial thickness anterior flaps apical to the cementoenamel junction of the anterior teeth with 5-0 monofilament nylon sutures (5-0 Ethilon; Ethicon, Raritan, New Jersey, NJ, USA) (Figure 4C–E).

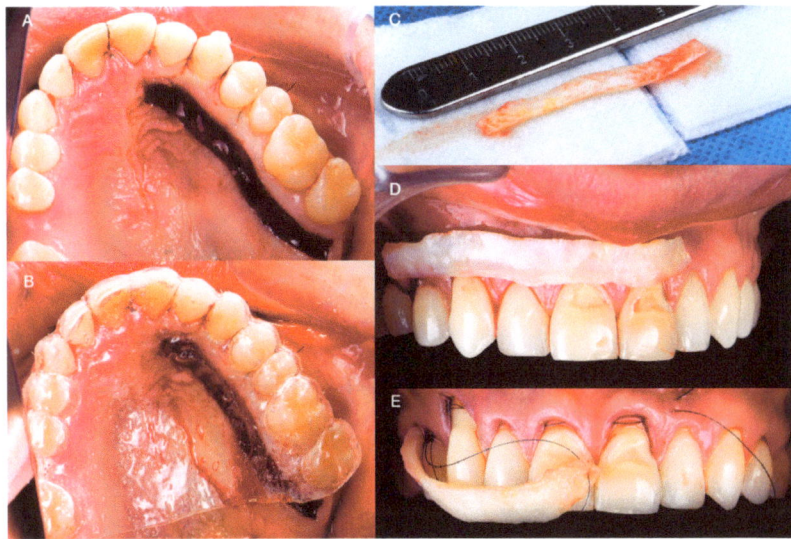

Figure 4. (**A**) Intraoral image of the donor site. (**B**) Donor site protected with plastic sheet. (**C**) Connective tissue graft. (**D**) Connective tissue graft over gingival recessions. (**E**) Insertion of the connective tissue graft under detached interdental papilla and marginal gingiva.

Additional vertical suspensory extending from the base of each interdental papilla to coronal anchorage points were created using flowable composite (3M Filtek Supreme Flowable Composite; 3M ESPE, St Paul, MN, USA). The suspensory sutures were carefully placed to secure the gingival graft, maximize graft coverage, and maintain the height of the interdental papillae (Figure 5A,B).

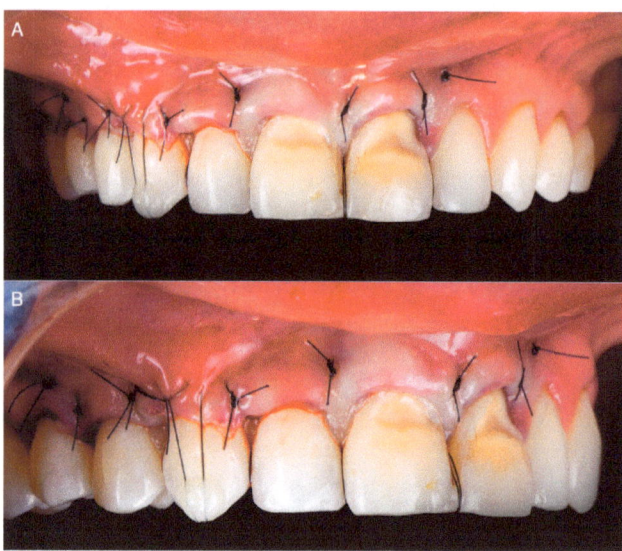

Figure 5. (**A**) Frontal intra-oral image after tunneling procedure. (**B**) Lateral intra-oral image after tunneling procedure.

A home maintenance regime consisting of a soft diet, careful cleaning of the sites with a soft bristle brush (GUM Post-Surgical Toothbrush; Sunstar Americas, Schaumburg, IL, USA), and oral rinses with 0.12% Chlorhexidine Gluconate (Peridex Oral Rinse; 3M ESPE, St Paul, MN, USA) twice a day for 7 days was established after surgery.

The surgical sites were reevaluated 48 h, 2 weeks, and 1 month after surgery. At this stage, satisfactory root coverage and adequate healing with complete reepithelization of the donor site were observed clinically (Figure 6A–C).

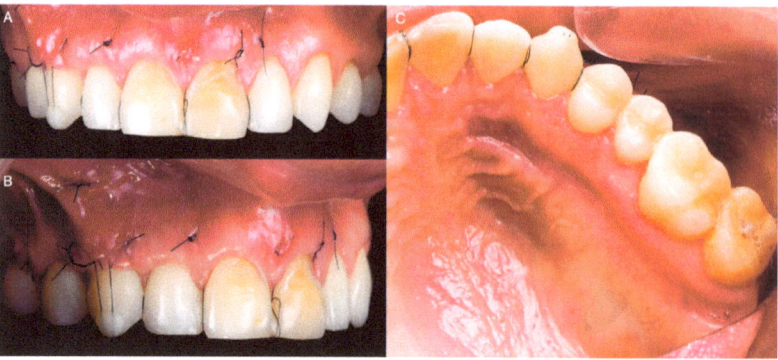

Figure 6. (**A**) Frontal image 1 month after surgery. (**B**) Lateral image 1 month after surgery. (**C**) Image of donor site 1 month after surgery.

Additionally, the patient denied any discomfort or complication during healing related to the surgical procedures performed. After 6 months of healing, the tissues were reassessed and deemed adequate to restore the anterior teeth with ceramic veneers (Figure 7A,B).

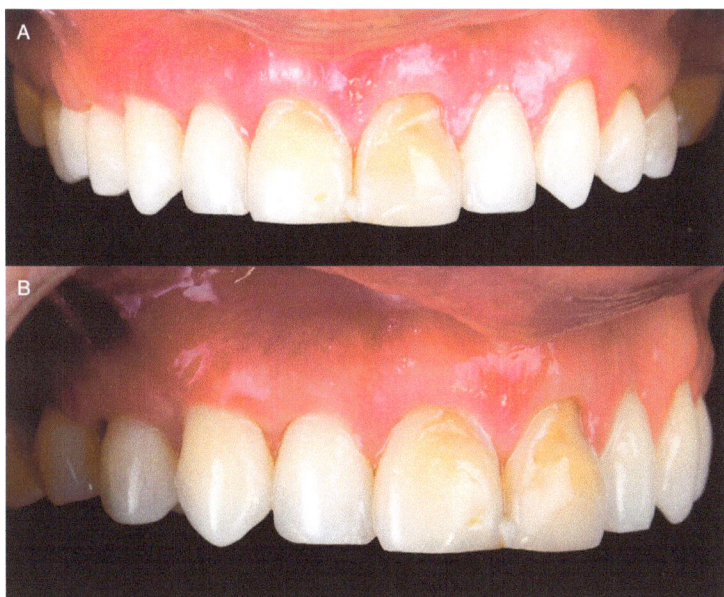

Figure 7. (**A**) Frontal image after 6 months of healing. (**B**) Lateral image after 6 months of healing.

An additive diagnostic wax-up of the anterior teeth was performed and used as a reference for fabricating a reduction guide using heavy-bodied condensation silicone (Zetaplus, Putty Zhermack; Rome, Italy). Subsequently, the labial erosive lesion on the maxillary left lateral tooth was blocked out using resin-modified glass ionomer cement (GC Fuji 2: GC America, Alsip, IL, USA), and conservative laminate veneer preparations extending 0.2 below the free gingival margin were performed. Using the reduction guide as a reference, careful attention was paid to keep the preparation on enamel, ensuring a reduction of approximately 0.5 mm in the labial surfaces, anterior line angles, and incisal edges (Figure 8A–C). The patient was offered either CAD/CAM or traditional hand-made intraorally made provisionals, and due to costs the patient selected traditional provisional restorations. Temporary restorations were fabricated with bisacryl-based composite resin (ProTemp Plus; 3M ESPE, St Paul, MN, USA) and retained using the spot-etch technique [17] (Figure 8D).

Subsequently, impressions were made with irreversible hydrocolloid (Geltrate, Dentsply Sirona, Fair Lawn, NJ, USA) and diagnostic casts were fabricated with type III dental stone (Buff Stone; Whip Mix Corp, Louisville, KY, USA). Using the contours of the diagnostic casts as reference, 6 lithium disilicate (E.max CAD; Ivoclar Vivadent, Schaan, Liechtenstein, Switzerland) ceramic veneers were fabricated using a professional computer-aided design and computer-aided manufacturing (CAD-CAM) dental software (Exocad, Exocad GmbH; Darmstadt, Germany) (Figure 8A,B). Subsequently, the restorations were tried intraorally and the interproximal contact and margins were assessed and carefully adjusted. After complete seating was achieved, the restorations were etched for 20 s with hydrofluoric acid (IPS Ceramic Etching Gel; Ivoclar Vivadent, Schaan, Liechtenstein, Switzerland), primed (MonoBond Plus; Ivoclar Vivadent, Schaan, Liechtenstein, Switzerland), and cemented with resin-based cement (MultiLink Automix; Ivoclar Vivadent, Schaan, Liechtenstein, Switzerland) (Figure 9A,B).

The patient was provided with instructions for proper maintenance including brushing teeth with a soft-bristled toothbrush thoroughly twice a day, flossing daily between teeth to remove food and plaque, and dental cleanings twice a year. The patient was reassessed 1 week, 1 month, and 6 months after delivery. During the 1-year follow-up appointments, the patient denied any discomfort or issues related to the restorations provided (Figure 10A,B).

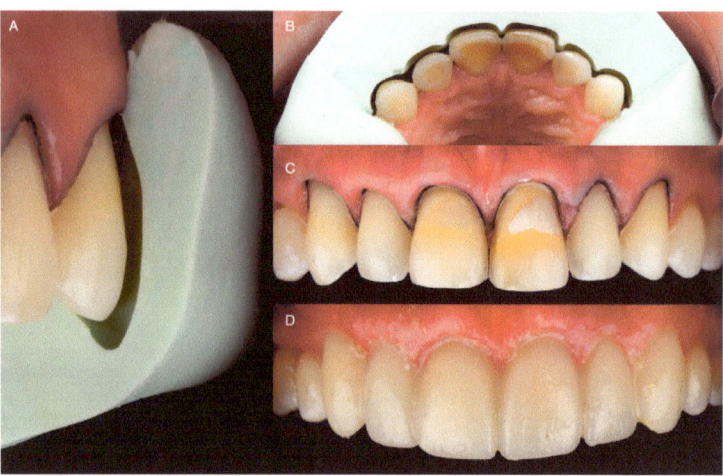

Figure 8. (**A**) Lateral image of minimally invasive veneer preparation with silicone reduction guide. (**B**) Occlusal image of minimally invasive veneer preparation. (**C**) Frontal image of final preparations. (**D**) Provisional restorations.

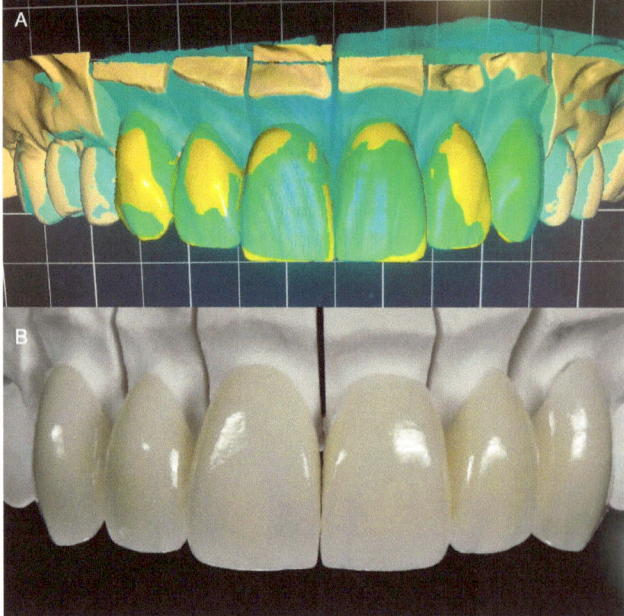

Figure 9. (**A**) Digital design of the veneers. (**B**) Finished ceramic veneers.

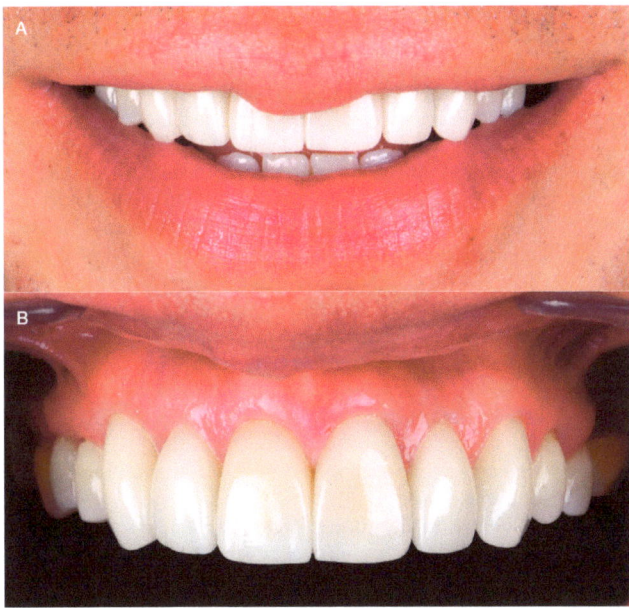

Figure 10. One-year follow-up. (**A**) Smile. (**B**) Intra-oral.

3. Results

The case study describes a 32-year-old male patient who presented to the clinic with esthetic concerns regarding his anterior teeth and severe root sensitivity. Generalized clinical attachment loss and gingival recessions were observed, along with cervical non-carious lesions and significant loss of facial enamel. The endodontic condition of the teeth was assessed and found to be positive. The patient was presented with a treatment plan consisting of plastic mucogingival surgery involving tunneling connective tissue grafts and anterior ceramic laminate veneers. The patient agreed to proceed with the proposed treatment. A unilateral (left) side was used for the donor site and the amount was able to cover the receptor sites. Bilateral anterior superior alveolar, nasopalatine, and left greater palatine blocks were performed, followed by tunneling and connective tissue grafting. The surgical sites were reevaluated at different intervals and adequate root coverage and healing were observed clinically. Conservative veneer preparations were performed using a reduction guide as a reference and the patient was re-assessed after delivery and during a 1-year follow-up period with no reported issues.

4. Discussion

An attractive smile plays a significant role in contemporary society [1], and with the advances in dental material science and CAD-CAM technologies, highly esthetic ceramic restorations [26–28] can now be designed and manufactured consistently and predictably [18]. To achieve satisfactory results, gingival esthetics must be established to provide a pleasing "frame" for dental restorations [1]. Successful plastic surgery periodontal procedures have been used to correct deficiencies related to gingival recession [11,13]. Connective tissue grafts have been reported to provide satisfactory root surface coverage, ranging from 76.6% to 100%, depending on the size and configuration of the recession, the location, and the number of teeth treated [7,9]. Research suggests that connective tissue grafts and tunneling techniques offer advantages over other periodontal procedures, such as coronally and horizontally repositioned flaps, as the forces exerted by intraoral muscle insertions can be circumvented [7] and the integrity of fragile interproximal tissues can be preserved [9]. Moreover, this treatment modality permits predictably enhancing the amount of keratinized tissue available, thus creating a more maintainable periodontal environment [8]. Both elements are crucial to ensure the satisfactory esthetic integration of restorations with equigingival or subgingival finish lines [14]. Previous case reports treating multiple recessions in the esthetic zone have shown positive outcomes. Case series treating 22 patients with a total of 73 recessions with a mean depth of 2.8 mm were treated with the coronally advanced flap technique and reevaluated at 1 year, resulting in an average of 97% root surface coverage, and a complete root coverage was achieved in 16 out of the 22 patients [29]. Patients were treated with a similar approach in another case series with a longer follow-up treating 22 patients with 73 gingival recessions in the esthetic zone Miller Class I and II [30]. The results displayed 94% of root coverage at 5 years of examination and complete coverage was obtained in 15 out of the 22 patients [30]. Moreover, a systematic review from the American Academy of Periodontology (AAP) evaluated the success of soft tissue root coverage procedures. This review evaluated 234 clinical trials on class I, II III, and IV gingival recessions, and it demonstrated that all clinical procedures provided a significant reduction in recession depth, concluding that connective tissue grafts provide the best outcome for clinical practice [31]. Due to the positive clinical reports, soft tissue grafting procedures can be considered in the anterior region to fulfill the patient's esthetic demands.

Traditionally, root surfaces are cleaned with compounds such as citric acid or tetracycline hydrochloride preceding root coverage procedures to remove the smear layer, open the dentinal tubules, and decrease the microbial load and bacterial cytotoxic byproducts [7–9]. In the present clinical report, 24% EDTA gel (Straumann PrefGel; Straumann, Basel, Switzerland) was applied for 2 min before the connective tissue graft application. Ethylenediaminetetraacetic acid is an organic compound widely used in endodontics as an adjuvant irrigation agent due to its effectiveness in removing calcium by means of chelation [18]. Highly concentrated gel preparations of this compound are advantageous since their viscosity permits the selective treatment of the intended surfaces only, thus avoiding the highly concentrated formulation's unnecessary demineralization of other dental tissues and substances. Some studies have recommended the results obtained with EDTA gel. A clinical trial evaluating EDTA gel conditioning during periodontitis assessed the surface topography and periodontal ligament cell adhesion with and without the application of EDTA gel, and the results concluded that it provides the most desirable root surface to which maximum periodontal ligament cells can adhere and on which they can grow [32].

Ceramic restorations are a well-supported treatment that can improve the patient's self-esteem and social interactions [1,14]. Modern dental ceramics possess mechanical and chemical properties, making them excellent restorative materials. Feldspathic and glass-infiltrated ceramics can be bonded to the enamel using an adhesive hybrid layer [18] and have a modulus of elasticity similar to the enamel, making them a suitable "biomimetic" alternative to replace lost enamel [14]. In the present clinical report, the teeth were minimally prepared using the desired restorative contours established with a diagnostic wax-up as a reference. This step was critical to ensure that the tooth preparations preserved as much enamel as possible to guarantee adequate union between the restoration and the substrate, and to provide enough space to fabricate esthetic and structurally durable restorations.

Further studies with larger sample sizes and longer follow-up periods are needed to confirm the effectiveness of the connective tissue grafting technique in combination with EDTA gel for root surface cleaning. Additionally, it would be valuable to compare the outcomes of this technique with other periodontal procedures to determine the most effective and efficient treatment for gingival recession.

5. Conclusions

A case with high esthetic demands can be treated successfully by an interdisciplinary approach including connective tissue grafts, CAD/CAM veneers, and a combination of periodontal and restorative treatments.

Author Contributions: Conceptualization, G.G.-P. and C.A.J.; methodology, F.X.A.-F.; validation, K.I.A., H.N. and G.G.-P.; formal analysis, H.M.-L.; investigation, F.X.A.-F.; resources, C.A.J.; data curation, H.M.-L.; writing—original draft preparation, F.X.A.-F.; writing—review and editing, C.A.J. and K.I.A.; visualization, H.N.; supervision, G.G.-P.; project administration, H.N.; funding acquisition, H.N. All authors have read and agreed to the published version of the manuscript.

Funding: This research received no external funding.

Institutional Review Board Statement: The study was conducted in accordance with the Declaration of Helsinki for studies involving humans.

Informed Consent Statement: Written informed consent has been obtained from the patient to publish this paper.

Data Availability Statement: Not applicable.

Acknowledgments: We thank A.T. Still Research Institute and the Universität Bern for partially supporting the open-access publication of this work.

Conflicts of Interest: The authors declare no conflict of interest.

References

1. Afrashtehfar, K.I.; Bryant, S.R. Understanding the Lived Experience of North American Dental Patients with a Single-Tooth Implant in the Upper Front Region of the Mouth: Protocol for a Qualitative Study. *JMIR Res. Protoc.* **2021**, *10*, e25767. [CrossRef]
2. Jurado, C.A.; Parachuru, V.; Tinoco, J.V.; Guzman-Perez, G.; Tsujimoto, A.; Javvadi, R.; Afrashtehfar, K.I. Diagnostic Mock-Up as a Surgical Reduction Guide for Crown Lengthening: Technique Description and Case Report. *Medicina* **2022**, *58*, 1360. [CrossRef]
3. Roe, P.; Rungcharassaeng, K.; Kan, J.Y.; Patel, R.D.; Campagni, W.V.; Brudvik, J.S. The influence of upper lip length and lip mobility on maxillary incisal exposure. *Am. J. Esthet. Dent.* **2012**, *2*, 115–125.
4. Del Monte, S.; Afrashtehfar, K.I.; Emami, E.; Nader, S.A.; Tamimi, F. Lay preferences for dentogingival esthetic parameters: A systematic review. *J. Prosthet. Dent.* **2017**, *118*, 717–724. [CrossRef] [PubMed]
5. Alikhasi, M.; Yousefi, P.; Afrashtehfar, K.I. Smile Design. *Dent. Clin. N. Am.* **2022**, *66*, 477–487. [CrossRef] [PubMed]
6. Tinoco, J.V.; Jurado, C.A.; Sayed, M.E.; Cortes, J.O.G.; Kaleinikova, Z.; Hernandez, A.; Alshabib, A.; Tsujimoto, A. Conservative approach for management of fractured maxillary central incisors in young adults. *Clin. Case Rep.* **2020**, *8*, 2692–2700. [CrossRef] [PubMed]
7. Langer, B.; Langer, L. Subepithelial Connective Tissue Graft Technique for Root Coverage. *J. Periodontol.* **1985**, *56*, 715–720. [CrossRef]
8. Salama, H.; Salama, M.; Garber, D. The Tunnel Technique in the Periodontal Plastic Treatment of Multiple Adjacent Gingival Recession Defects: A Review. *Inside Dent.* **2008**, *4*, 79–81.
9. Afrashtehfar, K.I.; Jurado, C.A.; Wang, H.-L. For peri–implant soft tissue augmentation, soft tissue substitutes may improve patients' surgical and postoperative experience compared to autogenous grafts. *J. Évid. Based Dent. Pract.* **2023**, *23*, 101835. [CrossRef]
10. Hürzeler, M.B.; Weng, D. A single-incision technique to harvest subepithelial connective tissue grafts from the palate. *Int. J. Periodontics Restor. Dent.* **1999**, *19*, 279–287.
11. Monnet-Corti, V.; Santini, A.; Glise, J.-M.; Fouque-Deruelle, C.; Dillier, F.-L.; Liébart, M.-F.; Borghetti, A. Connective Tissue Graft for Gingival Recession Treatment: Assessment of the Maximum Graft Dimensions at the Palatal Vault as a Donor Site. *J. Periodontol.* **2006**, *77*, 899–902. [CrossRef] [PubMed]
12. Moore, R.L.; Hill, M. Suturing techniques for periodontal plastic surgery. *Periodontology* **2000**, *11*, 103–111. [CrossRef] [PubMed]
13. Park, J.-B. Clinical showcase. Treatment of gingival recession with subepithelial connective tissue harvested from the maxillary tuberosity by distal wedge procedure. *J. Can. Dent. Assoc.* **2009**, *75*, 643–646.
14. Chambrone, L.; Ortega, M.A.S.; Sukekava, F.; Rotundo, R.; Kalemaj, Z.; Buti, J.; Prato, G.P.P. Root coverage procedures for treating single and multiple recession-type defects: An updated Cochrane systematic review. *J. Periodontol.* **2019**, *90*, 1399–1422. [CrossRef] [PubMed]
15. Veneziani, M. Ceramic laminate veneers: Clinical procedures with a multidisciplinary approach. *Int. J. Esthet. Dent.* **2017**, *12*, 426–448.
16. Jurado, C.A.; AlResayes, S.; Sayed, M.E.; Villalobos-Tinoco, J.; Llanes-Urias, N.; Tsujimoto, A. A customized metal guide for controllable modification of anterior teeth contour prior to minimally invasive preparation. *Saudi Dent. J.* **2020**, *33*, 518–523. [CrossRef]
17. Anterior Veneer Restorations–An Evidence-based Minimal-Intervention Perspective. *J. Adhes. Dent.* **2021**, *23*, 91–110. [CrossRef]
18. Villalobos-Tinoco, J.; Fischer, N.G.; Jurado, C.A.; Sayed, M.E.; Feregrino-Mendez, M.; Garcia, O.D.L.M.; Tsujimoto, A. Combining a single implant and a veneer restoration in the esthetic zone. *Int. J. Esthet. Dent.* **2020**, *15*, 428–439.
19. Anusavice, K.J.; Shen, C.; Rawls, H.R. *Philips Science of Dental Materials*, 12th ed.; Elsevier: Amsterdam, The Netherlands, 2012.

20. Czigola, A.; Abram, E.; Kovacs, Z.I.; Márton, K.; Hermann, P.; Borbely, J. Effects of substrate, ceramic thickness, translucency, and cement shade on the color of CAD/CAM lithium-disilicate crowns. *J. Esthet. Restor. Dent.* **2019**, *31*, 457–464. [CrossRef]
21. Jurado, C.A.; Afrashtehfar, K.I.; Hyer, J.; Alhotan, A. Effect of sintering on the translucency of CAD–CAM lithium disilicate restorations: A comparative in vitro study. *J. Prosthodont.* **2023**, *7*, 1–6. [CrossRef]
22. Peumans, M.; van Meerbeek, B.; Yoshida, Y.; Lambrechts, P.; Vanherle, G. Porcelain veneers bonded to tooth structure: An ul-tra-morphological FE-SEM examination of the adhesive interface. *Dent. Mater.* **1999**, *15*, 105–119. [CrossRef] [PubMed]
23. Morita, R.K.; Hayashida, M.F.; Pupo, Y.M.; Berger, G.; Reggiani, R.D.; Betiol, E.A.G. Minimally Invasive Laminate Veneers: Clinical Aspects in Treatment Planning and Cementation Procedures. *Case Rep. Dent.* **2016**, *2016*, 1839793. [CrossRef] [PubMed]
24. Nanda, T.; Jain, S.; Kaur, H.; Kapoor, D.; Nanda, S.; Jain, R. Root conditioning in periodontology-Revisited. *J. Nat. Sci. Biol. Med.* **2014**, *5*, 356–358. [CrossRef]
25. Jurado, C.A.; Amarillas-Gastelum, C.; Afrashtehfar, K.I.; Argueta-Figueroa, L.; Fischer, N.G.; Alshabib, A. Ceramic and Composite Polishing Systems for Milled Lithium Disilicate Restorative Materials: A 2D and 3D Comparative In Vitro Study. *Materials* **2022**, *15*, 5402. [CrossRef]
26. Santos, G.C., Jr.; Boksman, L.L.; Santos, M.J. CAD/CAM technology and esthetic dentistry: A case report. *Compend. Contin. Educ. Dent.* **2013**, *34*, 764.
27. Jurado, C.A.; Villalobos-Tinoco, J.; Watanabe, H.; Sanchez-Hernandez, R.; Tsujimoto, A. Novel translucent monolithic zirconia fixed restorations in the esthetic zone. *Clin. Case Rep.* **2022**, *10*, e05699. [CrossRef]
28. Poticny, D.; Conrad, R. Predictable aesthetic replacement of a metal-ceramic crown using CAD/CAM technology: A case report. *Pract. Proced. Aesthetic Dent. PPAD* **2005**, *17*, 491–496. [PubMed]
29. Zucchelli, G.; De Sanctis, M. Treatment of Multiple Recession-Type Defects in Patients With Esthetic Demands. *J. Periodontol.* **2000**, *71*, 1506–1514. [CrossRef]
30. Zucchelli, G.; De Sanctis, M. Long-Term Outcome Following Treatment of Multiple Miller Class I and II Recession Defects in Esthetic Areas of the Mouth. *J. Periodontol.* **2005**, *76*, 2286–2292. [CrossRef]
31. Chambrone, L.; Tatakis, D.N. Periodontal Soft Tissue Root Coverage Procedures: A Systematic Review From the AAP Regeneration Workshop. *J. Periodontol.* **2015**, *86*, S8–S51. [CrossRef]
32. Gamal, A.Y.; Mailhot, J.M. The effects of EDTA gel conditioning exposure time on periodontitis-affected human root surfaces: Surface topography and PDL cell adhesion. *J. Int. Acad. Periodontol.* **2003**, *5*, 11–22. [PubMed]

Disclaimer/Publisher's Note: The statements, opinions and data contained in all publications are solely those of the individual author(s) and contributor(s) and not of MDPI and/or the editor(s). MDPI and/or the editor(s) disclaim responsibility for any injury to people or property resulting from any ideas, methods, instructions or products referred to in the content.

Article

Assessment and Correlation of Salivary Ca, Mg, and pH in Smokers and Non-Smokers with Generalized Chronic Periodontitis

Saad Mohammad Alqahtani [1,*], Shankar T. Gokhale [1], Mohamed Fadul A. Elagib [1], Deepti Shrivastava [2,*], Raghavendra Reddy Nagate [1], Badar Awadh Mohammad Alshmrani [1], Abduaziz Mohammed Abdullah Alburade [1], Fares Mufreh Abdullah Alqahtani [1], Anil Kumar Nagarajappa [3], Valentino Natoli [4,5] and Kumar Chandan Srivastava [3,6,*]

1. Department of Periodontics and Community Sciences (PCS), College of Dentistry, King Khalid University, Abha 62529, Saudi Arabia
2. Department of Preventive dentistry, College of Dentistry, Jouf University, Sakaka 72345, Saudi Arabia
3. Department of Oral Maxillofacial Surgery & Diagnostic Sciences, College of Dentistry, Jouf University, Sakaka 72345, Saudi Arabia
4. Department of Dentistry, School of Biomedical and Health Sciences, European University of Madrid, 28670 Madrid, Spain
5. Private Dental Practice, 72015 Fasano, Italy
6. Department of Oral Medicine and radiology, Saveetha Dental College, Saveetha Institute of Medical and Technical Sciences, Saveetha University, Chennai 602105, India
* Correspondence: s.alqahtani@kku.edu.sa (S.M.A.); sdeepti20@gmail.com (D.S.); drkcs.omr@gmail.com (K.C.S.)

Abstract: *Background and Objectives*: Diagnostic evaluation with the aid of biomarkers has reached newer heights to assess disease activity. Salivary calcium, magnesium, and pH are one of the biochemical parameters which can be helpful in assessing the progression of periodontal disease. Smokers are at topnotch threat for having oral diseases, predominantly periodontal diseases. The aim of this study was to assess the salivary calcium, magnesium, and pH levels in smokers compared with non-smokers with chronic periodontitis. *Materials and Methods*: The current study was conducted on 210 individuals affected with generalized chronic periodontitis, with the age group between 25 and 55 years. Based on their smoking habit, an equal number of patients were categorized into two groups; namely, group I consisted of non-smokers and group II consisted of smokers. The clinical parameters that were measured included Plaque Index (PI), Gingival Index (GI), Probing Pocket Depth (PPD), and Clinical Attachment Loss (CAL). The biochemical variables that were evaluated in the current study included salivary calcium, magnesium, and pH using an AVL9180 electrolyte analyzer (Roche, Germany). The gathered data were analyzed with an unpaired t test was using SPSS 20.0. *Results*: A statistically significant higher PPD ($p < 0.01$), CAL ($p < 0.05$), and salivary calcium levels ($p < 0.001$) were observed in the smokers' compared with their non-smoking counterparts. Among the biochemical parameters, calcium showed a significantly ($p < 0.001$) higher level in smokers (5.79 ± 1.76) in contrast to non-smokers (3.87 ± 1.03). Additionally, a significant negative correlation ($p < 0.05$) between calcium and PPD was observed in non-smokers, whereas a non-significant inverse relation ($p > 0.05$) was seen in smokers. *Conclusions*: The present study indicates that the salivary calcium level can be a potential biochemical parameter to assess the progression of periodontal disease in smokers and non-smokers. Within the limitations of the current study, the salivary biomarkers appear to have an essential role in the identification and indication of the status of periodontal diseases.

Keywords: periodontology; periodontitis; smokers; salivary calcium; probing pocket depth; salivary biomarkers; salivary magnesium; salivary pH; clinical dentistry

1. Introduction

The metabolic profiles of human biofluids have been used for a long time to evaluate and differentiate an individual's condition in terms of health or disease. Fluctuations have been observed in the volume and compositions of these fluids by virtue of a change in activity, drug usage, nutrition, or disease progression [1].

Oral cavities possess two prominent fluids including gingival crevicular fluid (GCF) and saliva. GCF, being in the closest proximity to gingival tissues, exhibits great potential in detecting periodontal disease and differentiating it from a healthy state [2]. Saliva has an indispensable role in various biological activities in the oral cavity and plays a pivotal role in its defense mechanism [3]. The whole saliva is a combination of fluids consisting of secretions from the major and minor salivary glands; gingival crevicular fluids; and oral mucosa transudate [4]. Thus, saliva is loaded with a variety of molecules and trace elements which make it a promising disease biomarker. Furthermore, it is easy to collect and store, as well as being easily resampled [5].

Ionomics is the study of the ionome, which is defined as a "mineral nutrient and trace element composition of an organism representing the inorganic component of the cellular and organ systems." In recent years, salivary ionomes have emerged as a promising biomarker and thus have been projected as a vital diagnostic means to observe oral and systemic diseases. As a medium for clinical diagnosis, salivary biomarkers have a number of benefits over serum, such as the non-invasive nature of sample collection and the cost-effective approach, especially when targeting a large population [6,7].

As the main constituent, water comprises 99% of saliva, whereas the remaining 1% is made up of organic and inorganic constituents. The predominant electrolytes present in saliva include calcium, magnesium, potassium, sodium chloride, bicarbonate, and phosphate [8]. Salivary calcium has a close affinity for plaque formation that eventually influences the calculus formation. Since plaque and calculus are considered the main culprit in the etiopathogenesis of periodontal disease [9], the presence of an increased amount of calcium in saliva is known to influence plaque formation and its maturation. It has been observed that periodontally healthy participants with no marginal alveolar bone loss have a lesser potential for plaque and calculus mineralization in contrast to the patients who have been previously treated for periodontitis [10–13]. Magnesium is a known physical antagonist to calcium; however, the exact functional reciprocation in periodontitis or other risk factors associated with periodontitis, such as smoking, have not been explored. Nevertheless, there are a few studies that have shown the association of magnesium with periodontitis [14], and calcium and magnesium with periodontitis [15,16].

According to various cross-sectional and longitudinal studies, smoking is a significant risk factor for the development of periodontal disease [17,18]. Epidemiological as well as clinical studies are in alignment with the detrimental effects of smoking on periodontal tissues and, eventually, in the progression of periodontal disease that manifests as alveolar bone loss, increased probing depth, and tooth loss [19]. Additionally, it has been observed that smokers have poor oral hygiene and increased supragingival calculus formation [20]. It is well-documented that smoking induces a significant increase in the salivary flow rate as a spontaneous reflex action, which may explain the observation of increased calculus in smokers [21]. According to other research, smoking improves the mineralizing potential of saliva thus facilitating calculus formation [18].

Several studies have reported that patients with reduced bone mineral density, heavy smokers, and women in their menopausal ages have greater salivary calcium levels than age-matched peers [8,22,23]. The normal range of salivary calcium is 0.5–2.7 mmol/L [24]. In smokers, a higher level of salivary calcium is produced, which is linked to more bone loss and, accordingly, lower bone mineral density compared with non-smokers [25,26]. Salivary pH is normally between 6.2 and 7.6, with 6.7 being the average [25]. However, the pH of the oral cavity does not dip below 6.3 during rest and it is kept near neutral (6.7–7.3) by saliva [27]. Since smokers have a higher oral pH than non-smokers, there is more room for this pH to remove calcium and deposit it on teeth, perhaps resulting in high amounts of salivary calcium [28].

There are a few studies that have stated the role of calcium, magnesium, and pH in the progression of periodontal disease [1,11,12,17]. However, there is a lack of data about the appraisal and evaluation of salivary calcium and magnesium levels in smokers and non-smokers with chronic periodontitis. Hence, the present study aims to evaluate the effect of salivary calcium and magnesium in addition to the pH levels in smoking and non-smoking chronic periodontitis patients.

2. Materials and Methods

2.1. Study Characteristics

A cross-sectional study was conducted at the College of Dentistry, King Khalid University, Abha, Saudi Arabia in the year 2019, after approval from the Institutional Ethical committee (SRC/ETH/2018-19/075). This study followed the protocol of the Declaration of Helsinki (1975) revised in 2002.

2.2. Sample Characteristics

A priori sample size calculation was performed using G* power software (Universität Düsseldorf: Psychologie—HHU) [29]. Considering t-test for comparing means of two independent study groups with equal allocation (Allocation ratio $N_2/N = 1$), an effect size (Cohen's d value) of 0.5, and a confidence interval (1-β error) of 95% and 0.05 α, a total sample of 210 was calculated. With this sample size, the power of the study was estimated to be 0.95.

Based on the inclusion and exclusion criteria, a total of 210 chronic generalized periodontitis patients were recruited from outpatient department. Later, based on smoking status, an equal number of patients (105) were divided into the two study groups, namely Group I, consisting of non-smokers, and Group II, of smokers. The patients who smoked at least one cigarette per day in the last year were considered active smokers and were included in the study group [14]. After explaining the purpose of the study, informed consent was obtained from all the patients participating in the study.

The patients included were in the age range from 25 to 55 years, with at least 20 permanent teeth. Patients who were clinically diagnosed with chronic periodontitis presented with an evident bone loss on radiographical assessment and with a Probing Pocket Depth (PPD) of ≥4 mm with a Clinical Attachment Loss (CAL) of ≥1 mm. Patients who gave a history of periodontal therapy in last 6 months and had taken antibiotic coverage in last 3 months were excluded. Along with this, the patients on medications who were affected with a chronic disease which has influence on periodontal parameters were excluded from the study. Patients having xerostomia, either due to systemic or local conditions, were also excluded, as this could influence the periodontal conditions.

2.3. Study Protocol and Clinical Parameters Measured in the Study

A pre-designed data extraction sheet was used to collect information regarding demographic data and details such as medical history and oral hygiene practices. The clinical parameters including Loe and Silness Gingival Index (GI) [30], Bleeding on probing (BOP), Probing Pocket Depth (PPD), and Clinical Attachment Loss (CAL) were used for the assessment of the clinical condition. To lessen the bias, the measurements of all clinical parameters were documented and taken by a single examiner, who was initially calibrated. The intra-examiner reliability of the examiner for all the coding was 0.88, which was of good agreement. Plaque Index was measured after giving erythrosine in the form of a chewing tablet. BOP and CAL were assessed using a specific periodontal probe (UNC-15, Hu-friedy, Chicago, IL, USA). PPD was recorded from the gingival margin to the gingival sulcus base, while CAL was recorded from cemento-enamel junction (CEJ) to the base of the gingival sulcus.

2.4. Collection of Salivary Sample and Its Laboratory Analysis

A saliva sample was obtained after clinical recordings. A 2 mL of unstimulated whole saliva was collected by the "spitting method" as described by Navazesh M. (1993) [31]. To correspond to the circadian rhythm, salivary samples were collected 2 h after the last meal, after rinsing with water for 5 min. Patient was instructed to spit the saliva gathered in the floor of the mouth into the collecting unit. To avoid time-related alteration in pH of saliva, it was collected immediately. The samples were then sent to the laboratory within 24 h, with temperatures maintained at 2 to 4 degrees Celsius. Salivary pH was measured using pH litmus test paper. AVL9180 electrolyte analyzer (Roche, Germany) was used for measuring calcium and magnesium ions.

2.5. Data Analysis

The data collected were analyzed using statistical package of social sciences (SPSS) 20.0 version (IBM; Chicago, IL, USA). The gathered data were initially checked for normality with Kolmogorov–Smirnov test and visualization methods including histogram and Q-Q plots. All the variables tested in the current study were found to be normally distributed ($p > 0.05$). Results were expressed as means and standard deviation. Based on the normality distribution of the data, parametric test–Unpaired t test was used to compare the clinical and biochemical parameters between the study groups. Correlation among the clinical and biochemical were analyzed using Pearson's and Spearman correlations for parametric and categorial type of variable, respectively.

3. Results

3.1. Sample Characteristics

There was no significant difference ($p > 0.05$) in the age and gender distribution between the groups, with smokers having a mean age of 42.1 ± 2.3 years and non-smokers having a mean age of 45.8 ± 3.4 years (Table 1).

Table 1. Sample Characteristics.

Variable	Categories	Study Group		p Value
		Group I (Non-Smoker) n = 105	Group II (Smoker) n = 105	
Age (Mean ± SD)		45.80 ± 3.46	42.08 ± 6.19	0.573
Gender [†]	Male	57 (54)	59 (56)	0.62
	Female	48 (46)	46 (44)	

Note: [†]—results expressed in Number (%); SD—Standard Deviation.

3.2. Comparative Analysis of Clinical Parameters between the Study Groups

There is a significantly higher PPD ($p < 0.05$) and CAL ($p < 0.01$) in the smoker group compared with the non-smoker patients. However, non-significant ($p > 0.05$) differences in PI and GI were observed in the study group when compared with the control group patients. (Table 2).

Table 2. Comparative analysis of clinical parameters among the study group.

Clinical Parameter	Group I	Group II	p Value
Plaque Index	1.71 ± 0.48	1.51 ± 0.34	0.109
Gingival Index	1.55 ± 0.38	1.67 ± 0.29	0.222
Periodontal Probing Depth	5.57 ± 1.02	6.16 ± 0.77	0.025 *
Clinical Attachment Level	5.08 ± 0.73	5.70 ± 0.67	0.003 **

Note: results expressed in Mean ± Standard Deviation; * $p < 0.05$; ** $p < 0.01$.

3.3. Comparative Analysis of Biochemical Parameters between the Study Groups

Among the biochemical parameters, significantly ($p < 0.001$) raised calcium levels (5.79 ± 1.76 mmol/L) were observed in smokers when compared with non-smokers (3.86 ± 1.03 mmol/L). However, magnesium did not show any difference between the groups. (Table 3)

Table 3. Comparative analysis of biochemical parameters among the study group.

Parameter	Group I	Group II	*p* Value
pH	6.44 ± 0.86	6.80 ± 0.91	0.160
Calcium	3.86 ± 1.03	5.79 ± 1.76	0.000 ***
Magnesium	0.54 ± 0.18	0.49 ± 0.24	0.413

Note: results expressed in Mean ± Standard Deviation; *** $p < 0.001$.

3.4. Correlational Analysis of Biochemical and Clinical Parameter in the Study Groups

Depending on the type of variable (parameteric Vs. non-parametric), Pearson and Spearman correlation analysis was carried out for all variables in both study groups.

The two crucial periodontal clinical indicators, namely PPD and CAL, showed a highly significant ($p < 0.001$) positive correlation in both study groups. Additionally, PPD and CAL were later analyzed with calcium and magnesium. Similarly, the gingival parameters, namely PI and GI, showed a significant ($p < 0.001$) positive correlation in Group I and a positive but non-significant ($p > 0.05$) correlation in Group II. These correlation results reaffirm the presentation of periodontal diseases.

Another key parameter, the pH of the saliva, showed a significant ($p < 0.05$) negative correlation with magnesium in Group I and a significant ($p < 0.05$) negative correlation with calcium in Group II.

The correlation analysis between salivary calcium and periodontal clinical parameters such as CAL and PPD was carried out in each study group. In the control group (Non-smoker), a significant ($p < 0.05$) negative correlation was found between calcium and PPD and CAL. However, a non-significant ($p > 0.05$) positive correlation was seen between the parameters in the study group (Tables 4 and 5) (Figures 1 and 2).

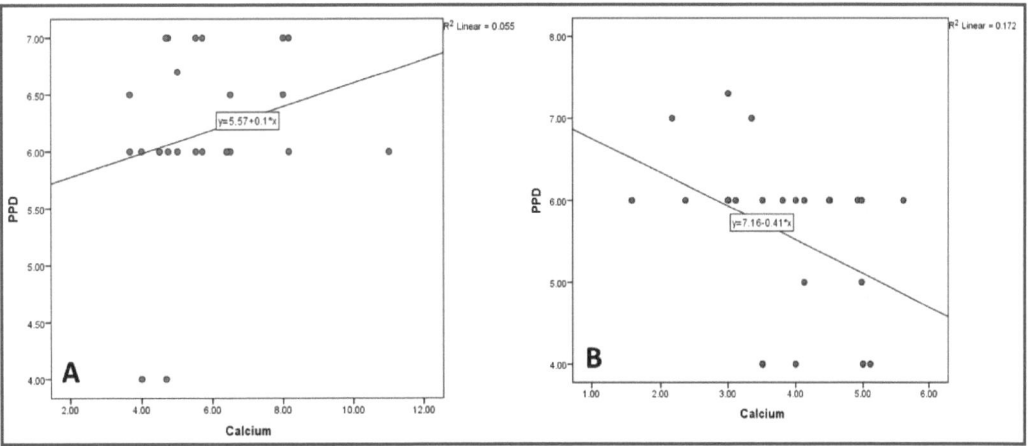

Figure 1. Correlational analysis of Calcium with Periodontal Probing Depth in (**A**) Smokers and (**B**) Non-Smokers.

Table 4. Correlation analysis of parameters in Group I.

	Ca	Mg	pH	PI	GI	PPD	CAL	Age	Gender [¶]
Ca	-	0.985 (0.004)	0.243 (0.237)	0.978 (−0.006)	0.994 (0.002)	0.039 * (−0.415)	0.043 * (−0.407)	0.415 (−0.171)	0.490 (−0.145)
Mg	0.985 (0.004)	-	0.037 * (−0.419)	0.306 (0.213)	0.671 (0.089)	0.855 (−0.038)	0.789 (−0.056)	0.176 (0.280)	0.853 (−0.039)
pH	0.243 (0.237)	0.037 * (−0.419)	-	0.105 (0.332)	0.068 (0.371)	0.423 (0.168)	0.370 (0.187)	0.616 (0.105)	0.688 (0.084)
PI	0.978 (−0.006)	0.306 (0.213)	0.105 (0.332)	-	0.000 *** (0.783)	0.521 (0.135)	0.570 (0.119)	0.677 (0.088)	0.739 (0.070)
GI	0.994 (0.002)	0.671 (0.089)	0.068 (0.371)	0.000 *** (0.783)	-	0.902 (0.026)	0.865 (−0.036)	0.064 (0.376)	0.711 (0.078)
PPD	0.039 * (−0.415)	0.855 (−0.038)	0.423 (0.168)	0.521 (0.135)	0.902 (0.026)	-	0.000 *** (0.937)	0.834 (0.044)	0.725 (0.074)
CAL	0.043 * (−0.407)	0.789 (−0.056)	0.370 (0.187)	0.570 (0.119)	0.865 (−0.036)	0.000 *** (0.937)	-	0.791 (−0.056)	0.669 (0.090)
Age	0.415 (−0.171)	0.176 (0.280)	0.616 (0.105)	0.677 (0.088)	0.064 (0.376)	0.834 (0.044)	0.791 (−0.056)	-	0.811 (0.050)
Gender	0.490 (−0.145)	0.853 (−0.039)	0.688 (0.084)	0.739 (0.070)	0.711 (0.078)	0.725 (0.074)	0.669 (0.090)	0.811 (0.050)	-

Note: results are expressed as p value (correlation coefficient); * $p < 0.05$; *** $p < 0.001$; [¶]—Spearman Correlation; Ca—Calcium; Mg—Magnesium; PI—Plaque Index; GI—Gingival Index; PPD—Probing Pocket Depth; CAL—Clinical Attachment Loss.

Table 5. Correlation analysis of parameters in Group II.

	Ca	Mg	pH	PI	GI	PPD	CAL	Age	Gender [¶]
Ca	-	0.614 (−0.106)	0.003 ** (−0.572)	0.403 (0.175)	0.343 (0.198)	0.260 (0.234)	0.385 (0.182)	0.058 (0.385)	0.692 (0.083)
Mg	0.614 (−0.106)	-	0.488 (−0.145)	0.580 (0.116)	0.426 (−0.167)	0.667 (−0.090)	0.693 (−0.083)	0.473 (0.151)	0.145 (0.300)
pH	0.003 ** (−0.572)	0.488 (−0.145)	-	0.089 (0.347)	0.201 (0.265)	0.850 (−0.040)	0.976 (−0.006)	0.772 (−0.061)	0.286 (−0.222)
PI	0.403 (0.175)	0.580 (0.116)	0.089 (0.347)	-	0.068 (0.371)	0.444 (0.160)	0.327 (0.204)	0.270 (0.229)	0.453 (0.157)
GI	0.343 (0.198)	0.426 (−0.167)	0.201 (0.265)	0.068 (0.371)	-	0.632 (0.101)	0.492 (0.144)	0.033 * (0.427)	0.689 (0.084)
PPD	0.260 (0.234)	0.667 (−0.090)	0.850 (−0.040)	0.444 (0.160)	0.632 (0.101)	-	0.000 *** (0.963)	0.386 (0.181)	0.098 (−0.338)
CAL	0.385 (0.182)	0.693 (−0.083)	0.976 (−0.006)	0.327 (0.204)	0.492 (0.144)	0.000 *** (0.963)	-	0.388 (0.180)	0.054 (−0.390)
Age	0.058 (0.385)	0.473 (0.151)	0.772 (−0.061)	0.270 (0.229)	0.033 * (0.427)	0.386 (0.181)	0.388 (0.180)	-	0.222 (0.253)
Gender [¶]	0.692 (0.083)	0.145 (0.300)	0.286 (−0.222)	0.453 (0.157)	0.689 (0.084)	0.098 (−0.338)	0.054 (−0.390)	0.222 (0.253)	-

Note: results are expressed as p value (correlation coefficient); [¶]—Spearman Correlation; * $p < 0.05$; ** $p < 0.01$; *** $p < 0.001$; Ca—Calcium; Mg—Magnesium; PI—Plaque Index; GI—Gingival Index; PPD—Probing Pocket Depth; CAL—Clinical Attachment Loss.

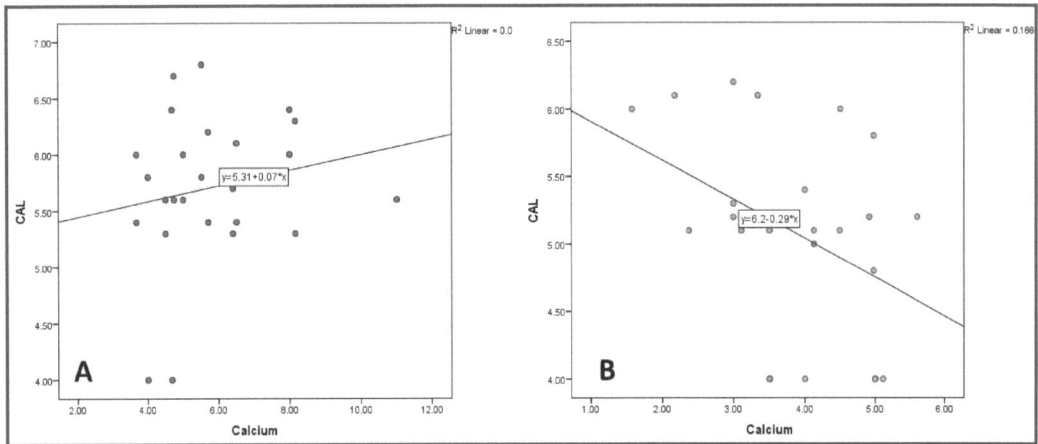

Figure 2. Correlational analysis of Calcium with Clinical Attachment Loss in (**A**) Smokers and (**B**) Non-Smokers.

4. Discussion

With the advancement of research, the metabolites profiling of a biological system has been commonly utilized to provide insight into the normal and disconcert metabolic processes [32]. Salivary metabolites can act as a biomarker to understand the complex biochemical interaction of host and bacteria in periodontal diseases [33–35]. It has been proven with various studies that tobacco smoke can alter the biochemical composition, and subsequently the function, of saliva [36,37].

Salivary Ca and Mg can be considered imperative in periodontal health concerning their influence on plaque mineralization. Magnesium may play an important role in preventing periodontal disease as it has a unique ability to reduce inflammation caused by bacterial toxins [18]. A group of studies reported that reduced magnesium concentrations are associated with an enhanced inflammatory response to bacterial challenges, thus promoting periodontitis [15,38]. Conversely, Manea et al. reported that salivary Mg concentrations were significantly higher in the periodontitis group compared with the controls. In another study, it was observed that salivary Mg concentrations were higher in smokers with periodontitis than in non-smokers who were also affected by periodontitis [38]. Although in the present study reduced Mg levels were reported in the smoker group compared with the non-smokers, the difference was non-significant. Similarly, Mg levels showed a non-significant negative correlation with PPD and CAL in both groups. A similar correlation was reported between Mg and periodontal parameters in the study conducted by Erdemir EO et al. [39].

Smokers have been classified as light smokers who smoke one–ten cigarettes a day; moderate smokers who smoke eleven–twenty cigarettes a day; and heavy smokers who smoke more than twenty cigarettes a day [14,40]. Smoking is thought to increase salivary Ca levels independently by reducing skeletal bone density [40]. The literature highlights the increased Ca levels in periodontitis patients [31,35]. However, it is important to note that dietary calcium intake and overall calcium turnover can influence salivary calcium levels [41]. In addition, the continuous exposure of taste receptors to tobacco products such as nicotine probably affects salivary flow rate [42], salivary reflex, and also salivary Ca levels [8]. Smokers have fairly eminent levels of salivary calcium, which is allied with a greater degree of bone loss and lower bone mineral density than non-smokers. The present study showed significantly elevated Ca levels in smokers when compared with non-smokers. A study by Megha Varghese et al. and Kolte et al. reported analogous findings in a sample of periodontitis patients, with salivary calcium ranging higher in the smoker group than in non-smokers [43,44]. Gupta VV et al. also observed concordant findings in their study, wherein calcium level was increased in smokers diagnosed with aggressive periodontitis [45]. This was contradictory to the study of Ivana Sutej et al. and Shashikanth et al. who found no difference in calcium levels between smokers and non-smokers [28,46]. A study conducted by Zuabi et al. observed a reduction in calcium levels post treatment of periodonitis patients [47]. A higher calcium level was observed in the stimulated saliva of smokers in studies conducted by Sevon et al. [48] and Mc Gregor et al. [25]. According to sevon et al., the decreased bone mineral density, a side effect of smoking, could be a reason for high salivary calcium [48].

The normal salivary pH ranges from 6.2 to 7.6. The buffering capacities of saliva and salivary flow both have an impact on salivary pH [37]. It was observed in one of the studies that salivary pH was lower in periodontitis patients compared with healthy controls. There was no significant difference in pH readings amongst the groups, although it was more acidic in the smokers' group [27]. Similar findings were observed in a study conducted by Kumar et al. which found a lower pH in smokers with periodontitis [49]. In contrast, the study of Gupta VV et al. showed a significant increase in pH levels in smokers against healthy controls [45] which could be due to the different technique adopted for the collection of saliva. However, the present study did not establish any significant difference in pH between the groups. The current study utilized the unstimulated saliva collection procedure as it bathes the oral cavity predominantly and moistens the oral cavity round the clock. Furthermore, it also represents the pooled sub-gingival plaque sample [50]; whereas, in other studies, stimulated saliva was collected [45]. Additionally, in a study conducted to evaluate the pH of smokers with traditional smoking and e-cigarette smoking and non-smokers, it was found that the traditional smokers and e-cigarette smokers had a lower pH than non-smokers [37].

On comparing the clinical parameters, such as PPD and CAL, smokers had more PPD and CAL compared with non-smokers with periodontitis. A similar observation was noticed by Haffajee AD et al. [51], Shashikanth H et al. [46], and Velidandla S et al. [52]. On comparing the Plaque Index, no difference was found between the groups. A similar observation was noticed in a study conducted by Sreedevi et al. [53]. When the Gingival Index was compared between the groups, no statistically significant difference was found. A similar finding was reported in other studies [54]. However, this result is contradictory to another study conducted by Zuabi et al. [47]. In a study conducted by Erdemir et al., they found that, in smokers, there was a positive correlation between the levels of Ca, Mg, and CAL. Whereas, in the non-smoker group, there was a negative correlation between the mean level of sodium and the Plaque Index ($p < 0.05$) [39]. In our study, we found that, in the non-smokers, there was a significant negative correlation between calcium and PPD and CAL. However, a non-significant ($p > 0.05$) positive correlation was seen between the parameters in the smokers' group. The difference in the study could be because of the assessment method as in the previous study inductively coupled plasma–atomic emission spectrophotometry was used. However, in the present study, an AVL9180 electrolyte analyzer was used for assessment.

Limitations and Future Directions

Within the limitations of this study, confounding factors such as the presence of calcium in the diet and differences in age were not addressed in this study. Therefore, longitudinal studies are recommended for establishing the causal relationship between the parameters. This will also aid the scientific society in winding up the judgment against the role of saliva in the initiation and progression of periodontal disease.

5. Conclusions

Among all the constituents of saliva, salivary calcium is one of the most extensively studied potential markers for the identification of periodontal diseases. The present study draws attention towards the specific risk factors that could influence the pathogenesis of periodontal disease, amid which smoking is a prompt factor. Smoking also serves as an indirect biomarker for periodontal lesion predilection. The results of the current study indicate that smokers have significantly higher PPD, CAL, and calcium than their non-smoking counterparts. Importantly, salivary calcium was found to be elevated in smokers with chronic generalized periodontitis, thus the attempts to signify that calcium levels in saliva act as both a risk factor and imminent biochemical marker for the assessment of periodontal lesions.

Author Contributions: Conceptualization, S.M.A., S.T.G., M.F.A.E. and R.R.N.; methodology, S.M.A., S.T.G., M.F.A.E., R.R.N. and B.A.M.A.; software, B.A.M.A., A.M.A.A., F.M.A.A. and D.S.; validation, B.A.M.A., A.M.A.A., F.M.A.A. and D.S.; formal analysis, D.S. and K.C.S.; investigation, S.M.A., S.T.G., M.F.A.E., R.R.N. and B.A.M.A.; data curation, K.C.S., V.N. and A.K.N.; writing—original draft preparation, S.M.A., S.T.G., D.S. and K.C.S.; writing—review and editing, S.M.A., S.T.G., M.F.A.E., R.R.N., B.A.M.A., A.M.A.A., F.M.A.A., D.S.; A.K.N., V.N. and K.C.S.; visualization, R.R.N., B.A.M.A., A.M.A.A. and F.M.A.A.; supervision, S.M.A.; project administration, S.M.A., K.C.S. and A.K.N.; funding acquisition, B.A.M.A., A.M.A.A., F.M.A.A., A.K.N., V.N. and K.C.S. All authors have read and agreed to the published version of the manuscript.

Funding: This research received no external funding.

Institutional Review Board Statement: This study was conducted in accordance with the Declaration of Helsinki and approved by the Institutional Review Board of King Khalid University, College of Dentistry (SRC/ ETH/2018-19/075). Date of access: 19/3/2019.

Informed Consent Statement: Informed consent was obtained from all subjects involved in the study.

Data Availability Statement: The data are available on a reasonable request from the corresponding author.

Acknowledgments: The authors extend their appreciation to the Deanship of Scientific Research at King Khalid University for funding this work through Small Groups Project under grant number RGP.1/351/43.

Conflicts of Interest: The authors declare no conflict of interest.

References

1. Velsko, I.M.; Overmyer, K.A.; Speller, C.; Klaus, L.; Collins, M.J.; Loe, L.; Frantz, L.A.; Sankaranarayanan, K.; Lewis, C.M.; Martinez, J.B.; et al. The dental calculus metabolome in modern and historic samples. *Metabolomics* **2017**, *13*, 134. [CrossRef] [PubMed]
2. Bibi, T.; Khurshid, Z.; Rehman, A.; Imran, E.; Srivastava, K.; Shrivastava, D. Gingival Crevicular Fluid (GCF): A Diagnostic Tool for the Detection of Periodontal Health and Diseases. *Molecules* **2021**, *26*, 1208. [CrossRef] [PubMed]
3. Dawes, C.; Pedersen, A.L.; Villa, A.; Ekström, J.; Proctor, G.B.; Vissink, A.; Aframian, D.; McGowan, R.; Aliko, A.; Narayana, N.; et al. The functions of human saliva: A review sponsored by the World Workshop on Oral Medicine VI. *Arch. Oral. Biol.* **2015**, *60*, 863–874. [CrossRef] [PubMed]
4. Castagnola, M.P.M.P.; Picciotti, P.M.; Messana, I.; Fanali, C.; Fiorita, A.; Cabras, T.; Calo, L.; Pisano, E.; Passali, G.C.; Iavarone, F.; et al. Potential application of human saliva as diagnostic fluid. *Acta Otorhinolaryngol. Ital.* **2011**, *31*, 347–357. [PubMed]
5. Dame, Z.T.; Aziat, F.; Mandal, R.; Krishnamurthy, R.; Bouatra, S.; Borzouie, S.; Guo, A.C.; Sajed, T.; Deng, L.; Lin, H.; et al. The human saliva metabolome. *Metabolomics* **2015**, *11*, 1864–1883. [CrossRef]
6. Sonalee, S.; Manpreet, K. A study of analytical indicators of saliva. *Ann. Essences Dent.* **2012**, *4*, 9–18.
7. Al Kawas, S.; Rahim, Z.H.; Ferguson, D.B. Potential uses of human salivary protein and peptide analysis in the diagnosis of disease. *Arch. Oral. Biol.* **2012**, *57*, 1–9. [CrossRef]
8. Tjahajawati, S.; Rafisa, A.; Lestari, E.A. The Effect of Smoking on Salivary Calcium Levels, Calcium Intake, and Bleeding on Probing in Female. *Int. J. Dent.* **2021**, *2021*, 2221112. [CrossRef]
9. Shrivastava, D.; Srivastava, K.C.; Ganji, K.K.; Alam, M.K.; Al Zoubi, I.; Sghaireen, M.G. Quantitative Assessment of Gingival Inflammation in Patients Undergoing Nonsurgical Periodontal Therapy Using Photometric CIELab Analysis. *BioMed Res. Int.* **2021**, *2021*, 6615603. [CrossRef]
10. Giannobile, W.V.; Beikler, T.; Kinney, J.S.; Ramseier, C.A.; Morelli, T.; Wong, D.T. Saliva as a diagnostic tool for periodontal disease: Current state and future directions. *Periodontol. 2000* **2009**, *50*, 2–64. [CrossRef]
11. Acharya, A.; Kharadi, M.D.; Dhavale, R.; Deshmukh, V.L.; Sontakke, A.N. High salivary calcium level associated with periodontal disease in Indian subjects—A pilot study. *Oral. Health Prev. Dent.* **2011**, *9*, 195–200. [PubMed]

12. Sudhir, S. Quantitative evaluation of salivary calcium, phosphorous, protein and Ph in health and diseased periodontium. *Ann. Essences Dent.* **2010**, *2*, 21–24. [CrossRef]
13. Shrivastava, D.; Srivastava, K.C.; Dayakara, J.K.; Sghaireen, M.G.; Gudipaneni, R.K.; Al-Johani, K.; Baig, M.N.; Khurshid, Z. BactericidalActivity of Crevicular Polymorphonuclear Neutrophils in Chronic Periodontitis Patients and Healthy Subjects under the Influence of Areca Nut Extract: An In Vitro Study. *Appl. Sci.* **2020**, *10*, 5008. [CrossRef]
14. Wijaya, T.K.; Susanto, A.; Hendiani, I. Comparison of gingival health status and salivary magnesium levels in smokers and nonsmokers. *Sci. Dent. J.* **2021**, *5*, 79.
15. Rajesh, K.S.; Zareena, S.H.; Kumar, M.A. Assessment of salivary calcium, phosphate, magnesium, pH, and flow rate in healthy subjects, periodontitis, and dental caries. *Contemp. Clin. Dent.* **2015**, *6*, 461.
16. Patel, R.M.; Varma, S.; SuRaGiMath, G.; ZoPe, S. Estimation and comparison of salivary calcium, phosphorous, alkaline phosphatase and pH levels in periodontal health and disease: A cross-sectional biochemical study. *J. Clin. Diagn. Res. JCDR* **2016**, *10*, ZC58. [CrossRef]
17. Sewón, L.; Söderling, E.; Karjalainen, S. Comparative study on mineralization related intraoral parameters in periodontitis affected and periodontitis-free adults. *Scand. J. Dent. Res.* **1990**, *98*, 305–312. [CrossRef]
18. Calsina, G.; Ramón, J.M.; Echeverría, J.J. Effects of smoking on periodontal tissues. *J. Clin. Periodontol.* **2002**, *29*, 771–776. [CrossRef]
19. Nociti, F.H., Jr.; Casati, M.Z.; Duarte, P.M. Current perspective of the impact of smoking on the progression and treatment of periodontitis. *Periodontol. 2000* **2015**, *67*, 187–210. [CrossRef]
20. Bergstrom, J. Tobacco smoking and supragingival dental calculus. *J. Clin. Periodontol.* **1999**, *26*, 541–547. [CrossRef]
21. Petrovic, M.; Kesic, L.; Obradovic, R.; Savic, Z.; Mihailovic, D.; Obradovic, I.; Avdic-Saracevic, M.; Janjic-Trickovic, O.; Janjic, M. Comparative analysis of smoking influence on periodontal tissue in subjects with periodontal disease. *Mater. Sociomed.* **2013**, *25*, 196–198. [CrossRef] [PubMed]
22. Wasti, A.; Wasti, J.; Singh, R. Estimation of salivary calcium level as a screening tool for the osteoporosis in the post-menopausal women: A prospective study. *Indian J. Dent. Res.* **2020**, *31*, 252. [PubMed]
23. Saha, M.K.; Agrawal, P.; Saha, S.G.; Vishwanathan, V.; Pathak, V.; Saiprasad, S.V.; Dhariwal, P.; Dave, M. Evaluation of correlation between salivary calcium, alkaline phosphatase and osteoporosis-a prospective, comparative and observational study. *J. Clin. Diagn. Res. JCDR* **2017**, *11*, ZC63. [PubMed]
24. Rockenbach, M.I.; Marinho, S.A.; Veeck, E.B.; Lindemann, L.; Shinkai, R.S. Salivary flow rate, pH, and concentrations of calcium, phosphate, and sIgA in Brazilian pregnant and non-pregnant women. *Head Face Med.* **2006**, *2*, 44. [CrossRef]
25. MacGregor, I.D.M.; Edgar, W.M. Calcium and phosphate concentrations and precipitate formation in whole saliva from smokers and non-smokers. *J. Periodontal Res.* **1986**, *21*, 429–433. [CrossRef]
26. Sevon, L.A.; Laine, M.A. Effect of age on flow rate, protein and electrolyte composition of stimulated whole saliva in healthy, non-smoking women. *Open Dent. J.* **2008**, *2*, 89–92. [CrossRef]
27. Baliga, S.; Muglikar, S.; Kale, R. Salivary pH: A diagnostic biomarker. *J. Indian Soc. Periodontol.* **2013**, *17*, 461–465. [CrossRef]
28. Ivana, S.; Kristina, P.; Anica, B.; Krunoslav, C.; Kresimir, B.; Kata, R.G. Salivary calcium concentration and periodontal health of young adults in relation to tobacco smoking. *Oral. Health Prev. Dent.* **2012**, *10*, 397–403.
29. Faul, F.; Erdfelder, E.; Lang, A.-G.; Buchner, A. G*Power 3: A flexible statistical power analysis program for the social, behavioral, and biomedical sciences. *Behav. Res. Methods* **2007**, *39*, 175–191. [CrossRef]
30. Loe, H. The Gingival Index, the Plaque Index and Retention Index systems. *J. Periodontol.* **1967**, *38*, 610–616. [CrossRef]
31. Navazesh, M. Methods for collecting saliva. *Ann. N. Y Acad. Sci.* **1993**, *694*, 72–77. [CrossRef] [PubMed]
32. Clarke, C.J.; Haselden, J.N. Metabolic profiling as a tool for understanding mechanisms of toxicity. *Toxicol Pathol.* **2008**, *36*, 140–147. [CrossRef]
33. Kuboniwa, M.; Sakanaka, A.; Hashino, E.; Bamba, T.; Fukusaki, E.; Amano, A. Prediction of periodontal inflammation via metabolic profiling of saliva. *J Dent Res.* **2016**, *95*, 1381–1386. [CrossRef] [PubMed]
34. Gardner, A.; Carpenter, G.; So, P.W. Salivary metabolomics: From diagnostic biomarker discovery to investigating biological function. *Metabolites* **2020**, *10*, 47. [CrossRef]
35. Liebsch, C.; Pitchika, V.; Pink, C.; Samietz, S.; Kastenmüller, G.; Artati, A.; Suhre, K.; Adamski, J.; Nauck, M.; Völzke, H.; et al. The saliva metabolome in association to oral health status. *J. Dent. Res.* **2019**, *98*, 642–651. [CrossRef] [PubMed]
36. Macgregor, I.D. Smoking, saliva and salivation. *J. Dent.* **1988**, *16*, 14–17. [CrossRef]
37. Cichońska, D.; Kusiak, A.; Kochańska, B.; Ochocińska, J.; Świetlik, D. Influence of Electronic Cigarettes on Selected Physicochemical Properties of Saliva. *Int. J. Environ. Res. Public. Health* **2022**, *19*, 3314. [CrossRef]
38. Manea, A.; Nechifor, M. Research on plasma and saliva levels of some bivalent cations in patients with chronic periodontitis (salivary cations in chronic periodontitis). *Rev. Med. Chir. Soc. Med. Nat. Iasi* **2014**, *118*, 439–449.
39. Erdemir, E.O.; Erdemir, A. The detection of salivary minerals in smokers and non-smokers with chronic periodontitis by the inductively coupled plasma-atomic emission spectrophotometry technique. *J. Periodontol.* **2006**, *77*, 990–995. [CrossRef]
40. Sewon, L.A.; Karjalainen, S.M.; Sainio, M.; Seppä, O. Calcium and other salivary factors in periodontitis-affected subjects prior to treatment. *J. Clin. Periodontol* **1995**, *22*, 267–270. [CrossRef]
41. Najeeb, S.; Zafar, M.S.; Khurshid, Z.; Zohaib, S.; Almas, K. The Role of Nutrition in Periodontal Health: An Update. *Nutrients* **2016**, *8*, 530. [CrossRef]

42. Sewon, L.A.; Karjalainen, S.M.; Söderling, E.; Lapinlaimu, H.; Simell, O. Association between salivary calcium and oral health. *J. Clin. Periodontol.* **1998**, *25*, 915–919. [CrossRef] [PubMed]
43. Varghese, M.; Hegde, S.; Kashyap, R.; Maiya, A.K. Quantitative assessment of calcium profile in whole saliva from smokers and non-smokers with chronic periodontitis. *J. Clin. Diagn. Res.* **2015**, *9*, ZC54–ZC57. [CrossRef] [PubMed]
44. Kolte, A.P.; Kolte, R.A.; Laddha, R.K. Effect of smoking on salivary composition and periodontal status. *J. Indian Soc. Periodontol.* **2012**, *16*, 350–353. [CrossRef] [PubMed]
45. Gupta, V.V.; Chitkara, N.; Gupta, H.V.; Singh, A.; Gambhir, R.S.; Kaur, H. Comparison ofsalivary calcium level and ph in patients with aggressive periodontitis and healthy individuals: A clinico-biochemical study. *Oral. Health Dent. Manag.* **2016**, *15*, 122–126.
46. Shashikanth, H.; Raghavendra, U.; Naveena, N.; Rajesh, K.S. Assessment of Salivary Composition in Smokers and Non Smokers with Chronic Periodontitis. *J. Dent. Med. Sci.* **2016**, *15*, 84–88.
47. Zuabi, O.; Machtei, E.E.; Ben-Aryeh, H.; Ardekian, L.; Peled, M.; Laufer, D. The effect of smoking and periodontal treatment on salivary composition in patients with established periodontitis. *J. Periodontol.* **1999**, *70*, 1240–1246. [CrossRef]
48. Sewon, L.; Laine, M.; Karjalanien, S.; Dorpguinskania, A.; Lentonen-Veromaa, M. Salivary calcium concentration reflects skeletalosteoporotic changes in heavy smokers. *Arch. Oral. Biol.* **2004**, *49*, 335–358. [CrossRef]
49. Kumar, C.N.; Rao, S.M.; Jethlia, A.; Linganna, C.S.; Bhargava, M.; Palve, D.H. Assessment of salivary thiocyanate levels and pHin the saliva of smokers and nonsmokers with chronic periodontitis—A comparative study. *Indian J. Dent. Res.* **2021**, *32*, 74–78.
50. Rane, M.V.; Suragimath, G.; Varma, S.; Zope, S.A.; Ashwinirani, S.R. Estimation and comparison of salivary calcium levels in healthy controls and patients with generalized gingivitis and chronic periodontitis. *J. Oral. Res. Rev.* **2017**, *9*, 12.
51. Haffajee, A.D.; Socransky, S.S. Relationship of smoking to attachment level profiles. *J. Clin. Periodontol.* **2001**, *28*, 283–295. [CrossRef]
52. Velidandla, S.; Bodduru, R.; Birra, V.; Jain, Y.; Valluri, R.; Ealla, K.K. Distribution of periodontal pockets among smokers and Nonsmokers in patients with chronic periodontitis: A cross-sectional study. *Cureus J. Med. Sci.* **2019**, *11*, e5586. [CrossRef] [PubMed]
53. Sreedevi, M.; Ramesh, A.; Dwarakanath, C. Periodontal status in smokers and nonsmokers: A clinical, microbiological, and histopathological study. *Int. J. Dent.* **2012**, *2012*, 571590. [CrossRef] [PubMed]
54. Haber, J.; Wattles, J.; Crowley, M.; Mandell, R. Evidence for cigarette smoking as a major risk factor for periodontitis. *J. Periodontol.* **1993**, *64*, 16–23. [CrossRef] [PubMed]

Disclaimer/Publisher's Note: The statements, opinions and data contained in all publications are solely those of the individual author(s) and contributor(s) and not of MDPI and/or the editor(s). MDPI and/or the editor(s) disclaim responsibility for any injury to people or property resulting from any ideas, methods, instructions or products referred to in the content.

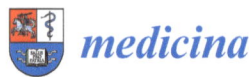 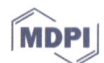

Systematic Review

Gaucher: A Systematic Review on Oral and Radiological Aspects

Giuseppe Minervini [1,*], Rocco Franco [2], Maria Maddalena Marrapodi [3,*], Vini Mehta [4], Luca Fiorillo [5,*], Almir Badnjević [6], Gabriele Cervino [5] and Marco Cicciù [7]

1. Multidisciplinary Department of Medical-Surgical and Odontostomatological Specialties, University of Campania "Luigi Vanvitelli", 80121 Naples, Italy
2. Department of Biomedicine and Prevention, University of Rome "Tor Vergata", 00100 Rome, Italy
3. Department of Woman, Child and General and Specialist Surgery, University of Campania "Luigi Vanvitelli", 80100 Naples, Italy
4. Department of Public health Dentistry, Dr. D. Y. Patil Dental College and Hospital, Dr. D. Y. Patil Vidhyapeeth University, Pune 411014, India
5. Department of Biomedical and Dental Sciences and Morphofunctional Imaging, School of Dentistry, University of Messina, 98125 Messina, Italy
6. Verlab Research Institute for Biomedical Engineering, Medical Devices and Artificial Intelligence, 71000 Sarajevo, Bosnia and Herzegovina
7. Department of General Surgery and Medical-Surgical Specialties, School of Dentistry, University of Catania, 95131 Catania, Italy

* Correspondence: giuseppe.minervini@unicampania.it (G.M.); mariamaddalena.marrapodi@studenti.unicampania.it (M.M.M.); lfiorillo@unime.it (L.F.)

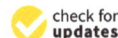

Citation: Minervini, G.; Franco, R.; Marrapodi, M.M.; Mehta, V.; Fiorillo, L.; Badnjević, A.; Cervino, G.; Cicciù, M. Gaucher: A Systematic Review on Oral and Radiological Aspects. *Medicina* 2023, 59, 670. https://doi.org/10.3390/medicina59040670

Academic Editor: Vita Maciulskiene

Received: 7 March 2023
Revised: 16 March 2023
Accepted: 23 March 2023
Published: 28 March 2023

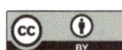

Copyright: © 2023 by the authors. Licensee MDPI, Basel, Switzerland. This article is an open access article distributed under the terms and conditions of the Creative Commons Attribution (CC BY) license (https://creativecommons.org/licenses/by/4.0/).

Abstract: *Background and Objectives*: Gaucher disease (GD) is a lysosomal storage disorder with the genetic autosomal recessive transmission. Bone involvement is a prevalent finding in Gaucher disease. It causes deformity and limits daily activities and the quality of life. In 75% of patients, there is bone involvement. This review aims to evaluate the principal findings in the jaw by a Cone-beam computed tomography (CBTC) and X-ray orthopantomography; *Materials and Methods*: PubMed, Web of Science, Lilacs and Scopus were systematically searched until 31 December 2022. In addition, a manual search was performed using the bibliography of selected articles and a Google Scholar search. Clinical studies were selected that considered principal radiographic findings in radiography in a group of patients affected by GD. *Results*: Out of 5079 papers, four studies were included. The main findings are generalized rarefaction and enlarged narrow space, anodontia. *Conclusions*: The exact mechanism of bone manifestation is probably due to the infiltration of Gaucher cells in the bone marrow and, consequently, the destruction of bone architecture. All long bones are a potential means of skeletal manifestation. The jaw is more affected than the maxilla, and the principal features are cortical thinning, osteosclerosis, pseudocystic lesions, mental demineralization, flattening in the head of the condyle, effacement of anatomical structures, thickening of maxillary sinus mucosa. The dentist plays a crucial role in diagnosing and treating these patients. Sometimes the diagnosis can be made by a simple panoramic radiograph. All long bones are affected, and the mandible is particularly involved.

Keywords: Gaucher disease; bone; oral health; congenital disorders

1. Introduction

Gaucher disease (GD) is a lysosomal storage disorder with genetic autosomal recessive transmission [1–4]. The mutation of the β-glucocerebrosidase gene causes the malfunction of the lysosomal enzyme glucocerebrosidase. Cells, especially macrophages, that undergo glucocerebrosidase accumulation are called Gaucher cells. These cells, called Gaucher cells, become dilated and have a cytoplasm with an engorged, wrinkled tissue paper appearance and are displaced around the nuclei [5–7]. GD has an incidence of 1 in 50,000 to 100,000 people in the general population. Still, there is an increase among communities with consanguineous marriages, inbreeding, or geographically limited groups with an expected birth rate of 1:850 among the Ashkenazi Jewish population [8]. In some geographical areas, such as the Norrbottnian region of Northern Sweden, there is a higher incidence of GD with a particular form of the disease [1,9]. The main features of the disorder are due to the infiltration of Gaucher cells into the principal organs of the reticuloendothelial system, such as spleen, liver, and bone marrow [10,11]. The mutated gene is located on chromosome 1q22 and is inherited paternally. It is formed by ten introns and 11 exons [12–15]. Nowadays, 300 mutations are discovered as the cause of GD [16]. N370S, L444P, 84GG, and IVS2 are several gene loci most frequently involved in mutation for the onset of GD, with a prevalence of 98% [17,18]. The first two influence clinical manifestations, as some others several genetic diseases [13,14]. GD causes significant morbidity and disability; in types 1 and 3 many organs of the skeletal system are involved, while in type two the visceral and neurological blood system are involved so as in others many several oro-craniofacial diseases. [19–22]. The skeletal manifestations include osteopenia, pathological fractures, growth retardation, osteoporosis, focal lytic or sclerotic lesions, bone pain, painful or bone crisis, decreased mineralization [23–26], osteonecrosis or vascular necrosis, cortical and medullary infarcts [21,27,28]. Anemia and thrombocytopenia are the early signs of the most common hematologic manifestations [7,9,11,15]. The infiltration of engorged macrophages in the spleen, liver, and bone marrow causes a depression of hematopoiesis, leading to thrombocytopenia [11,29]. Other hematologic manifestations include monoclonal and polyclonal gammopathies, which are risk factors for neoplasms as multiple myeloma [7,30,31]. The most affected organs in Gaucher disease are the liver and spleen, which increased in volume due to macrophage accumulation in Kupffer cells [11]. Nevertheless, portal hypertension is rare due to cirrhosis and fibrosis [4]. Spleen volume is normally 5–15 times greater in type 1; however, it can sometimes significantly increase and exceed 50 times normal. Massive splenomegaly may cause fibrosis and increase the risk of rupture and malignancies. In type 1 GD, the most frequent neurological manifestation is Parkinson's disease, while in type 2 and 3, central nervous system (CNS) manifestations, including dementia and epilepsy, are more frequent, so a multidisciplinary approach it is necessary [7,13,21,30,32]. Recently, a new manifestation of myoclonic epilepsy has been connected to Gaucher's disease. Bleeding is an important sign and manifests itself as frequent epistaxis, easy bruising, and hemorrhaging after surgical/or dental procedures or during pregnancy or childbirth, so that the clinician must be prepared in the management of these various possible unexpected events in the different fields of medicine and dentistry [9,13,33–37]. The abnormal bleeding is caused by hypersplenism and the infiltration of bone marrow by Gaucher cells. GD is associated with some abnormal platelet function or malfunction of clotting [10]. The diagnosis is made through the measurement of low levels of enzyme activity in peripheral blood cells. Sometimes, molecular genotype analyses are important to evaluate the possible evolution of the disease [27]. There is no cure for Gaucher's disease; in 1991, intravenous infusions of enzyme replacement therapy (ERT) were approved. However, it only treats symptomatic episodes, while asymptomatic episodes are untreated. Early ERT improves hepatosplenomegaly, hematologic manifestations, bone pain, and bone mineral density [10,11,38]. The symptomatic Gaucher Disease commonly involves the bones. The bone manifestation causes pain, difficulty in motility, and skeletal abnormalities, and it is a very limiting factor for the life of the individual, a differential diagnosis with other diseases must to be carefully obtained, thanks to the use of technologies and specific diagnostics methods [9,21,39]. The epidemiologic study of Germain estimated that 75% of patients with type 1 Gaucher Disease have a bone manifestation of the disease. With the improvement of radiologic and diagnostic techniques [40,41], 90% of patients have one or more bone manifestations [8,21]. The exact mechanism of bone manifestation is probably due to the infiltration of Gaucher cells in the bone marrow and, consequently, the destruction of bone architecture [7]. All long bones are a potential means of skeletal manifestation [21]. All long bones, including the mandible, are potential infiltration sites [28]. In the literature, about 100 cases describe the infiltration of the maxillo-mandibular complex noted on radiographs.

The most common finding is the presence of radiolucent honeycomb areas in the premolar-molar region. The most common radiographic observation in an affected mandible is the presence of radiolucent pseudocystic or honeycomb lesions, mainly in the premolar-molar regions. There is also a loss of normal bone trabeculae [9]. Other findings include generalized osteoporosis, widening, and widening of bone marrow spaces, endosseous scallops and, in some cases, apical root resorption, all presumably due to Gaucher cell density in the apical regions. Cortical bone, however, remains intact. It has been hypothesized that the sclerotic areas are not empty, and this process is completely reversible [34,40]. In regard to the jaw, it is a possible focus on Gaucher cells infiltration [21]. In the literature, only 100 cases with jaw manifestations have been documented. The discovery is often accidental during a dental or panoramic X-ray [13,16]. The study aims to identify the principal bone jaw features involved in GD. This is a review that evaluates jawbone manifestations, which helps the dentist to make an early diagnosis.

2. Materials and Methods

2.1. Eligibility Criteria

All documents were assessed for eligibility based on the following population (including animal species), Exposure, Comparator, and Outcomes (PECO) [42]:

(P) Participants consisted of patients.

(E) The exposure consists of patients with GD and bone manifestations.

(C) The comparison was healthy patients with no GD history and other bone-related systemic diseases.

(O) The result is to evaluate the frequency and incidence of bone lesions detected by radiology in GD patients compared with healthy patients. The secondary purpose is to assess the differences in oral health (caries index and periodontal disease) between the GD and healthy patient groups.

Only papers providing data at the end of the intervention were included. Exclusion criteria were the following: (1) Studies on GD with no radiographic exams; (2) Studies with groups of patients suffering from other systemic diseases; (3) deals with bone manifestations in other anatomical districts; (4) cross-over study design; (5) studies written in a language different from English; (6) full-text unavailability (i.e., posters and conference abstracts); (7) studies involving animals; (8) review articles; (9) case reports.

2.2. Search Strategy

The study used the main scientific databases (PUBMED, WEB of SCIENCE, LILACS, SCOPUS). The time window considered for the electronic search was from 1 March 1990 to 31 December 2022. The term "Gaucher disease" was first combined with "bone" and then independently with "oral health" using the Boolean connector "OR". The web search was assisted using MESH (Medical Subjects Headings) (Table 1). The keywords used in the search engine using MeSh are as follows: ("Gaucher disease" [MeSH Terms] OR ("gaucher" [All Fields] AND "disease" [All Fields] OR "gaucher disease" [All Fields] AND ("bone and bones" [MeSH Terms] OR ("bone" [All Fields] AND "bones" [All Fields] OR "bone and bones" [All Fields] OR "bone" [All Fields] OR ("oral health" [MeSH Terms] OR ("oral" [All Fields] AND "health" [All Fields] OR "oral health" [All Fields]). In addition, a manual search was performed using the bibliography of found articles and a free search on Google Scholar.

This systematic review was conducted according to Preferred Reporting Items for Systematic Reviews (PRISMA) guidelines and the Cochrane Handbook for Systematic Reviews of Interventions. The systematic review protocol was registered on the International Prospective Register of Systematic Reviews (PROSPERO) with the following number CRD42022333235 on 21 April 2022.

Table 1. Search strategy.

PubMed
(gaucher disease) AND ((bone) OR (oral health))
Web of Science
TITLE-ABS-KEY (gaucher disease) AND ((bone) OR (oral health))
Lilacs
(gaucher disease) AND ((bone) OR (oral health))
Scopus
TITLE-ABS-KEY (((gaucher AND disease) AND ((bone) OR (oral AND health))))

2.3. Data Extraction

Two reviewers (GM and RF) independently extracted data from the included studies using a customized data extraction on a Microsoft Excel sheet. In disagreement, a consensus was reached through a third reviewer (MC).

The following data were extracted: (1) First author; (2) Year of publication; (3) Nationality; (4) Age of study participants; (5) Sample; (6) Radiographic signs; (7) Evaluation of oral health.

2.4. Quality Assessment

The risk of bias in papers was assessed by two reviewers using Version 2 of the Cochrane risk-of-bias tool for randomized trials (RoB 2) (Cochrane Corp., Fredericksburg, VA, USA). Any disagreement was discussed until a consensus was reached with a third reviewer.

3. Results

3.1. Study Characteristics

After searching the three search motors, 5079 articles were selected. The exclusion criteria automatically removed the review and non-English articles via the Boolean operator NOT. Specifically, 25 articles from LILACS, 261 from Web of Science, 273 from PubMed, and 350 from Scopus were deleted. A fourth search engine on Scopus was used, given the specificity of the topic. In addition, 1226 articles were eliminated as duplicates. During the first screening phase, 2953 articles were considered; however, according to the inclusion criteria, clinical trials and randomized controlled trials were considered, and so 2902 articles were excluded. One article was excluded because the full text could not be found.

Therefore, 50 articles were after this screening stage; the abstracts were read to assess eligibility. According to the PRISMA 2020 flowchart in Figure 1, only four were chosen for this review. The articles were excluded because they were either off-topic and did not meet PECO or were systematic literature reviews. Figure 1 shows the screening process and why articles were excluded from this systematic review. A total of 46 articles were excluded: 32 were eliminated because do not answer the question posed in Section 2 by PECO and therefore were included in this review (assessing the frequency of bone lesions in patients with GD and evaluating their oral health), and 14 were off-topic. According to the PECO model, four papers were chosen for title and abstract screening. The included studies have been published over the past 20 years (1983 to 2022). In parallel, a manual bibliography search of the selected articles and a search of the main sites were performed. From this it emerged that ten papers were selected. However, six were excluded because they were off-topic, and the remaining four articles coincided with those found in the databases. The studies analyzed were conducted in various parts of the world: South America (Brazil) and Israel. A total of 430 subjects with GD were analyzed. Regarding the study designs, there were four clinical studies. Among these four studies, three included a control group; all used DMFT to evaluate caries and Gingival Index (GI) to assess periodontal status. All studies evaluated radiographic evidence in the oral cavity by either orthopanoramic or Tc Cone Beam. Table 2 summarizes the main characteristics of all the study included in the present systematic review.

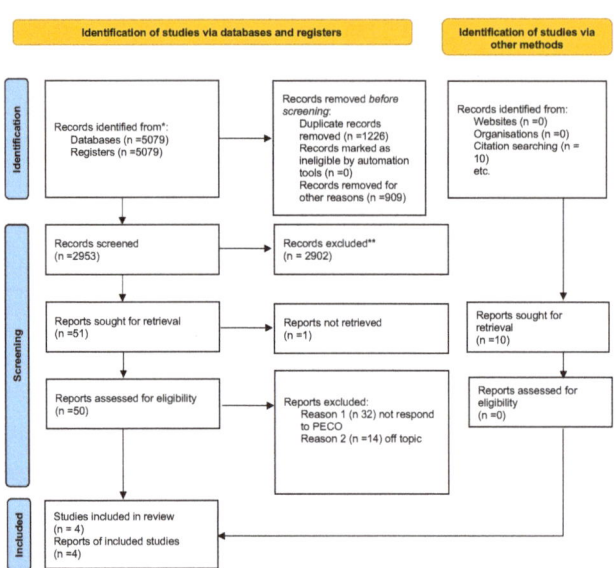

Figure 1. Prisma Flowchart. * papers identified by search methods; ** papers removed because systematic reviews of the literature.

Table 2. Main characteristics of the studies included in the present systematic review.

Authors	Year	Sample	Age	Radiographic Signs	Evaluation of Oral Health	Nationality
Norbre et al.	2012	10 with GD compared with 20 healthy	23.2 years	Generalized rarefaction and enlarged narrow space	No difference	Brazil
Mohamed et al.	2020	42 with GD compared with 84 healthy	11.37 years	Generalized rarefaction, pseudocysts radiolucent lesion, anodontia	No difference	Egypt
Fischman et al.	2003	350 with GD and 31 control	30.7 years	Bone involvement is frequent. The finding in the ortho-panoramic is always frequent	No statistical significance between DMFT, Gingival Index	Israel
Carter et al.	1998	28 with GD	32.4 years	The most common findings are enlargement of medullary spaces	No dental findings in oral health	Israel

3.2. Main Findings

The study of Nobre et al. analyses the principal bone abnormalities of 10 GP. The study comprises a group of 10 patients affected by GD (4 males; 6 females) and a control group of 20 healthy patients. The patients underwent radiographic analysis (Cone Beam Tc and orthopantomography). All patients underwent an anamnestic control, intra- and extra-oral examination, and a CBCT and panoramic radiography. Although there was radiological evidence of bone involvement in all ten patients, only four had pathological fractures or delays in tooth eruption. During CBCT analysis, the jaw showed pathological features in all ten patients and the maxilla in six. The radiographic analysis revealed the presence of generalized rarefaction and enlarged marrow spaces in all patients. Other radiographic signs were cortical thinning, osteosclerosis (five patients), pseudocystic lesions (nine patients), mental demineralization (seven patients), flattening in the head of the condyle (one patient), effacement of anatomical structures (eight patients), thickening of maxillary sinus mucosa (three patients). The orthopantomography revealed signs in the mandible and in 8 maxillae. Afterwards, the author compared the radiographic findings in CBCT and orthopantomography with the study and control groups against a Fisher's exact test. CBCT has more predictability to evaluate the following signs: generalized bone rarefaction ($p = 0.0001$) and TMJ involvement ($p = 0.0002$). CBCT is not an important tool to reveal other bone signs with statistical relevance. CBCT is more effective in highlighting differences between GD and control groups, thus proving an essential tool for evaluating patients with GD [15]. The second study by Mohamed et al. focuses on jaw involvement and radiographic features. The case-control study evaluates a panel of 42 GP (26 males and 16 females with an average age of 9.54 ± 4.25 years) and a control group of 84 (45 males and 39 females with a mean age of 11.37 ± 1.83 years). The patients all had Gaucher type 1 and type 3. The following features in the radiographic images were examined: generalized bone rarefaction, localized rarefaction and enlarged bone marrow spaces thinning of the cortex, pseudocystic radiolucent lesions, anodontia and dental anomalies. Cyst-like radiolucent lesions were defined as a pseudocyst. The biopsy was not performed due to the lack of symptoms of the lesions. Generalized rarefaction is a radiographic finding in type I and type 3. GD type III presents a localized rarefaction, but type I widens the bone marrow. The following signs are more frequent in type III: pseudocysts radiolucent lesions, cortex thinning, anodontia, and dental anomalies. Chi-squared test showed an association between types I and III and generalized rarefaction, wide bone marrow spaces, pseudocyst radiolucency, cortex thinning, dental abnormalities, and absence of abnormal radiographic features with a p-value < 0.05. Generalized rarefaction, wide bone marrow spaces, and cortex thinning are more frequent in type I GD, but pseudocysts are not associated with type I. The radiological features are not essential signs in type I (95% CI 0.03–0.39, p-value = 0.0009). On the other hand, type III is associated with some radiological features (generalized rarefaction, pseudocysts radiolucent lesions, thinning of the cortex, and dental anomalies). The widening of bone marrow is not a radiological feature of type III (p-value = 0.3464). In conclusion, the radiological features are associated with type III (odds ratio of 0.13, 95% CI 0.05–0.37, p-value = 0.0001) [21]. Fischman's study analyzed a cohort of 350 patients who underwent a periodontal examination and radiological analysis. After the statistical analysis, the control patients showed a worse periodontal health status than those with this pathology. Affected patients showed better DMFS levels than carriers (36.8 vs. 49.4), with a $p = 0.048$. The most significant difference was found between MS (missing surfaces). Affected patients showed a halving of the missing surfaces, 9.5 versus 18.9, with a p-value of 0.008. The DMFS index between the two categories did not show large statistically significant differences. Therefore, this study showed no significant differences between periodontal health [18]. The study of Carter analyses 25 patients, and 25 of the 28 patients showed radiographic evidence of bone resorption. The most common finding is the enlargement of the medullary spaces. The most common result is the gross enlargement of the medullary spaces and the radiolucency and displacement of the mandibular canal. It has also been shown that delayed eruption of permanent teeth is present. Therefore, the alterations at the bone level are very significant and very frequent (Table 2) [17].

3.3. Quality Assessment and Risk of Bias

Using RoB 2, the risk of bias was estimated and reported in Figure 2. Regarding the randomization process, 75% of the studies ensured a low risk of bias. However, 50% of the studies excluded a performance bias, but 75% reported all outcome data, 50% of the included studies adequately excluded bias in the selection of reported outcomes, and 75%

excluded bias in self-reported outcomes. Overall, all four studies were shown to have a low risk of experiencing bias.

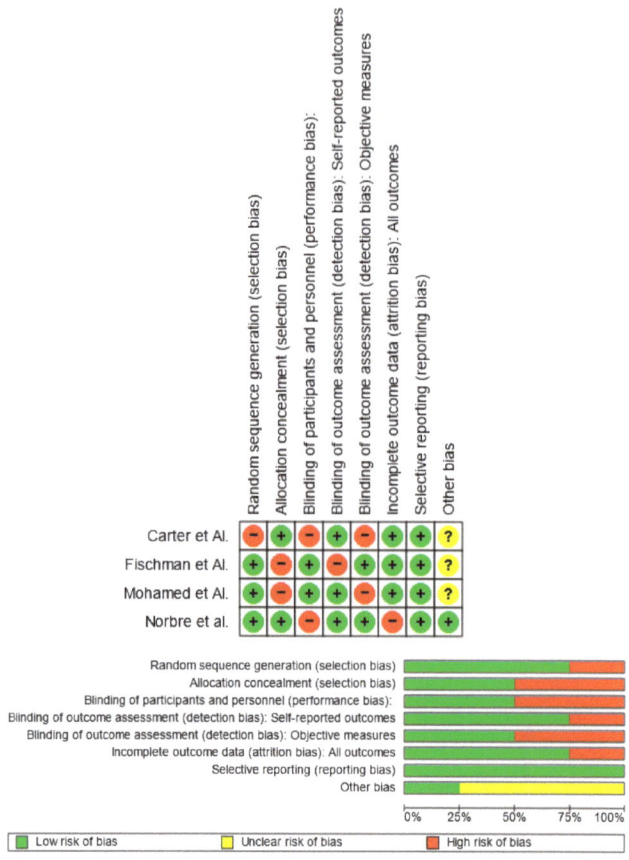

Figure 2. Risk-of-bias domains of included studies.

4. Discussion

The involvement of bones is a prevalent finding in Gaucher disease. It causes deformity and limits daily activities and patients' quality of life. In 75% of patients, there is bone involvement. Recent advances in diagnostic and imaging modalities have revealed that 90% of patients with type I or III Gaucher disease have one or more bone manifestations. Orthopedic prostheses are the only solution to replace the necrosis of bone and lytic changes [13,17,18,30,43]. The exact mechanism of bone manifestations is still uncertain, but the infiltration of Gaucher cells in the bone marrow is the most important feature [34,40]. All long bones are possible Gaucher cell targets. The mandible is classified as a long bone and is, therefore, involved. About 100 cases with maxilla-facial involvement are described and documented in the literature database. This is occasionally discovered during a radiographic survey [11,29]. Regarding oral symptoms, GD is frequently asymptomatic, but clinical examinations and regular radiographic exams can detect the disease's early warning signs. Spontaneous gingival bleeding, yellowish skin pigmentation, petechiae on the oral mucosa, [11,15,16] and delayed tooth eruption are some of the most typical oral symptoms. In young GD patients, Fischman et al. 7 found a significant correlation between the delayed eruption of the permanent teeth and mild to severe bone involvement.

Asymptomatic mandibular bone disorders are common. The lamina dura has thinned, there is pervasive osteopenia with loss of trabecular bone structure, and the mandibular canal has been displaced by pseudocysts lesions, among other recorded radiographic abnormalities of this area. It has also been shown that nearby teeth, mostly molars and premolars, undergo apical root resorption. The maxilla is less frequently impacted when it primarily comprises resorption in the maxillary sinus region. The possible mechanism of the bone lesion and the presence of radiolucent areas are osteosclerotic reactions or abnormal bone regeneration in the post-extraction area. Bender et al. [7] assert that a dental panoramic X-ray is essential for diagnosis. The region between premolars is rich in bone marrow. Therefore, the presence of 12 cases with radiographic signs in the premolar region indicates that jawbone marrow is infiltrated by Gaucher cells [7,8,21]. Some cases have later shown a possible apices reabsorption without pulpal necrosis. The accumulation of Gaucher cells causes a scalloped appearance in the endosteal bone region [7,11,29,41]. The mandible and the maxilla manifest diffuse osteoporosis like the radiographic signs of other conditions such as thalassemia major and sickle cell anemia. Dental X-rays can often provisionally detect GD [9,15,21]. In the soft tissue, there are no important signs. In some cases, platelet dysfunction, oral pigmentation, or petechiae are to be interpreted as clinical findings, as highlighted in the study of Givol et al. [3,30], which evaluates the risk of bleeding after oral surgery in GD patients. Givol treated a group of GD patients undergoing hematologic analysis and a platelet function exam [30]. The study showed the following results: patients with Gaucher disease who suffer from platelet dysfunction must be treated by performing an accurate hemostasis. Platelet transfusions are recommended if there is a high risk of bleeding. The first study showed that the main features of GD generalized rarefaction in the CBCT are enlarged marrow, cortical thinning, osteosclerosis, pseudocysts lesion, and dental demineralization in seven. This study confirms that the mandible is more affected than the maxilla [15]. The second study analyzed the prevalence of radiographic features in the different types of GD [21,44]. Generalized rarefaction has a similar incidence in two kinds of GD; localized rarefaction is a clinical finding of type III, and widening of the bone marrow spaces is a clinical finding of type I [8,21]. Pseudocysts radiolucent lesions, cortex thinning, anodontia and dental anomalies are clinical findings in type III [21]. According to the previous study by Bender, Saranjam et al. [7,45], the above features are mainly found in the mandible due to the infiltration of GD cells in the marrow. According to Bender et al. [10] and Michanowiz et al. [46], the common radiological features in the premolar-molar region are the presence of pseudocystic or honeycombed radiolucent lesions. Bone manipulation creates a bone turnover and improves the radiolucent lesions [34,40]. The jaw is more affected than the maxilla. The delayed eruption of the teeth is widespread in GD, except if amyloidosis and other pathology take over [17]. GD is a risk factor for mucosal disease such as amyloidosis; the literature described only five cases, according to Elstein et al. [41,44]. The salivary flow is lower compared to the control. Spontaneous or surgically induced bleeding is widespread due to thrombocytopenia and the alteration of the coagulation cascade. According to the DMFS index, the patient's dental health was equal to the controls. Compared to the control group, the patients had roughly half as many carious surfaces and half as many missing surfaces. Given that the carriers and the patients come from the same households, it is reasonable to presume that their socioeconomic circumstances and access to oral healthcare are similar. The negligible variation in filled surfaces, a measure of dental therapy, supports this notion. Though the patients may have had better health awareness, including greater concern for their dental health, they were aware of their Gaucher disease status. The observed differences between the DS and MS scores could be attributed to a healthier diet and improved dental hygiene. There was expected to be a connection between Gaucher disease and gingival disease because both conditions are characterized by anemia, a propensity to bleed, and poor healing. The patients may have adhered to better oral hygiene practices because they were aware of their "at risk" status, as was previously suggested. ERT helps the patient to control bleeding against the increase in platelets. In conclusion, the presence of a lesion, especially in the jaw, is a constant feature in dental radiography [7,30,47]. The dentist and must intercept this lesion to obtain a diagnostic suspicion and diagnose the disease. Today, thanks to new technologies that allow early diagnosis, it is possible to start therapy early in order to be able to reduce the adverse effects of the disease [48–51]. In this study, we analyzed the main radiographic features present radiographically in GD patients and oral health in this type of patient. Statistics showed that GD patients have radiographic manifestations that allow early diagnosis. Furthermore, the only study by Fischman et al. evaluated oral health and stated no statistically significant differences in periodontal and carious health. The limitations of the studies are that there has not been a classification and a study comparing the radiographic differences among the three subtypes and also a study analyzing whether any of these three subtypes have worse oral health. This is mainly due to the condition's rarity, which does not allow for a statistically significant sample. Patients with Gaucher disease frequently report excruciating pain in different skeletal regions but rarely in the jawbones or craniofacial region. With 13 and 60 years of follow-up, Bender and Bender reported two instances of Gaucher disease; in the first case, mandibular lesions were present in the premolar-molar region, and the affected teeth were essential. These results matched the description of our patient. Additionally, Bender and Bender found that ERT improved the mandibular rarefaction bilaterally without showing any signs of osteolysis. However, according to some research, orthopedic intervention such as joint (hip, knee, or shoulder replacement) replacement is advised because ERT cannot reverse the necrotic and lytic changes in long bones. Additionally, our patient had a history of having a hip joint replaced and long bones affected by Gaucher disease. Bender and Bender claimed that without clinical and laboratory testing and in light of radiographic findings, it is impossible to make a conclusive diagnosis of Gaucher disease involving the jawbone without biopsy; however, other studies have only recommended biopsy in situations where other conditions are suspected in the differential diagnosis, such as in the case described here.

5. Conclusions

This review analyzed Gaucher's disease's primary clinical and radiological signs and symptoms. Although a rare pathology, all radiological and clinical signs must direct the dental specialist to a correct diagnosis. In addition, this study showed no variation in the oral health of patients with GD. Therefore, the dentist's role is to establish and maintain a healthy periodontium and teeth. In addition, sometimes the dentist's role in the early diagnosis of the disease may be necessary.

Author Contributions: Conceptualization, R.F., G.M. and M.C.; methodology, L.F. and G.C.; formal analysis, M.M.M. and V.M.; investigation, M.C.; data curation, L.F.; writing—original draft preparation, G.M., R.F., A.B., M.C. and M.M.M.; writing—review and editing, G.M., R.F., M.C. and M.M.M.; visualization, M.C. and G.C.; All authors have read and agreed to the published version of the manuscript.

Funding: This research received no external funding.

Institutional Review Board Statement: Not applicable.

Informed Consent Statement: Not applicable.

Data Availability Statement: Not applicable.

Conflicts of Interest: The authors declare no conflict of interest.

Abbreviations

GD	Gaucher disease
CNS	Central nervous system
ERT	Enzyme replacement therapy
PECO	Patients, Exposure, Comparison, Outcome
MeSH	Medical subjects headings
PRISMA	Preferred Reporting Items for Systematic Reviews and Meta-Analyses
GI	Gingival index
DMFT	Decayed, missing and filled teeth
CBCT	Cone beam tc
TMJ	Temporomandibular joint
MS	Missing surface
DMFS	Decayed, missing and filled surface

References

1. Huang, W.J.; Zhang, X.; Chen, W.W. Gaucher disease: A lysosomal neurodegenerative disorder. *Eur. Rev. Med. Pharm. Sci.* **2015**, *19*, 1219–1226.
2. Stirnemann, J.; Belmatoug, N.; Camou, F.; Serratrice, C.; Froissart, R.; Caillaud, C.; Levade, T.; Astudillo, L.; Serratrice, J.; Brassier, A.; et al. A Review of Gaucher Disease Pathophysiology, Clinical Presentation and Treatments. *Int. J. Mol. Sci.* **2017**, *18*, 441. [CrossRef] [PubMed]
3. Mikosch, P.; Hughes, D. An overview on bone manifestations in Gaucher disease. *Wien. Med. Wochenschr. 1946* **2010**, *160*, 609–624. [CrossRef] [PubMed]
4. Adar, T.; Ilan, Y.; Elstein, D.; Zimran, A. Liver involvement in Gaucher disease—Review and clinical approach. *Blood Cells Mol. Dis.* **2018**, *68*, 66–73. [CrossRef]
5. Moch, W.S. Gaucher's disease with mandibular bone lesions. *Oral Surg. Oral Med. Oral Pathol.* **1953**, *6*, 1250–1254. [CrossRef] [PubMed]
6. Kumar, N.S.; John, R.R.; Rethish, E. Relatively rare entity of avascular necrosis of maxillary bone caused by Gaucher's disease—A case report. *J. Oral Maxillofac. Surg.* **2012**, *70*, 2590–2595. [CrossRef] [PubMed]
7. Bender, I.B.; Bender, A.L. Dental observations in Gaucher's disease: Review of the literature and two case reports with 13-and 60-year follow-ups. *Oral Surg. Oral Med. Oral Pathol. Oral Radiol. Endod.* **1996**, *82*, 650–659. [CrossRef]
8. Becquemont, L. Type 1 Gaucher disease (CYP2D6-eliglustat). *Therapies* **2017**, *72*, 323–326. [CrossRef]
9. Lehrer, S.; Montazem, A.; Ramanathan, L.; Pessin-Minsley, M.; Pfail, J.; Stock, R.G.; Kogan, R. Bisphosphonate-induced osteonecrosis of the jaws, bone markers, and a hypothesised candidate gene. *J. Oral Maxillofac. Surg.* **2009**, *67*, 159–161. [CrossRef]
10. Komada, N.; Fujiwara, T.; Yoshizumi, H.; Ida, H.; Shimoda, K.A. Japanese Patient with Gaucher Disease Treated with the Oral Drug Eliglustat as Substrate Reducing Therapy. *Case Rep. Gastroenterol.* **2021**, *15*, 838–845. [CrossRef]
11. Mitsui, J.; Matsukawa, T.; Sasaki, H.; Yabe, I.; Matsushima, M.; Dürr, A.; Brice, A.; Takashima, H.; Kikuchi, A.; Aoki, M.; et al. Variants associated with Gaucher disease in multiple system atrophy. *Ann. Clin. Transl. Neurol.* **2015**, *2*, 417–426. [CrossRef] [PubMed]
12. Poll, L.W.; Koch, J.A.; Vom Dahl, S.; Loxtermann, E.; Sarbia, M.; Niederau, C.; Häussinger, D.; Mödder, U. Extraosseous manifestation of Gaucher's disease type I: MR and histological appearance. *Eur. Radiol.* **2000**, *10*, 1660–1663. [CrossRef] [PubMed]
13. Saccomanno, S.; Quinzi, V.; D'andrea, N.; Albani, A.; Paskay, L.C.; Marzo, G. Traumatic events and eagle syndrome: Is there any correlation? A systematic review. *Healthcare* **2021**, *9*, 825. [CrossRef]
14. Peterschmitt, M.J.; Freisens, S.; Underhill, L.H.; Foster, M.C.; Lewis, G.; Gaemers, S.J.M. Long-term adverse event profile from four completed trials of oral eliglustat in adults with Gaucher disease type 1. *Orphanet J. Rare Dis.* **2019**, *14*, 128. [CrossRef]
15. Nobre, R.M.; Ribeiro, A.L.R.; Alves-Junior, S.M.; Tuji, F.M.; Rodrigues Pinheiro, M.D.G.; Pinheiro, L.R.; Pinheiro, J.J.V. Dentomaxillofacial manifestations of Gaucher's disease: Preliminary clinical and radiographic findings. *Dentomaxillofac. Radiol.* **2012**, *41*, 541–547. [CrossRef] [PubMed]
16. Mistry, P.K.; Cappellini, M.D.; Lukina, E.; Özsan, H.; Pascual, S.M.; Rosenbaum, H.; Solano, M.H.; Spigelman, Z.; Villarrubia, J.; Watman, N.P.; et al. Consensus Conference: A reappraisal of Gaucher disease-diagnosis and disease management algorithms. *Am. J. Hematol.* **2011**, *86*, 110–115. [CrossRef]
17. Carter, L.C.; Fischman, S.L.; Mann, J.; Elstein, D.; Stabholz, A.; Zimran, A. The nature and extent of jaw involvement in Gaucher disease: Observations in a series of 28 patients. *Oral Surg. Oral Med. Oral Pathol. Oral Radiol. Endod.* **1998**, *85*, 233–239. [CrossRef] [PubMed]
18. Fischman, S.L.; Elstein, D.; Sgan-Cohen, H.; Mann, J.; Zimran, A. Dental profile of patients with Gaucher disease. *BMC Oral Health* **2003**, *3*, 4. [CrossRef]
19. Femiano, F.; Femiano, R.; Femiano, L.; Nucci, L.; Minervini, G.; Antonelli, A.; Bennardo, F.; Barone, S.; Scotti, N.; Sorice, V.; et al. A New Combined Protocol to Treat the Dentin Hypersensitivity Associated with Non-Carious Cervical Lesions: A Randomized Controlled Trial. *Appl. Sci.* **2020**, *11*, 187. [CrossRef]

20. Minervini, G.; Franco, R.; Marrapodi, M.M.; Mehta, V.; Fiorillo, L.; Badnjević, A.; Cervino, D.; Cicciu, M. The Association between COVID-19 Related Anxiety, Stress, Depression, Temporomandibular Disorders, and Headaches from Childhood to Adulthood: A Systematic Review. *Brain Sci.* **2023**, *13*, 481. [CrossRef]
21. Mohamed, Y.S.A.; Zayet, M.K.; Omar, O.M.; El-Beshlawy, A.M. Jaw bones' involvement and dental features of type I and type III Gaucher disease: A radiographic study of 42 paediatric patients. *Eur. Arch. Paediatr. Dent.* **2020**, *21*, 241–247. [CrossRef] [PubMed]
22. Fiorillo, L.; De Stefano, R.; Cervino, G.; Crimi, S.; Bianchi, A.; Herford, A.S.; Laino, L.; Cicciù, M.; Campagna, P. Oral and psychological alterations in haemophiliac patients. *Biomedicines* **2019**, *7*, 33. [CrossRef] [PubMed]
23. Spagnuolo, G.; Sorrentino, R. The Role of Digital Devices in Dentistry: Clinical Trends and Scientific Evidences. *J. Clin. Med.* **2020**, *9*, 1692. [CrossRef]
24. Chakraborty, T.; Jamal, R.F.; Battineni, G.; Teja, K.V.; Marto, C.M.; Spagnuolo, G. A review of prolonged post-covid-19 symptoms and their implications on dental management. *Int. J. Environ. Res. Public Health* **2021**, *18*, 5131. [CrossRef]
25. Cicciù, M.; Herford, A.S.; Cervino, G.; Troiano, G.; Lauritano, F.; Laino, L. Tissue fluorescence imaging (VELscope) for quick non-invasive diagnosis in oral pathology. *J. Craniofacial Surg.* **2017**, *28*, e112–e115. [CrossRef] [PubMed]
26. Spagnuolo, G. Cone-Beam Computed Tomography and the Related Scientific Evidence. *Appl. Sci.* **2022**, *12*, 7140. [CrossRef]
27. Weinreb, N.J. Encore! Oral therapy for type 1 Gaucher disease. *Blood J. Am. Soc. Hematol.* **2017**, *129*, 2337–2338. [CrossRef] [PubMed]
28. Cervino, G.; Fiorillo, L.; Arzukanyan, A.V.; Spagnuolo, G.; Campagna, P.; Cicciù, M. Application of bioengineering devices for stress evaluation in dentistry: The last 10 years FEM parametric analysis of outcomes and current trends. *Minerva Stomatol.* **2020**, *69*, 9. [CrossRef]
29. Chis, B.A.; Chis, A.F.; Dumitrascu, D.L. Gaucher disease—Therapeutic aspects in Romania. *Med. Pharm. Rep.* **2021**, *94* (Suppl. 1), S51–S53.
30. Givol, N.; Goldstein, G.; Peleg, O.; Shenkman, B.; Zimran, A.; Elstein, D.; Kenet, G. Thrombocytopenia and bleeding in dental procedures of patients with Gaucher disease. *Haemophilia* **2012**, *18*, 117–121. [CrossRef]
31. Mehta, V.; Sarode, G.S.; Obulareddy, V.T.; Sharma, T.; Kokane, S.; Cicciù, M.; Minervini, G. Clinicopathologic Profile, Management and Outcome of Sinonasal Ameloblastoma—A Systematic Review. *J. Clin. Med.* **2023**, *12*, 381. [CrossRef] [PubMed]
32. Minervini, G.; Mariani, P.; Fiorillo, L.; Cervino, G.; Cicciù, M.; Laino, L. Prevalence of temporomandibular disorders in people with multiple sclerosis: A systematic review and meta-analysis. *CRANIO®* **2022**, 1–9. [CrossRef] [PubMed]
33. Quinzi, V.; Paskay, L.C.; Manenti, R.J.; Giancaspro, S.; Marzo, G.; Saccomanno, S. Telemedicine for a multidisciplinary assessment of orofacial pain in a patient affected by eagle's syndrome: A clinical case report. *Open Dent. J.* **2021**, *15*, 102–110. [CrossRef]
34. D'Amore, S.; Kumar, N.; Ramaswami, U. Jaw involvement in Gaucher disease: A not-so-uncommon feature of a rare disease. *BMJ Case Rep.* **2021**, *14*, e244298. [CrossRef]
35. Nahidh, M.; Al-Khawaja, N.F.K.; Jasim, H.M.; Cervino, G.; Cicciù, M.; Minervini, G. The Role of Social Media in Communication and Learning at the Time of COVID-19 Lockdown—An Online Survey. *Dent. J.* **2023**, *11*, 48. [CrossRef]
36. Minervini, G.; Del Mondo, D.; Russo, D.; Cervino, G.; D'Amico, C.; Fiorillo, L. Stem Cells in Temporomandibular Joint Engineering: State of Art and Future Persetives. *J. Craniofacial Surg.* **2022**, *33*, 2181–2187. [CrossRef]
37. Minervini, G.; Basili, M.; Franco, R.; Bollero, P.; Mancini, M.; Gozzo, L.; Romano, G.L.; Marrapodi, M.M.; Gorassini, F.; D'Amico, C. Periodontal Disease and Pregnancy: Correlation with Underweight Birth. *Eur. J. Dent.* **2022**. [CrossRef]
38. Temelci, A.; Yılmaz, H.G.; Ünsal, D.; Uyanik, L.O.; Yazman, D.; Ayali, A.; Minervini, G. Investigation of the Wetting Properties of Thalassemia Patients' Blood Samples on Grade 5 Titanium Implant Surfaces: A Pilot Study. *Biomimetics* **2023**, *8*, 25. [CrossRef]
39. Rathi, S.; Chaturvedi, S.; Abdullah, S.; Rajput, G.; Alqahtani, N.M.; Chaturvedi, M.; Gurumurthy, V.; Saini, R.; Bavabeedu, S.; Minervini, G. Clinical Trial to Assess Physiology and Activity of Masticatory Muscles of Complete Denture Wearer Following Vitamin D Intervention. *Medicina* **2023**, *59*, 410. [CrossRef]
40. Vu, L.; Cox, G.F.; Ibrahim, J.; Peterschmitt, M.J.; Ross, L.; Thibault, N.; Turpault, S. Effects of paroxetine, ketoconazole, and rifampin on the metabolism of eliglustat, an oral substrate reduction therapy for Gaucher disease type 1. *Mol. Genet. Metab. Rep.* **2020**, *22*, 100552. [CrossRef]
41. Elstein, D.; Itzchaki, M.; Mankin, H.J. Skeletal involvement in Gaucher's disease. *Baillière's Clin. Haematol.* **1997**, *10*, 793–816. [CrossRef]
42. Morgan, R.L.; Whaley, P.; Thayer, K.A.; Schünemann, H.J. Identifying the PECO: A framework for formulating good questions to explore the association of environmental and other exposures with health outcomes. *Environ. Int.* **2018**, *121*, 1027–1031. [CrossRef] [PubMed]
43. La Torre, G.; Shivkumar, S.; Mehta, V.; Kumar Vaddamanu, S.; Shetty, U.A.; Hussain Alhamoudi, F.; Ali Alwadi, M.; Ibrahim Aldosari, L.; Ali Alshadidi, A.; Minervini, G. Surgical Protocols before and after COVID-19-A Narrative Review. *Vaccines* **2023**, *11*, 439. [CrossRef]
44. Bollero, P.; Carmine, P.P.; D'Addona, A.; Pasquantonio, G.; Mancini, M.; Condò, R.; Cerroni, L. Oral management of adult patients undergoing hematopoietic stem cell transplantation. *Eur. Rev. Med. Pharmacol. Sci.* **2018**, *22*, 876–887. [PubMed]
45. Saranjam, H.R.; Sidransky, E.; Levine, W.Z.; Zimran, A.; Elstein, D. Mandibular and dental manifestations of Gaucher disease. *Oral Dis.* **2012**, *18*, 421–429. [CrossRef]
46. Michanowicz, A.E.; Michanowicz, J.P.; Stein, G.M. Gaucher's disease: Report of a case. *Oral Surg. Oral Med. Oral Pathol.* **1967**, *23*, 36–42. [CrossRef]

47. Aşantoğrol, F.; Dursun, H.; Canger, E.M.; Bayram, F. Clinical and radiological evaluation of dentomaxillofacial involvement in Type I Gaucher disease. *Oral Radiol.* **2022**, *38*, 210–223. [CrossRef]
48. Gurbeta, L.; Alic, B.; Dzemic, Z.; Badnjevic, A. Testing of infusion pumps in healthcare institutions in Bosnia and herzegovina. In Proceedings of the Joint Conference of the European Medical and Biological Engineering Conference (EMBEC) and the Nordic-Baltic Conference on Biomedical Engineering and Medical Physics (NBC), Tampere, Finland, 11–15 June 2017; pp. 390–393.
49. Badnjevic, A.; Koruga, D.; Cifrek, M.; Smith, H.J.; Bego, T. Interpretation of pulmonary function test results in relation to asthma classification using integrated software suite. In Proceedings of the 36th International Convention on Information and Communication Technology, Electronics and Microelectronics (MIPRO 2013), Opatija, Croatia, 20–24 May 2013; pp. 140–144.
50. Granulo, E.; Bećar, L.; Gurbeta, L.; Badnjević, A. Telemetry system for diagnosis of asthma and chronical obstructive pulmonary disease (COPD). In *Lecture Notes of the Institute for Computer Sciences, Social-Informatics and Telecommunications Engineering, Proceedings of the Third International Conference, HealthyIoT 2016, Västerås, Sweden, 18–19 October 2016*; Springer: Cham, Switzerland, 2016; Volume LNICST 187, pp. 113–118.
51. Stokes, K.; Castaldo, R.; Franzese, M.; Salvatore, M.; Fico, G.; Pokvic, L.G.; Badnjevic, A.; Pecchia, L. A machine learning model for supporting symptom-based referral and diagnosis of bronchitis and pneumonia in limited resource settings. *Biocybern. Biomed. Eng.* **2021**, *41*, 1288–1302. [CrossRef]

Disclaimer/Publisher's Note: The statements, opinions and data contained in all publications are solely those of the individual author(s) and contributor(s) and not of MDPI and/or the editor(s). MDPI and/or the editor(s) disclaim responsibility for any injury to people or property resulting from any ideas, methods, instructions or products referred to in the content.

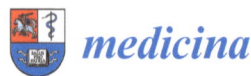

Article

Different Designs of Deep Marginal Elevation and Its Influence on Fracture Resistance of Teeth with Monolith Zirconia Full-Contour Crowns

Ali Robaian [1,*], Abdullah Alqahtani [1], Khalid Alanazi [2], Abdulrhman Alanazi [2], Meshal Almalki [2], Anas Aljarad [2], Refal Albaijan [3], Ahmed Maawadh [4], Aref Sufyan [5] and Mubashir Baig Mirza [1]

1. Conservative Dental Science Department, College of Dentistry, Prince Sattam bin Abdulaziz University, Al Kharj 11942, Saudi Arabia
2. Dental Intern, College of Dentistry, Prince Sattam bin Abdulaziz University, Al Kharj 11942, Saudi Arabia
3. Department of Prosthodontics, College of Dentistry, Prince Sattam bin Abdulaziz University, Al Kharj 11942, Saudi Arabia
4. Department of Restorative Dental Sciences, College of Dentistry, King Saud University, Riyadh 11545, Saudi Arabia
5. Department of Dental Biomaterials, College of Dentistry, King Saud University, Riyadh 11545, Saudi Arabia
* Correspondence: ali.alqahtani@psau.edu.sa; Tel.: +966-500010908

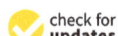

Citation: Robaian, A.; Alqahtani, A.; Alanazi, K.; Alanazi, A.; Almalki, M.; Aljarad, A.; Albaijan, R.; Maawadh, A.; Sufyan, A.; Mirza, M.B. Different Designs of Deep Marginal Elevation and Its Influence on Fracture Resistance of Teeth with Monolith Zirconia Full-Contour Crowns. *Medicina* 2023, 59, 661. https://doi.org/10.3390/medicina59040661

Academic Editors: Giuseppe Minervini, Stefania Moccia and João Miguel Marques dos Santos

Received: 14 February 2023
Revised: 23 March 2023
Accepted: 24 March 2023
Published: 27 March 2023

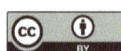

Copyright: © 2023 by the authors. Licensee MDPI, Basel, Switzerland. This article is an open access article distributed under the terms and conditions of the Creative Commons Attribution (CC BY) license (https://creativecommons.org/licenses/by/4.0/).

Abstract: *Background and objectives:* Even with the demand for high esthetics, the strength of the material for esthetic applications continues to be important. In this study, monolith zirconia (MZi) crowns fabricated using CAD/CAM were tested for fracture resistance (FR) in teeth with class II cavity designs with varying proximal depths, restored through a deep marginal elevation technique (DME). *Materials and Methods:* Forty premolars were randomly divided into four groups of ten teeth. In Group A, tooth preparation was conducted and MZi crowns were fabricated. In Group B, mesio-occluso-distal (MOD) cavities were prepared and restored with microhybrid composites before tooth preparation and the fabrication of MZi crowns. In Groups C and D, MOD cavities were prepared, differentiated by the depth of the gingival seat, 2 mm and 4 mm below the cemento-enamel junction (CEJ). Microhybrid composite resin was used for DME on the CEJ and for the restoration of the MOD cavities; beforehand, tooth preparations were conducted and MZi crowns were and cemented using resin cement. The maximum load to fracture (in newtons (N)) and FR (in megapascals (MPa)) were measured using the universal testing machine. *Results:* The average scores indicate a gradual decrease in the load required to fracture the samples from Groups A to D, with mean values of 3415.61 N, 2494.11 N, 2108.25 N and 1891.95 N, respectively. ANOVA revealed highly significant differences between the groups. Multiple group comparisons using the Tukey HSD post hoc test revealed that Group D had greater DME depths and showed significant differences compared with Group B. *Conclusions:* FR in teeth decreased when more tooth structure was involved, even with MZi crowns. However, DME up to 2 mm below the CEJ did not negatively influence the FR. Strengthening the DME-treated teeth with MZi crowns could be a reasonable clinical option, as the force required to fracture the samples far exceeded the maximum recorded biting force for posterior teeth.

Keywords: computer-aided designing; computer-aided manufacturing; dental crowns; deep marginal elevation; fracture resistance; zirconia

1. Introduction

Dental caries, or tooth fractures, which extend subgingivally complicate the restorative treatment approach [1]. They are challenging to restore and could result in the violation of the supracrestal connective tissue attachment (STA), leading to gingival inflammation and loss of periodontal supporting tissues [2]. Different techniques and procedures have been used to restore this critical area, keeping in mind the STA [3]. In fact, up to 10% of all periodontal surgical procedures are conducted to increase the crown length [4]. However, osteotomy itself is not without its shortcomings, such as being invasive with reduced patient acceptance, and if is not cautiously carried out, it can alter the crown–root ratio [5].

Deep marginal elevation (DME) is an alternative restorative technique suggested by Dietschi and Spreafico in 1998 [6]. It involves raising the deep margins to supragingival levels, noninvasively, to counter the difficulties encountered with subgingival margins [7]. This is achieved by using special matrix bands of shortened heights, which are secured subgingivally and tightened. Various materials have been presented to elevate the margins; however, DME conducted with composite resin seems to be well tolerated by the periodontium, even allowing the binding of epithelial fibers [8].

When the marginal ridge/s are involved in large lesions, it is wise to plan for indirect restorations (IRs), as the strength of the tooth is directly proportional to the integrity of the marginal ridges [9]. Depending on the extent of tooth structure loss, the need for cuspal coverage and the amount of reinforcement needed, IRs such as inlays, onlays, overlays and full-contour crowns are recommended [10]. Historically, IRs fabricated using gold alloys were considered the gold standard. However, due to increased demand for more natural and esthetic restorations, the use of composites and ceramics have more or less overhauled the use of metals [11].

With the advent of CAD/CAM technology and the ever-evolving choice in esthetic materials, more customizable and predictable restorations are being fabricated, minimizing the laboratory steps or eliminating them completely [12]. Zirconia (Zi) is usually the material of choice when posterior crowns are fabricated through CAD/CAM technology [13,14]. In lieu of the higher chipping rate of veneering porcelains on the Zi copings, full-contour zirconia crowns/monolith zirconia crowns (MZi) were developed [15]. MZi fabricated by CAD/CAM has been proven to be precise, stable and homogenous and has improved qualities compared to its predecessors [15]. Furthermore, Zi has been shown to achieve higher bond strengths if proper connections are achieved with resin adhesives by following the manufacturers' guidelines regarding surface pretreatment [16,17]. Studies related to the fracture resistance (FR) of teeth with monolith inlays, onlays and endocrowns exist in the literature. However, a dearth of information regarding the effect of DME on the FR of teeth with full-contour crowns led the authors to initiate the present study. Thus, by conducting this research, the authors aimed to evaluate the maximum load and resistance to fracture in teeth with different designs of DME, which were reinforced by MZi crowns. The null hypothesis is that there would be no difference in the FR of DME-treated teeth with MZi crowns.

2. Materials and Methods

2.1. Study Design

This experimental study was performed in the College of Dentistry, Prince Sattam bin Abdulaziz University (PSAU), Al Kharj, and the College of Dentistry, King Saud Bin Abdulaziz University (KSAU), Riyadh, after obtaining ethical approval from the Institutional Review Board, PSAU, IRB No (PSAU2021011), and the College of Dentistry Research Center, KSAU, CDRC No (FR0626).

2.2. Sample Collection

Non-carious maxillary premolars with all cusps and walls intact, freshly extracted for orthodontic reasons, were collected from the specialist clinic, PSAU. These teeth were inspected using a stereomicroscope (RX-100, Hirox, Tokyo, Japan) at 16× magnification for the presence of any deformities, craze lines or indications of fractures, which if found were excluded. Forty teeth which met the inclusion criteria were disinfected with 5.25% sodium hypochlorite for 30 min and stored in normal saline at room temperature until further use.

2.3. Description of the Experimental Groups

Selected teeth were divided into four groups, A–D, comprising of ten teeth each, allotted in a random order. All the teeth received full-contour crowns using CAD-CAM technology; however, groups would be differentiated based on the depth of DME from crown margins (Figure 1). Group A: Teeth with full-contour crowns without cavity preparation (control group). Group B: Teeth with mesio-occluso-distal (MOD) preparation/restoration with full-contour crowns (gingival seat 2 mm above the crown margin). Group C: Teeth with MOD preparation/restoration with DME and full-contour crowns (2 mm DME to crown margin). Group D: Teeth with MOD preparations with DME and full-contour crowns (4 mm DME to crown margin). The tooth-preparation scheme is shown in Figure 1.

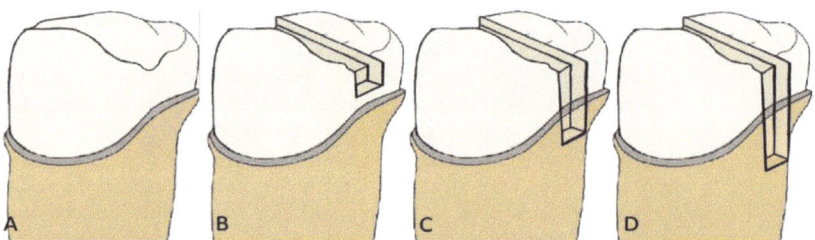

Figure 1. Schematic representation of groups. Group (**A**): Teeth with full-contour crowns without cavity preparation (control group). Group (**B**): Teeth with mesio-occluso-distal (MOD) preparation/restoration with full-contour crowns (gingival seat 2 mm above the crown margin). Group (**C**): Teeth with MOD preparation/restoration with DME and full-contour crowns (2 mm DME to crown margin). Group (**D**): Teeth with MOD preparations with DME and full-contour crowns (4 mm DME to crown margin).

2.4. Tooth Preparation

Orthodontic resin (Ortho-Resin, DeguDent GmbH, Hanau, Germany) was used to cover the roots of the teeth up to 5 mm below the CEJ. The preparation of samples was performed by one investigator to maintain uniformity. The proximal box preparations (mesial or/and distal) were conducted using a using a high-speed contra-angle handpiece Ti-Max Z900L (NSK, Nakanishi Inc., Tochigi, Japan) at a speed range of 320,000–400,000 rpm with a round-end tapered diamond (Bur # TR-14, ISO 198/022, Mani Inc., Tokyo, Japan), which was replaced by a new one for each tooth. The final tooth preparations had the following dimensions: 3 mm wide isthmus; 2 mm wide box at the gingival third and 4 mm occlusal width. The apical depth of the boxes in Group B was prepared 2 mm above the level of CEJ, and for Groups C and D, it was prepared 2 mm and 4 mm below the CEJ, respectively. For etching the dentin, 37% phosphoric acid gel (Prime-Dent, Chicago, IL, USA) was used for 15 s and rinsed with water. The excess water was then carefully removed by a brief burst of air, leaving the dentine and enamel surface slightly moist with a shiny surface. A fully saturated brush was used to apply the bonding agent (Bonding resin, Prime-Dent, Chicago, IL, USA) on the etched surface in two consecutive coats; it was air dried for 10 s and light-cured using an LED curing light (Smart lite max, Dentsply Caulk, Milford, DE, USA) for another 10 s on both the occlusal and proximal surfaces. The rest of the cavity in all samples was filled incrementally using a microhybrid composite, Filtek Z250 (3M ESPE, St. Paul, MN, USA), followed by light curing for 20 s.

Based on current principles of tooth preparation, for all-ceramic zirconia crowns, the occlusal surfaces were reduced by 2.0 mm, with a function-cusp bevel. A circumferential reduction by 1.0 mm was conducted, with the margins terminating at the CEJ. The final preparation had an axial wall taper of 6 to 8 degrees. The preparations were carried out using a flat-end long tapered diamond (Bur # TF-14, ISO 172/023, Mani Inc., Japan) with a highspeed contra-angle handpiece Ti-Max Z900L (NSK, Nakanishi Inc., Tochigi, Japan).

2.5. Fabrication of Crowns

All samples were digitally scanned using the Cercon eye scanner (DeguDent GmbH, Hanau, Germany) and designed by the software of Cercon art 3.2 (DeguDent GmbH,

Germany) to receive Cercon HT full-contoured crowns. The milling process was accomplished with a Cercon Xpert machine (DeguDent GmbH, Germany) after selecting a zirconia bur and a Cercon disc (DeguDent GmbH, Germany) containing 94.5% pure zirconium. To attain full strength, sintering was accomplished in the dental lab in a Cercon heat plus P8 machine (Dentsply Sirona, NC, USA) set at 8 h and 30 min by a dental technician with a sintering device Cercon Heat (DeguDent GmbH, Germany). The visually unacceptable teeth and those with margin damages were rejected, and another coping was made as needed. The intaglio surface of the Zi crowns were pretreated, mechanically, through air blasting with alumina oxide and cleaned with an alkaline agent, Ivoclean (ivoclar vivadent, Schaan, Liechtenstein), before cementation.

2.6. Cementation

The cementation of the crowns was conducted using an A2 shade, dual-cure, self-adhesive resin cement, RelyX U200 (3M, St. Paul, MN, USA), under a constant load of 20 N. The load was applied using a surveyor assembly machine to ensure equal pressure over the crowns, which were then light-cured for 20 secs per surface after cleaning the excess cement beyond the margins.

2.7. Aging

The aging of the samples to stimulate clinical conditions was conducted in a thermocycling machine (SD Mechnotronik THE 1100, Feldkirchen-Westerham, Germany). The samples were placed in a 10 × 10 open specimen basket and subjected to 5000 cycles in a water bath at (5 to 55 °C) for 30 s/cycle and a 5 s transfer time.

2.8. Fracture Test

Samples were subjected to a fracture test using the MTS 810 Universal Testing Machine (Eden Prairie, MN, USA). After mounting the samples on a metal base at a vertical angle, a stainless-steel flat-load cell was used, making sure that it contacted both the cusps before the force was applied in a vertical direction along the long axis of the tooth (Figure 2). The maximum force until fracture (1 mm/1 min) of the sample was recorded.

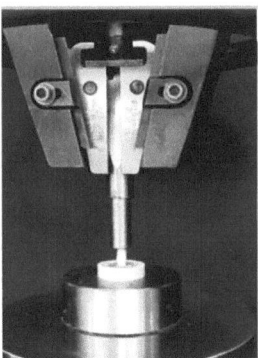

Figure 2. Fracture resistance test using Universal Testing Machine.

2.9. Statistical Analysis

ANOVA was used for the statistical analysis of the data. The comparative evaluation of the means was performed using the Tukey HSD post hoc test. A calculated p-value of less than 0.05 was considered significant.

3. Results

The maximum load-to-fracture values in newtons (N) and fracture-resistance values in megapascals (MPa) for the samples in all groups are listed in Table 1.

Table 1. Maximum load and fracture-resistance scores of samples in different groups.

Sample	Control		Mesio-Occluso-Distal (MOD) Tooth Preparation					
	A		B		C		D	
	Maximum Load (N)	FR (MPa)	Maximum Load (N)	FR (MPa)	Maximum Load (N)	FR (MPa)	Maximum Load (N)	FR (MPa)
1	3436.55	72.65	2040.66	56.06	1460.13	34.97	1368.39	30.23
2	3586.65	75.82	2072.61	45.22	2012.64	42.62	2285.31	40.88
3	3479.02	73.55	1801.64	49.57	2253.41	51.77	2168.52	45.84
4	3219.50	68.06	2222.84	48.38	2704.48	57.17	2103.77	41.80
5	3357.72	70.98	2959.94	62.57	2173.11	45.94	2180.15	43.61
6	3485.54	73.69	3170.40	67.02	2452.58	51.85	1358.02	32.16
7	3411.18	72.11	2737.58	57.87	1582.64	47.36	1883.83	48.56
8	3393.20	71.73	2654.50	56.12	2014.36	42.58	1979.91	45.99
9	3436.22	72.64	2773.51	58.63	2597.09	54.90	1854.38	41.00
10	3350.55	70.83	2507.50	53.01	1832.15	49.87	1737.28	36.72

N, Newtons; FR, Fracture resistance; MPa, Megapascals. Group A: Tooth preparation to receive full-contour crowns. Group B: Tooth preparation to receive full-contour crowns and mesio-occluso-distal (MOD) cavity preparation. Group C: Tooth preparation to receive full-contour crowns and MOD cavity preparation with DME (2 mm DME to crown margin). Group D: Tooth preparation to receive full-contour crowns and MOD tooth preparation with DME (4 mm DME to crown margin).

To compare and interpret the results of the experimental data seen in Table 1, analysis of variance (ANOVA) was performed using the mean values of each group, as seen in Table 2 and represented as bar diagrams in Figures 3 and 4.

Table 2. Comparison between groups using one-way ANOVA.

Units	Groups	n	Mean	Std. Deviation	95% Confidence Interval		p-Value
					Lower Bound	Upper Bound	
Max load(N)	A	10	3415.61	97.52	3345.8503	3485.3757	<0.00001 ***
	B	10	2494.11	443.97	2176.5202	2811.7158	
	C	10	2108.25	412.15	1813.4246	2403.0934	
	D	10	1891.95	325.14	1659.3600	2124.5520	
FR (MPa)	A	10	72.21	2.06	70.737	73.687	<0.00001 ***
	B	10	55.45	6.63	50.701	60.199	
	C	10	47.90	6.64	43.157	52.659	
	D	10	40.68	6.00	36.391	44.979	

***, Very high levels of significance with p value ≤ 0.05.

The results showed very high levels of significance among the groups, with the highest load and resistance to fracture seen in the control group, where the Zi crown was cemented on the prepared tooth without any cavity preparation or use of DME. On the other hand, the crowned teeth in Group D, which had MOD restorations and DME with a depth of 4 mm on either side, displayed the least load and resistance to fracture.

In order to compare and assess the significance between individual groups, the Tukey HSD post hoc test was performed, Table 3.

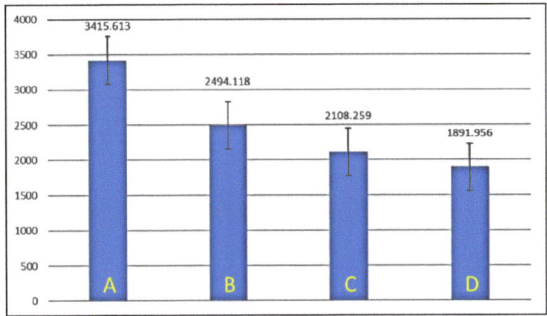

Figure 3. Mean values of maximum load to fracture expressed in newtons (N). A, Group A; B, Group B; C, Group C; D, Group D.

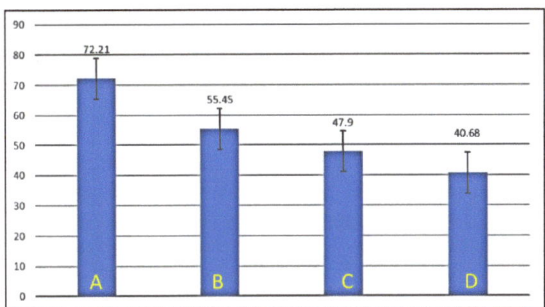

Figure 4. Mean values of fracture resistance in megapascals (MPa). A, Group A; B, Group B; C, Group C; D, Group D.

Table 3. Dependance of variable; Tukey HSD intergroup comparison.

Groups	Comparative Groups	Mean Difference	p	95% Confidence Interval	
				Lower Bound	Upper Bound
A	Group B	921.49500	<0.001 ***	465.0409	1377.9491
	Group C	1307.35400	<0.001 ***	850.8999	1763.8081
	Group D	1523.65700	<0.001 ***	1067.2029	1980.1111
B	Group C	385.85900	0.133	−70.5951	842.3131
	Group D	602.16200	0.004 **	145.7079	1058.6161
C	Group D	216.30300	0.664	−240.1511	672.7571

*** very highly significant; ** highly significant; with p value ≤ 0.05.

Very high levels of significance were seen when the control, Group A, was compared to all the other groups. Values of Group B also showed a very significant difference compared to Group D. Although the difference in means was noticeable between all the other groups, the results were not of significance.

Table 4 shows the percentages of failed patterns grouped under "restorable" for those samples with the presence of fracture lines or cracks on the Zi crowns, and "unrestorable" for those which failed below the CEJ.

Table 4. Failure patterns.

Groups	n	R (%)	U (%)
A	10	1 (10)	9 (90)
B	10	1 (10)	9 (90)
C	10	1 (10)	9 (90)
D	10	2 (20)	8 (80)

n, number of samples; R, restorable, with crack lines in the Zi crowns; U, unrestorable, with fractures below the CEJ.

4. Discussion

Modern restorative dentistry aims to preserve healthy dentition and replace missing tooth structures conservatively [18]. However, some clinical situations dictate excessive removal, compromising the strength of the remaining tooth structure, especially when the marginal ridges are removed [7,9]. Reeh et al. demonstrated that the tooth loses 63% of its stiffness if MOD preparations are made, and its FR was found to be lower than those teeth in which access opening was performed with intact walls [19]. More recently, a finite-element analysis (FEA) study demonstrated the least resistance to fracture in teeth where both the marginal ridges were removed, re-establishing the concept that the loss of tooth structure adversely affects the strength of the tooth [4]. The consolidation of such teeth should be accomplished by using IRs such as onlays or overlays, and in teeth which are compromised, full-coverage restorations are preferred [20].

Additionally, complete caries removal can also lead to the establishment of deep subgingival margins, which are often difficult to restore [21,22]. Surgical crown lengthening (SCL) is often the recommended treatment in such situations, where the cavity margins are relocated by apically displacing the periodontal attachment [23]. Despite its advantages, SCL is not always acceptable, due to delayed healing, loss of bony support, the elongation of clinical crowns, the development of black triangles and difficulties in estimating the final position of the margins [24].

Studies on the effect of DME on the periodontium indicate that it is well tolerated, both clinically and histologically [25]. In a long-term study comparing the survival rate of teeth, Mugri et al. suggested that the teeth in which DME was performed had a better rate of survival than those in which SCL was performed [24]. Dablanca-Blanco, in a case series, suggested the use of DME in teeth where the subgingival margins are limited in the epithelial tissue attachment, and SCL in teeth where the margins have reached the connective tissue attachment or the crestal bone level [2]. Ghezzi et al. proposed a new classification designed for choosing the line of treatment, based on the ability to isolate the tooth after caries removal and cavity preparation into class 1: nonsurgical DME, class 2a: surgical DME (gingival approach) and class 2b: surgical DME osseous approach [26].

In the present study, a traditional hybrid composite was used for the DME, as it is known to reduce marginal gap formation. The use of other materials such as glass ionomers, resin-modified glass ionomers and smart dentin replacement (SDR) bulk-fill composites for DME have also provided acceptable results with regards to FR, marginal adaptation and microleakage [27,28]. However, contrasting reports on the use of flowable composites have been reported in other studies [29]. The choice in hybrid composite in this study for DME and simultaneous restoration of the cavity was believed to eliminate the development of different interfaces.

The comparison of IRs such as onlays, overlays/partial crowns and full crowns have been extensively studied in the literature, with the majority of these studies reporting them to have clinical efficacy in excess of 93% [20,24]. Full-contour crowns continue to be used widely throughout the world, particularly in teeth which are extensively worn or severely destroyed [30]. A study comparing them to partial crowns found that the full crowns performed better from a technical, biologic and esthetic point of view [31]. Their use is time-tested and successful, regardless of the material and technique used to fabricate them [32]. However, with the use of CAD/CAM technology, monolith crowns fabricated entirely with Zi have gained popularity for use in posterior teeth due to their high strength and esthetics [20]. More recent studies on the clinical service of MZi crowns have shown a clinical success rate of more than 98% [14,33,34].

The FR of posterior teeth was determined previously to be in the range of 1120–2500 N [35]. In this study, the mean value for the maximum load required to fracture the teeth with MZi crowns, without being influenced by the effects of prior cavity preparations or DME, was found to be 3415.613 N (Group A). A 27% reduction in load to fracture was seen in Group B, which had mean values of 2494.118 N. This could be explained by the reduction in strength seen in teeth due to the effects of MOD cavity preparation/restoration. However, unlike in the teeth without crowns, where the effects of MOD preparations are severe, a less drastic reduction in strength was noticed due to the use of MZi crowns, which are known to provide cushioning and protection to the underlying tooth structures [36]. The mean values in this study were lower than those described by Nakamura et al., who reported that a load of 5000 N was required to fracture the crowns, slightly higher when than in another study which reported a mean value of 2337 N [37,38]. These differences could be due to the use of molar dyes fabricated using a hybrid polymer resin in the study by Nakamura, who also reported that the heights of axial walls could influence the FR of teeth under all ceramic crowns [37].

Research on the effects of DME on FR among indirect CAD/CAM restorations have generally focused on teeth with inlays, onlays, overlays and endocrowns. Most of these studies reported that the use of DME did not significantly impact the FR of teeth [21,22,39]. Grubbs et al., comparing the use of 2 mm-deep DME to CEJ in MOD cavities restored with onlays, displayed mean FR values between 1700 and 2029 N, which are slightly lower than in our study [28]. Furthermore, Zhang et al. demonstrated improved FR on root-canal-treated teeth, restored with CAD/CAM endocrowns following the use of DME [27,40]. Despite many such studies on IRs, the effect of DME on teeth under full-contour crowns have rarely been reported. Only one study could be partially compared to our study, in which the authors used CAD-/CAM-based monolith lithium–disilicate crowns over MOD prepared/restored premolars with DME [35]. The results showed fracture forces in the range of 1638–2253 N, comparable to values achieved in the experimental groups of this study where cavities (Groups B-D) were prepared, 1891.956–2494.118 N [41].

The type and site of fracture was visually evaluated. Failure type was classified based on the adaptation and modification from previous studies, as "restorable" for those with visible cracks and fracture lines on the zirconia crowns and "unrestorable" for those in which the fractures were seen below the CEJ [27,42,43]. In most of the samples in the present study, the teeth were unrestorably fractured below the CEJ. The results were expected due to the fact that MZi crowns usually fracture at higher loads and present with complete cohesive fractures, unlike the veneered zirconia crowns, which tend to chip [15]. Similar high percentages of unrestorable failure were seen in other in vitro studies [28,41,44]. The rationale for this could be the transmission of forces to the underlying natural teeth abutments, resulting in their fractures at high loads [15]. However, the choice in natural teeth in the present study was necessary to evaluate the effects of DME on FR, to better replicate the clinical scenario based on adhesive characteristics, strength and modulus of elasticity. The occurrence of restorable failures seen in the study could be related to fabrication defects compromising the integrity of MZi [45].

Under the limitations of this study, DME under normal depths (2 mm) rarely influenced the FR of teeth, except when the tooth structure was severely compromised, as in Group D. However, the load required to fracture the crowned teeth decreased as the extension of DME apical to the CEJ increased, thus rejecting the null hypothesis. Most of the samples failed unfavorably under maximum load. Nevertheless, more importantly, from a clinical point of view, the load required to fracture these samples far exceeded the maximum recorded biting force in posterior teeth, which is in the range of 800–1000 N [15].

In spite of the perceived advantages in this study, it has some limitations; a. The ease in performing the DME, especially where the distance to the crown margins is greater than 2 mm, might not be established in clinical settings without STA violations. b. Natural teeth variances in strength and morphology when compared to the dyes used in some of the other studies could have an influence on the results. c. The fracture of the teeth/MZi crown assembly was evaluated visually in this study; a more detailed fractographic evaluation would have provided precise details regarding the initiation and causes of cracks. The future trends in research will change the ever-evolving material choices for direct restorations and the development of monolith crowns using newer CAD/CAM technologies, which will help establish an ideal restorative choice, esthetically and functionally.

5. Conclusions

The loss of tooth structure, especially the marginal ridges, adversely affects the strength of teeth, even if supported by high-strength full-contour Zi crowns. The DME technique is suitable for use when deep margins are encountered, and the length of the DME-to-crown margins does not significantly impact its fracture resistance. However, caution should be undertaken in MOD preparations where the distance between the DME and the crown margins reaches 4 mm. Although unfavorable failures were common in this study, the load required to fracture all the samples, regardless of the DME margins, far exceeded the maximum recorded biting force.

Author Contributions: Conceptualization, A.R., A.A. (Abdullah Alqahtani), A.A. (Abdulrhman Alanazi) and A.M.; methodology, A.M., A.R., A.A. (Abdullah Alqahtani), A.M. and K.A.; software, A.M.; validation, A.R., K.A. and A.M.; formal analysis, R.A., A.S. and A.A. (Anas Aljarad); investigation, A.S. and M.A.; resources, A.A. (Abdullah Alqahtani); data curation, M.B.M.; writing—original draft preparation, M.B.M.; writing—review and editing, M.B.M., M.A., A.R. and A.A. (Anas Aljarad); visualization, R.A. and A.A. (Abdulrhman Alanazi); supervision, A.R.; project administration, A.S. and A.M. All authors have read and agreed to the published version of the manuscript.

Funding: This study is supported via funding from the Prince Sattam bin Abdulaziz University project number (PSAU/2023/R/1444).

Institutional Review Board Statement: This research was conducted in accordance with the Declaration of Helsinki and approved by the Institutional review board, PSAU, IRB No (PSAU2021011)) dated November 2021 and KSAU, CDRC No (FR0626).

Informed Consent Statement: Not applicable.

Data Availability Statement: Available on request.

Acknowledgments: The authors would like to acknowledge the Prince Sattam bin Abdulaziz University for their support in funding the study via project number (PSAU/2023/R/1444).

Conflicts of Interest: The authors declare no conflict of interest.

Abbreviations

CEJ, Cemento-enamel junction; DME, Deep marginal elevation; FEA, Finite-element analysis; FR, Fracture resistance; IR, Indirect restorations; LED, Light-emitting diode; MOD, Mesio-occluso-distal; MPa, Megapascals; MZi, Monolith Zirconia; N, Newtons; SCL, Surgical crown lengthening; SDR, Smart dentin replacement; STA, Supracrestal connective tissue attachment; Zi, Zirconia.

References

1. Serin Kalay, T.; Yildirim, T.; Ulker, M. Effects of different cusp coverage restorations on the fracture resistance of endodontically treated maxillary premolars. *J. Prosthet. Dent.* **2016**, *116*, 404–410. [CrossRef] [PubMed]
2. Dablanca-Blanco, A.B.; Blanco-Carrión, J.; Martín-Biedma, B.; Varela-Patiño, P.; Bello-Castro, A.; Castelo-Baz, P. Management of large class II lesions in molars: How to restore and when to perform surgical crown lengthening. *Restor. Dent. Endod.* **2017**, *42*, 240–252. [CrossRef] [PubMed]

3. Veneziani, M. Adhesive restorations in the posterior area with subgingival cervical margins: New classification and differentiated treatment approach. *Eur. J. Esthet. Dent.* **2010**, *5*, 50–76.
4. Magne, P.; Spreafico, R.C. Deep margin elevation: A paradigm shift. *Am. J. Esthet. Dent.* **2012**, *2*, 86–96.
5. Ferrari, M.; Koken, S.; Grandini, S.; Ferrari Cagidiaco, E.; Joda, T.; Discepoli, N. Influence of cervical margin relocation (CMR) on periodontal health: 12-month results of a controlled trial. *J. Dent.* **2018**, *69*, 70–76. [CrossRef]
6. Dietschi, D.; Spreafico, R. Current clinical concepts for adhesive cementation of tooth-colored posterior restorations. *Pract. Periodontics Aesthet. Dent.* **1998**, *10*, 47–56. [PubMed]
7. Juloski, J.; Köken, S.; Ferrari, M. Cervical margin relocation in indirect adhesive restorations: A literature review. *J. Prosthodont. Res.* **2018**, *62*, 273–280. [CrossRef]
8. Martins, T.M.; Bosco, A.F.; Nóbrega, F.J.; Nagata, M.J.; Garcia, V.G.; Fucini, S.E. Periodontal tissue response to coverage of root cavities restored with resin materials: A histomorphometric study in dogs. *J. Periodontol.* **2007**, *78*, 1075–1082. [CrossRef]
9. Shahmoradi, M.; Wan, B.; Zhang, Z.; Swain, M.; Li, Q. Mechanical failure of posterior teeth due to caries and occlusal wear- A modelling study. *J. Mech. Behav. Biomed. Mater.* **2022**, *125*, 104942. [CrossRef]
10. Abu-Awwad, M. Dentists' decisions regarding the need for cuspal coverage for endodontically treated and vital posterior teeth. *Clin. Exp. Dent. Res.* **2019**, *5*, 326–335. [CrossRef]
11. Irusa, K.; Al-Rawi, B.; Donovan, T.; Alraheam, I.A. Survival of cast gold and ceramic onlays placed in a school of Dentistry: A Retrospective Study. *J. Prosthodont.* **2020**, *29*, 693–698. [CrossRef]
12. Miyazaki, T.; Nakamura, T.; Matsumura, H.; Ban, S.; Kobayashi, T. Current status of zirconia restoration. *J. Prosthodont. Res.* **2013**, *57*, 236–261. [CrossRef] [PubMed]
13. Skjold, A.; Schriwer, C.; Olio, M. Effect of margin design on fracture load of zirconia crowns. *Eur. J. Oral Sci.* **2019**, *127*, 89–96. [CrossRef]
14. Kim, S.-H.; Yeo, M.-Y.; Choi, S.-Y.; Park, E.-J. Fracture resistance of monolith zirconia crowns depending on different marginal thicknesses. *Materials* **2022**, *15*, 4861. [CrossRef]
15. Sadeqi, H.A.; Baig, M.R.; Al-Shammari, M. Evaluation of marginal/internal fit and fracture load of monolithic zirconia and zirconia lithium silicate (ZLS) CAD/CAM crown systems. *Materials* **2021**, *14*, 6346. [CrossRef] [PubMed]
16. Raszewski, Z.; Brzakalski, D.; Derpenski, L.; Jalbrzykowski, M.; Przekop, R.E. Aspects and principles of material connections in Restorative dentistry—A comprehensive review. *Materials* **2022**, *15*, 7131. [CrossRef] [PubMed]
17. Thammajaruk, P.; Inokoshi, M.; Chong, S.; Guazzato, M. Bonding of composite cements to zirconia: A systematic review and meta-analysis of in vitro studies. *J. Mech. Behav. Biomed. Mater.* **2018**, *80*, 258–268. [CrossRef] [PubMed]
18. Grassi, E.D.A.; de Andrade, G.S.; Tribst, J.P.M.; Machry, R.V.; Valandro, L.F.; Ramos, N.D.C.; Bresciani, E.; Saavedra, G.D.S.F.A. Fatigue behavior and stress distribution of molars restored with MOD inlays with and without deep margin elevation. *Clin. Oral Investig.* **2021**, *26*, 2513–2526. [CrossRef]
19. Reeh, E.S.; Messer, H.H.; Douglas, W.H. Reduction in tooth stiffness as a result of endodontic and restorative procedures. *J. Endod.* **1989**, *15*, 512–516. [CrossRef]
20. Wang, B.; Fan, J.; Wang, L.; Xu, B.; Wang, L.; Chai, L. Onlays/partial crowns versus full crowns in restoring posterior teeth: A systematic review and meta-analysis. *Head Face Med.* **2022**, *18*, 36. [CrossRef]
21. Ilgenstein, I.; Zitzmann, N.; Bühler, J.; Wegehaupt, F.; Attin, T.; Weiger, R.; Krastl, G. Influence of proximal box elevation on the marginal quality and fracture behavior of root-filled molars restored with CAD/CAM ceramic or composite onlays. *Clin. Oral Investig.* **2014**, *19*, 1021–1028. [CrossRef]
22. Bresser, R.; van de Geer, L.; Gerdolle, D.; Schepke, U.; Cune, M.; Gresnigt, M. Influence of deep margin elevation and preparation design on the fracture strength of indirectly restored molars. *J. Mech. Behav. Biomed. Mater.* **2020**, *110*, 103950. [CrossRef] [PubMed]
23. Roggendorf, M.J.; Krämer, N.; Dippold, C.; Vosen, V.E.; Naumann, M.; Jablonski-Momeni, A.; Frankenberger, R. Effect of proximal box elevation with resin composite on marginal quality of resin composite inlays in vitro. *J. Dent.* **2012**, *40*, 1068–1073. [CrossRef]
24. Mugri, M.H.; Sayed, M.E.; Nedumgottil, B.M.; Bhandi, S.; Raj, A.T.; Testarelli, L.; Khurshid, Z.; Jain, S.; Patil, S. Treatment Prognosis of Restored Teeth with Crown Lengthening vs. Deep Margin Elevation: A Systematic Review. *Materials* **2021**, *14*, 6733. [CrossRef] [PubMed]
25. Bertoldi, C.; Monari, E.; Cortellini, P.; Generali, L.; Lucchi, A.; Spinato, S.; Zaffe, D. Clinical and Histological Reaction of Periodontal Tissues to Subgingival Resin Composite Restorations. *Clin. Oral Investig.* **2019**, *24*, 1001–1011. [CrossRef]
26. Ghezzi, C.; Brambilla, G.; Conti, A.; Dosoli, R.; Ceroni, F.; Ferrantino, L. Cervical margin relocation: Case series and new classifica-tion system. *Int. J. Esthet. Dent.* **2019**, *14*, 272–284. [PubMed]
27. Zhang, H.; Li, H.; Cong, Q.; Zhang, Z.; Du, A.; Wang, Y. Effect of proximal box elevation on fracture resistance and microleakage of premolars restored with ceramic endocrowns. *PLoS ONE* **2021**, *16*, e0252269. [CrossRef]
28. Grubbs, T.D.; Vargas, M.; Kolker, J.; Teixeira, E.C. Efficacy of direct restorative materials in proximal box elevation on the margin quality and fracture resistance of molars restored with CAD/CAM onlays. *Oper. Dent.* **2020**, *45*, 52–61. [CrossRef]
29. Scotti, N.; Baldi, A.; A Vergano, E.; Tempesta, R.M.; Alovisi, M.; Pasqualini, D.; Carpegna, G.C.; Comba, A. Tridimensional evaluation of the interfacial gap in deep cervical margin restorations: A micro-CT study. *Oper. Dent.* **2020**, *45*, E227–E236. [CrossRef]
30. Christensen, G.J. The case for onlays versus tooth-colored crowns. *J. Am. Dent. Assoc.* **2012**, *143*, 1141–1144. [CrossRef]

31. Al-Haj Husain, N.; Özcan, M.; Molinero-Mourelle, P.; Joda, T. Clinical performance of partial and full-coverage fixed dental restorations fabricated from hybrid polymer and ceramic CAD/CAM materials: A systematic review and meta-analysis. *J. Clin. Med.* **2020**, *9*, 2107. [CrossRef] [PubMed]
32. Larsson, C.; Wennerberg, A. The clinical success of zirconia-based crowns: A systematic review. *Int. J. Prosthodont.* **2014**, *27*, 33–43. [CrossRef] [PubMed]
33. Sulaiman, T.A.; Abdulmajeed, A.A.; Delgado, A.; Donovan, T.E. Fracture rate of 188695 lithium disilicate and zirconia ceramic restorations after up to 7.5 years of clinical service: A dental laboratory survey. *J. Prosthet. Dent.* **2020**, *123*, 807–810. [CrossRef]
34. Sola-Ruiz, M.F.; Baixauli-Lopez, M.; Roig-Vanaclocha, A.; Amengual-Lorenzo, J.; Agustin-Panadero, R. Prospective study of monolith zirconia crowns: Clinical behavior and survival rate at a 5-year follow-up. *J. Prosthodont. Res.* **2021**, *65*, 284–290. [CrossRef]
35. Göktürk, H.; Karaarslan, E.Ş.; Tekin, E.; Hologlu, B.; Sarıkaya, I. The effect of the different restorations on fracture resistance of root-filled premolars. *BMC Oral Health* **2018**, *18*, 196. [CrossRef] [PubMed]
36. Rekow, E.D.; Harsono, M.; Janal, M.; Thompson, V.P.; Zhang, G. Factorial analysis of variables influencing stress in all-ceramic crowns. *Dent. Mater.* **2006**, *22*, 125–132. [CrossRef] [PubMed]
37. Nakamura, K.; Harada, A.; Inagaki, R.; Kanno, T.; Niwano, Y.; Milleding, P.; Örtengren, U. Fracture resistance of monolithic zirconia molar crowns with reduced thickness. *Acta. Odontol. Scand.* **2015**, *73*, 602–608. [CrossRef]
38. Jassim, Z.M.; Majeed, M.A. Comparative evaluation of the fracture strength of monolithic crowns fabricated from different all-ceramic CAD/CAM materials (an in vitro study). *Biomed. Pharmacol. J.* **2018**, *11*, 1689–1697. [CrossRef]
39. Chen, Y.C.; Lin, C.L.; Hou, C.H. Investigating inlay designs of class II cavity with deep margin elevation using finite element method. *BMC Oral Health* **2021**, *21*, 264. [CrossRef]
40. Zhang, H. Fracture resistance of endodontically treated premolar with deep class II: In vitro evaluation of different restorative procedures. *Investig. Clin.* **2019**, *60*, 154–161.
41. Alahmari, N.M.; Adawi, H.A.; Moaleem, M.M.A.; Alqahtani, F.M.; Alshahrani, F.T.; Aldhelai, T.A. Effects of the cervical marginal relocation technique on the marginal adaptation of lithium disilicate CAD/CAM ceramic crowns on premolars. *J. Contemp. Dent. Pract.* **2021**, *22*, 900–906. [CrossRef] [PubMed]
42. Sorrentino, R.; Nagasawa, Y.; Infelise, M.; Bonadeo, G.; Ferrari, M. In vitro analysis of the fracture resistance of CAD-CAM monolithic lithium disilicate molar crowns with different occlusal thickness. *J. Osseointegr.* **2018**, *10*, 50–56. [CrossRef]
43. Yildiz, C.; Vanlıoğlu, B.A.; Evren, B.; Uludamar, A.; Ozkan, Y.K. Marginal-internal adaptation and fracture resistance of CAD/CAM crown restorations. *Dent. Mater. J.* **2013**, *32*, 42–47. [CrossRef] [PubMed]
44. Sorrentino, R.; Triulzio, C.; Tricarico, M.G.; Bonadeo, G.; Gherlone, E.F.; Ferrari, M. In vitro analysis of the fracture resistance of CAD-CAM monolithic zirconia molar crowns with different occlusal thickness. *J. Mech. Behav. Biomed. Mater.* **2016**, *61*, 328–333. [CrossRef]
45. Zhang, Y.; Mai, Z.; Barani, A.; Bush, M.; Lawn, B. Fracture-resistant monolithic dental crowns. *Dent. Mater.* **2016**, *32*, 442–449. [CrossRef]

Disclaimer/Publisher's Note: The statements, opinions and data contained in all publications are solely those of the individual author(s) and contributor(s) and not of MDPI and/or the editor(s). MDPI and/or the editor(s) disclaim responsibility for any injury to people or property resulting from any ideas, methods, instructions or products referred to in the content.

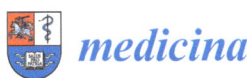

Article

The Impact of Anemia-Related Early Childhood Caries on Parents' and Children's Quality of Life

Dila Özyılkan [1], Özgür Tosun [2] and Aylin İslam [3,*]

1 Pediatric Dentistry Department, Faculty of Dentistry, Near East University, Nicosia 99138, Cyprus
2 Department of Biostatistics, Faculty of Medicine, Near East University, Nicosia 99138, Cyprus
3 Pediatric Dentistry Department, Faculty of Dentistry, European University of Lefke, Lefke 99010, Cyprus
* Correspondence: aislam@eul.edu.tr; Tel.: +90-392-660-2000; Fax: +90-392-727-7528

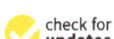

Citation: Özyılkan, D.; Tosun, Ö.; İslam, A. The Impact of Anemia-Related Early Childhood Caries on Parents' and Children's Quality of Life. *Medicina* 2023, 59, 521. https://doi.org/10.3390/medicina59030521

Academic Editors: Giuseppe Minervini and Stefania Moccia

Received: 19 January 2023
Revised: 27 February 2023
Accepted: 28 February 2023
Published: 7 March 2023

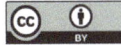

Copyright: © 2023 by the authors. Licensee MDPI, Basel, Switzerland. This article is an open access article distributed under the terms and conditions of the Creative Commons Attribution (CC BY) license (https://creativecommons.org/licenses/by/4.0/).

Abstract: *Background and Objectives*: Today, oral diseases are well-known for their effects, not only on daily life but also on quality of life (QoL). Dental caries, especially early childhood caries (ECC), are considered a public health concern as regards their impact on the life quality of children and parents from multiple aspects. The present research was conducted to assess the effect of anemia on oral-health-related quality of life (OHRQoL) in terms of children and parents. *Materials and Methods*: The current study was performed in two independent stages. In the first stage, the Turkish version of the Early Childhood Oral Health Impact Scale (ECOHIS), and in the second stage, the Turkish version of the Parental-Caregivers Perceptions Questionnaire (P-CPQ) were used to measure the effect of anemia-related dental caries among children and parents. SPSS and Jamovi software were used for all calculations, graphs and comparisons. *Results*: A total of 204 participants (child–parent pairs) were incorporated in the present study. A considerable number of children (81.5%) reported occasional or more frequent oral/dental pain. Secondly, the subscale scores were determined for child symptoms (2.25 ± 0.067), child function (6.8 ± 0.22), child psychology (3.87 ± 0.128), self-image and social interaction (1.74 ± 0.063), parental distress (3.82 ± 0.143), and family function (3.5 ± 0.121). Additionally, more than half of the parents (56.3%) responded "fair" for the health of their children's teeth, lips, jaws and mouth. Similarly, the child's overall well-being was stated as being affected "a lot" by the condition of their child's teeth, lips, jaws or mouth by half of the parents (49.5%). *Conclusions*: Anemia-related dental caries has a highly negative impact on the quality of life of children and parents according to both of the questionnaires. Therefore, children with high scores should be prioritized for preventive procedures and timely dental treatments.

Keywords: anemia; quality of life; children; parent

1. Introduction

Today, oral diseases are well-known for their effects not only on daily life but also on quality of life (QoL), as oral health exhibits the main physiological, social and psychological characteristics that are fundamental for quality of life [1,2]. In this sense, the evaluation of oral health related to quality of life (OHRQoL) has come into prominence. The existence of dental disease, treatment experience, and oral health issues can cause unfavorable effects on the quality of daily life of children and parents [3–5]. Dental caries, especially early childhood caries (ECC), sre considered a public health concern due to their impact on the quality of life of children and parents through multiple aspects such as pain, eating disorders, sleeping problems, taking time off from school, social embarrassment for children, and financial problems related to treatment fees and time off work for parents [6–8]. Evaluating and measuring the child's OHRQoL to help display the priority of care and the interpretation of treatment outcomes have gained popularity [9].

Even though various studies have mentioned the multifactorial etiology of ECC, including behavioral, socioeconomic, biological, and environmental factors, the relationship between anemia (particularly associated with malnutrition, iron deficiency, and vitamin D deficiency) and ECC has recently been highlighted. According to recent studies, it has been shown that there is a correlation between ECC and anemia, which is defined as the number of red blood cells or the oxygen-carrying capacity of blood being below normal levels [10–13]. Particularly, the possible mechanism of iron deficiency anemia (IDA) in the development of dental caries is the potential inhibitory effect of iron on cariogenic microorganisms [14]. The clinical and practical significance of iron and ferritin deficiency on dental caries was identified by the findings of a recent meta-analysis, which reported that children with caries had significantly lower levels of salivary and serum iron and ferritin [15]. Previous cross-sectional and case studies have also demonstrated that children with anemia or IDA have a higher risk of caries development. Additionally, the anticariogenic potential of iron in *Streptococcus mutans (S. mutans)* has been shown through the following mechanisms: (1) prevention of enamel demineralization in an acidic environment; (2) decreasing the level of dental plaque acidity, and (3) disinfectant and bacteriostatic capacity in *S. mutans*; and (4) inhibition of the glycosyltransferase activity [16–21]. Although the reasons regarding the theoretical basis for the link between anemia and ECC are described and discussed, there has been no research reported in the literature that underlines the effect of anemia-related dental caries on the OHRQoL of children and families. To date, numerous questionnaires have been developed in order to evaluate the OHRQoL for children, adults, and for families. However, self-reports of very young children on their oral health tend to be unreliable, and the reports are inefficient for different age groups [22]. Hence, the Early Childhood Oral Health Impact Scale (ECOHIS) was designed to measure the relationship between parents' perceptions of their children's quality of life and their oral health [23] together with the Parental-Caregivers Perceptions Questionnaire (P-CPQ), which is another scale that is used to evaluate oral health quality of the child from the perception of the parental/caregiver by providing good evidence of responsiveness [24].

In the current literature research, no study was found showing the effect of the presence of anemia on OHRQoL. The present research was conducted to assess the effect of anemia on oral-health-related quality of life (OHRQoL) in terms of children and parents.

2. Materials and Methods

2.1. Ethical Approval

The present cross-sectional study was conducted between June 2022 and August 2022 and performed at the Dr. Burhan Nalbantoğlu Government Hospital located in Northern Cyprus. The current research was approved by the Dr. Burhan Nalbantoğlu Government Hospital (YTK 1.01-30/22).

2.2. Data Collection and Participants

All data were collected following ethical approval. Firstly, all parents (mother/father) of children attending the Dr. Burhan Nalbantoğlu Government Hospital and diagnosed with anemia were analyzed and detected from the hospital's archive. Later, the children aged between 2 and 18 years who presented at the dental clinic (Dr. Burhan Nalbantoğlu Government Hospital) with the complaint of dental caries, and without any accompanying systemic disease or an otherwise noncontributory medical history (except for anemia), were determined as meeting the inclusion criteria of the current study. Children with no anemia diagnosis or dental caries, parents living outside of Northern Cyprus, uncooperative children and families, children with a mental disorder, children who applied to the dental clinic with signs that constituted advanced infection (dental trauma/cellulitis), and children undergoing long-term antibiotic treatment were excluded from the study. Parents who enrolled in the study did so on a voluntary basis and received an informed-consent form to answer their questions.

The children who participated in the present study were screened by two of the pediatric dentists for the presence or absence of S-ECC, according to the AAPD guidelines [25], the first time they applied at the dental clinic. Five percent of all inspection objects were randomly selected and repeated for each day. Repeat checks were carried out in agreement with inter-investigator agreement.

2.3. Sample Size Determination and Questionnaire Design

G* power software (Ver.3.1.9.4) was used for the calculation of sample size. With a confidence level of 95% and a confidence interval of 7.5%, the targeted statistical power of 80% was calculated as 190. The current study was performed in two independent stages. In the first stage, the Turkish version of the ECOHIS was used, and in the second stage, the Turkish version of the P-CPQ was used to measure the effect of anemia-related dental caries among children and parents [26,27].

The questionnaire consisted of 61 questions divided into three parts: demographic information, ECOHIS questionnaire, and P-CPQ. Questions about parents' relationship to the child, age, education level, occupation, marital status, number of children, income level, and their duties are asked in the demographic information section. Medication prescribed for the anemia, age of diagnosis, and age of starting medication questions were determined, and responses were recorded in the demographic information. The second part of the questionnaire includes the Early Childhood Oral Health Impact Scale (ECOHIS), which assesses Oral Health Related Quality of Life (OHRQoL). In the present study, the accepted and reliable Turkish form of the ECOHIS was used (26). The scale includes two parts, child impact and family impact, with 13 questions. The child impact part has subscales of child symptoms (1 question), child function (4 questions), child psychology (2 questions), and child self-image and social interaction (2 questions). The family impact part includes parental distress (2 questions) and family function (2 questions). Response classes for every question were rated on a five-point Likert scale: 0 = never; 1 = hardly ever; 2 = occasionally; 3 = often; 4 = very often; 5 = don't know. For the child impact section, the score for children can vary from 0 to 36, and for the family impact section, the score can vary from 0 to 16, and so the system creates a total score range of 0 to 52. ECOHIS scores were calculated separately as a straightforward addition of the response codes for the child impact and family impact sections. According to the scale, higher scores demonstrate greater impact. For the ECOHIS scale, all "don't know" (DK) responses were coded as missing. For the third part, the Turkish-accepted validity and reliability version of the Parental-Caregiver Perceptions Questionnaire (P-CPQ) was used to evaluate the QoL of children [20]. The scale includes 31 questions with 4 subscales of oral symptoms (6 questions), functional limitations (8 questions), emotional well-being (7 questions), and social well-being (10 questions). As with the ECOHIS, the P-CPQ was also rated on a 5-point Likert scale of never: 0; once/twice: 1; sometimes: 2; often: 3; and every day/almost every day: 4. General well-being was scored as follows: not at all = 0; very little = 1; somewhat = 2; a lot = 3; and very much = 4. For subscales, scores can vary for oral symptoms from 0–24, for functional limitations from 0–32, for emotional well-being from 0–28, and for social well-being from 0–40. Total scores were added, and a total-scale score was obtained. Similarly to the ECOHIS scale, a higher score represents a worse effect on quality of life. Parents who enrolled in the study did so on a voluntary basis and received the informed consent form of the study. Before the participating parents were selected, children were confirmed to have dental ECC.

2.4. Statistical Analysis

Descriptive statistics for qualitative variables (frequency and percentage) and quantitative variables (arithmetic mean ± standard deviation) were calculated. Parametric test assumptions were controlled for the data, and the Shapiro–Wilk or Kolmogorov–Smirnov normality test was applied where appropriate. Non-parametric hypothesis tests were accordingly performed due to the distribution characteristics. For two independent groups, the Mann–Whitney U test was applied to evaluate the significance of the differences. In the case of more than two independent groups, the Kruskal–Wallis test was performed. In the case of significance, the Dwass–Steel–Critchlow–Fligner test was further performed to assess the pairwise significance. To investigate the associations between scale scores, the

Pearson correlation test was performed. Cronbach's alpha was calculated for each scale and subscale score to evaluate the reliability of the surveys. The level of significance was accepted to be 0.05. SPSS (Demo version 25.0 for Mac) and Jamovi (Version 2.2.0) software were used for all calculations, graphs, and comparisons.

3. Results

3.1. Sociodemographic Characteristics of Parents and Children

A total of 204 participants (child–parent pairs) were incorporated in the present study. Among the participants, 146 (71.6%) were mothers, and 58 (24.8%) were fathers, while 94 (46%) of children were male, and 110 (54%) were female. The age of parents ranged between 21 and 30 (26/12.7%), 31 and 40 (104/51%), and >40 (74/36.3%). Furthermore, the majority of respondents (79.3%) were well-educated (graduate–postgraduate level). Anemia type and medical treatment for this disease were also assessed. Responses related to anemia type were as follows: 54.5% for iron deficiency anemia, 29.5% for 25-hydroxyvitamin D deficiency anemia, and 9.3% for vitamin B12 deficiency anemia. Additionally, 151 (74%) of children had received medical treatment, and 53 (26%) of them had received no medical treatment for anemia. All details related to sociodemographic characteristics of parents and children are given in Table 1.

Table 1. Sociodemographic characteristics of parents and children.

Characteristics	Number (*n*)	Percentage (%)
Demographic characteristics of parents		
Parental Relationship		
Mother	146	71.6
Father	58	28.4
Age (Years)		
21–30	26	12.7
31–40	104	51.0
>40	74	36.3
Educational Level		
Primary–high school	42	20.7
Graduate–postgraduate	161	79.3
Employment Status and Occupation		
Non-health professional	103	50.5
Health professional	78	38.2
Unemployed	23	11.3
Marital Status		
Married	176	86.3
Single	28	13.7
Family Income (Monthly/EUR) *		
333 (minimum wage)	45	22.3
334–555	57	28.2
>555	100	49.5
Demographic characteristics of children		

Table 1. *Cont.*

Characteristics	Number (n)	Percentage (%)
Gender		
Male	94	46.1
Female	110	53.9
Anemia type		
Iron deficiency anemia	111	54.4
25-hydroxyvitamin D deficiency anemia	60	29.4
Vitamin B12 deficiency anemia	19	9.3
Other	13	6.4
Medical treatment for anemia		
Yes	151	74.0
No	53	26.0

* Monthly family income measured in TRY (Turkish lira, EUR 1 = TRY 18).

3.2. Results of P-CPQ

The answers to two general questions which were asked to parents before the Turkish version of the P-CPQ, "How would you rate the health of your child's teeth, lips, jaws and mouth?" and "How much is your child's overall well-being affected by the condition of his/her teeth, lips, jaws or mouth?" are shown in Table 2.

Table 2. Child's oral health and well-being from Parental Caregiver Perception Questionnaire (P-CPQ).

Health of Your Child's Teeth, Lips, Jaws and Mouth	Number (n)	Percentage (%)
Excellent	11	5.4
Very good	14	6.9
Good	52	25.5
Fair	115	56.4
Poor	12	5.9
Child's oral well-being affected by the condition of his/her teeth, lips, jaws or mouth		
Not at all	14	6.9
Very little	20	9.8
Some	51	25
A lot	101	49.5
Very much	18	8.8

More than half of parents (56.3%) responded *"fair"* for the health of their children's teeth, lips, jaws and mouth. Similarly, the child's overall well-being was stated as being affected *"a lot"* by the condition of their child's teeth, lips, jaws or mouth by half of parents (49.5%).

Besides the abovementioned two general questions, the descriptive statistical analyses (the values of mean, standard error, and percentage) of each item in all four subscales with general impacts are given in Table 3.

The subscale scores for oral symptoms (OS), functional limitations (FL), emotional well-being (EWB), and social well-being (SWB) domains were calculated as 12 ± 0.413, 10.36 ± 0.385, 7.75 ± 0.412 and 7.13 ± 0.513, respectively. Moreover, the P-CPQ total score (TS), which was determined by summing up the scores of all 31 items, was 36 ± 1.36. The highest percentages of impacts were reported as *"often"* in the oral symptoms subscale for the items of *"pain in teeth and mouth/45.1%"*, *"bleeding gums/38.2%"*, *"mouth sores/37.3%"*, *"bad breath/40.4%"*, and *"food caught between teeth/39.7%"* by parents. Furthermore, few *"don't know (DK)"* responses, which were accepted as *"missing"*, were recorded. Only 11 parents ticked DK as an answer in one item of oral symptoms and three items of emotional and social well-being.

The results of association between overall and subscale scores of the P-CPQ with demographic factors are given in Table 4, and more than one statistically significant comparisons were obtained in the subscale scores regarding demographic factors. Firstly, the scores of functional limitations between parental relationship were detected to be significant ($p = 0.032$). Mothers (10.01 ± 0.44) reported less functional limitation compared to fathers (12.05 ± 0.749). Another statistically-significant difference was detected between the educational level of parents in the oral symptoms subscale ($p = 0.002$). The parents with higher educational levels reported a higher impact in comparison to parents with lower education levels (8.38 ± 0.866, 11.43 ± 0.419, respectively). When the responses for medical treatment for anemia (yes/no) were analyzed, all differences in each subscale and total score were observed as significant ($p = 0.006$ for OS, $p < 0.001$ for FL, $p = 0.008$ for EWB, $p = 0.03$ for SWB, and $p < 0.001$ for TS). To elaborate on this further, the parents whose children take medical treatment for anemia reported a larger effect on children in all subscale scores. Another significant difference was observed for the sensitive analysis conducted between health professionals and unemployed groups in the oral symptom subscale. Health professional groups responded that their children were more affected in the oral symptom subscale compared to those of unemployed parents ($p = 0.04$).

3.3. Results of ECOHIS

The responses to each item in the ECOHIS questionnaire are represented in Table 5 by giving detailed descriptive statistical analyses (the values of mean, standard error and percentage). First of all, a large number of children (81.5%) reported occasional or more frequent oral/dental pain. Secondly, the subscale scores were determined for child symptoms (2.25 ± 0.067), child function (6.8 ± 0.22), child psychology (3.87 ± 0.128), self-image and social interaction (1.74 ± 0.063), parental distress (3.82 ± 0.143), and family function (3.5 ± 0.121). The values of child impact, family impact and total score were calculated according to responses to each item (16.3 ± 0.486, 7.32 ± 0.242, 23.6 ± 0.701, respectively). Moreover, a detailed analysis on descriptive statistics of the ECOHIS further showed that several children (160, 79.2%) had difficulty drinking and that 152 (76.7%) children had trouble eating food occasionally or more frequently. According to family impact section responses, the majority of parents reported that they felt upset (142/70.6%) and guilty (138/69.3%) occasionally or more frequently. Likewise, 73.1% of parents stated that they take time off from work, and 69% of parents reported that their child's dental procedures occasionally or more frequently had a financial impact on the family.

The association between overall and subscale scores of the ECOHIS and demographic data is given in Table 6.

The statistically-significant results were observed in groups of educational level and medical treatment for anemia. The most dramatic results were seen in the medical treatment group for parents with children taking medical treatment for anemia, who reported a much larger impact on the child and family and larger total scores in comparison to parents with children not taking medical treatment ($p < 0.001$ for all comparisons). Regarding parental education level, the results for primary–high-school graduated parents for child impact and total score were lower than those for graduate–postgraduate parents ($p < 0.016$, $p < 0.025$ respectively). An additional pairwise comparison regarding employment status and occupations of parents revealed that the comparison between non-health professional and unemployed parents had a statistically significant value in the total score ($p = 0.028$).

Table 3. Descriptive statistics and summary of Parental Caregiver Perception Questionnaire (P-CPQ) responses (n = 204).

Impacts	Mean	SE *	Never: 0	Once/Twice: 1	Sometimes: 2	Often: 3	Every Day/Almost Every Day: 4	Missing
Oral symptoms subscale (6 items)								
Pain in teeth and mouth	1.917	0.082	36(17.6)	41(20.1)	33(16.2)	92(45.1)	2(1)	0
Bleeding gums	1.667	0.087	56(27.5)	34(16.7)	36(17.6)	78(38.2)	0(0)	0
Mouth sores	1.735	0.0845	46(22.5)	42(20.6)	38(18.6)	76(37.3)	2(1)	0
Bad breath	2.005	0.0767	27(13.3)	35(17.2)	55(27.1)	82(40.4)	4(2)	1
Food stuck to roof of mouth	1.461	0.07	51(25)	31(15.2)	101(49.5)	19(9.3)	2(1)	0
Food caught between teeth	1.995	0.075	26(12.7)	36(17.6)	58(28.4)	81(39.7)	3(1.5)	0
General	12	0.413						
Functional limitation subscale (8 items)								
Difficulty chewing firm food	1.922	0.0823	38(18.6)	30(14.7)	51(25)	80(39.2)	5(2.5)	0
Breathing through mouth	0.956	0.0787	102(50)	36(17.6)	43(21.1)	19(9.3)	4(2)	0
Trouble sleeping	1.495	0.0686	47(23)	30(14.7)	110(53.9)	13(6.4)	4(2)	0
Unclear speech	0.701	0.071	127(62.3)	25(12.3)	41(20.1)	8(3.9)	3(1.5)	0
Slow eating	1.451	0.0619	40(19.6)	44(21.6)	110(53.9)	8(3.9)	2(1)	0
Difficulty drinking/eating hot/cold foods	1.265	0.0636	40(19.6)	92(45.1)	52(25.5)	18(8.8)	2(1)	0
Difficulty eating preferred foods	1.564	0.0649	39(19.1)	31(15.2)	117(57.4)	14(6.9)	3(1.5)	0
Restricted diet	1.235	0.0627	49(24)	70(34.3)	75(36.8)	8(3.9)	2(1)	0
General	10.6	0.385						
Emotional well-being subscale (7 items)								
Upset	2	0.0789	33(16.2)	29(14.2)	48(23.5)	93(45.6)	1(0.5)	0
Irritable/frustrated	0.971	0.0839	111(54.4)	25(12.3)	32(15.7)	35(17.2)	1(0.5)	0
Anxious/fearful	1.851	0.0893	49(24.3)	31(15.3)	24(11.9)	97(48)	1(0.5)	2
Worried about being different from other people	0.716	0.0757	131(64.2)	24(11.8)	26(12.7)	22(10.8)	1(0.5)	0
Worried he or she is less attractive than others	0.775	0.0792	127(62.3)	25(12.3)	25(12.3)	25(12.3)	2(1)	0
Shy (embarrassed)	0.833	0.0803	120(59.1)	27(13.3)	28(13.8)	26(12.8)	2(1)	1
Worried about having few friends	0.522	0.0703	150(73.9)	19(9.4)	19(9.4)	11(5.4)	4(2)	1

Table 3. Cont.

Impacts	Mean	SE *	n (%)					Missing
			Never: 0	Once/Twice: 1	Sometimes: 2	Often: 3	Every Day/Almost Every Day: 4	
General	7.75	0.412						
Social well-being subscale (10 items)								
Missed school	1.328	0.0679	50(24.5)	58(28.4)	77(37.7)	17(8.3)	2(1)	0
Had hard time paying attention in school	0.824	0.0804	122(59.8)	26(12.7)	29(14.2)	24(11.8)	3(1.5)	0
Not wanting to speak/read aloud in class	0.74	0.0773	128(62.7)	24(11.8)	35(17.2)	11(5.4)	6(2.9)	0
Not wanting to talk other children	0.611	0.0674	134(66)	27(13.3)	30(14.8)	11(5.4)	1(0.5)	1
Avoiding smiling when around other children	1.118	0.0683	65(32)	67(33)	55(27.1)	14(6.9)	2(1)	1
Teased/called names by other children	0.348	0.0578	163(79.9)	24(11.8)	7(3.4)	7(3.4)	3(1.5)	0
Left out by other children	0.324	0.0507	162(79.4)	25(12.3)	10(4.9)	7(3.4)	0	0
Not wanting/unable to be with other children	0.539	0.0615	137(67.2)	33(16.2)	26(12.7)	7(3.4)	1(0.5)	0
Not wanting/unable to take part in activities	0.529	0.0686	149(73)	19(9.3)	21(10.3)	13(6.4)	2(1)	0
Asked by other children about the condition	0.705	0.0763	127(63.5)	29(14.5)	23(11.5)	18(9)	3(1.5)	4
General	7.13	0.523						
Total Score	36	1.36						

* Standard error.

Table 4. Association between overall and subscale scores of Parental Caregiver Perception Questionnaire (P-CPQ) with demographic factors.

	Subscale Scores																			Total Score (TS)			
	Oral Symptoms (OS)				Functional Limitations (FL)				Emotional Well-Being (EWB)				Social Well-Being (SWB)									
	Mean	Median	SE*	p value	Mean	Median	SE*	p value	Mean	Median	SE*	p value	Mean	Median	SE*	p value	Mean	Median	SE*	p value			
Parental Relationship																							
Mother	10.47	11.00	0.488	0.237	10.01	11.00	0.440	0.032	7.71	6.00	0.502	0.628	6.87	3.00	0.624	0.222	34.84	37.00	1.639	0.143			
Father	11.52	12.00	0.775		12.05	12.00	0.749		7.83	6.00	0.716		7.75	4.00	0.962		39.07	38.00	2.380				
Age (Years)																					Pairwise comparisons	OS	FL	EWB	SWB	TS
21–30	8.04	8.00	1.050	0.002	9.88	9.50	1.310	0.532	7.12	4.50	1.250	0.390	8.60	5.00	1.610	0.177	33.30	32.00	4.440	0.696	21–30/31–40	0.002	0.402	0.445	0.905	0.613
31–40	12.00	13.00	0.547		11.30	11.00	0.453		8.07	6.00	0.574		6.82	3.00	0.689		37.90	37.00	1.690		21–30/>40	0.314	0.993	0.799	0.684	0.992
>40	10.00	10.00	0.714		9.88	12.00	0.711		7.53	6.00	0.673		7.04	3.50	0.908		34.40	37.00	2.440		31–40/>40	0.064	0.703	0.854	0.784	0.574
Educational Level																										
Primary–high school	8.38	8.50	0.866	0.002	11.02	12.00	0.939	0.076	8.17	7.00	0.817		8.54	6.00	1.167		35.98	38.00	2.906							
Graduate–postgraduate	11.43	12.00	0.419		10.40	11.00	0.416		7.59	6.00	0.476		6.76	3.00	0.584		35.93	37.00	1.543							
Employment Status and Occupation																					Pairwise comparisons	OS	FL	EWB	SWB	TS
Non-health professional	10.70	11.00	0.579		10.40	12.00	0.555		8.17	6.00	0.607		7.94	4.00	0.784		37.00	38.00	1.980		Non-health professional/health professional	0.711	0.872	0.801	0.34	0.766
Health professional	11.60	13.00	0.670		11.60	11.00	0.558		7.52	6.00	0.661		6.23	3.00	0.794		35.70	37.00	2.110		Non-health professional/unemployed	0.153	0.916	0.599	0.69	0.795
Unemployed	8.30	8.00	1.140		11.40	11.00	1.410		6.61	6.00	0.903		6.52	5.00	1.380		32.80	37.00	4.070		Health professional/unemployed	0.04	0.928	0.881	0.996	0.928
Marital Status																										
Married	10.87	12.00	0.437	0.661	10.32	11.00	0.395	0.198	7.67	6.00	0.443	0.570	6.89	3.00	0.553	0.188	35.48	37.00	1.452	0.216						
Single	10.14	10.00	1.244		12.29	12.00	1.281		8.21	6.50	1.128		8.63	5.00	1.564		39.57	39.00	3.818							
Family Income (Monthly/EUR)*																					Pairwise comparisons	OS	FL	EWB	SWB	TS
333 (minimum wage)	11.50	13.00	0.951		10.90	12.00	0.782		7.38	6.00	0.677		6.95	4.00	1.030		36.50	38.00	2.440		333/334–555	0.76	0.691	0.891	0.863	0.779
334–555	10.80	11.00	0.832		10.40	11.00	0.720		6.93	6.00	0.736		7.02	3.00	1.050		35.00	37.00	2.560		333/>555	0.317	0.895	0.798	0.984	0.701
>555	10.40	11.00	0.549		10.60	11.00	0.573		8.46	6.00	0.659		7.32	3.00	0.756		36.50	37.00	2.100		334–555/>555	0.828	0.942	0.507	0.904	0.987
Gender of child																										
Male	9.91	10.00	0.606	0.090	10.15	11.00	0.545	0.849	7.57	6.00	0.592	0.493	7.59	4.00	0.775	0.358	35.03	37.00	1.986							
Female	11.30	12.00	0.565		10.92	12.00	0.553		7.94	6.00	0.589		6.83	3.00	0.721		36.84	38.00	1.913							
Anemia type																					Pairwise comparisons	OS	FL	EWB	SWB	TS
Iron deficiency anemia (IDA)	11.40	12.00	0.551		10.40	11.00	0.467		7.00	6.00	0.518		5.90	3.00	0.633		34.40	37.00	1.680		IDA/DA	0.908	0.145	0.041	0.003	0.038
25-hydroxyvitamin D-deficiency anemia (DA)	10.80	12.00	0.734		11.80	12.00	0.740		9.95	7.00	0.826		10.20	8.50	1.080		42.60	40.00	2.620		IDA/B12A	0.956	0.551	0.714	0.599	0.401

Table 4. Cont.

	Subscale Scores																	
	Oral Symptoms (OS)				Functional Limitations (FL)				Emotional Well-Being (EWB)				Social Well-Being (SWB)				Total Score (TS)	
Vitamin B12 deficiency anemia (B12A)	10.50	11.00		0.370	1.510	12.00	12.00		1.280	8.21	7.00			1.740	4.50	4.00		39.60	40.00		4.390	DA/B12A	0.999	0.824	0.836	0.974
Medical treatment for anemia																			
Yes	11.52	12.00	0.006	0.452	0.426	11.50	12.00	<0.001	0.499	8.48	6.00	0.008	0.640	7.82	4.00	0.030	39.10	38.00	<0.001	1.540					
No	8.64	8.00		0.878	0.762	8.13	8.00		0.611	5.61	6.00		0.812	5.17	3.00		27.30	30.00		2.470					

* Standard error.

Table 5. Descriptive statistics and summary of Early Childhood Oral Health Impact Scale Responses (ECOHIS) (n = 204).

			n (%)				
Impacts	Mean	SE *	Never/0	Hardly Ever/1	Occasionally/2	Often/3	Very Often/4	Don't Know (Missing)/0
Child Impacts	16.3	0.486						
Child symptoms subscale (1 item)								
Oral/Dental Pain	2.245	0.0678	15(7.5)	22(11)	68(34)	89(44.5)	6(3)	4(0)
General Score	2.25	0.0678						
Child function subscale (4 items)								
Difficulty Drinking	2.262	0.0714	18(8.9)	24(11.9)	53(26.2)	101(50)	6(3)	2(0)
Difficulty Eating	2.242	0.0738	18(9.1)	28(14.1)	46(23.2)	100(50.5)	6(3)	6(0)
Difficulty Pronouncing Words	0.851	0.0768	109(50.4)	38(18.8)	35(17.3)	16(7.9)	4(2)	2(0)
Missed Preschool or School	1.575	0.0651	34(17)	41(20)	103(51.5)	20(10)	2(1)	4(0)
General Score	6.8	0.22						
Child psychology subscale (2 items)								
Trouble Sleeping	2.005	0.0774	27(13.4)	37(18.4)	47(23.4)	88(43.8)	2(1)	3(0)
Irritable or Frustrated	1.94	0.0667	16(8)	30(15.1)	119(59.8)	18(9)	16(8)	5(0)
General Score	3.87	0.128						
Self-image and social interaction subscales (2 items)								
Avoided Smiling or Laughing	1.739	0.0635	27(13.3)	29(14.3)	123(66.6)	18(8.9)	6(3)	1(0)

Table 5. Cont.

Impacts	Mean	SE *	Never/0	Hardly Ever/1	Occasionally/2	Often/3	Very Often/4	Don't Know (Missing)/0
Avoided Talking	1.7	0.07	31(15.3)	38(18.7)	104(51.2)	21(10.3)	9(4.4)	1(0)
General Score	1.74	0.0635						
Family Impacts	7.32	0.242						
Parental distress subscale (2 items)								
Being upset	1.801	0.0691	25(12.4)	34(16.9)	109(54.2)	22(10.9)	11(5.5)	3(0)
Felt guilty	2.095	0.0851	31(15.6)	30(15.1)	38(19.1)	89(44.7)	11(5.5)	5(0)
General Score	3.82	0.143						
Family function subscale (2 items)								
Time off from Work	1.846	0.0662	22(10.9)	32(15.9)	110(54.7)	29(14.4)	8(4)	3(0)
Financial Impact	1.715	0.0674	29(14.5)	33(16.5)	111(55.5)	20(10)	7(3.5)	4(0)
General Score	3.5	0.121						
Total Score	23.6	0.701						

* Standard error.

Table 6. Association between overall and subscales scores of Early Childhood Oral Health Impact Scale Responses (ECOHIS) and demographic data.

	Subscale Scores								Total Score		
	Child Impact				Family Impact							
	Mean	Median	p value	SE *	Mean	Median	p value	SE *	Mean	Median	p value	SE *
Parental Relationship												
Mother	16.14	19.00	0.860	0.613	7.20	9.00	0.685	0.300	23.34	27.50	0.857	0.885
Father	16.67	19.50		0.742	7.62	9.00		0.393	24.29	2800.00		1.061

p value

Table 6. Cont.

	Child Impact				Subscale Scores Family Impact				Total Score			Pairwise comparisons	Child Impact	Family Impact	TS
Age (Years)															
21–30	12.90	12.00	1.300	6.12	6.00	0.662	19.00	19.50	1.850			21–30/31–40	<0.001	0.009	<0.001
31–40	17.70	20.00	0.609	8.10	9.00	0.299	25.80	29.00	0.869			21–30/>40	0.141	0.661	0.217
>40	15.50	16.00	0.878	6.65	8.00	0.441	22.10	24.50	1.280			31–40/>40	0.102	0.012	0.028
Educational Level															
Primary–high school	14.74	15.00	0.813	6.64	7.00	0.416	21.38	22.00	1.150	0.016	0.096	0.025			
Graduate–postgraduate	16.75	20.00	0.573	7.45	9.00	0.283	24.20	29.00	0.830						
													Child Impact	Family Impact p value	TS
Employment Status and Occupation												Pairwise comparisons			
Non-health professional	17.10	20.00	0.676	7.66	9.00	0.314	24.70	29.00	0.967			Non-health professional/health professional	0.680	0.633	0.674
Health professional	16.10	20.00	0.815	7.18	9.00	0.425	23.30	29.00	1.180			Non-health professional/unemployed	0.014	0.141	0.028
Unemployed	13.30	15.00	1.210	6.26	6.00	0.728	19.70	21.00	1.780			Health professional/unemployed	0.062	0.503	0.128
Marital Status															
Married	16.20	19.00	7.040	7.23	9.00	0.268	23.40	28.50	0.774	0.939	0.563	0.900			
Single	16.80	19.00	6.400	7.89	8.50	0.530	23.60	27.00	1.570						
													Child Impact	Family Impact p value	TS
Family Income (Monthly/EUR) *												Pairwise comparisons			
333 (minimum wage)	15.90	20.00	0.926	7.730	9.00	0.461	23.60	29.00	1.310			333/334–555	0.794	0.448	0.765
334–555	15.30	19.00	0.908	7.000	9.00	0.426	22.30	27.00	1.290			333/>555	0.730	0.780	0.943
>555	17.00	19.00	0.734	7.310	8.00	0.377	24.30	26.50	1.070			334–555/>555	0.368	0.883	0.517

Table 6. Cont.

	Subscale Scores										
	Child Impact			Family Impact			Total Score				
		*	p value		*	p value		*	p value		

Gender of child											
Male	15.24	16.00	0.758	0.052	7.05	8.00	0.385	0.472	22.30	25.00	1.107	0.112
Female	17.06	20.00	0.638		7.49	9.00	0.316		24.55	29.00	0.912	

									p value		
								Pairwise comparisons	Child Impact	Family Impact	TS
Anemia type											
Iron deficiency anemia (IDA)	16.60	20.00	0.628		7.39	9.00	0.317		24.00	29.00	0.906	IDA/B12A	0.999	0.834	0.999
25-hydroxyvitamin D deficiency anemia (DA)	16.80	18.50	0.963	<0.001	7.70	9.00	0.452	<0.001	24.50	26.50	1.380	IDA/DA	0.649	0.991	1.000
Vitamin B12 deficiency anemia (B12A)	17.50	19.00	1.360		8.16	9.00	0.735		25.60	27.00	1.840	B12A/D2A	1.000	0.942	0.995

Medical treatment for anemia											
Yes	17.50	20.00	0.538	<0.001	7.91	9.00	0.274	<0.001	25.50	29.00	0.771	<0.001
No	12.70	13.00	0.918		5.64	6.00	0.439		18.40	18.00	1.330	

* Standard error.

3.4. Internal Consistency Evaluation

The examination of the internal consistency of each questionnaire was performed by determining Cronbach's alpha. Cronbach's alpha values of the ECOHIS were 0.918, 0.859, and 0.946 for the sections of child impact, family impact and total score, respectively.

In terms of the P-CPQ, Cronbach's alpha values ranged from 0.844 to 0.941. Cronbach's alpha for the oral symptoms, functional limitation, emotional well-being, social well-being, and total scale was calculated as 0.932, 0.844, 0.853, 0.916 and 0.941, respectively.

All details for Cronbach's alpha evaluation are given in Table 7.

Table 7. Cronbach's alpha results.

Impacts	Validity Percentage (%)	Number of Items	Cronbach's α
P-CPQ impacts			
Oral symptoms subscale	99.5	6	0.932
Functional limitation subscale	100	8	0.844
Emotional well-being subscale	98	7	0.853
Social well-being subscale	97.1	10	0.916
Total score	94.5	31	0.941
ECOHIS impacts			
Impacts			
Child impacts	92.5	9	0.918
Family impacts	95.6	4	0.859
Total score	89.7	13	0.946

4. Discussion

The objective of the present study was to evaluate oral-health-related quality of life (OHRQoL) for children and for parents regarding the dental effects of anemia. Within the study, Turkish versions of the P-CPQ and ECOHIS were preferred to measure the OHRQoL of parents and children. Assessing the parental opinion of children's OHRQoL is important from different perspectives, since the child's health and their parents'/caregivers' opinion are correlated and reveal the treatment needs of the child. Moreover, the reports of parents/caregivers provide more comprehensive analysis of the child's OHRQoL [28]. Hence, a strength of the current study was that it followed the Turkish version of the P-CPQ that was adapted cross-culturally, with a good internal consistency and reliability of subscales regarding parents [27]. The impact of anemia on OHRQoL was measured using the reliable and valid Turkish version of the ECOHIS questionnaire to expose the effects of anemia-related dental caries and to create a strategy for oral health improvement for children and their families [26]. To the best of our knowledge, there are no similar studies regarding OHRQoL of anemia-related dental caries in the literature.

Turning back to the present findings of the P-CPQ, it is clear that more than half of the parents stated their children's oral health and well-being was affected substantially by the presence of anemia. The perceptions of parents of oral QoL could be associated with oral symptoms of their child, including the complaints of pain in the teeth and mouth, bad breath, and food caught between teeth. Hence, the results of questions which were answered prior to the P-CPQ showed greater agreement with the study of Gültekin et al. [27]. When the parental relationship is evaluated within the subscale scores, fathers reported a more negative impact on the functional limitations of their child compared to mothers. The mentioned result has been clarified by better mother–child communication, which allows mothers to more reliably monitor their child's difficulties during drinking and eating. Even though the results of the current study could not be directly compared with the study of Fernandes et al. [29]. due to different points of investigation, their featured results concerning parental monitorization of their child were partially consistent with the present results. Moreover, families with higher education level (graduate–postgraduate) reported greater negative impact on the oral symptoms subscale of their child in comparison with primary–high school-educated families. A possible reason for this is the better knowledge of the anemia–oral effect relationship of families with higher education level.

According to the latest report of the World Health Organization (WHO), it was estimated that 42% of children aged less than five years are anemic. Iron deficiency, including deficiencies in folate and vitamins B12 and A, is considered the main cause of anemia. In addition, hemoglobinopathies and infectious diseases, such as malaria, tuberculosis, and HIV, and parasitic infections, are reported as important etiological factors of anemia [30]. Iron deficiency is the predominant etiological factor of anemia, showing numerous oral manifestations (e.g., angular cheilitis, angular stomatitis, erythematous stomatitis, atrophic glossitis) across countries [31]. Similarly, iron-deficiency anemia was detected at a high level in the current study. Besides the beforementioned oral symptoms of anemia, black-stain formations on tooth surfaces are also among the most common oral manifestations due to iron supplementation during anemia treatment [32]. Strikingly, however, medical treatment for anemia significantly affected all subscales of the P-CPQ consisting of oral symptoms, functional limitations, emotional well-being, social well-being, and overall well-being in the present study. Therefore, the negative impact of medical treatment for anemia on children's well-being in all attitudes may be associated with the pharmacological side effects of anemia syrups, especially iron supplements, in our study.

When the results of the ECOHIS questionnaire were evaluated, there was a correlation between anemia and oral-health impact. Generally, the most negative impacts were revealed on the functions of children during drinking/eating, and their symptoms related to oral/dental pain in a similar vein to the studies of Farsi et al. [33] and Hashim et al. [34]. The ECOHIS findings also were comparatively evaluated from the standpoint of each sociodemographic factor. Even though a weak and non-significant relationship was observed between parental relationship and all subscale scores of the ECOHIS, a strong correlation was observed between education level of parents and the child-impact section. Moreover, similar to the answers to the P-CPQ, parents with graduate—postgraduate education level reported that anemia created greater negative effects on their child. Besides the similarity in educational levels of two different questionnaires, medical treatment for anemia showed powerful adverse impacts on all subscales of the ECOHIS along with the P-CPQ.

The reliability and Internal consistency of each questionnaire were evaluated by using Cronbach's alpha. Cronbach's alpha values for both questionnaires were satisfactory for the current study. For the ECOHIS, Cronbach's alpha values were close to those of Turkish version of the ECOHIS (0.981, 0.859, 0.946 for child impact section, family impact, and total score, respectively) [26]. For the P-CPQ, Cronbach's alpha estimation showed high internal consistency reliability and parallelism with the original Turkish version (0.932, 0.844, 0.853, 0.916, 0.941 for oral symptoms, functional well-being, emotional well-being, social well-being, and total score, respectively) [27].

Lastly, the lack of data on age of anemia diagnosis was the major limitation in the present research. However, importantly, the age at which anemia was diagnosed could not be the exact age of disease onset. It was therefore possible that data related to age of anemia diagnosis were not always reliable.

The clinical significance of this work is that understanding the adverse relationship between anemia-related ECC and quality of life of children and parents may lead to the design of cost-effective and approachable international preventive programs, especially for infants and preschool children.

The most important findings of the study are as follows:

- Anemia-related dental caries leads to negative impacts on the quality of life of children and families.
- A large number of children (81.5%) reported occasional or more frequent oral/dental pain.

- More than half of parents (56.3%) responded *"fair"* for the health of their children's teeth, lips, jaws, and mouth. Similarly, children's overall well-being was stated as being affected *"a lot"* by the condition of their child's teeth, lips, jaws or mouth by half of parents (49.5%).
- The age of anemia diagnosis is a very significant issue in analyzing the main mechanism of anemia in ECC development.
- Further investigations must be designed to determine the exact oral adverse effects of anemia related to ECC.

5. Conclusions

Within the limitations of the present study, it may be concluded that anemia-related dental caries has a highly negative impact on the quality of life of children and parents, according to both questionnaires. Therefore, it could be possible to prioritize children with high scores for preventive procedures and timely dental treatments. However, further investigations must be developed to understand the exact oral effects of anemia by further evaluation of each subscale.

Author Contributions: Conceptualization, A.İ.; Methodology, A.İ., Ö.T. and D.Ö.; Software, A.İ. and Ö.T.; Validation, A.İ., Ö.T. and D.Ö.; Formal Analysis, A.İ., Ö.T. and D.Ö.; Investigation; A.İ. and D.Ö.; Resources, A.İ. and D.Ö.; Data Curation, A.İ. and Ö.T.; Writing—Original Draft Preparation, A.İ. and D.Ö.; Writing—Review and Editing, A.İ.; Visualization, A.İ. and D.Ö.; Supervision, A.İ.; Project Administration, A.İ. and D.Ö.; Funding Acquisition, A.İ., Ö.T. and D.Ö. All authors have read and agreed to the published version of the manuscript.

Funding: This research received no external funding.

Institutional Review Board Statement: The study was conducted according to the guidelines of the Declaration of Helsinki and approved by the Institutional Review Board of Dr. Burhan Nalbantoğlu Government Hospital (YTK 1.01-30/22 1 June 2022). Witten informed consent was obtained from the parents to publish this paper.

Informed Consent Statement: Written informed consent was obtained from the parents to publish this paper.

Data Availability Statement: The data presented in this study are openly available.

Acknowledgments: No financial support was received from funding agencies in this study.

Conflicts of Interest: The authors declare no conflict of interest.

References

1. Zucoloto, M.L.; Maroco, J.; Campos, J.A. Impact of oral health on health-related quality of life: A cross-sectional study. *BMC Oral Health* **2016**, *16*, 55. [CrossRef] [PubMed]
2. Glick, M.; Williams, D.M.; Kleinman, D.V.; Vujicic, M.; Watt, R.G.; Weyant, R.J. A new definition for oral health developed by the FDI World Dental Federation opens the door to a universal definition of oral health. *Int. Dent. J.* **2016**, *66*, 322–324. [CrossRef]
3. Er-Sabuncuoğlu, M.; Diken, I.H. Early Childhood Intervention in Turkey: Current situation, challenges and suggestions. *Int. J. Early Child. Spec. Educ.* **2011**, *2*, 149–160.
4. Vieira-Andrade, R.G.; Siqueira, M.B.; Gomes, G.B.; D'Avila, S.; Pordeus, I.A.; Paiva, S.M.; Granville-Garcia, A.F. Impact of traumatic dental injury on the quality of life of young children: A case-control study. *Int. Dent. J.* **2015**, *65*, 261–268. [CrossRef] [PubMed]
5. Sun, L.; Wong, H.M.; McGrath, C.P. Relationship between the severity of malocclusion and oral health related quality of life: A systematic review and meta-analysis. *Oral Health Prev. Dent.* **2017**, *15*, 503–517.
6. Nora, Â.D.; da Silva Rodrigues, C.; de Oliveira Rocha, R.; Soares, F.Z.M.; Minatel Braga, M.; Lenzi, T.L. Is caries associated with negative impact on oral health-related quality of life of pre-school children? A systematic review and meta-analysis. *Pediatr. Dent.* **2018**, *40*, 403–411.
7. Martins-Júnior, P.A.; Vieira-Andrade, R.G.; Corrêa-Faria, P.; Oliveira-Ferreira, F.; Marques, L.S.; Ramos-Jorge, M.L. Impact of early childhood caries on the oral health- related quality of life of preschool children and their parents. *Caries Res.* **2013**, *47*, 211–218. [CrossRef] [PubMed]
8. Bönecker, M.; Abanto, J.; Tello, G.; Oliveira, L.B. Impact of dental caries on preschool children's quality of life: An update. *Braz. Oral Res.* **2012**, *26*, 103–107. [CrossRef]

9. McGrath, C.; Pang, H.N.; Lo, E.C.; King, N.M.; Hägg, U.; Samman, N. Translation and evaluation of a Chinese version of the child Oral health-related quality of life measure. *Int. J. Paediatr. Dent.* **2008**, *18*, 267–274. [CrossRef] [PubMed]
10. Meyer, F.; Enax, J. Early Childhood Caries: Epidemiology, Aetiology, and Prevention. *Int. J. Dent.* **2018**, *2018*, 1415873. [CrossRef]
11. Hajishengallis, E.; Parsaei, Y.; Klein, M.I.; Koo, H. Advances in the microbial etiology and pathogenesis of early childhood caries. *Mol. Oral Microbiol.* **2017**, *32*, 24–34. [CrossRef]
12. Ji, S.; Guan, X.; Ma, L.; Huang, P.; Lin, H.; Han, R. Iron deficiency anemia associated factors and early childhood caries in Qingdao. *BMC Oral Health* **2022**, *22*, 104. [CrossRef]
13. Folayan, M.O.; El Tantawi, M.; Schroth, R.J.; Vukovic, A.; Kemoli, A.; Gaffar, B.; Obiyan, M.; Early Childhood Caries Advocacy Group. Associations between early childhood caries, malnutrition and anemia: A global perspective. *BMC Nutr.* **2020**, *6*, 16. [CrossRef]
14. Asgari, I.; Soltani, S.; Sadeghi, S.M. Effects of Iron Products on Decay, Tooth Microhardness, and Dental Discoloration: A Systematic Review. *Arch. Pharm. Pract.* **2020**, *11*, 60–72.
15. Sharifi, R.; Tabarzadi, M.F.; Choubsaz, P.; Sadeghi, M.; Tadakamadla, J.; Brand, S.; Sadeghi-Bahmani, D. Evaluation of Serum and Salivary Iron and Ferritin Levels in Children with Dental Caries: A Meta-Analysis and Trial Sequential Analysis. *Children* **2021**, *8*, 1034. [CrossRef]
16. Mohamed, W.E.; Abou El Fadl, R.K.; Thaber, R.A.; Helmi, M.; Kamal, S.H. Iron deficiency anaemia and early childhood caries: A cross-sectional study. *Aust. Dent. J.* **2021**, *66*, S27–S36. [CrossRef]
17. Bansal, K.; Goyal, M.; Dhingra, R. Association of severe early childhood caries with iron deficiency anemia. *J. Indian Soc. Pedod. Prev. Dent.* **2016**, *34*, 36–42. [CrossRef] [PubMed]
18. Torell, P. Iron and dental caries. *Swed. Dent. J.* **1988**, *12*, 113–124.
19. Oppermann, R.V.; Rölla, G. Effect of some polyvalent cations on the acidogenicity of dental plaque in vivo. *Caries Res.* **1980**, *14*, 422–427. [CrossRef] [PubMed]
20. Dunning, J.C.; Ma, Y.; Marquis, R.E. Anaerobic killing of oral streptococci by reduced, transition metal cations. *Appl. Environ. Microbiol.* **1998**, *64*, 27–33. [CrossRef] [PubMed]
21. Wunder, B.; Bowen, W.H. Action of agents on glucosyltransferases from Streptococcus mutans in solution and adsorbed to experimental pellicle. *Arch. Oral Biol.* **1999**, *44*, 203–214. [CrossRef] [PubMed]
22. Thomson, W.M.; Broder, H.L. Oral–Health–Related Quality of Life in Children and Adolescents. *Pediatr. Clin. N. Am.* **2018**, *65*, 1073–1084. [CrossRef]
23. Abanto, J.; Paiva, S.M.; Sheiham, A.; Tsakos, G.; Mendes, F.M.; Cordeschi, T.; Vidigal, E.A.; Bönecker, M. Changes in preschool children's OHRQoL after treatment of dental caries: Responsiveness of the B-ECOHIS. *Int. J. Paediatr. Dent.* **2016**, *26*, 259–265. [CrossRef] [PubMed]
24. Razanamihaja, N.; Boy-Lefèvre, M.L.; Jordan, L.; Tapiro, L.; Berdal, A.; de la Dure-Molla, M.; Azogui-Levy, S. Parental–Caregivers Perceptions Questionnaire (P-CPQ): Translation and evaluation of psychometric properties of the French version of the questionnaire. *BMC Oral Health* **2018**, *18*, 211. [CrossRef] [PubMed]
25. American Academy of Pediatric Dentistry (AAPD). Policy on early childhood caries (ECC): Classifications, consequences, and preventive strategies. *Pediatr. Dent.* **2020**, 79–81.
26. Peker, K.; Uysal, Ö.; Bermek, G. Cross-cultural adaptation and preliminary validation of the Turkish version of the Early Childhood Oral Health Impact Scale among 5–6-year-old children. *Health Qual. Life Outcomes* **2011**, *9*, 118. [CrossRef]
27. Mergen Gultekin, I.; Ozsin Ozler, C.; Serdar Eymirli, P.; Unal, F.; Atac, A.S. Cross-cultural adaptation of Turkish version of Parental-Caregiver Perceptions Questionnaire (P-CPQ). *Int. J. Dent. Hyg.* **2021**, *20*, 519–526. [CrossRef]
28. Barbosa Tde, S.; Gavião, M.B. Validation of the Parental-Caregiver Perceptions Questionnaire: Agreement between parental and child reports. *J. Public Health Dent.* **2015**, *75*, 255–264. [CrossRef]
29. Fernandes, M.L.; Kawachi, I.; Corrêa-Faria, P.; Paiva, S.M.; Pordeus, I.A. The impact of the oral condition of children with sickle cell disease on family quality of life. *Braz. Oral Res.* **2016**, *30*. [CrossRef]
30. World Health Organisation (WHO). Health Topics: Anaemia, Latest Report. Available online: https://www.who.int/health-topics/anaemia#tab=tab_1 (accessed on 1 September 2021).
31. Nirmala, S.V.S.G.; Saikrishna, S. Dental Considerations of Children with Anemias—An Overview. *J. Dent. Oral Disord.* **2019**, *5*, 1113.
32. Żyła, T.; Kawala, B.; Antoszewska-Smith, J.; Kawala, M. Black stain and dental caries: A review of the literature. *BioMed Res. Int.* **2015**, *2015*, 469392. [CrossRef] [PubMed]
33. Farsi, N.J.; El-Housseiny, A.A.; Farsi, D.J.; Farsi, N.M. Validation of the Arabic version of the early childhood oral health impact scale (ECOHIS). *BMC Oral Health* **2017**, *17*, 60. [CrossRef] [PubMed]
34. Hashim, A.N.; Yusof, Z.Y.; Esa, R. The Malay version of the Early Childhood Oral Health Impact Scale (Malay-ECOHIS)–assessing validity and reliability. *Health Qual. Life Outcomes* **2015**, *13*, 190. [CrossRef] [PubMed]

Disclaimer/Publisher's Note: The statements, opinions and data contained in all publications are solely those of the individual author(s) and contributor(s) and not of MDPI and/or the editor(s). MDPI and/or the editor(s) disclaim responsibility for any injury to people or property resulting from any ideas, methods, instructions or products referred to in the content.

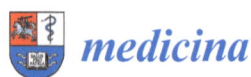

Systematic Review

The Effect of Dentine Desensitizing Agents on the Retention of Cemented Fixed Dental Prostheses: A Systematic Review

Mohammed E. Sayed

Department of Prosthetic Dental Sciences, College of Dentistry, Jazan University, Jazan 45142, Saudi Arabia; drsayed203@gmail.com or mesayed@jazanu.edu.sa; Tel.: +966-506529134

Abstract: *Background and Objectives:* The use of desensitizing agents (DA) after tooth preparation to prevent hypersensitivity is well documented in the literature. A fixed dental prosthesis (FDP) should have good retention to be successful. Inadequate retention may result in microleakage, secondary caries, and, eventually, dislodgement of the FDP. The effect of DAs on the retention of FDPs has been widely studied in the literature, but the results are conflicting. Thus, this study aimed to conduct a systematic review to assess the effect of dentine desensitizing agents, used to prevent post-cementation hypersensitivity, on the retention of cemented FDPs. The null hypothesis framed was that there is no effect of dentine desensitizing agents on the retention of cemented FDPs. The focused PICO question was as follows: "Does the application of dentine desensitizing agents (I) affect the retention (O) of cemented fixed dental prosthesis (P) when compared to non-dentine desensitizing groups (C)"? *Materials and Methods:* Four electronic databases were systematically searched and, on the basis of the predefined inclusion and exclusion criteria, 23 articles were included in this systematic review. A modified CONSORT scale for in vitro studies was used to assess the quality of the selected studies, as all included studies were in vitro studies. *Results:* Most of the studies compared the effect of more than one type of DA on retention. The results of the selected studies varied due to differences in the composition of tested dentine DAs and types of luting cements. *Conclusions:* Within the limitations of this study, it can be concluded that the retention values of FDPs cemented using zinc phosphate cement were reduced with most of the DAs, whereas retention values increased when GIC, resin-modified GIC, and resin cements were used with the majority of DAs. These findings are important, as they can guide dentists in selecting the DA before cementing the crowns with the luting agent of their choice, without compromising the retention of the crowns.

Keywords: dentin hypersensitivity; desensitizing agent; retention; luting cements; bond strength; GLUMA; glass ionomer cement; resin cement; tooth preparation

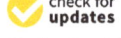

Citation: Sayed, M.E. The Effect of Dentine Desensitizing Agents on the Retention of Cemented Fixed Dental Prostheses: A Systematic Review. *Medicina* 2023, 59, 515. https://doi.org/10.3390/medicina59030515

Academic Editor: Giuseppe Minervini

Received: 7 February 2023
Revised: 28 February 2023
Accepted: 3 March 2023
Published: 6 March 2023

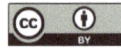

Copyright: © 2023 by the author. Licensee MDPI, Basel, Switzerland. This article is an open access article distributed under the terms and conditions of the Creative Commons Attribution (CC BY) license (https://creativecommons.org/licenses/by/4.0/).

1. Introduction

A fixed dental prosthesis (FDP) is a common treatment modality for replacing missing teeth and for transforming unhealthy teeth into functional and esthetically pleasing ones [1]. To prepare a tooth for an FDP, the coronal tooth structure is prepared, which involves the removal of 1–2 mm of the tooth structure [1]. This procedure leads to the opening of millions of dentinal tubules [2–4]. Preparation also reduces the thickness of the dentine (depending upon the type of preparation and location of preparation), which increases the permeability of the dentine [3–7]. This causes pulpal irritation and post-operative hypersensitivity [7,8].

Heat generation [9–11], desiccation [9–11], aggressive tooth preparation [9], microleakage underneath provisional restoration [11,12], and the acidic pH of many luting agents [10,11,13] lead to irritation of the dentinal tubules, which in turn irritate the pulp and cause discomfort to the patient in the form of sensitivity.

The use of desensitizing agents (DA) after tooth preparation to prevent hypersensitivity has been well documented in the literature [14–17]. Various generations of DAs have been used in the past, and they have shown promising results in reducing post-preparation sensitivity [14–20]. These include 2-hydroxyethyl-methacrylate (HEMA), urethane dimethacrylate (UDMA), Tolnyl ethyl glycidal dimethacrylate (TEGMA), N-Olyglycine glycidyl methacrylate (NTG-GMA), biphenyl dimethacrylate (BPDM), 5% glutaraldehyde + HEMA, Low and highly filled resins, etc. [14–20]. Recent studies have demonstrated that new types of DAs have comparable desensitizing effects on dentine. These include nano-hydroxyapatite (n-HAp) [21–23], photobiomodulation therapy (PBM) with a low-level infrared laser [24], nano-sized carbonate apatite (n-CAP) [25], zinc-containing desensitizer [26], etc. Most of the DAs block the opening of the bulk of the dentinal tubules and make the dentinal surface smooth by filling the irregularities, thereby decreasing the sensitivity [14–17].

For an FDP to be successful, it should have good retention. Multiple factors affect the retention of FDP, including adequacy of tooth preparation, impression-making, fit and precision of the retainer, space and type of luting agent [27–31]. Inadequate retention may result in microleakage, secondary caries, and dissolution of luting agent [30–33]. A dislodged FDP is considered to be a failure from the patient's perspective, and he/she may doubt the reliability of the treatment provided by the dentist.

The effect of DAs on retention of FDPs has been widely studied in the literature, but the results are conflicting. Studies by Johnson et al. [34], Jalandar et al. [18], Chandavarkar et al. [8] and Himashilpa et al. [35] have reported higher retention values when GIC was used with Gluma DA, whereas lower retention values were reported by Swift et al. [36], Yim et al. [37] and Sipahi et al. [38]. Similarly, studies by Chandavarkar et al. [8] and Pilo et al. [39] reported higher retention values when GIC was used with pro-argenine-based DAs, whereas Himashilpa et al. [29] reported lower retention values for the same combination. Retention of FDP was reported to be affected by the combined effect of the type of luting agent and DA.

To the best of our knowledge, this is the first systematic review to assess the effect of DAs on the retention of cemented FDPs. The findings are important, as they can guide dentists in selecting the DA before cementing the FDPs with the luting agent of their choice, without compromising retention. Thus, the objective of this study is to conduct a systematic review to assess the effect of dentine desensitizing agents, used to prevent post-cementation hypersensitivity, on the retention of cemented FDPs. The null hypothesis framed is that there is no effect of dentine desensitizing agents on the retention of cemented FDPs.

2. Materials and Methods

2.1. Permission and Registration

For the planning of this systematic review, registration in the International Prospective Register of Systematic Reviews (PROSPERO) was applied for (CRD388403). The preferred reporting items for systematic reviews and meta-analyses (PRISMA) guidelines were used to structure this systematic review [40].

2.2. Search Criteria

Studies were selected based on the following inclusion and exclusion criteria. All published in vitro and in vivo studies in the English language that compared the effect of dentine desensitizers on the retention of full- and partial-coverage FDPs after cementation were included in this systematic review. Studies that were under trial, unpublished abstracts, commentaries, letters to editors, case reports, or dissertations were excluded. Exclusion criteria also included studies in languages other than English, animal studies, studies comparing the sensitivity or bond strength of luting agents to dentine after the application of dentine desensitizers, and studies evaluating materials under trial.

The focused PICO question was as follows: "Does the application of dentine desensitizing agents (I) affect the retention (O) of cemented fixed dental prosthesis (P) when compared to non-dentine desensitizing groups (C)"?

P: Cemented fixed dental prosthesis

I: Dentine desensitizer application
C: Non-dentine desensitizer application
O: Retention of crowns

Four electronic databases (MEDLINE/PubMed, Scopus, Cochrane Library, and Web of Science–Core Collection) were systematically searched in October 2022 for relevant titles with respect to the formulated PICO question. Details of the keywords and Boolean operators used in the search strategy are listed in Supplementary Table S1. On the basis of the requirements of each electronic database, slight amendments were made to the search strategy. A reference list of articles was searched manually for further relevant titles.

2.3. Screening, Selection of Studies, and Data Extraction

After performing the search on the selected electronic databases, the collected titles and their abstracts were independently examined by two reviewers (MES and MM). Duplicate titles were removed, and the titles and abstracts of the remaining studies were assessed against the preset inclusion and exclusion criteria. Full texts of the selected titles were reviewed and the studies that met the inclusion criteria were collected. Two reviewers (MES and MM) discussed the selected studies, and any disputed studies were discussed with third reviewer (S.J.) to resolve disagreements. The reference list of the selected studies was searched manually to check for any supplementary relevant studies that met the requirements. Relevant data were extracted from the studies that fulfilled the inclusion criteria and were tabulated in a self-designed table. Table 1 is a self-designed master table containing information related to Author, Year and Country; Study Design; Sample Size; Abutment Type; Specimen Fabrication Technique; Type of Framework (Single Crown/3 Unit FPD); Crown/FPD Fabrication Technique; Control; Intervention; Name of DA (Manufacturer); Main Chemical Composition of DA; Type of Cement, Trade Name and Manufacturer; Test and Machine Used; Mean Tbs/Retentive Strength; Primary Outcomes; Secondary Outcomes; and Authors' Suggestions/Conclusions/Inferences.

2.4. Quality Assessment of the Included Studies

A modified CONSORT scale for in vitro studies [50,51] was used to assess the quality of the selected studies. The standards of different sections of the published studies can be assessed using the checklist, which includes 14 items. The items included were as follows: "Item 1: Abstract containing structured summary of study design, methodology, results, and conclusions; Item 2a: Introduction should have scientific background and detailed explanation of rationale; Item 2b: Introduction should have study objectives with a defined hypothesis; Item 3: Methodology should contain approach used in the experiment with sufficient details to enable replication; Item 4: Precisely stated primary and secondary outcomes to enable comparison; Item 5: Details of how sample size was determined; Item 6: Details of how random allocation sequence was generated; Item 7: Method used for random allocation concealment; Item 8: Who implemented randomization? Item 9: If randomization is performed, how was blinding followed? Item 10: Statistical assessment; Item 11: Results outcome and estimation; Item 12: Study limitations; Item 13: Details related to funding; Item 14: Details related to the availability of study protocol, if available" (Table 2).

Table 1. General characteristics and specific results of the included studies.

Author, Year and Country	Study Design	Sample Size	Abutment Type	Specimen Fabrication Technique	Type of FDP (Single Crown, 3 Unit FPD) and Fabrication Technique	Control	Intervention	Name of DA (Manufacturer)	Main Chemical Composition	Type of Cement, Trade Name and Manufacturer	Test and Machine Used	Mean TBS (N)/ Retentive Strength (MPa)	Primary Outcomes	Secondary Outcomes	Authors' Suggestions/Conclusions/Inferences
Mausner et al., 1996, USA [41]	In vitro	n = 96 (16 per group)	Human Third molars	Finish line: rounded shoulder/bevel Axial height: 5 mm Taper: 6–10° Spacer: 3 coats Ageing: No	Full metal silver-palladium alloy copings (Ceradela 2, Metalor, Neuchatel, Switzerland) Fabrication technique: lost wax casting	No DA applied	Application of DA before final cementation	(A) Imperva bonding agent (IBA) (Shofu Dental Corp., Menlo Park, CA, USA) (B) All-Bond (AB) desensitizing agent (Bisco Inc., Itasca, IL, USA)	(A) HEMA & UDMA & TEGMA (B) NTG-GMA & BPDM	(i) ZPC (Flecks Mizzy, Mizzy, Inc., Cherry Hill, NJ, USA) (ii) PCC (Duralon, Espe-Premier, Norristown, PA, USA) (iii) GIC (Ketac-Gem Maxicaps, Espe-Premier, St. Paul, MN, USA) (iv) RC (NM)	Retention values, UTM	Retention values (N) (A) ZPC: 383.28 ± 62.17 (B) ZPC + IBA DA: 354.89 ± 84.06 (C) ZPC + AB DA: 187.48 ± 50.18 (D) PCC: 335.97 ± 54.29 (E) PCC + IBA DA: 388.26 ± 34.53 (F) PCC + AB DA: 42.85 ± 14.24 (G) GIC: 234.74 ± 64.70 (H) GIC+IBA DA: 135.73 ± 41.39 (I) GIC + AB DA: 211.37 ± 39.43 (J) RC: 289.25 ± 116.10 (K) RC + IBA DA: 485.05 ± 117.21 (L) RC + AB DA: 406.06 ± 132.61	Retention values: RC + IBA DA > RC + AB DA > PCC + IBA DA > ZPC > ZPC + IBA DA > PCC > RC > GIC > GIC + AB DA > ZPC + AB DA > GIC + IBA DA > PCC + AB DA	Retention values: ZPC > PCC > RC > GIC	In general, application of DA reduced the retention in most of the tested specimens when cemented with ZPC, PCC or GIC, whereas retention increased when RC was used.
Swift et al., 1997, USA [36]	In vitro	n = 30 (10 per group)	Human molars	Finish line: NM Axial height: 4 mm Taper: 2.4° per wall Spacer: NM Ageing: No	Full metal silver-palladium copings (Ney-Oro 76, Ney Dental International) Fabrication technique: lost wax casting	No DA applied	Application of DA before final cementation	(A) One step (Bisco Dental Products, Schaumburg, IL, USA) (B) Gluma (Heraeus Kulzer, South Bend, IN, USA)	(A) phosphoric acid with Benzalkonium Chloride (B) glutaraldehyde and HEMA	(i) ZPC (Hy-Bond, Shofu Inc., Koyoto, Japan) (ii) GIC (Fuji I, GC America Inc., Alsip, IL, USA) (iii) RMGIC (Vitremer Luting Cement, 3M Dental Products Division, St. Paul, MN, USA)	Mean force for removing crown, UTM	Mean force for removing crown (N) (A) ZPC: 587 ± 400 (B) ZPC + One step DA: 479 ± 215 (C) ZPC + Gluma DA: 449 ± 277 (D) GIC: 788 ± 401 (E) GIC + One Step DA: 872 ± 342 (F) GIC + Gluma DA: 653 ± 234 (G) GIC + Gluma DA: 685 ± 156 (H) RMGIC + One Step DA: 713 ± 191 (I) RMGIC + Gluma DA: 748 ± 306	Mean force for removing crown GIC + One Step DA > GIC > RMGIC + Gluma DA + One-Step DA > RMGIC > GIC + Gluma DA > ZPC > ZPC + One step DA > ZPC + Gluma DA	Retention GIC > RMGIC > ZPC	Use of DA does not affect the retentive properties of the three tested luting cements.
Johnson et al., 1998, USA [34]	In vitro	n = 60 (10 per group)	Human molars	Finish line: chamfer Axial height: 4 mm Taper: 20° Spacer: 3 coats Ageing: No	Full base metal alloy copings (Olympia porcelain metal alloy, Jelenko Dental Products, Armonk, NY, USA) Fabrication technique: lost wax casting	No DA applied	Application of DA before final cementation	Gluma Desensitizer (Heraeus/Kulzer, Dental Products Division, South Bend, IN, USA)	5% glutaraldehyde + HEMA	(i) ZPC (Fleck's, Mizzy Inc., Cherry Hill, NJ, USA) (ii) GIC (Ketac-Cem Maxicap, ESPE GmbH, Seefeld, Germany) (iii) Modified RC (Resinomer, Bisco, Inc., Schaumburg, IL, USA)	Failure stress, UTM	Failure stress (MPa) (A) ZPC: 6.3 (B) ZPC + Gluma DA: 6.4 (C) GIC: 9.1 (D) GIC + Gluma DA: 10.1 (E) Modified RC: 12.1 (F) Modified RC + Gluma DA: 12.6	Failure stress: RC + DA > RC > GIC + DA > GIC > ZPC + DA > ZPC	RC > GIC > ZPC	Application of Gluma DA for desensitizing treatment does not affect retention of crowns cemented with the tested luting agents.
Yim et al., 2000, Georgia [37]	In vitro	n = 144 (12 per group)	Human molars	Finish line: Chamfer Axial height: 4 mm Taper: 26° Spacer: 2 coats Ageing: No	Full metal Ni-Cr Fabrication technique: lost wax casting	No DA	Application of DA before final cementation	(A) PD (All-Bond 2, BISCO Dental Products, Schaumburg, IL, USA) (B) NPD (Gluma Desensitizer, Heraeus Kulzer, South Bend, IN, USA)	(A) Photopolymerizable, resin-based DA (B) Nonpolymerizing, protein-precipitating, resin-based DA	(i) ZPC (Fleck's Cement, Mizzy Inc., Cherry Hill, NJ, USA) (ii) GIC (Ketac-Cem, ESPE GmbH, Seefeld, Germany) (iii) RMGIC (Fuji Plus, GC Corporation, Tokyo, Japan) (iv) RC (Panavia 21, J. Morita, Tustin, CA, USA)	Debond Stress; UTM	Debond Stress (MPa): (A) ZPC + PD DA: 0.67 ± 0.14 (B) ZPC + NPD DA: 0.81 ± 0.11 (C) ZPC: 1.68 ± 0.08 (D) GIC + PD DA: 2.23 ± 0.20 (E) GIC + NPD DA: 1.98 ± 0.23 (F) GIC: 2.36 ± 0.20 (G) RMGIC + PD DA: 3.46 ± 0.26 (H) RMGIC + NPD DA: 2.81 ± 0.15 (I) RMGIC: 2.96 ± 0.18 (J) RC + PD DA: 5.68 ± 0.70 (K) RC + NPD DA: 4.12 ± 0.37 (L) RC: 4.67 ± 0.48	Debond Stress RC + PD DA > RC > RMGIC + PD DA > RMGIC > RMGIC + NPD DA > GIC + PD DA > GIC > GIC + NPD DA > ZPC + NPD DA > ZPC + PD DA	Debond Stress RC > RMGIC > GIC > ZPC	Application of NPD DA significantly decreased the retention strength when RC, GIC and ZPC were used. Application of PD DA significantly increased retention strength when RC and RMGIC were used. DA when used with ZPC significantly decreased retention strength.

131

Table 1. Cont.

Author, Year and Country	Study Design	Sample Size	Abutment Type	Specimen Fabrication Technique	Type of FDP (Single Crown, 3 Unit FPD) and Fabrication Technique	Control	Intervention	Name of DA (Manufacturer)	Main Chemical Composition	Type of Cement, Trade Name and Manufacturer	Test and Machine Used	Mean TBS (N)/Retentive Strength (MPa)	Primary Outcomes	Secondary Outcomes	Authors' Suggestions/Conclusions/Inferences
Wolfart et al., 2003, Germany [12]	In vitro	n = 80 (10 per group)	Human premolars	Finish line: Chamfer Axial height: 4 mm Taper: 11° Spacer: yes Ageing: 3 days and 150 days (37,500 cycles)	Full metal nickel chromium alloy (Wiron 99, Bego, Germany) copings Fabrication technique: lost wax casting	Calcium Hydroxide DA applied	Application of DA before final cementation	(A) Gluma (Heraeus Kulzer) (B) Prompt L-Pop (3M-Espe, Seefeld, Germany) (C) Optibond FL (Kerr, Orange County, CA, USA) (D) Calcium hydroxide suspension (Merck, Darmstadt, Germany)	(A) 5% Glutaraldehyde and HEMA (B) Low filled resin sealer (C) Highly filled resin sealer	GIC (Ketac-Cem Maxicap, 3M-Espe, Seefeld, Germany)	Failure Stress, UTM	Failure Stress (MPa) After 3 days ageing: ## (A) GIC + Calcium hydroxide:6.92 (B) GIC + Gluma: 6.20 (C) GIC + Prompt L-Pop: 6.62 (D) GIC + Optibond: 4.91 After 150 days ageing: ## (A) GIC + Calcium hydroxide: 6.02 (B) GIC + Gluma: 5.60 (C) GIC + Prompt L-Pop: 6.9 (D) GIC + Optibond:5.01	Failure stress After 3 days ageing: GIC + Calcium hydroxide > GIC + Prompt L-Pop > GIC + Gluma > GIC + Optibond After 150 days ageing: GIC + Prompt L-Pop > GIC + Calcium hydroxide > GIC + Gluma > GIC + Optibond	-	Gluma and Prompt L-Pop DA does not affect the retention of crowns cemented with GIC when compared to calcium hydroxide application.
Johnson et al., 2004; USA [42]	In vitro	n = 55 (11 per group)	Human molars	Finish line:—N/A Axial height: 4 mm Taper: 20° Spacer: 1 layer Ageing: 2500 cycles	Full ceramometal high noble alloy (Olympia) copings Fabrication technique: lost wax casting	No DA applied	Application of DA before final cementation	(A) One step (Bisco Dental Products, Schaumburg, IL, USA)	Phosphoric acid with Benzalkonium Chloride	(A) ZPC (Fleck's, Keystone Industries GmbH, Singen, Germany), (B) GIC (Ketac-Cem, ESPE Gmbh, Seefeld, Germany) (C) Modified-RC (Resinomer, Schaumburg, IL, USA)	Dislodgment stresses, UTM	Mean dislodgment stress (MPa) (A) ZPC: 3.7 ± 1.0 (B) ZPC + One step DA:2.2 ± 0.8 (C) GIC: 2.7 ± 1.2 (D) GIC + One step DA: 4.2 ± 0.9 (E) Modified-RC: 6.4 ± 1.7	Mean dislodgment stress Modified RC > GIC + One step > ZPC > GIC > ZPC + One step	dislodgment stress: Modified RC > ZPC > GIC	Resin sealers reduced retention when used with ZPC and increased retention when used with GIC.
Sipahi et al., 2007, Turkey [38]	In vitro	n = 50 (10 per group)	Human molars	-	Full metal base metal alloy copings Fabrication technique: lost wax casting	No DA applied	Application of DA before final cementation	(A) Laser group (LAS), (B) sodium fluoride group (C) Oxagel (D) Gluma primer group	-	GIC	TS, UTM	TS (N) (A) GIC: 261 (B) GIC + Laser DA: 223 (C) GIC + sodium fluoride DA: 208 (D) GIC + Oxagel DA: 147 (E) GIC + Gluma DA: 161	Ts: GIC > GIC + Laser > GIC + sodium fluoride > GIC + Gluma > GIC + Oxagel	-	Laser negative effect of laser treatment on retention for crowns cemented with GIC, as compared to other DA.
Jalandar et al., 2012, India [18]	In vitro	n = 90 (10 per group molars)	Human molars	Finish line: Chamfer Axial height: 4 mm Taper: 6° Spacer: 35–40 μ Ageing: No	Full metal Ni-Cr crown Fabrication technique: lost wax casting	No DA	Application of DA before final cementation	(A) GC Tooth Mousse (GC International, Itabashiku, Tokyo, Japan) (B) GLUMA desensitizer (Heraeus Kulzer, Hanau, Germany).	(A) CPP-ACP-based (B) GLU-based	(i) ZPC (Harvard cement Quick setting, Harvard Dental International GmbH, Hoppegarten, Germany) (ii) GIC (GC Fuji I Tokyo, Japan) (iii) RMGIC (RelyX™ Luting, 3M ESPE, St. Paul, MN, USA)	TBS; UTM	TBS (kg) (A) ZPC + TM DA: 25.27 ± 4.60 (B) ZPC + GLUMA DA: 27.92 ± 3.20 (C) ZPC:27.69 ± 3.39 (D) GIC + TM DA: 40.32 ± 3.89 (E) GIC + GLUMA DA: 41.14 ± 2.42 (F) GIC: 39.09 ± 2.80 (G) RMGIC + TM DA: 48.34 ± 2.94 (H) RMGIC + GLUMA DA: 49.02 ± 3.32 (I) RMGIC: 48.61 ± 3.54	TBS: RMGIC + GLUMA DA > RMGIC > RMGIC + TM DA > GLUMA DA > GIC + TM DA > GIC > ZPC + GLUMA DA > ZPC + TM DA	TBS: RMGIC > GIC > ZPC	GLUMA DA improves retention of cast crowns with ZPC, GIC, RMGIC. Tooth Mousse DA improves retention of cast crowns with GIC, RMGIC and reduces retention for ZPC.

Table 1. Cont.

Author, Year and Country	Study Design	Sample Size	Abutment Type	Specimen Fabrication Technique	Type of FDP (Single Crown, 3 Unit FPD) and Fabrication Technique	Control	Intervention	Name of DA (Manufacturer)	Main Chemical Composition	Type of Cement, Trade Name and Manufacturer	Test and Machine Used	Mean TBS (N)/ Retentive Strength (MPa)	Primary Outcomes	Secondary Outcomes	Authors' Suggestions/Conclusions/ Inferences
Stawarczyk et al., 2012, Switzerland [19]	In vitro	n = 144 (12 per group)	Human molars	Finish line: Shoulder Axial height: 3 mm Taper: 10° Spacer: 35–40 μ Ageing: half specimens were aged–chewing machine, 6000 cycles	Zirconia crowns Fabrication technique: CAD/CAM milled	No DA	Application of DA before final cementation	Gluma Desensitizer (Haereus Kulzer, Hanau, Germany)	HEMA, glutaraldehyde	(i) Panavia 21 (Kurrary Dental Co. Ltd., Osaka, Japan) (ii) RelyX Unicem (3M ESPE, Seefeld, Germany) (iii) G-Cem (GC, Leuven, Belgium)	TS; UTM	Tensile strength (MPa) Initial: (A) Panavia 21 + Gluma DA: 2.6 ± 1.4 (B) Panavia 21: 14.1 ± 3.5 (C) RelyX Unicem + Gluma DA: 13.1 ± 2.9 (D) RelyX Unicem: 12.8 ± 2.9 (E) G-Cem + Gluma DA: 13.7 ± 4.2 (F) G-Cem: 10.7 ± 2.9 After Ageing (A) Panavia 21: 7.3 ± 1.7 (B) RelyX Unicem + Gluma DA: 0.9 ± 0.6 (C) RelyX Unicem + Gluma DA: 12.8 ± 4.3 (D) RelyX Unicem: 9.1 ± 3 (E) G-Cem + Gluma DA: 13.4 ± 6.2 (F) G-Cem: 8.6 ± 2.2	Tensile strength Initial: Panavia 21 > G-Cem + Gluma DA > RelyX Unicem + Gluma DA > RelyX Unicem > G-Cem > Panavia 21 + Gluma DA After Ageing G-Cem + Gluma DA > RelyX Unicem > G-Cem > Panavia 21 > Panavia 21 + Gluma DA	TS: Panavia 21 > RelyX Unicem > G-Cem	RelyX Unicem & G-Cem (self-adhesive Resins) when used with Gluma DA displayed better long-term stability.
Patel et al., 2013, India [20]	In vitro	n = 55 (11 per group)	Human molars	Finish line: Chamfer Axial height: 4 mm Taper: 20° Spacer: 3 layer Ageing: 2500 cycles	base metal porcelain metal alloy (Wirobond 280, BEGO, Fabrication technique: lost wax casting	No DA applied	Application of DA before final cementation	One-Step—Resinomer, (Bisco)	phosphoric acid with Benzalkonium Chloride	(A) ZPC (Harvard, Harvard Dental International GmbH, Hoppegarten, Germany) (B) GIC (Vivaglass; Ivoclar vivadent Inc., Buffalo, NY, USA) (C) Modified RC (Resinomer, Bisco Inc., Schaum-burg, IL, USA)	Removal stress, UTM	Removal stress (MPa) (A) ZPC: 3.5682 ± 0.2135 (B) ZPC + DA: 1.9209 ± 0.152 (C) GIC: 2.4082 ± 0.2581 (D) GIC + DA: 4.2609 ± 0.1963 (E) Modified RC: 6.9591 ± 0.5883	Removal stress: Modified RC > GIC + DA > GIC > ZPC + DA > ZPC	Removal stress: RC > GIC > ZPC	DA reduces retention with ZPC and increases retention with GIC.
Chandrasekaran et al., 2014, India [43]	In vitro	n = 81 (9 per group)	Human maxillary first premolars	Finish line: Chamfer Axial height: 4 mm Taper: 6–10° Spacer: NM Ageing: No	Full metal Ni-Cr crown Fabrication technique: lost wax casting	No DA	(A) & (B) Application of DA before final cementation	(A) Seal and protect (dentsply) (B) Tooth Mousse (GC)	(A) D-TMR & PENTA (B) CPP-ACP	(i) ZPC (Harvard cement, Harvard Dental International GmbH, Hoppegarten, Germany) (ii) GIC (GC Fuji I, Tokyo, Japan) (iii) RMGIC (GC Fuji Plus, GC Corporation, Tokyo, Japan)	Bond strength; UTM	Mean Bond strength (MPa) (A) ZPC + SP DA: 249.25 ± 65.65 (B) ZPC + TM DA: 219 ± 49.30 (C) ZPC: 295.12 ± 31.16 (D) GIC + SP DA: 345.49 ± 109.86 (E) GIC + TM DA: 421.46 ± 96.52 (F) GIC: 416.21 ± 113.10 (G) RMGIC + SP DA: 379.26 ± 114.59 (H) RMGIC + TM DA: 528.5 ± 67.65 (I) RMGIC: 537.2 ± 73.83	Mean Bond strength: RMGIC > RMGIC + TM DA > GIC + TM DA > GIC > RMGIC + SP DA > ZPC > ZPC + SP DA > ZPC + TM DA	Mean Bond strength: RMGIC > GIC > ZPC	Retentive strength: RMGIC: Control > TM > SP GIC: TM > Control > SP ZPC: Control > SP > TM TM & SP Can be used before crown cementation using GIC or RMGIC, but not with ZPC.
Kumar et al., 2015, India [44]	In vitro	n = 48 (12 per group)	Human maxillary first premolars	NM	Full metal Ni-Cr crown Fabrication technique: lost wax casting	No DA	laser treatment Er, Cr: YSGG laser at 0.5 W potency for 15 s	Desensitising Laser: Er, Cr: YSGG laser (NM)	NA	(i) GIC (ii) self-adhesive RC	TBS; UTM	TBS (N): GIC: 170 ± 7519 GIC + DA: 119.08 ± 5.350 RC: 244.33 ± 11.865 RC + DA: 269.16 ± 5.184	TBS: RC + DA > RC > GIC > GIC_DA	TBS: RC > GIC	The luting agent of choice for laser DA treated dentine: self-adhesive RC.

Table 1. Cont.

Author, Year and Country	Study Design	Sample Size	Abutment Type	Specimen Fabrication Technique	Type of FDP (Single Crown, 3 Unit FPD) and Fabrication Technique	Control	Intervention	Name of DA (Manufacturer)	Main Chemical Composition	Type of Cement, Trade Name and Manufacturer	Test and Machine Used	Mean TBS (N)/ Retentive Strength (MPa)	Primary Outcomes	Secondary Outcomes	Authors' Suggestions/Conclusions/Inferences
Chandavarkar et al., 2015 India [8]	In vitro	n = 50 (10 per group)	human premolars	Finish line: Chamfer Axial height: 4 mm Taper: 20° Spacer: 25 µ Ageing: No	Full metal Ni-Cr crown Fabrication technique: lost wax casting	No DA	(A), (B), (D): Application of DA before final cementation (C) laser treatment Er, Cr: YSGG laser at 0.5 W potency for 45 s	(A) Gluma Desensitizer, (Haereus Kulzer, Hanau, Germany) (B) GC Tooth Mousse, Recaldent Tooth Mousse, GC Corporation, Tokyo, Ja-pan) (C) Waterlase MD Turbo, Biolase Inc, Foothill Ranch, CA, USA) (D) Colgate Pro-Relief in-office polishing paste, New York, NY, USA)	(A) GLU-based (B) CPP-ACP-based (C) Er, Cr: YSGG laser (D) Pro-Argin	GIC	Tensile stress; UTM	Tensile stress (MPa): (A) GLU DA + GIC: 3.87 (B) CPP-ACP DA + GIC: 4.01 (C) Laser DA + GIC: 3.37 (D) Pro-Argin DA + GIC: 4.10 (E) GIC: 3.65	Tensile stress: Pro-Argin DA + GIC > CPP-ACP DA + GIC > GLU DA + GIC > GIC > Laser DA + GIC	-	Pro-Argin and CPP-ACP-based DA can be used safely without compromising the retention of cast crowns cemented with GIC. Laser as DA reduces the tensile stress when used with GIC.
Janapala et al., 2015, India [45]	In vitro	n = 40 (10 per group)	Human maxillary first premolars	Finish line: NM Axial height: 4 mm Taper: 20° Spacer: NM Ageing: No	Full metal nickel chromium alloy copings (Bellabond, BEGO) Fabrication technique: lost wax casting	No DA applied	Application of DA before final cementation	(A) Cavity varnish (Namuvar, Deepti Dental Products, Maharashtra, India) (B) Glutaraldehyde (Gluma Heraeus Kulzer, Hanau, Germany), (C) Resin (AdheSil bond, Ivoclar Vivadent, Buffalo, NY, USA)	(A) Dissolved solids (B) 5% Glutaraldehyde & HEMA (C) HEMA, dimethacrylate, silicon dioxide	RMGIC (FujiCEM, GC Corporation, Tokyo, Japan)	TS; UTM	Tensile strength (N) (A) RMGIC: 2.627 ± 1.1867 (B) RMGIC + Varnish: 1.968 ± 0.751 (C) RMGIC + GLUMA: 3.304 ± 0.762 (D) RMGIC + AdheSE: 4.042 ± 0.742	Tensile strength RMGIC + AdheSE > RMGIC + GLUMA > RMGIC > RMGIC + Varnish	-	Recommends use of resin-based and glutaraldehyde-based sealers with RMGIC before crown cementation.
Lawaf et al., 2016, Iran [31]	In vitro	n = 20 (10 per group)	Human premolars	Finish line: Deep chamfer Axial height: 4 mm Taper: 6° Spacer: 3 coats Ageing: No	Full base metal alloy copings Fabrication technique: lost wax casting	No DA applied	Application of DA before final cementation	GLUMA (Heraeus-Kulzer, Hanau, Germany)	5% Glutaraldehyde & HEMA	Self-adhesive RC (RelyX U200, 3M ESPE, St. Paul, MN, USA)	TBS; UTM	Tensile Bond Strength (N) (A) RC: 164.45 ± 39.3 (B) RC + GLUMA DA: 230.63 ± 63.8	TBS RC + GLUMA DA > RC	-	Application of GLUMA DA on Hypersensitive prepared teeth before final cementation using self-adhesive RC
Pilo et al., 2016, Israel [10]	In vitro	n = 40 (10 per group)	Human Mandibular molars	Finish line: Chamfer Axial height: 5 mm Taper: 10° Spacer: 50 µ Ageing: 10,000 cycles	Zirconia crowns (Lava frame Y-TZP blocks, 3M ESPE, Seefeld, Germany) Fabrication technique: CAD/CAM milling	No DA applied	Application of DA before final cementation	Colgate Sensitive Pro-Relief Desensitizing Paste (Colgate Palmolive Company, New York, NY, USA)	8% arginine and calcium carbonate	(i) RMGIC (RelyX Luting 2, 3M ESPE) (ii) Self Adhesive RC (RelyX U-200, 3M ESPE)	Retentive strength; UTM	Retentive strength (MPa) (A) RMGIC + DA: 2.92 ± 0.84 (B) RMGIC: 3.16 ± 0.73 (C) Self Adhesive RC + DA: 2.27 ± 0.64 (D) Self Adhesive RC: 2.29 ± 0.55	Retentive strength RMGIC > RC > RC + DA	Retentive strength RMGIC > RC	Retentive strengths of zirconia crowns cemented by either RMGIC or RC remain unaltered when 8% A-C-C is used as DA.

Table 1. Cont.

Author, Year and Country	Study Design	Sample Size	Abutment Type	Specimen Fabrication Technique	Type of FDP (Single Crown, 3 Unit FPD) and Fabrication Technique	Control	Intervention	Name of DA (Manufacturer)	Main Chemical Composition	Type of Cement, Trade Name and Manufacturer	Test and Machine Used	Mean TBS (N)/ Retentive Strength (MPa)	Primary Outcomes	Secondary Outcomes	Authors' Suggestions/Conclusions/Inferences
Mapkar et al., 2018, India [11]	In vitro	n = 33 (11 per group)	Human maxillary first premolars	Finish line: shoulder Axial height: 4 mm Taper: 20° Spacer: 1 layer Ageing: 2500 cycles	Full metal base metal alloy copings Fabrication technique: lost wax casting	No DA applied	Application of DA before final cementation	(A) Gluma (Heraeus Kulzer, hanau, Germany) (B) Ultraseal (Ultradent, South Jordan, UT USA)	(A) 5% Glutaraldehyde & HEMA (B) Non polymerizable, high-molecular-weight resin	ZPC (MEDIcept, Middlesex, UK).	Dislodgement force, UTM	Dislodgement force (N): (A) ZPC:345.01 (B) ZPC + Gluma:556.41 ZPC + Ultraseal: 320.22	Dislodgement force: ZPC + Gluma > ZPC + Ultraseal	-	Significant increase in retention after application of Gluma DA, whereas non-significant decrease after Ultraseal application.
Pilo et al., 2018 Israel [39]	In vitro	n = 40 (10 per group)	Human Mandibular molars	Finish line: Chamfer Axial height: 5 mm Taper: 10° Spacer: 50 μ Ageing: 5000 cycles	Full metal Co-Cr alloy Fabrication technique: selective laser melting (SLM) technology	No DA applied	Application of DA before final cementation	Colgate Sensitive Pro-Relief Desensitizing Paste (Colgate-Palmolive Company, New York, NY, USA)	8% arginine and calcium carbonate	(i) GIC (ii) ZPC	Retentive strength, UTM	Retentive strength (MPa) GIC + DA: 6.39 ± 1.06 GIC: 5.73 ± 1.10 ZPC + DA: 2.39 ± 0.99 ZPC: 3.10 ± 1.44	Retentive strength: GIC + DA > GIC > ZPC > ZPC + DA	Retentive strength: GIC > ZPC	Application of 8% arginine and calcium carbonate can be used safely without reducing the retentive strength of crowns cemented with GIC and/or ZPC.
Asadullah et al., 2018, India [46]	In vitro	n = 33 (11 per group)	Human maxillary first premolars	Finish line: shoulder Axial height: 4 mm Taper: 20° Spacer: 1coat Ageing: 2500 cycles	Full base metal alloy copings Fabrication technique: lost wax casting	No DA applied	Application of DA before final cementation	(A) ULTRASEAL (Ultradent, South Jordan, UT, USA) (B) GLUMA (Heraeus-Kulzer, Hanau, Germany)	(A) non polymerizable, high-molecular-weight resin (B) 5% Glutaraldehyde & HEMA	RC (RelyX, 3M ESPE)	Dislodgement force, UTM	Dislodgement force (N) (A) RC: 228.892 ## (B) RC + Ultra seal DA: 173.353 ## (C) RC + GLUMA DA: 339.098 ##	Dislodgement force: RC + GLUMA > RC > RC + Ultra seal	-	GLUMA DA can be safely used with RC, whereas, Ultraseal DA should not be used with RC.

Table 1. Cont.

Author, Year and Country	Study Design	Sample Size	Abutment Type	Specimen Fabrication Technique	Type of FDP (Single Crown, 3 Unit FPD) and Fabrication Technique	Control	Intervention	Name of DA (Manufacturer)	Main Chemical Composition	Type of Cement, Trade Name and Manufacturer	Test and Machine Used	Mean TBS (N)/Retentive Strength (MPa)	Primary Outcomes	Secondary Outcomes	Authors' Suggestions/Conclusions/Inferences
Himashilpa et al., 2019, India [35]	In vitro	n = 420 (10 per group)	Human maxillary premolars	Finish line: Shoulder Axial height: 4 mm Taper: 12° Spacer: NM Ageing: No	Full metal nickel chromium alloy copings Fabrication technique: lost wax casting	No DA applied	Application of DA before final cementation	(A) Systemp (ivoclar vivadent, Liechtenstein) (B) Gluma (Heraeus Kulzer, Hanau, Germany) (C) GC tooth Mousse (GC International, Itabashi-ku, Tokyo, Japan) (D) Colgate Sensitive Pro-Relief Desensitizing Paste (Colgate-Palmolive Company, New York, NY, USA) (E) Sensodyne rapid action repair and protect (F) Sensodyne rapid action repair and protect	(A) Poly(ethylene gy-col)dim-ethacrylate and glutaraldehyde (B) 5% Glutaraldehyde & HEMA (C) CPP-ACP (D) 8% arginine and calcium carbonate (E) Novamin (F) Fluoride	(A) GIC (Fuji luting GC, G.C. Corporation, Tokyo, Japan) (B) RMGIC (RelyX Luting Cement 3M ESPE) (C) self-adhesive RC (Maxcem Elite, Kerr, Orange County, CA, USA)	TBS, UTM	TBS (N) Thermocycling (A) GIC: 6.79 ± 0.74 (B) GIC + Systemp: 7.75 ± 0.67 (C) GIC + Gluma: 6.89 ± 0.66 (D) GIC + Mousse: 6.88 ± 0.65 (E) GIC + Arginine: 6.40 ± 0.86 (F) GIC + Novamin: 6.39 ± 0.36 (G) GIC + Flouride: 6.59 ± 1.32 (H) RMGIC: 8.26 ± 0.64 (I) RMGIC + Systemp: 8.44 ± 0.51 (J) RMGIC + Gluma: 8.13 ± 0.49 (K) RMGIC + Mousse: 7.80 ± 0.59 (L) RMGIC + Arginine: 8.15 ± 0.96 (M) RMGIC + Novamin: 8.05 ± 0.42 (N) RMGIC + Flouride: 7.37 ± 1.10 (O) RC: 9.85 ± 0.85 (P) RC + Systemp: 10.80 ± 0.91 (Q) RC + Gluma: 10.06 ± 0.77 (R) RC + Mousse: 9.97 ± 0.82 (S) RC + Novamin: 9.63 ± 0.80 (T) RC + Flouride: 9.17 ± 0.64 Non-thermocycling (A) GIC: 5.41 ± 1.02 (B) GIC + Systemp: 6.15 ± 0.49 (C) GIC + Gluma: 5.61 ± 0.89 (D) GIC + Arginine: 6.85 ± 0.71 (F) GIC + Arginine: 6.29 ± 0.43 (F) GIC + Novamin: 5.86 ± 0.49 (G) GIC + Flouride: 6.15 ± 1.10 (H) RMGIC: 6.58 ± 1.32 (I) RMGIC + Systemp: 7.54 ± 0.77 (J) RMGIC + Gluma: 7.47 ± 0.98 (K) RMGIC + Mousse: 7.35 ± 1.10 (L) RMGIC + Arginine: 6.54 ± 0.89 (M) RMGIC + Novamin:7.54 ± 0.34 (N) RMGIC + Flouride: 6.97 ± 0.61 (O) RC: 9.17 ± 0.52 (P) RC + Systemp: 9.25 ± 0.78 (Q) RC + Gluma: 9.12 ± 0.59 (R) RC + Mousse: 8.80 ± 0.78 (S) RC + Arginine: 8.64 ± 0.60 (T) RC + Flouride: 8.75 ± 0.58 (U) RC + Flouride: 8.74 ± 0.64	TBS: Thermocycling Resin Cement: RC + Systemp > RC + Gluma > RC + Mousse > RC + Arginine > RC + Novamin > RC + Flouride RMGIC: RMGIC + Systemp > RMGIC > RMGIC + Arginine > RMGIC + Gluma > RMGIC + Novamin > RMGIC + Mousse > RMGIC + Flouride GIC: GIC + Systemp > GIC + Gluma > GIC + Mousse > GIC + Flouride > GIC + Arginine > GIC + Novamin	TBS: RC > RMGIC > GIC	Highest TBS displayed by use of systemp DA, and lowest by Pro-Arginine in all groups. Thermocycling increased TBS
Supraja et al., 2020, India [47]	In vitro	n = 45 (5 per group)	Human Maxillary premolars	Finish line: Chamfer Axial height: 4 mm Taper: 6° Spacer: NM Ageing: No	Full metal Co-Cr alloy Fabrication technique: additive manufacturing (direct metal laser sintering).	No DA applied	Application of DA before final cementation	(A) A-CCF DA (custom made) (B) CPP-ACP-F DA (custom made)	(A) Arginine, Calcium Carbonate, Fluoride (B) Casein Phosphopeptide, Amorphous Calcium Phosphate, Fluoride	(i) GIC (NM) (ii) RMGIC (NM) (iii) RC (NM)	TBS; UTM	TBS (N): GIC + A-CC-F DA: 90.26 ± 10.68 GIC + CPP-ACP-F DA: 272.32 ± 30.5 GIC: 308.62 ± 58.84 RMGIC + A-CC-F DA: 85.07 ± 18.82 RMGIC + CPP-ACP-F DA: 203.47 ± 60.57 RMGIC: 176.89 ± 35.46 RC + A-CC-F DA: 226.05 ± 43.62 RC + CPP-ACP-F DA: 158.66 ± 25.32 RC-: 300.35 ± 27.9	TBS: GIC: GIC > GIC + A-CC-F DA > GIC + CPP-ACP-F DA RMGIC: RMGIC > CPP-ACP-F DA > A-CC-F DA RC: RC > RC + A-CC-F DA > RC + CPP-ACP-F DA	TBS: RC > RMGIC > GIC	Application of both types of DA decreased TBS for GIC to dentin Application of CPP-ACP-F DA increased, while A-CC-F DA decreased the TBS for RMGIC to dentin Application of both types of DA decreased TBS for RC to dentin

136

Table 1. Cont.

Author, Year and Country	Study Design	Sample Size	Abutment Type	Specimen Fabrication Technique	Type of FDP (Single Crown, 3 Unit FPD) and Fabrication Technique	Control	Intervention	Name of DA (Manufacturer)	Main Chemical Composition	Type of Cement, Trade Name and Manufacturer	Test and Machine Used	Mean TBS (N)/ Retentive Strength (MPa)	Primary Outcomes	Secondary Outcomes	Authors' Suggestions/Conclusions/Inferences
Hanijk et al., 2021, Syria [48]	In vitro	n = 40 (10 per group)	Human Maxillary premolars	Finish line: Chamfer Axial height: 4 mm Taper: 6° Spacer: 2 layer, 1 mm above the finish line. Ageing: No	Full metal Ni-Cr crown Fabrication technique: lost wax casting	No DA applied	Application of DA before final cementation	Systemp desensitizer (Ivoclar vivadent, Schaan, Liechtenstein)	Polyethylene gly-coldimethacrylate and glutaraldehyde in an aqueous solution	(i) GIC (Cavex, CJ Haarlem, The Netherlands) (ii) RMGIC (GC Fuji plus, Tokyo Japan)	TBS: UTM	TBS (N): RMGIC + DA: 829.95 ± 104.29 RMGIC + No DA: 604.03 ± 127.20 GIC + DA: 415.74 ± 139.92 GIC + No DA: 433.74 ± 177.73	TBS: DA + RMGIC > RMGIC > GIC > DA + GIC	TBS: RMGIC > GIC	Application of DA increase TBS for RMGIC to dentin Application of DA decrease TBS for GIC to dentin
Dewan et al., 2022, Saudi Arabia [49]	In vitro	n = 40 (10 per group)	Human molars	Finish line: Chamfer Axial height: 4 mm Taper: 10° Spacer: NM Ageing: 3000 cycles	Zirconia copings (Ceramill ZI, Austria) Fabrication technique: CAD/CAM milling	No DA applied	Application of DA before final cementation	(A) Gluma (Heraeus Kulzer, Hanau, Germany) (B) Telio CS (Ivoclar Vivadent, Schaan, Liechtenstein) (C) Shield Force Plus (Tokuyama Dental, Encinitas, CA, USA)	(A) 5% Glutaraldehyde & HEMA (B) PEGDMA, Glutaraldehyde (C) HPDMA & PA	RC (Rely X U200, 3M ESPE, St. Paul, MN, USA)	TS, UTM	TS (MPa) (A) RC: 0.22 ± 0.03 (B) RC + Gluma: 0.53 ± 0.08 (C) RC + Telio CS: 0.35 ± 0.10 (D) RC + Shield force: 0.36 ± 0.14	TS: RC + Gluma > RC + Shield force > RC + Telio CS > RC	-	Advocates using the tested DAs before cementing Zirconia crowns.

TBS: tensile bond strength; DA: desensitizing agent; RMGIC: resin-modified glass ionomer cement; Ni-Cr: nickel chromium; Co-Cr: cobalt chromium; A-C-C-F: arginine–calcium carbonate–fluoride; A-C-C: arginine–calcium carbonate; CPP-ACP-F: casein phosphopeptide–amorphous calcium phosphate–fluoride; NM: not mentioned; RC: resin cement; ZPC: zinc phosphate cement; UTM: universal testing machine; Er, Cr: YSCG: erbium, chromium:yttrium, selenium, galium, garnet; NM: not mentioned; GLU: glutaraldehyde; D-TMR: di- and trimethacrylate resin; SP: seal and protect; TM: tooth MousseMousse; PENTA: dipentaerythritol penta acrylate monophosphate; HEMA: 2-hydroxyethyl-methacrylate; PCC: polycarboxylate cement; NTG-GMA: N-olyglycine glycidyl methacrylate; BPDM: biphenyl dimethacrylate; UDMA: urethane dimethacrylate; TEGMA: tohnyl ethyl glycidal dimethacrylate; PEGDMA: polyethylene glycol dimethacrylate; HPDMA: hydroxy propoxy dimethacrylate; PA: phosphoric acid; ##: data retrieved from plot digitizer app.

Table 2. Quality analyses of the included studies using the modified CONSORT scale.

Item → Studies	1	2a	2b	3	4	5	6	7	8	9	10	11	12	13	14
Mausner et al., 1996 [41]	Y	Y	Y	Y	Y	N	Y	N	N	N	Y	Y	N	N	N
Swift et al., 1997 [36]	Y	Y	Y	Y	Y	N	Y	N	N	N	Y	Y	N	N	N
Johnson et al., 1998 [34]	Y	Y	Y	Y	Y	N	N	N	N	N	Y	Y	N	N	N
Yim et al., 2000 [37]	Y	Y	Y	Y	Y	N	Y	N	N	N	Y	Y	Y	Y	N
Wolfart et al., 2003 [12]	Y	Y	Y	Y	Y	N	Y	N	N	N	Y	Y	Y	N	N
Johnson et al., 2004 [42]	Y	Y	Y	Y	Y	N	N	N	N	N	Y	Y	N	N	N
Sipahi et al., 2007 [38]	Y	Y	Y	Y	Y	N	N	N	N	N	Y	Y	N	N	N
Jalandar et al., 2012 [18]	Y	Y	Y	Y	Y	N	N	N	N	N	Y	Y	Y	N	N
Stawarczyk et al., 2012 [19]	Y	Y	Y	Y	Y	N	Y	N	N	N	Y	Y	Y	N	N
Patel et al., 2013 [20]	Y	Y	Y	Y	Y	N	N	N	N	N	Y	Y	Y	N	N
Chandrasekaran et al., 2014 [43]	Y	Y	Y	Y	Y	N	Y	Y	N	N	Y	Y	Y	N	N
Kumar et al., 2015 [44]	Y	Y	Y	Y	Y	N	N	N	N	N	Y	Y	N	N	N
Chandavarkar et al., 2015 [8]	Y	Y	Y	Y	Y	N	N	N	N	N	Y	Y	Y	Y	N
Janapala et al., 2015 [45]	Y	Y	Y	Y	Y	Y	N	N	N	N	Y	Y	Y	Y	N
Lawaf et al., 2016 [31]	Y	Y	Y	Y	Y	N	N	N	N	N	Y	Y	Y	N	N
Pilo et al., 2016 [10]	Y	Y	Y	Y	Y	N	N	N	N	N	Y	Y	N	N	N
Mapkar et al., 2018 [11]	Y	Y	Y	Y	Y	N	N	N	N	N	Y	Y	Y	Y	N
Pilo et al., 2018 [39]	Y	Y	Y	Y	Y	N	N	N	N	N	Y	Y	Y	Y	N
Asadullah et al., 2018 [46]	Y	Y	Y	Y	Y	N	N	N	N	N	Y	Y	N	Y	N
Himashilpa et al., 2019 [35]	Y	Y	Y	Y	Y	N	N	N	N	N	Y	Y	N	N	N
Supraja et al., 2020 [47]	Y	Y	Y	Y	Y	Y	N	N	N	N	Y	Y	Y	Y	N
Hanjik et al., 2021 [48]	Y	Y	Y	Y	Y	N	N	N	N	N	Y	Y	N	N	N
Dewan et al., 2022 [49]	Y	Y	Y	Y	Y	N	N	N	N	N	Y	Y	Y	Y	Y

3. Results

3.1. Identification and Screening

An electronic search in PubMed, Scopus, Cochrane, and Web of Sciences resulted in 1454 hits. Of these, 202 articles were duplicates and, hence, were removed. After screening the titles and abstracts of these articles, 1234 articles were removed. The full texts of the remaining 18 articles were reviewed by two authors and, after discussion, all 18 articles were selected for final inclusion in the study. Five articles were added after manual search of the references of the selected articles. Thus, finally, a total of 23 articles were included that satisfied all the selection criteria and addressed the PICO question (Figure 1).

3.2. Characteristics of the Selected Studies

A total of 23 in vitro studies were assessed via a selection process in this systematic review. Out of the 23 total studies, 10 studies were conducted in India, 4 in the USA, 2 in Israel, and 1 each in Georgia, Iran, Saudi Arabia, Syria, Turkey, Germany, and Switzerland. The most recent studies were published in 2022, and the oldest was published in 1996 (Table 1). All 23 studies demonstrated comparative analysis of the test and control groups and assessed the effect of desensitizing agents on the retention of cemented crowns. The sample size in the selected studies ranged from $n = 20$ [31] to $n = 420$ [35].

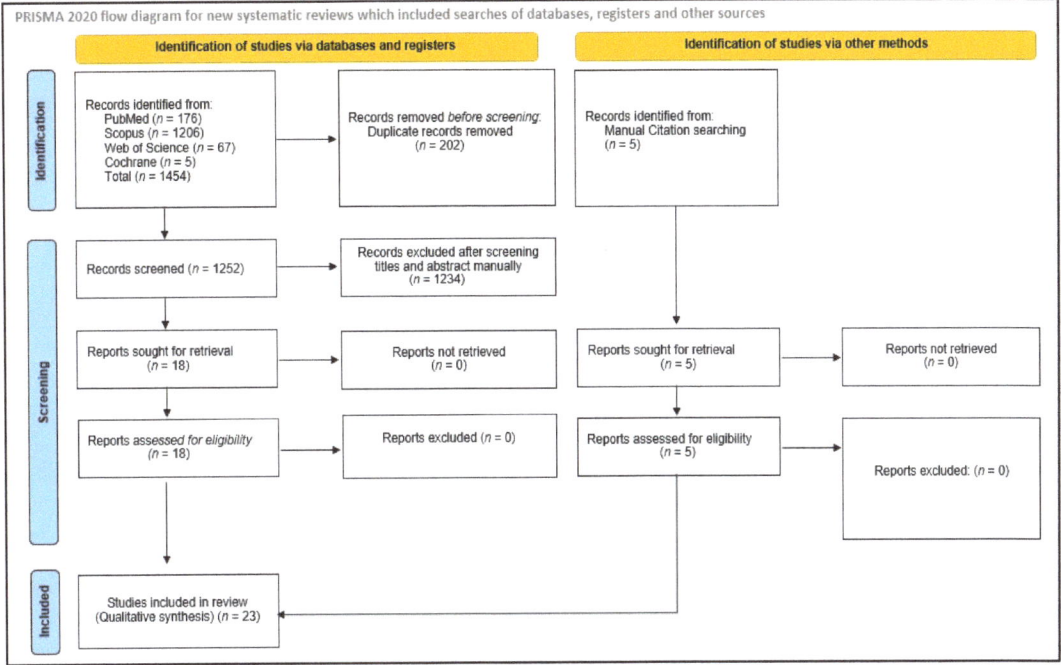

Figure 1. PRISMA flow-chart demonstrating the article selection strategy, preferred reporting items for systematic reviews and meta-analyses.

Twelve out of the twenty-three studies used human molars, whereas eleven studies used human premolars for evaluating the bond strength of the cemented crowns/copings. In most of the studies, the taper for preparation of the tooth was kept between 6° and 20°. All studies used full-coverage crowns/copings for retention assessment. The materials used to fabricate these full-coverage retainers were base metal alloys in seventeen studies [8,11,12,18,20,31,34,35,37–39,43–48], noble/high noble alloys in three studies [36,43,45], and zirconia ceramic in three studies [10,19,49]. In most of the studies involving metal alloys, the fabrication technique of crowns/copings was lost wax casting, whereas in two studies, an additive manufacturing technique (3D printing) was used [39,47]. In all of the studies using zirconia crowns/copings, the subtractive manufacturing technique (CAD/CAM milling) was used for fabrication [10,19,49]. (Table 1).

The majority of the studies compared the effect of liquid-based DAs on retention, whereas three studies compared the effect of lasers as DA along with liquid-based DAs [8,38,44]. Most of the studies compared the effect of more than one type of DA on retention. Nearly thirteen studies used glutaraldehyde-based DAs [8,11,12,18,19,31,34–36,45,46,48,49], six used arginine-based DAs [8,10,35,39,46], five used CPP-ACP-based DAs [8,18,35,43,47], and three studies each used phosphoric acid-based [20,36,42] and resin-based [11,12,37] DAs. Few studies assessed the effect of other types of DAs (D-TMR-based, HEMA NTG-GMA-based, etc.) on the retention of cemented crowns. (Table 1).

Most of the studies compared the bond strength using different types of luting cement [10–12,18–20,34–37,39,41–44,47–49]. Commonly used cements include zinc phosphate, glass ionomer cement, resin-modified GIC, and resin cement. Only one study also compared polycarboxylate cement along with the above-mentioned cements [41]. (Table 1).

3.3. Findings of Quality Analysis

As all of the studies selected in this systematic review were in vitro studies, the modified CONSORT scale [50,51] for in vitro studies was used to perform quality analysis of the selected studies, on the basis of which 61.7% (213/345) of the entries were positively rated (Table 2). Entries related to the quality of the abstract (Item 1), the introduction (Item 2a, 2b), the intervention (Item 3), the outcomes (Item 4), the statistical methods used (Item 10) in the methodology section, and the results section (Item 11) were rated positively for all of the selected articles. Thirteen studies reported their limitations (Item 12), eight reported details related to the sources of funding (Item 13), six briefly reported details on the randomization method (Item 6), only two reported of the method used for sample size calculation (Item 5), and one study made the full study protocol accessible (Item 14). One study reported steps taken to conceal the random allocation (Item 7), but none of the studies reported having taken steps necessary to prevent bias, such as who made the random distribution sequence (Item 7) and how blinding was performed (Item 9). Overall, the quality of the selected articles was good, with a moderate risk of bias.

3.4. Results of Individual Studies

The results of the selected studies varied due to differences in the composition of the tested dentine DAs and the types of luting cements. After the application of liquid-based DAs, the studies reported an increase in the retention of crowns when cemented with resin cements [19,31,36,37,41,46,49], when cemented with GIC [8,18,20,39,42,43], and when cemented with RMGIC [18,37,45,47,48]. However, the use of DAs with ZPC was reported in almost all of the studies to decrease the retention of cemented crowns [11,18,20,37,39,41–43]. The studies also reported a reduction in retention when GIC or resin cements were used with specific DAs [35,37,41,46–48]. The use of a laser as a DA was reported to reduce the retention of crowns when cemented using GIC [8,38,44]. However, Kumar et al. [44] reported that retention increased when laser was used as a DA and resin cement was used for the cementation of retainers (Table 1).

4. Discussion

Tooth preparation for full-coverage FDP involves reduction of the coronal tooth structure. Hypersensitivity is commonly reported after cementation of crowns/FPDs on prepared vital teeth [52]. Dentine desensitizing agents are commonly applied on the teeth before cementation to prevent this hypersensitivity, but their effect on the retention of cemented crowns is still debatable [8,10–12,18–20,31,34–39,41–49]. The current systematic review is the first of its kind to evaluate the quality of the published literature assessing the effect of DAs on the bond strength of cemented crowns. All 23 included articles were in vitro prospective randomized controlled trials [8,10–12,18–20,31,34–39,41–49]. The findings of the 23 included studies suggest that the use of DAs affects the bond strength of cemented crowns, and that the results vary according to the type of DA and the cement used for cementation, thereby rejecting the proposed null hypothesis.

Multiple reasons for post-cementation hypersensitivity have been postulated in the literature, including the opening of dentinal tubules, the chemical composition and the initial low pH of the luting cements, microleakage and bacterial leakage due to polymerization shrinkage of luting agents, desiccation of the tooth, hydraulic pressure on tubules during luting, higher permeability due to smear layer removal, etc. [47,53–56]. To minimize this post-cementation hypersensitivity, DAs are commonly used before cementation. These DAs can be in the form of liquids or lasers [8,12,38,42–47]. They act in multiple ways, which include blocking the opening of dentinal tubules, reducing inflammation, depolarization of the nerves, etc. [11,47]. The protective layer formed by DA can affect the retention of cemented crowns by reducing the micromechanical retention tags [15,16,44].

When evaluating the retention of crowns cemented with ZPC, most studies report a decrease in retention values after the application of DAs. [11,18,20,35,37,39,41–43]. ZPC uses irregularities on the dentine surface to attain mechanical retention. Application of most of the DAs blocked these irregularities, thus making the surface smooth and causing a decrease in retention. Meanwhile, in three studies, the retention values were slightly higher [11,18,34]. All three studies used the GLUMA desensitizer, which has been reported to obliterate the bulk of dentinal tubules and infiltrate into them as plugs [57]. This does not alter the irregularities on the dentine and, thus, does not reduce the retention of cemented crowns [18,57].

With GIC as a luting agent, studies have reported contrasting results for retention values with the application of DAs. The type of DA used affected the retention values to a great extent. The retention values were reported to be higher in all studies that used GC Tooth Mousse [8,18,35,43] and One Step [20,36,42] as a DA before cementation. The mechanism of bonding of GIC is chemico-mechanical. The use of GC Tooth Mousse makes the dentine surface smooth, thus helping to increase retention values, as GIC bonds better on smoother surfaces [18,35]. Higher retention values with the application of One Step DA may be due to the chemical affinity of GIC towards HEMA monomers of resin DAs. Thus, after the interface of GIC and resin has been set, it is reported to be like that of RMGIC [20,36,42]. Four studies reported higher retention values when Gluma DA was used [8,18,34,35], whereas three studies reported lower retention values [36–38]. The increase in retention values was proposed to be due to the chemical affinity of GIC towards resin sealers containing glutaraldehyde and HEMA [18], whereas the reduction in retention values was proposed to be due to GLUMA being a non-polymerizing resin-based sealer that fills the irregularities of dentine, thus preventing the formation of chelating bonds with dentine [37]. The use of Colgate Sensitive Pro-Relief was reported in two studies to increase retention values [8,39] and in one study to reduce retention values [35]. Chelation between polyalkenoic chains in GIC and calcium carbonate in Pro-Arging-based DAs was presumed to be a possible cause of higher retention values [39], whereas interference in bonding due to the delicate plugs formed by the DAs was presumed to be the cause of poor retention values [35]. Systemp DA increased the retention values in one study [35] and reduced them in the other [48]. The binding of calcium and fluoride minerals released from GIC with the system protein plugs was proposed to be the cause of higher retention values [35]. All Bond [37,41] and lasers [8,38,44] reduced retention values in all of the studies that used them as DAs. Lasers were reported to cause desiccation of the collagen fibrils, as well as producing micro-explosions on the top surface of the dentinal tubules, leading to smear layer formation. These changes interfere with the chemical bonding of GIC with dentine, thus reducing the retention values [44,58].

Retention values when RMGIC is used as a luting agent after DA application varied in different studies. In general, the use of Systemp DA increased retention values [35,48]. Gluma as DA increased retention values in three studies [18,36,45] and decreased them in two studies [35,37]. The use of Tooth Mousse [18,43] or Colgate Sensitive Pro-Relief [10,35] as DAs had no effect on retention values. The binding of protein plugs formed by Systemp with resin tags was proposed to be the cause of higher retention values when Systemp DA was used with RMGIC [35,48]. The increase in retention values with Gluma was proposed to be due to the chemical affinity of RMGIC towards resin sealers containing HEMA [18,45].

Most of the studies reported higher retention values for crowns cemented using resin cements after the application of different DAs [19,31,34,35,37,41,46,49]. Polymerization between the HEMA complex (at the dentine–DA junction) and resin cement [31,59,60], the rewetting properties of HEMA, the buffering capacity of resins [61], and micro-mechanical bonding between protein plugs formed by DAs and resin tags [35,62] may be possible reasons for increased retention values when RC is used with DAs. The use of Pro-Argenine [10] and lasers [44] as DAs was reported to cause no change in retention values when RC was used. It has been proposed that lasers increase the calcium ions on the surface of the dentine, which may increase chelating reactions and resin cements, partially decalcifying the smear layer (formed after laser treatment), thus forming resin tags [44,63].

In the absence of DAs, the retention values were reported to be highest for RC, followed by RMGIC and GIC, while ZPC displayed lowest retention values [18,20,34,35,37,39,41–44,47,48].

Adhesive bonding between calcium ions and monomers in resin cement was shown to possess increased retention values compared to other cements [64,65].

The type of dentine desensitizing agent used in the selected studies influenced the outcome of this systematic review. With time, new generations of DAs have evolved that have better handling and properties. The comprehensive search and selection protocol is a key feature of this systematic review. Limitations of this systematic review include a moderate to high risk of bias in the selected studies, the wide variety of tested materials, and the differences in testing conditions. The current systematic review aimed to discuss the effects of DAs on the retention of crowns. The effect of these DAs on hypersensitivity also needs to be addressed, as this is an important parameter when selecting the best DA for patients before crown cementation to minimize post-operative sensitivity.

5. Conclusions

The following conclusions can be drawn on the basis of this systematic review:
1. The type of dentine desensitizing agent and luting agent used affect the retention values of the cemented FDPs.
2. In general, the retention values of FDPs cemented using zinc phosphate cement are reduced with most of the DAs, whereas retention values increase when GIC, resin-modified GIC, and resin cements are used with the majority of DAs.
3. Blinding protocols should be followed in future in vitro studies to avoid bias.
4. Dentists should have knowledge regarding the compatibility of DAs and luting cements in order to provide the best treatment to their patients.

Supplementary Materials: The following supporting information can be downloaded at: https://www.mdpi.com/article/10.3390/medicina59030515/s1, Table S1: Search strategy for the electronic databases.

Funding: This research received no external funding.

Institutional Review Board Statement: Not applicable.

Informed Consent Statement: Not applicable.

Data Availability Statement: The data that support the findings of this study are available from the corresponding author upon reasonable request.

Acknowledgments: Author would like to thank Maryam H. Mugri (M.M.) and Saurabh Jain (S.J.) for their help in the screening and selection of the reviewed articles.

Conflicts of Interest: The authors declare no conflict of interest.

References

1. Shillingburg, H.T.; Hobo, S.; Whit, L.D. *Fundamentals of Fixed Prosthodontics*, 2nd ed.; Quintessence: Chicago, IL, USA, 1981.
2. Krauser, J.T. Hypersensitive teeth. Part I: Etiology. *J. Prosthet. Dent.* **1986**, *56*, 153–156. [CrossRef] [PubMed]
3. Richardson, D.; Tao, L.; Pashley, D.H. Dentin permeability: Effects of crown preparation. *Int. J. Prosthodont.* **1991**, *4*, 219–225. [PubMed]
4. Watson, T.F.; Flanagan, D.; Stone, D.G. High and low torque handpieces: Cutting dynamics, enamel cracking and tooth temperature. *Br. Dent. J.* **2000**, *188*, 680–686. [CrossRef] [PubMed]
5. Outhwaite, W.C.; Livingston, M.; Pashiey, D.H. Effects of changes in surface area, thickness, temperature and postextraction time on human dentin permeability. *Arch. Oral Biol.* **1976**, *21*, 599–603. [CrossRef]
6. Reeder, O.W.; Walton, R.E.; Livingston, M.J.; Pashley, D.H. Dentin permeability: Determinants of hydraulic conductance. *J. Dent. Res.* **1978**, *57*, 187–193. [CrossRef]
7. Fogei, H.M.; Marshall, F.; Pashley, D.H. Effects of distance from the pulp and thiciiness on the permeability of human radicular dentin. *J. Dent. Res.* **1991**, *67*, 1381.
8. Chandavarkar, S.M.; Ram, S.M. A comparative evaluation of the effect of dentin desensitizers on the retention of complete cast metal crowns. *Contemp. Clin. Dent.* **2015**, *6* (Suppl. 1), S45–S50. [CrossRef]
9. Garberoglio, R.; Brännström, M. Scanning electron microscopic investigation of human dentinal tubules. *Arch. Oral Biol.* **1976**, *21*, 355–3562. [CrossRef]
10. Pilo, R.; Harel, N.; Nissan, J.; Levartovsky, S. The retentive strength of cemented zirconium oxide crowns after dentin pretreatment with desensitizing paste containing 8% arginine and calcium carbonate. *Int. J. Mol. Sci.* **2016**, *17*, 426. [CrossRef]

11. Mapkar, M.A.; Jagtap, A.; Asadullah, S.R.S. Effect of two desensitizing agents on crown retention using zinc phosphate cement. *Int. J. Oral Care Res.* **2018**, *6*, 64–68.
12. Wolfart, S.; Linnemann, J.; Kern, M. Crown retention with use of different sealing systems on prepared dentine. *J. Oral Rehabil.* **2003**, *30*, 1053–1061. [CrossRef] [PubMed]
13. Smith, D.C.; Ruse, N.D. Acidity of glass ionomer cements during cementation and its relation to pulp sensitivity. *JADA* **1986**, *112*, 654–657.
14. Watanabe, T.; Sano, M.; Itoh, K.; Wakumoto, S. The effects of primers on the sensitivity of dentin. *Dent. Mater.* **1991**, *7*, 148–150. [CrossRef] [PubMed]
15. Dhondi dall'Orologio, G.; Malferrari, S. Desensitizing effects of Gluma and Gluma 2000 on hypersensitive dentin. *Am. J. Dent.* **1993**, *6*, 283–286.
16. Felton, D.A.; Bergenholtz, G.; Kanoy, B.E. Evaluation of the desensitizing effect of Gluma dentin bond on teeth prepared for complete-coverage restorations. *Int. J. Prosthodont.* **1991**, *4*, 292–298.
17. Bergenholtz, G.; Jontell, M.; Tuttle, A.; Knutsson, G. Inhibition of serum albumin flux across exposed dentine following conditioning with GLUMA primer, glutaraldehyde or potassium oxalates. *J. Dent.* **1993**, *21*, 220–227. [CrossRef]
18. Jalandar, S.S.; Pandharinath, D.S.; Arun, K.; Smita, V. Comparison of effect of desensitizing agents on the retention of crowns cemented with luting agents: An in vitro study. *J. Adv. Prosthodont.* **2012**, *4*, 127–133. [CrossRef]
19. Stawarczyk, B.; Hartmann, L.; Hartmann, R.; Roos, M.; Ender, A.; Özcan, M.; Sailer, I.; Hämmerle, C.H.F. Impact of Gluma Desensitizer on the tensile strength of zirconia crowns bonded to dentin: An in vitro study. *Clin. Oral Investig.* **2012**, *16*, 201–213. [CrossRef]
20. Patel, P.; Thummar, M.; Shah, D.; Pitti, V. Comparing the effect of a resin based sealer on crown retention for three types of cements: An in vitro study. *J. Indian Prosthodont. Soc.* **2013**, *13*, 308–314. [CrossRef]
21. Fambrini, E.; Miceli, M.; Pasini, M.; Giuca, M.R. Clinical evaluation of the use of desensitizing agents in the management of dentinal hypersensitivity. *Appl. Sci.* **2022**, *12*, 11238. [CrossRef]
22. Najibfard, K.; Ramalingam, K.; Chedjieu, I.; Amaechi, B.T. Remineralization of early caries by a nano-hydroxyapatite dentifrice. *J. Clin. Dent.* **2011**, *22*, 139–143.
23. de Melo Alencar, C.; de Paula, B.L.F.; Guanipa Ortiz, M.I.; Barauna Magno, M.; Martins Silva, C.; Cople Maia, L. Clinical efficacy of nano-hydroxyapatite in dentin hypersensitivity: A systematic review and meta-analysis. *J. Dent.* **2019**, *82*, 11–21. [CrossRef] [PubMed]
24. Tolentino, A.B.; Zeola, L.F.; Fernandes, M.R.U.; Pannuti, C.M.; Soares, P.V.; Aranha, A.C.C. Photobiomodulation therapy and 3% potassium nitrate gel as treatment of cervical dentin hypersensitivity: A randomized clinical trial. *Clin. Oral. Investig.* **2022**, *26*, 6985–6993. [CrossRef] [PubMed]
25. Lee, S.; Kwon, H.; Kim, B. Effect of dentinal tubule occlusion by dentifrice containing nano-carbonate apatite. *J. Oral Rehabil.* **2008**, *35*, 847–853. [CrossRef]
26. Matsuura, T.; Mae, M.; Ohira, M.; Mihara, Y.; Yamashita, Y.; Sugimoto, K.; Yamada, S.; Yoshimura, A. The efficacy of a novel zinc-containing desensitizer CAREDYNE Shield for cervical dentin hypersensitivity: A pilot randomized controlled trial. *BMC Oral Health* **2022**, *22*, 294. [CrossRef] [PubMed]
27. Shillinberg, H.T., Jr.; Sumiya, H.; Whitsett, L.D.; Richard, J.; Brackette, S.E. *Fundamentals of Fixed Prosthodontics*, 3rd ed.; Quintessence: Chicago, IL, USA, 1997; pp. 119–128.
28. Rosenstiel, S.F.; Land, M.F.; Fujimoto, J. *Contemporary Fixed Prosthodontics*, 4th ed.; Mosby Inc.: St. Louis, MI, USA, 2006; pp. 226–243.
29. Tyllman, S.D.; Malone, W.F.; Koth, D.L.; Edmund, C., Jr.; Kaiser, D.A.; Margano, S.M. *Theory and Practice of Fixed Prosthodontics*, 8th ed.; Medico Dental Media International Inc.: New York, NY, USA, 2001; pp. 113–135.
30. Ayad, M.F.; Johnston, W.M.; Rosenstiel, S.F. Influence of tooth preparation taper and cement type on recementation strength of complete metal crowns. *J. Prosthet. Dent.* **2009**, *102*, 354–361. [CrossRef] [PubMed]
31. Lawaf, S.; Jalalian, E.; Roshan, R.; Azizi, A. Effect of GLUMA desensitizer on the retention of full metal crowns cemented with Rely X U200 self-adhesive cement. *J. Adv. Prosthodont.* **2016**, *8*, 404–410. [CrossRef]
32. Al-Omari, W.M.; Al-Wahadni, A.M. *Convergence Angle, Occlusal Reduction, and Finish Line Depth of Full-Crown Preparations Made by Dental Students*; Quintessence: Chicago, IL, USA, 2004; Volume 35, pp. 287–293.
33. Zidan, O.; Ferguson, G.C. The retention of complete crowns prepared with three different tapers and luted with four different cements. *J. Prosthet. Dent.* **2003**, *89*, 565–571. [CrossRef] [PubMed]
34. Johnson, G.H.; Lepe, X.; Bales, D.J. Crown retention with use of a 5% glutaraldehyde sealer on prepared dentin. *J. Prosthet. Dent.* **1998**, *79*, 671–676. [CrossRef] [PubMed]
35. Himashilpa, G.V.R.; Ravishankar, Y.; Srinivas, K.; Harikrishna, M.; Shameen Kumar, P.; Satyendra, T. Influence of desensitizing agents on the retention quality of Complete cast crowns cemented with various luting agents—An in-vitro study. *J. Sci. Res.* **2019**, *8*, 1–4.
36. Swift, E.J., Jr.; Lloyd, A.H.; Felton, D.A. The effect of resin desensitizing agents on crown retention. *JADA* **1997**, *128*, 195–200. [CrossRef] [PubMed]

37. Yim, N.H.; Rueggeberg, F.A.; Caughman, W.F.; Gardner, F.M.; Pashley, D.H. Effect of dentin desensitizers and cementing agents on retention of full crowns using standardized crown preparations. *J. Prosthet. Dent.* **2000**, *83*, 459–465. [CrossRef]
38. Sipahi, C.; Cehreli, M.; Ozen, J.; Dalkiz, M. Effects of precementation desensitizing laser treatment and conventional desensitizing agents on crown retention. *Int. J. Prosthodont.* **2007**, *20*, 289–292. [PubMed]
39. Pilo, R.; Agar-Zoizner, S.; Gelbard, S.; Levartovsky, S. The retentive strength of laser-sintered cobalt-chromium-based crowns after pretreatment with a desensitizing paste containing 8% arginine and calcium carbonate. *Int. J. Mol. Sci.* **2018**, *19*, 4082. [CrossRef]
40. Shamseer, L.; Moher, D.; Clarke, M.; Ghersi, D.; Liberati, A.; Petticrew, M.; Shekelle, P.; Stewart, L.A.; PRISMA-P Group. Preferred reporting items for systematic review and meta-analysis protocols (PRISMA-P) 2015: Elaboration and explanation. *BMJ* **2015**, *349*, g7647. [CrossRef] [PubMed]
41. Mausner, I.K.; Goldstein, G.R.; Georgescu, M. Effect of two dentinal desensitizing agents on retention of complete cast coping using four cements. *J. Prosthet. Dent.* **1996**, *75*, 129–134. [CrossRef]
42. Johnson, G.H.; Hazelton, L.R.; Bales, D.J.; Lepe, X. The effect of a resin-based sealer on crown retention for three types of cement. *J. Prosthet. Dent.* **2004**, *91*, 428–435. [CrossRef]
43. Chandrasekaran, A.P.; Deepan, N.; Rao, B.K.; Pai, S.; Sonthalia, A.; Bettanpalya, S.V. Evaluation of the effect of desensitizing agents on the retention of complete cast crowns: An in vitro study. *SRM J. Res. Dent. Sci.* **2014**, *5*, 174. [CrossRef]
44. Kumar, S.; Rupesh, P.L.; Kalekar, S.G.A.; Ghunawat, D.B.; Siddiqui, S. Effect of desensitising laser treatment on the bond strength of full metal crowns: An in vitro comparative study. *J. Int. Oral Health* **2015**, *7*, 36–41.
45. Janapala, S.D.R.; Reddy, P.S.; Jain, A.R.; Pradeep, R. The effect of three dentinal sealers on retention of crowns cemented with resin-modified glass ionomer cement: An in vitro study. *March World J. Dent.* **2015**, *6*, 10–15.
46. Syed Asadullah, S.R.; Rakhewar, P.; Mapkar, M.A. Comparison of effect of desensitizing agents on the retention of crowns cemented with resinomer cement: An in vitro study. *Int. J. Prev. Clin. Dent. Res.* **2018**, *5*, 5–9.
47. Kottem, S.; Dileep, N.V.; Divi, V.V.V.K.; Srinivas, R.P. Evaluation of freshly prepared "arginine-calcium carbonate-fluoride" and "casein phosphopeptide-amorphous calcium phosphate-fluoride" desensitizing agents on crown retention: An in vitro study. *World J. Dent.* **2020**, *11*, 355–360.
48. Seba, H.; Ebtisam, L. The influence of systemp desensitizer on the retention quality of Complete cast crowns cemented by glass ionomer and resin modified glass Ionomer cements (in-vitro study). *Int. J. Recent Sci. Res.* **2021**, *12*, 41662–41669.
49. Dewan, H.; Sayed, M.E.; Alqahtani, N.M.; Alnajai, T.; Qasir, A.; Chohan, H. The effect of commercially available desensitizers on bond strength following cementation of zirconia crowns using self-adhesive resin cement—An in vitro study. *Materials* **2022**, *15*, 514. [CrossRef] [PubMed]
50. Faggion, C.M., Jr. Guidelines for reporting pre-clinical in vitro studies on dental materials. *J. Evid. Based Dent. Pract.* **2012**, *12*, 182–189. [CrossRef]
51. Krithikadatta, J.; Datta, M.; Gopikrishna, V. CRIS guidelines (checklist for reporting in-vitro studies): A concept note on the need for standardized guidelines for improving quality and transparency in reporting in-vitro studies in experimental dental research. *J. Conserv. Dent.* **2014**, *17*, 301–304. [CrossRef]
52. Johnson, G.H.; Powell, L.V.; DeRouen, T.A. Evaluation and control of post-cementation pulpal sensitivity: Zinc phosphate and glass ionomer luting cements. *J. Am. Dent. Assoc.* **1993**, *124*, 38–46. [CrossRef]
53. Jackson, C.R.; Skidmore, A.E.; Rice, R.T. Pulpal evaluation of teeth restored with fixedprostheses. *J. Prosthet. Dent.* **1992**, *67*, 323–325. [CrossRef]
54. Brannstrom, M.; Linden, L.A.; Astrom, A. The hydrodynamics of the dental tubule and ofpulp fluid. *Caries Res.* **1967**, *1*, 310–317. [CrossRef]
55. Nicholson, J.W.; Croll, T.P. Glass-ionomer cements in restorative dentistry. *Quintessence* **1997**, *28*, 705–714.
56. Pace, L.L.; Hummel, S.K.; Marker, V.A.; Bolouri, A. Comparison of the flexural strength of five adhesive resin cements. *J. Prosthodont.* **2007**, *16*, 18–24. [CrossRef] [PubMed]
57. Arrais, C.A.; Chan, D.C.; Giannini, M. Effects of desensitizing agents on dentinal tubule occlusion. *J. Appl. Oral Sci.* **2004**, *12*, 144–148. [CrossRef]
58. Ceballo, L.; Toledano, M.; Osorio, R.; Tay, F.R.; Marshall, G.W. Bonding to Er-YAG-laser-treated dentin. *J. Dent. Res.* **2002**, *81*, 119–122. [CrossRef] [PubMed]
59. Munksgaard, E.C.; Asmussen, E. Bond strength between dentin and restorative resins mediated by mixtures of HEMA and glutaraldehyde. *J. Dent. Res.* **1984**, *63*, 1087–1089. [CrossRef]
60. Qin, C.; Xu, J.; Zhang, Y. Spectroscopic investigation of the function of aqueous 2-hydroxyethylmethacrylate/glutaraldehyde solution as a dentin desensitizer. *Eur. J. Oral Sci.* **2006**, *114*, 354–359. [CrossRef]
61. Acar, O.; Tuncer, D.; Yuzugullu, B.; Celik, C. The effect of dentin desensitizers and Nd: YAG laser pre-treatment on microtensile bond strength of self-adhesive resin cement to dentin. *J. Adv. Prosthodont.* **2014**, *6*, 88–95. [CrossRef] [PubMed]
62. Khalil, A.; Khalid, A.; Ziad, N.A.-D.; Hani, A.; Abdulrhman, A.; Abdulaziz, A.; Edward, L. Retention of zirconium oxide copings using different types of luting agents. *J. Dent. Sci.* **2013**, *8*, 392–398.
63. Monticelli, F.; Osorio, R.; Mazzitelli, C.; Ferrari, M.; Toledano, M. Limited decalcification/diffusion of self-adhesive cements into dentin. *J. Dent. Res.* **2008**, *87*, 974–979. [CrossRef]

64. Pathak, S.; Shashibhushan, K.K.; Poornima, P.; Reddy, V.V.S. In Vitro evaluation of stainless steel crowns cemented with resin-modified glass Ionomer and two new self-adhesive resin cements. *Int. J. Clin. Pediatr. Dent.* **2016**, *9*, 197–200. [CrossRef]
65. Sabatini, C.; Patel, M.; D'Silva, E. In Vitro shear bond strength of three self adhesive resin cements and a resin-modified glass ionomer cement to various prosthodontic substrates. *Oper. Dent.* **2013**, *38*, 186–196. [CrossRef]

Disclaimer/Publisher's Note: The statements, opinions and data contained in all publications are solely those of the individual author(s) and contributor(s) and not of MDPI and/or the editor(s). MDPI and/or the editor(s) disclaim responsibility for any injury to people or property resulting from any ideas, methods, instructions or products referred to in the content.

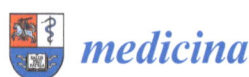

Article

The Impact of Simulated Bruxism Forces and Surface Aging Treatments on Two Dental Nano-Biocomposites—A Radiographic and Tomographic Analysis

Amelia Anita Boitor [1], Elena Bianca Varvară [1], Corina Mirela Prodan [1], Sorina Sava [2], Diana Dudea [1] and Adriana Objelean [2,*]

[1] Department of Dental Propaedeutics and Esthetics, Faculty of Dental Medicine, University of Medicine and Pharmacy "Iuliu Hatieganu", 400006 Cluj-Napoca, Romania
[2] Department of Dental Materials and Ergonomics, Faculty of Dental Medicine, University of Medicine and Pharmacy "Iuliu Hatieganu", 400083 Cluj-Napoca, Romania
* Correspondence: adriana.caracostea@umfcluj.ro

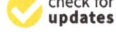

Citation: Boitor, A.A.; Varvară, E.B.; Prodan, C.M.; Sava, S.; Dudea, D.; Objelean, A. The Impact of Simulated Bruxism Forces and Surface Aging Treatments on Two Dental Nano-Biocomposites—A Radiographic and Tomographic Analysis. *Medicina* **2023**, *59*, 360. https://doi.org/10.3390/medicina59020360

Academic Editors: Giuseppe Minervini and Stefania Moccia

Received: 30 January 2023
Revised: 8 February 2023
Accepted: 11 February 2023
Published: 14 February 2023

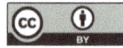

Copyright: © 2023 by the authors. Licensee MDPI, Basel, Switzerland. This article is an open access article distributed under the terms and conditions of the Creative Commons Attribution (CC BY) license (https://creativecommons.org/licenses/by/4.0/).

Abstract: *Background and Objectives*: Nowadays, indication of composite materials for various clinical situations has increased significantly. However, in the oral environment, these biomaterials are subjected (abnormal occlusal forces, external bleaching, consumption of carbonated beverages, etc.) to changes in their functional and mechanical behavior when indicated primarily for patients with masticatory habits. The study aimed to recreate in our lab one of the most common situations nowadays—in-office activity of a young patient suffering from specific parafunctional occlusal stress (bruxism) who consumes acidic beverages and is using at-home dental bleaching. *Materials and Methods*: Sixty standardized class II cavities were restored with two nanohybrid biocomposite materials (Filtek Z550, 3M ESPE, and Evetric, Ivoclar Vivadent); the restored teeth were immersed in sports drinks and carbonated beverages and exposed to an at home teeth bleaching agent. The samples were subjected to parafunctional mechanical loads using a dual-axis chewing simulator. A grading evaluation system was conducted to assess the defects of the restorations using different examination devices: a CBCT, a high-resolution digital camera, and periapical X-rays. *Results*: Before mechanical loading, the CBCT analysis revealed substantially fewer interfacial defects between the two resin-based composites ($p > 0.05$), whereas, after bruxism forces simulation, significantly more defects were identified ($p < 0.05$). Qualitative examination of the restorations showed more occlusal defects for the Evetric than the other nanohybrid composite. *Conclusions*: There were different behaviors observed regarding the studied nanocomposites when simulation of parafunctional masticatory forces was associated with aging treatments.

Keywords: CBCT; nanohybrid biocomposites; masticatory parafunction; surface aging treatment; dental bleaching; digital X-ray; two-body wear simulation; bruxism; imaging in dentistry

1. Introduction

It is known that the most resistant material that withstands the oral cavity environment is the natural tooth, with its biological tissues, enamel, and dentine [1]. However, due to possible tooth diseases or traumas, these naturally engineered tissues may be damaged by carious lesions, resulting in tooth decay and defects that need to be reconstructed with oral biomaterials. These materials must be biocompatible, with optimal physical, mechanical, chemical, and aesthetic properties. One of the most often indicated groups of restorative materials is resin composite, which has shown an acceptable survival rate in clinical and in vitro studies [2].

During recent decades, research and development of resin-based composites have generated different subcategories of restorative materials that include composites containing nano-sized filler particles [3–6]. Nano-filled composites have nanometric-sized particles, while nanohybrid ones contain finely ground glass fillers and nano-fillers in a pre-polymerized filler form [7,8]. Some professionals claim that the newly introduced materials [7] offer reduced polymerization contraction, enhanced mechanical properties, and improved aesthetics [7–9].

Aesthetics has always been an important topic for patients. Thus, for over two decades, bleaching treatments, especially those carried on at home, under a doctor's supervision, are often treatments of choice for improving dental color in adolescents and young adults, particularly those interested in their body image [8–11]. This group of patients is known to prioritize body aesthetics and practice sports regularly. Along with cutting-edge new technologies in sports coming into play, there are also various sports drinks, energy drinks, or soft drinks containing other sugary and mineral compounds [10].

It was reported in the literature that oral biofilm might induce surface changes in dental restorative materials, leading to their chemical degradation and thus a higher chance for the dental fillings to develop marginal percolation and other defects [12]. It was also reported that chewing gum might lead to leaching of chemical compounds of resin-based composites [13]. It is well known that any change in the architecture of the oral cavity may interfere with the whole oral equilibrium, disturbing it at different levels (e.g., muscles, teeth, TMJ) [8,9]. Consequently, parafunctional occlusal habits that generate increased forces on teeth are frequently encountered and reported to highly affect tooth-adhesive interface and tooth wear strength [1,8,9,14].

In this established environment, dramatic oral changes were observed due to low-pH drink consumption and at-home dental bleaching or other whitening pastes. This problem could be clinically translated with dental erosions and surface and interfacial failure of different dental fillings [12,13,15–20].

Micro-computer tomography is a non-destructive X-ray 3D image analyzer used mainly in laboratory investigations. Digital radiography is the most often clinically indicated imagistic analysis used by dental practitioners. This radiographic method uses 2D images, but new systems or devices can analyze a broader range of oral environment changes. One of these systems is cone-beam computed tomography (CBCT), which offers a three-dimensional view of oral tissues for different clinical indications (such as caries detection, TMJ disorders, or bone density) [21,22]. A few years ago, CBCT was proposed as a 3D image analyzer for in vitro studies [22–24].

The literature did not thoroughly analyze the consequences of combined patients' high aesthetic demands, sugar-added carbonated beverages, and parafunctional occlusal habits. Based on the research data on this subject, the present in vitro study aimed to assess behavior of two direct resin-based nanocomposites subjected to two surface aging treatments (external bleach and acid beverages) combined with simulated occlusal parafunctional forces.

The null hypothesis was that the two restorative nano-biocomposites had very similar mechanical, aesthetic, and functional behaviors regardless of type of surface aging and higher impact loads applied.

2. Materials and Methods

The study protocol was approved by the Research Ethics and Methodology Department, University of Medicine and Pharmacy "Iuliu Hatieganu", Cluj-Napoca, Romania (247/30.06.2021).

For this investigation, the sample size was determined based on a previous pilot study, for which the effect size was 1, power (1-β) of 0.8, and the level of significance = 0.05. The data were analyzed using a t-test family for matched pairs, with G*power software version 3.1.9.7 (Kiel University Software, Germany) for Windows software. The optimal sample size was calculated as up to 10 dental cavities based on the abovementioned assumptions.

Before the experimental test, the teeth were checked for cracks, fractures, or other surface defects using dental loupes (3× magnification) and a sharp explorer. Then, the teeth were cleaned, and any soft tissue was removed using an ultrasound scaler (U600 LED,

Woodpecker Medical Instruments Co. Ltd., Guilin, China). After the cleaning procedure, the teeth were kept in 1% Chloramine T, and, after a thorough rinse, they were stored in distilled water at 4 °C.

Sixty standardized class II cavities (mesio-occlusal, disto-occlusal) were prepared on intact human premolars extracted for periodontal or orthodontic reasons upon the patient's consent. Two proximal cavities were prepared for each tooth with the following dimensions: 3 mm occlusal depth, 4 mm in buccal-lingual width, 2 mm proximal depth, 4 mm width at the cervical area; all the proximal cavities had the gingival margin placed at 1 mm above the cementoenamel junction (CEJ). The teeth were randomly divided into two groups (n = 30 cavities/material) and restored using the following nanohybrid resin-based composites: Group 1, Evetric, Ivoclar Vivadent (Gr 1 EV); Group 2, Filtek Z550, 3M ESPE (Gr 2 FZ). A self-etch universal adhesive (Opti-bond XTR Universal Self-Etch, Kerr Corp, USA) was applied before the respective restorative composite (). The composites were applied based on the zig-zag technique (2 mm/layer/material). For polymerization of each increment (40 s/layer), we used a 2nd generation LED light-curing lamp (SDI, Radi-plus, light intensity = 1500 mW/cm^2; wavelength range = 440–480 nm). The tip of the curing lamp was placed in direct contact with the dental wall where the material increment was placed. Then, the restorations were finished and polished using oval carbide burs (SS White, T&F, Carbide burs, FG, 7406), Sof-Lex abrasive disk (3M ESPE), Occlubrush impregnated polishers (Kerr Co.), and Super Polish Paste (Kerr Co.).

The teeth were immersed twice a day for 28 days in a sports drink ((Gatorade Red Orange with a pH of 3.2) and then in a carbonated beverage (Coca-Cola, pH = 2.4)) [10]. The pH of the two beverages was tested using a pH meter HI-98103 (Hanna Instruments) three times for each. After immersion in each acid beverage, the teeth were thoroughly cleaned and rinsed. Then, they were subjected to external home bleaching treatment (Natural White 5 min Whitening) for 14 days, 5 min/day, according to the manufacturer's recommendations [25]. After external bleaching procedures, the samples were cleaned and rinsed with distilled water.

For high-impact occlusal forces simulation, a dual-axis chewing simulator was used (CS 4.2, SD Mechatronik, Germany). Before the simulation, the roots of the restored teeth were wax-sealed apically, covered with a type 3 polyvinyl siloxane (PVS), and then embedded in self-cured acrylic resin according to a previously published article [14]. While subjected to mechanical loading and surface treatments, the restored teeth were immersed in artificial saliva.

In the chewing simulator device, the restored teeth were placed side by side in the test chambers so that the stylus simultaneously touched the contact point between two opposed adjacent restorations. Thus, half of the samples from each nanocomposite were subjected to mechanical loads and surface aging treatments (ML + ST, n = 15 samples). Half of them were only subjected to surface treatments (ST, n = 15 sample restorations). The following parameters were used for parafunctional mechanical loading: 125,000 cycles at 7 kgf (70N) per stylus at 1.6 Hz frequency with lateral travel of ±3 mm.

The description of the setup protocol is shown in Figure 1.

The samples were covered with two layers of nail polish with 1 mm preservation around the margins of the restorations; then, the restored teeth were immersed in 50 wt% of silver nitrate solution. After a thorough rinse, the teeth were immersed in a photo-developer for eighth (Dental X-ray Developer, Kodak Co, Rochester, NY, USA) and analyzed with a digital X-ray and CBCT device.

Qualitative analysis was accomplished by one observer according to macro-morphological characteristics based on Modified Clinical parameters criteria [26,27] using dental loupes (3× magnification) and a high-resolution digital camera.

Using modified clinical parameters criteria, the restored teeth were observed and evaluated for the following characteristics based on a grading system (Gr 0–Gr 2) (Table 1):

1. Color match (CM)
2. Marginal adaptation (MA)

3. Surface roughness (SR)
4. Anatomical form (AF)

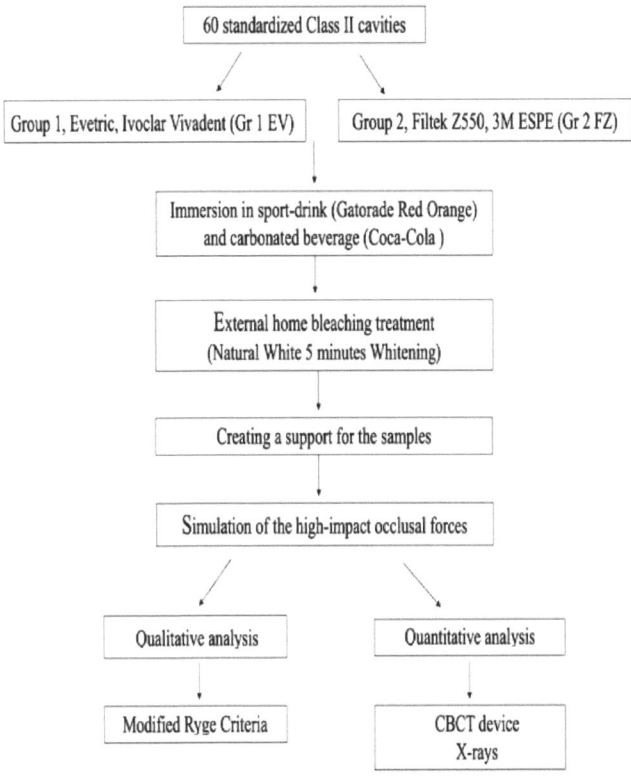

Figure 1. The workflow of the protocol used in the study.

Table 1. The grading system used based on modified clinical parameters criteria.

Grade	Color Match (CM)	Marginal Adaptation (MA)	Surface Roughness (SR)	Anatomical Form (AF)
GR 0	No change in color	The tooth-restoration margin is undetectable.	Smooth surface of the restoration	No change of the ana-tomical shape
GR 1	Slight change in color	Detectable tooth-restoration margins without any crevicular ditch	Slightly rough surface of the restoration	Detectible under- or over-contoured ana-tomical shape of the restoration
GR 2	Obvious change in color of the restoration	Detectable tooth-restoration margins with visible crevicular space	Rough surface of the restoration	

Detailed information on the materials used in the study appears in Tables 2 and 3.

Table 2. Chemical composition of the restorative materials used in the study [7,28].

Material [Lot Number]	Organic Matrix (+ Photo-Initiator) *	Inorganic Phase *	Medium Particle Size *	Particles' Distribution wt% (vol%) *	Manufacturer
Evetric (EV) [Z03XB7] A3 shade	-BisGMA -BisEMA -UDMA +Ivocerin®	-Barium glass -Ytterbium trifluoride -Oxides -Pre-polymerized particles	0.04–3 μm	80–81 (55–57)	Ivoclar, Vivadent, Schaan Liechtenstein
Filtek Z550 (FZ) [NC35371] A3 shade	-BisGMA -BisEMA -UDMA -PEGDMA -TEGDMA +Camphorquinone (CQ)	-Zirconium oxide silica -Silica particles	0.005–3 μm (Cluster 0.6–1.4 μm)	82 (68)	3M ESPE, St Paul, MN, USA

BisGMA: bisphenol A diglycidyl ether dimethacrylate; TEGDMA: triethylene-glycol dimethacrylate BisEMA6: bisphenol A polyethylene glycol diether dimethacrylate; UDMA: urethane dimethacrylate; PEGDMA: polyethylene glycol dimethacrylate; * in accordance with the information provided by the manufacturers.

Table 3. The chemical composition of the adhesive used in the study [29].

Material	Composition *	Manufacturer
Optibond eXTRa Universal two-step self-etch Adhesive [Primer: 7247705 Adhesive:7247706]	Primer: GPDM, hydrophilic co-monomers, water/ethanol, acetone Adhesive: resin monomers, inorganic fillers, ethanol	Kerr Corporation

* In accordance with the information provided by the manufacturers.

For quantitative assessment of the dental filling defects, the following devices were used: the digital X-rays device and the CBCT device (Planmeca USA Inc, Hoffman Estates, IL, USA) (the thickness of the smallest slice was established at 200 μm).

Statistical Analysis

For statistical analysis, the samples were evaluated by material, by grade of defects, and by mechanically loaded or not. Shapiro–Wilk test was performed to test the normal distribution of the results. The data were subjected to different non-parametric statistical tests (Kruskal–Wallis, Mann–Whitney U) using IBM SPSS software, version 21.0 (SPSS Inc, Chicago, IL, USA). The Spearman rho test was used to verify any statistical correlation between the extrinsic modified clinical parameters criteria system and the radiographic and tomographic intrinsic grading system. The level of statistical significance was established at $p < 0.05$.

3. Results

This study observed the restorations after surface aging treatments (ST) and after the mechanical loading and surface treatments were applied (ML + ST) and evaluated them based on qualitative and quantitative analysis.

3.1. Qualitative Analysis

When using the modified clinical parameters criteria to compare the two tested materials, the statistical analysis revealed the following:

(1) For color match parameters (CM) of Filtek Z550 and Evetric restorations, the Kruskal–Wallis test showed significant differences among the grades for both aging treatments (ML + ST and ST) ($p < 0.0000001$) (Table 4).

Table 4. Kruskal–Wallis test for color match parameter (CM).

	Test Statistics [a,b]			
	CM_ Filtek Z550 ST	CM_ Evetric ST	CM_ Filtek Z550 ML + ST	CM_ Evetric ML + ST
Chi-Square	22.880	35.787	9.387	12.320
df	2	2	2	2
Asymp. Sig.	0.000	0.000	0.009	0.002

a. Kruskal–Wallis test; b. grouping variable: grade CM.

The Mann–Whitney test indicated the following results: for ST and ML + ST aging groups, higher statistically significant differences for Gr 0 compared to Gr 1 and Gr 2 for both tested restorative materials ($p < 0.05$). Less statistically significant color changes were observed for Grade 2 compared with Grade 1 for tested materials and aging treatments ($p < 0.05$).

(2) When the Kruskal–Wallis test was applied, the marginal adaptation parameter (MA) for both resin-based composite materials had statistically significant differences among the grades for both aging treatment groups ($p < 0.05$). After being subjected to mechanical forces (ML + ST), both materials showed higher statistically significant values for Grade 2 (Figure 2). For the restorations that were only subjected to surface treatments (ST), the Mann–Whitney test showed a higher amount of Evetric samples without marginal adaptation defects (Gr 0) than the Filtek restorations.

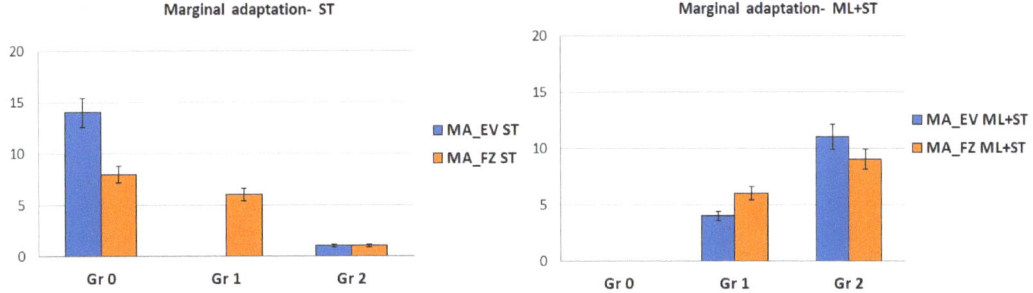

Figure 2. Error bars chart representing the 'grades' distribution of the marginal adaptation (MA) parameter.

(3) For the surface roughness parameter (SR), the Kruskal–Wallis statistical test revealed significant differences only for the Evetric ST group between the grades ($p < 0.000001$) (Table 5). At the same time, the Mann–Whitney U test showed significantly higher values for Gr 1 than Gr 0 ($p = 0.001$) for the same group. After the Evetric samples were subjected to mechanical loading treatment (ML + ST), a higher number of restorations with Gr 2 were observed ($p > 0.05$). Regarding Filtek Z550 samples, the statistical tests did not show significant differences among the tested groups (ST versus ML + ST) (Table 5).

Table 5. Kruskal–Wallis test for surface roughness (SR) parameter.

	Test Statistics [a,b]			
	SR_ Filtek Z550 ST	SR_ Evetric ST	SR_ Filtek Z550 ML + ST	SR_ Evetric ML + ST
Chi-Square	4.808	15.840	2.347	4.107
df	2	2	2	2
Asymp. Sig.	0.090	0.000	0.309	0.128

a. Kruskal–Wallis test; b. grouping variable: grade SR.

(4) For the anatomical form parameter (AF), the statistical tests indicated significant differences for both groups of restorations no matter whether they were subjected or not to simulated bruxism forces ($p < 0.05$) (Figure 3).

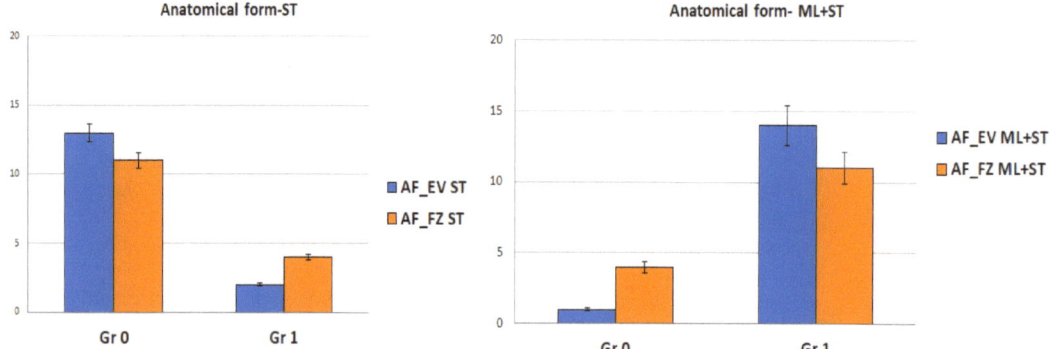

Figure 3. Error bars chart representing the 'grades' distribution of the anatomical form (AF) parameter.

When comparing the restorations by material, the Kruskal–Wallis test did not reveal any statistical difference in terms of color changes between the tested resin composites for both mechanically and non-mechanically loaded groups (ML + ST and ST) ($p > 0.05$). On the other hand, when comparing surface roughness (SR), a smoother surface (Gr 0) was observed for the samples restored with FZ material compared to EV after surface aging treatments (ST) ($p = 0.021$) (Figure 4).

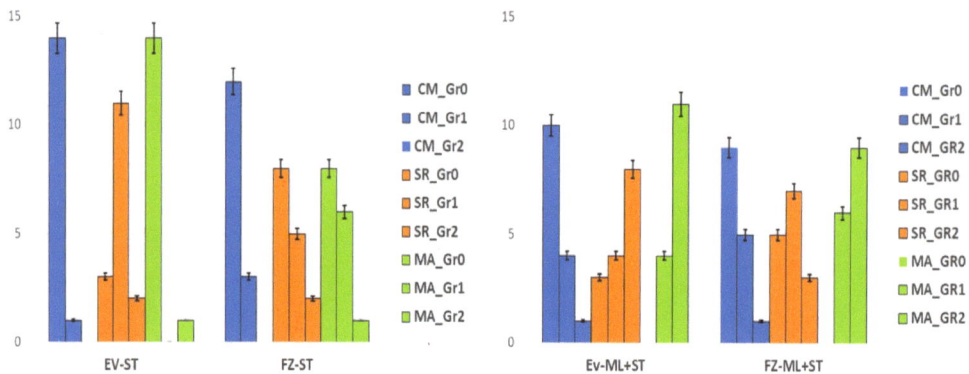

Figure 4. Error bars chart representing the restorative composite materials by applied aging methods among the modified Ryge criteria parameters.

The Kruskal–Wallis test revealed no defects of marginal adaptation for the EV restorations after surface treatments (ST) compared to FZ restorations ($p < 0.00001$). On the other hand, similar marginal adaptation defects were observed for both resin-based biocomposites subjected to ML + ST ($p > 0.05$) (Figure 4).

3.2. Quantitative Analysis

The quantitative evaluation was based on a grading system of the defects that appeared at the interface and occlusal level of the restorations, respectively (Tables 6 and 7). Importantly, all the restorations were assessed with the help of periapical X-ray and CBCT images.

Table 6. The grading system used in the study to assess occlusal defects of dental restorations.

Grade	Significance
0	-without occlusal defects
1	-occlusal defects

Table 7. The grading system used in the study to assess interfacial defects of dental restorations.

Grade	Significance
0	-without interfacial defects
1	-interfacial defects at the cervical
2	-interfacial defects at the cervical level and pulpal wall

It was observed that Evetric restorations were more radio-opaque than Filtek Z550 restorations (Figure 5). More cervical defects were observed radiographically for the Evetric nanohybrid material compared with the samples restored with Filtek Z550. When degree of impairment at the level of dental fillings was evaluated based on CBCT images, Filtek Z550 showed similar occlusal defects with Evetric biocomposite ($p > 0.05$). At the same time, for Filtek Z550 composite material, we observed a detachment line at the tooth-restoration interface after high-impact bruxism simulation.

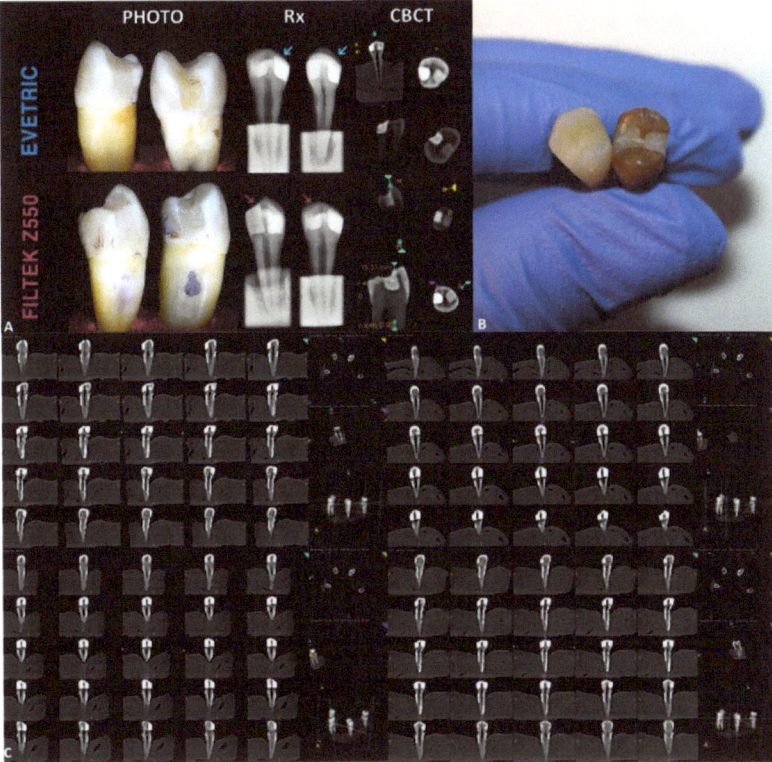

Figure 5. (**A**) Qualitative evaluation of the restorations based on high-resolution photos, digital X-rays, and CBCT images. (**B**) Restored teeth samples before and after immersion in sports drinks and carbonated beverages. (**C**) CBCT images of 200 μm slice evaluating the occlusal and interfacial defects after the bruxism forces simulation.

The Kruskal–Wallis test revealed statistically significant differences between grades of impairment for Evetric composite for both situations (with and without high occlusal forces simulation) ($p = 0.001$). For Filtek Z550 material, similar behavior was observed for samples were treated only with sports drink/carbonated juice and bleaching substance (ST) ($p = 0.56$). In contrast, for those that underwent high-impact occlusal force simulation (ML + ST), a statistically significant difference was observed between grades of impairment ($p = 0.017$) (Figure 5A).

Mann–Whitney U test showed a statistically significantly lower number of non-mechanically loaded restorations (ST) of Filtek Z550 composite material that presented Gr 0 interfacial defects compared with Evetric ($p = 0.029$). For Grade 2, there were not found any statistical differences between samples of materials that were not subjected to parafunctional simulation (ST) ($p > 0.05$).

For Evetric restorations, on one side, the non-mechanically simulated restorations (ST) did not present any interfacial defects compared with Filtek Z550 samples (Gr 0, $p < 0.000001$); on the other side, a statistically significant higher number of restorations graded at level 2 with interfacial defects after high-impact bruxism force simulation (ML + ST) was accomplished compared with Filtek Z550 samples ($p = 0.009$) (Figure 6). Both resin-based composite materials had statistically significant differences in Gr 2 interfacial defects after simulation of parafunctional occlusal forces (ML + ST) compared to non-mechanically loaded samples (ST) ($p < 0.05$).

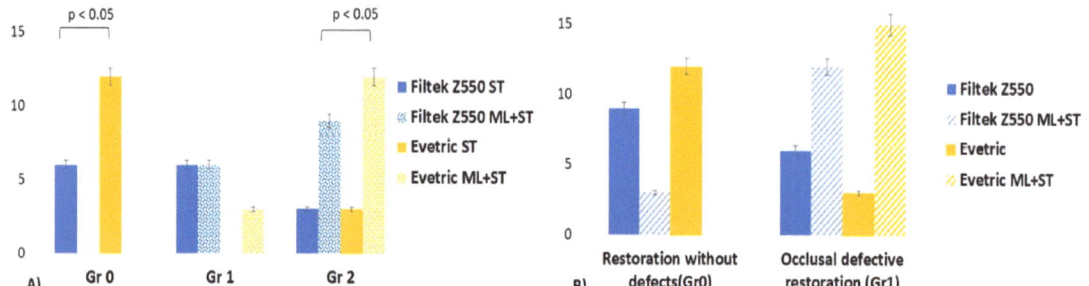

Figure 6. (**A**) Error bars chart representing the 'grades' distribution of interfacial defects for mechanically loaded (ML + ST) and non-mechanically loaded (ST) restorations of both resin-based materials. (**B**) Error bars chart representing the 'grades' distribution of occlusal defects for mechanically loaded (ML + ST) and non-mechanically loaded (ST) restorations of both tested materials.

When comparing by material, the Kruskal–Wallis test did not reveal any statistical difference between the tested resin composites for both mechanically and non-mechanically loaded groups no matter the presence of occlusal defects ($p > 0.05$). Regarding occlusal defects, there were statistically significant differences observed between Gr 0 and Gr1 among the samples restored with Evetric material subjected only to surface treatments (ST) ($p = 0.009$). In contrast, the samples restored with the same material subjected to high-impact parafunctional force simulation (ML + ST) showed a statistically significantly higher number of occlusal defects (Gr 1) compared with the Gr 0 mechanically simulated probes ($p < 0.000001$) (Figure 6B).

Importantly, Spearman's rho correlation coefficient revealed a strong relationship between anatomical form parameter (AF)—(our scoring system) occlusal defects and marginal adaptation parameter (MA)—interfacial defects, respectively (ST and ML + ST) groups) for both tested biocomposite restorative materials ($p < 0.05$).

4. Discussion

For many decades, indication of biocomposite materials for various clinical situations has increased significantly. However, these dental restorative biomaterials are subjected in the oral environment (abnormal occlusal forces, external bleaching, consumption of carbonated beverages) to changes in their functional and mechanical behavior when indicated primarily for patients with masticatory habits.

The study aimed to recreate one of the most common situations of a young patient suffering from specific parafunctional occlusal stress (bruxism) who consumes acidic beverages and uses at-home dental bleaching.

Dental aesthetics has always been a primary concern. Thus, home-use dental bleaching gels or other whitening pastes are now widely available online. Bleaching gels often advertise that 5 min home use is enough to whiten one's teeth [25]. The target audience for this type of product is teenagers and young adults ages 17 to 30. It is called into question whether these types of gels, indicated by the dentist, have a mild or strong effect only on natural teeth or dental restorations. Because the bleaching agent acts on the surface of the teeth or restorations, it was observed that it may affect fracture toughness of resin-based composite restorations [30,31]] and may lead to release of some organic matrix polymers in the oral environment [32]. According to Schuster L. et al., bleaching procedures may cause reduced or enhanced elution of chemicals from the composites [33].

Another critical issue nowadays is the high percentage of patients who consume large quantities of sports drinks (Gatorade, Isostar, etc.) and carbonated beverages (e.g., Coca-Cola, Pepsi, Fanta, etc.), who represent the same target audience mentioned above [10,11]. When these two extrinsic elements are combined with intrinsic ones, such as parafunctional occlusal forces, it is essential to understand the affected dental areas and what the practitioner can use to restore the teeth [15–20].

In our in vitro investigation, we combined two surface treatments (home-use dental bleaching gel and immersion in sports drinks and carbonated beverages) with high-parafunctional masticatory simulation to assess both qualitatively and quantitatively the behavior of two resin-based biocomposites. Thus, we used a dual-axis chewing simulator with the loading force established at 70N [8] corresponding to the non-physiological masticatory force of a bruxer human subject [34]. It must be pointed out that there are not enough studies on this specific subject—consumption of acidic beverages and simulated bruxism forces in association with uncontrolled at-home tooth whitening procedures and their effect on mechanical behavior of composite restorative materials.

Qualitative analysis revealed significantly rougher surfaces for Evetric biocomposite subjected to surface treatments compared to Filtek Z550. This result may be explained based on the chemical composition of the restorative materials: Evetric contains pre-polymerized particles and a distribution of 55–57% vol. of the inorganic fillers, while Filtek Z550 contains 68% vol. distribution (nanoparticles and nanoclusters). Given the values, it can be noted that the fillers protect the remaining organic matrix for Filtek Z550. Thus, it might be a higher chance for Evetric to wear its surface matrix much easier due to the low volume distribution of the filler particles [35]. (Table 2).

The slight color change observed is based on the size of the particles mentioned above. Filtek Z550 has smaller particles and, therefore, has a smoother surface and will have lower external coloration (Figure 7); the same results were obtained by Ozkanoglu S. et al. [35]. Although nanohybrid composite resins should be resistant to external coloration, Güler et al. and other researchers [36,37] reported that excess silane-binding agent and resin amount have a significant difference that increases coloration. Therefore, similar behavior of the color parameters of grades 1 and 2 was observed for the tested samples (Figures 4 and 7).

When discussing the materials' composition, two other aspects are worth mentioning: the influence of filler percentage and the photoinitiator. Dikova T et al. [38] conducted an in vitro study that analyzed three composites (Filtek One Bulk Fill, Evetric, and FC G-aenial Universal Flo) and concluded that the Filtek material (with a similar distribution of matrix and filler particles to Filtek Z550), due to its higher filler content and composition, has the highest microhardness in comparison to Evetric [39]. Similar results were also obtained in our study: Filtek Z550 showed better preservation than Evetric of the initial anatomical form after high parafunctional simulated forces (Figure 3).

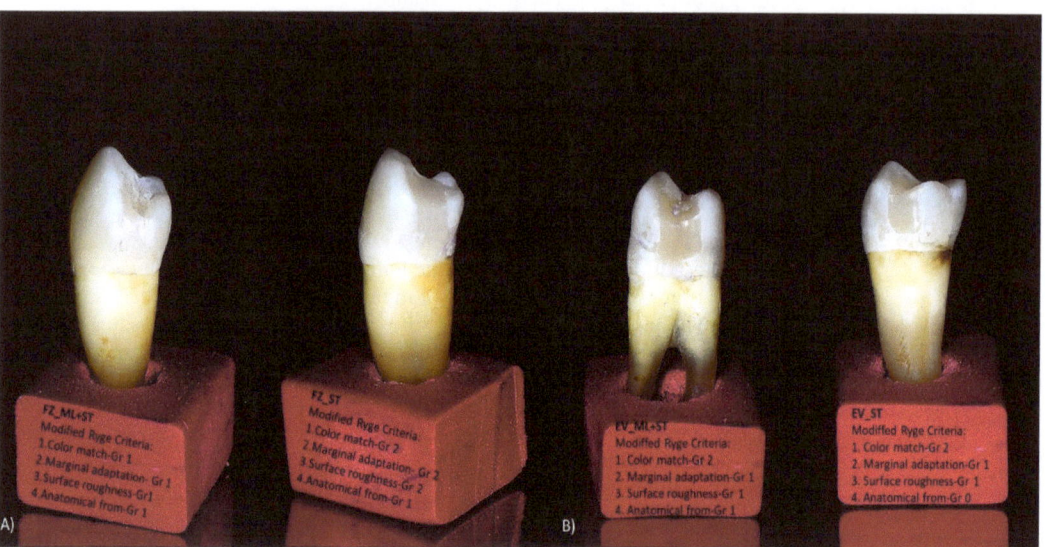

Figure 7. Photos of restored samples representing modified clinical parameters criteria for (**A**) Filtek Z550-ML + ST and ST groups and (**B**) Evetric ML + ST and ST groups.

It is essential to note that properties of composite materials are also influenced by a patient's diet (erosive factors), the materials' composition, and the polymerization method [40,41].

In our study, the tested nanohybrid composites had different photoinitiators: Ivocerin (390–445 nm wavelength), for Evetric and for Filtek Z550, camphorquinone (CQ; 360–510 nm wavelength). Kowalska A. et al. [39] demonstrated that the highest hardness and microhardness are associated with Filtek Z550, which contained CQ as a photoinitiator [35]. In our study, the LED light-curing unit had a very narrow range of wavelength (440–480 nm), which increased the possibility for Evetric to have a higher depth of cure and polymerization degree, even if the filler particles content was low [38,39]; on the other side, in the case of Filtek Z550, there was higher inorganic filler content and a wider range of the wavelength compared with that of the LED lamp. Our investigation observed similar changes ($p > 0.05$) in mechanical surface behavior related to anatomical form and occlusal defects of the tested composite materials when surface treatments (ST) were simulated (Figures 4, 5C, 6 and 7). Our findings are in accordance with other studies [8,18,38,39].

On the X-ray and CBCT images, it was observed that the samples restored with Evetric were more radio-opaque than those restored with Filtek Z550 (Figure 5A,C). This observation agrees with the results reported by other researchers [7,42,43]. Thus, the following possible explanation may be taken into consideration: within the inorganic phase composition, Evetric has different variants of filler particles (BaO glass, Ytterbium fluorides, oxides) and a low number of variants of organic polymers (Table 2) [28], while Filtek Z550 is highly represented by a variety of organic matrix monomers and only a few types of inorganic fillers (Zirconia and Silica particles) [7,43], so, the higher the variety of inorganic filler particles, the higher the radio-opacity.

Use of micro-CT is considered a "golden standard" non-destructive radiographic method for evaluating small areas for different human structures [23], especially detection of tooth-restorative material interfacial defects [22–24,44–46]. This method uses high radiation values for tiny areas and thus may be used only with a specific type of prepared samples along with laboratory investigations [23,44–46]. To better detect defects, dental samples are immersed in 50% silver nitrate solution [44–46]

For many years, cone beam computer tomography (CBCT) has been widely used for different dental specialties, especially surgical ones. This non-invasive investigation method was preferred in the past decade and is often indicated for endodontics and caries detection [21,24,47]. With CBCT, it is possible to explore dental tissues based on three-dimensional analysis, which can be completed from different plans and sectioning of the assessed tissues at different levels [21,23]. Thus, CBCT analysis on a daily dental basis may help a dental practitioner with more elements and information three-dimensionally evaluated than simple radiography at high resolution. Thus, both methods may be corroborated by the dental clinician to improve a single radiographic analysis.

The reason for using a cone beam CT device for our investigation was based on its clinical indication by dental practitioners [21,24,47]. This analysis was accomplished by respecting the conditions of clinical practice to identify its limits as correctly as possible. Our results have demonstrated similar detections with micro-CT images used by other investigators [44,45].

In our study, quantitative analysis completed with an X-ray and CBCT device showed significantly higher interfacial and occlusal defects for Evetric than Filtek Z550 (Gr 2, $p < 0.05$) after the samples were subjected to high-impact masticatory forces simulation (Figures 5 and 6). Other studies also reported similar results [14,20,44].

When interfacial defects were analyzed, based on silver nitrate infiltration, CBCT images revealed statistically significant higher differences between the samples of both materials when these were subjected to bruxism simulation compared with those samples that underwent only surface treatments (immersion in carbonated juice and dental bleaching gel) ($p < 0.05$). Other researchers also observed similar effects [19,44–46,48]; moreover, for interfacial microleakage analysis, they reported [44–46] immersion of the samples in silver nitrate 50%, which is the same tracer used in our study.

Summing up, the Spearman rho correlation coefficient revealed a relationship between the two variables, which may strengthen the reliability of our grading system. Moreover, there is a correlation between the clinical parameters that evaluate the restorations exteriorly (modified clinical parameters criteria) and the internal ones (X-rays and CBCT).

The present study was based on the hypothesis that there is no difference between the tested composites regarding their mechanical behavior, aesthetics, and functional behaviors regardless of type of surface aging treatment and bruxism simulation forces. After qualitative and quantitative analysis, the null hypothesis was rejected.

Our study had some limitations, such as laboratory setup, simulation of high parafunctional occlusal forces, type of restorative materials, and lack of elution chemical compounds collected for both assessment methods (ST and ML + ST), as well as the use of a thermocycler. Nevertheless, we want to emphasize some of the strong points of this investigation: simulation of the periodontal ligament for tooth mobility using a polyvinyl siloxane material along with the Willytec Chewing simulator type (C.S.-4.2, SD Mechatronik, Feldkirchen-Westerham, Germany); to our knowledge, this study design has not yet been reported by different groups of researchers from another academic university. Along with periodontal ligament simulation, the whole laboratory setup had the goal to implement a real clinical situation from a daily basis dental activity. The restored teeth were placed in contact proximally so that the ceramic stylus met both restored teeth. Another strong point is use of the assessment devices (high-resolution camera, digital X-rays, and CBCT device) recommended daily by dental practitioners. Moreover, to analyze the restored samples, we used loupes and digital images, enabling us to evaluate the dental restorations from an extrinsic and intrinsic 3D point of view.

However, more clinical and in vitro studies should analyze this vast domain of cone-beam computed tomography assessment and the effects of combined bruxism–acid beverages–dental bleaching on more types of dental restorative materials, other types of dental fillings, and different lab-simulated clinical setups.

5. Conclusions

Within the limits of this in vitro investigation, the following conclusions may be drawn:

- simulation of bruxism forces combined with surface treatments (immersion in carbonated juice and external bleaching) induced different mechanical and functional behavior patterns of the analyzed resin-based biocomposites.
- radiographic and CBCT evaluation revealed more details regarding the mechanical behavior of the tested restorative biomaterials compared with other analyzed methods (digital camera and loupes).
- use of different surface agents (carbonated juice and dental bleaching agent) dramatically impacts surface behavior of tested materials for simulated bruxism conditions.
- higher radio-opacity was observed for Evetric compared with Filtek Z550.
- more cervical defects were observed on radiographic and CBCT images for Evetric compared with Filtek Z550.
- color parameter indicated a slight color change between tested materials.
- aging treatments increased surface roughness of Evetric restorations compared with Filtek Z550 samples.

Author Contributions: Conceptualization, A.O. and A.A.B.; methodology, C.M.P. and A.A.B.; software, A.O., writing—original draft preparation, A.A.B., E.B.V. and C.M.P.; writing—review and editing, A.O., S.S. and D.D.; supervision, A.O. and D.D. All authors have read and agreed to the published version of the manuscript.

Funding: This research received no external funding.

Institutional Review Board Statement: The study was carried out in accordance with the Declaration of Helsinki and approved by the Research Ethics and Methodology Department, University of Medicine and Pharmacy "Iuliu Hatieganu," Cluj-Napoca, Romania (247/30.06.2021).

Informed Consent Statement: Informed consent was obtained from all subjects involved in the study.

Data Availability Statement: The data supporting this study's findings are available on request from the corresponding author.

Conflicts of Interest: The authors have no conflict of interest to declare.

References

1. Hardan, L.; Mancino, D.; Bourgi, R.; Cuevas-Suárez, C.E.; Lukomska-Szymanska, M.; Zarow, M.; Jakubowicz, N.; Zamarripa-Calderón, J.E.; Kafa, L.; Etienne, O.; et al. Treatment of Tooth Wear Using Direct or Indirect Restorations: A Systematic Review of Clinical Studies. *Bioengineering* **2022**, *9*, 346. [CrossRef] [PubMed]
2. Ferracane, J.L. Resin composite—State of the art. *Dent. Mater.* **2011**, *27*, 29–38. [CrossRef] [PubMed]
3. Burke, F.J.; Crisp, R.J.; James, A.; Mackenzie, L.; Pal, A.; Sands, P.; Thompson, O.; Palin, W.M. Two year clinical evaluation of a low-shrink resin composite material in UK general dental practices. *Dent Mater.* **2011**, *27*, 622–630. [CrossRef] [PubMed]
4. Wang, Y.; Zhu, M.; Zhu, X.X. Functional fillers for dental resin composites. *Acta Biomater.* **2021**, *122*, 50–65. [CrossRef]
5. Mok, Z.H.; Proctor, G.; Thanou, M. Emerging nanomaterials for dental treatments. *Emerg. Top. Life Sci.* **2020**, *4*, 613–625. [CrossRef] [PubMed]
6. Jandt, K.D.; Watts, D.C. Nanotechnology in dentistry: Present and future perspectives on dental nanomaterials. *Dent. Mater.* **2020**, *36*, 1365–1378. [CrossRef]
7. 3M Dental Products FiltekTM Supreme Universal Restorative System. Technical Product Profile St. Paul MN 55144-1000. 2019. Available online: https://multimedia.3m.com/mws/media/744411O/filtek-z550-technical-data-sheet-cee.pdf (accessed on 23 January 2021).
8. Ghazal, M.; Kern, M. Wear of human enamel and nano-filled composite denture teeth under different loading forces. *J. Oral Rehabil.* **2009**, *36*, 58–64. [CrossRef]
9. Lobbezoo, F.; Ahlberg, J.; Glaros, A.G.; Kato, T.; Koyano, K.; Lavigne, G.J.; de Leeuw, R.; Manfredini, D.; Svensson, P.; Winocur, E. Bruxism defined and graded: An international consensus. *J. Oral Rehabil.* **2013**, *40*, 2–4. [CrossRef]
10. Mettler, S.; Rusch, C.; Colombani, P.C. Osmolarity and pH of sport and other drinks available in Switzerland. *Schweiz. Z. Med. Traumatol.* **2006**, *54*, 92–95.

11. Frese, C.; Frese, F.; Kuhlmann, S.; Saure, D.; Reljic, D.; Staehle, H.J.; Wolff, D. Effect of endurance training on dental erosion, caries, and saliva. *Scand. J. Med. Sci. Sport.* **2015**, *25*, e319–e326. [CrossRef]
12. Park, J.W.; An, J.S.; Lim, W.H.; Lim, B.S.; Ahn, S.J. Microbial changes in biofilms on composite resins with different surface roughness: An in vitro study with a multispecies biofilm model. *J. Prosthet. Dent.* **2019**, *122*, 493. [CrossRef] [PubMed]
13. Favero, V.; Bacci, C.; Volpato, A.; Bandiera, M.; Favero, L.; Zanette, G. Pregnancy and Dentistry: A Literature Review on Risk Management during Dental Surgical Procedures. *Dent. J.* **2021**, *9*, 46. [CrossRef] [PubMed]
14. Caracostea (Objelean), A.; Labuneț, A.; Silaghi-Dumitrescu, L.; Moldovan, M.; Sava, S.; Badea, M. E In vitro chewing simulation model influence on the adhesive-tooth structure interface. *KEM* **2016**, *695*, 77–82. [CrossRef]
15. Kumar, N.; Amin, F.; Hashem, D.; Khan, S.; Zaidi, H.; Rahman, S.; Farhan, T.; Mahmood, S.J.; Asghar, M.A.; Zafar, M.S. Evaluating the pH of Various Commercially Available Beverages in Pakistan: Impact of Highly Acidic Beverages on the Surface Hardness and Weight Loss of Human Teeth. *Biomimetics* **2022**, *7*, 102. [CrossRef]
16. Zimmer, S.; Kirchner, G.; Bizhang, M.; Benedix, M. Influence of various acidic beverages on tooth erosion. Evaluation by a new method. *PLoS ONE* **2015**, *10*, e0129462. [CrossRef]
17. Pinelli, M.D.; Catelan, A.; de Resende, L.F.; Soares, L.E.; Aguiar, F.H.; Liporoni, P.C. Chemical composition and roughness of enamel and composite after bleaching, acidic beverages and toothbrushing. *J. Clin. Exp. Dent.* **2019**, *11*, e1175–e1180. [CrossRef]
18. Scribante, A.; Gallo, S.; Scarantino, S.; Dagna, A.; Poggio, C.; Colombo, M. Exposure of Biomimetic Composite Materials to Acidic Challenges: Influence on Flexural Resistance and Elastic Modulus. *Biomimetics* **2020**, *5*, 56. [CrossRef]
19. Féliz-Matos, L.; Hernández, L.M.; Abreu, N. Dental Bleaching Techniques; Hydrogen-carbamide Peroxides and Light Sources for Activation, an Update. Mini Review Article. *Open Dent. J.* **2015**, *8*, 264–268. [CrossRef]
20. Caracostea (Objelean), A.; Morar, N.; Florea, A.; Soanca, A.; Badea, M.E. Two-body wear simulation influence on some direct and indirect dental resin biocomposites—A qualitative analysis. *Acta Bioeng. Biomech.* **2016**, *18*, 61–72. [CrossRef]
21. Pauwels, R.; Araki, K.; Siewerdsen, J.H.; Thongvigitmanee, S.S. Technical aspects of dental CBCT: State of the art. *Dentomaxillofac. Radiol.* **2015**, *44*, 20140224. [CrossRef]
22. Wang, L.; Li, J.P.; Ge, Z.P.; Li, G. CBCT image based segmentation method for tooth pulp cavity region extraction. *Dentomaxillofac. Radiol.* **2019**, *48*, 20180236. [CrossRef]
23. Liang, X.; Zhang, Z.; Gu, J.; Wang, Z.; Vandenberghe, B.; Jacobs, R.; Yang, J.; Ma, G.; Ling, H.; Ma, X. Comparison of micro-CT and cone beam CT on the feasibility of assessing trabecular structures in mandibular condyle. *Dentomaxillofac. Radiol.* **2017**, *46*, 20160435. [CrossRef] [PubMed]
24. Kajan, Z.D.; Taromsari, M. Value of cone beam CT in the detection of dental root fractures. *Dentomaxillofac. Radiol.* **2012**, *41*, 3–10. [CrossRef]
25. Amazon.com: 5 Pack Natural White 5-Minute Teeth Whitening Kits: Health & Household. Available online: https://www.amazon.com/Natural-White-5-minute-Teeth-Whitening/dp/B00OQU4U88 (accessed on 15 January 2020).
26. Crisp, R.J.; Cowan, A.W.; Lamb, J.; Thompson, O.; Tulloch, N.; Burke, F.J.T. A clinical evaluation of all-ceramic bridges placed in UK general dental practices: First-year results. *Br. Dent. J.* **2008**, *205*, 477–482. [CrossRef] [PubMed]
27. Hickel, R.; Peschke, A.; Tyas, M.; Mjör, I.; Bayne, S.; Peters, M.; Hiller, K.A.; Randall, R.; Vanherle, G.; Heintze, S.D. FDI World Dental Federation: Clinical criteria for the evaluation of direct and indirect restorations-update and clinical examples. *Clin. Oral Investig.* **2010**, *14*, 349–366. [CrossRef] [PubMed]
28. Evetric. Instructions for Use (eIFU). Ivoclar Vivadent Products Shaan, Lichtenstein. Available online: https://www.ivoclar.com/en_li/eifu?ref-number=&brand=evetric (accessed on 23 January 2021).
29. OptiBond eXTRa Universal—Instructions for Use (IFU). Kerr Dental. Available online: https://www.kerrdental.com/en-eu/resource-center/optibond-extra-universal-instructions-use-ifu (accessed on 23 January 2021).
30. Bagheri, R.; Fani, M.; Barfi Ghasrodashti, A.R.; Nouri Yadkouri, N.; Mousavi, S.M. Effect of a Home Bleaching Agent on the Fracture Toughness of Resin Composites: Using short rod design. *J. Dent. Shiraz Univ. Med. Sci.* **2014**, *15*, 74–80.
31. Abdelaziz, K.M.; Mir, S.; Khateeb, S.U.; Baba, S.M.; Alshahrani, S.S.; Alshahrani, E.A.; Alsafi, Z.A. Influences of Successive Exposure to Bleaching and Fluoride Preparations on the surface Hardness and Roughness of the Aged Resin Composite Restoratives. *Medicina* **2020**, *56*, 476. [CrossRef]
32. Schuster, L.; Reichl, F.-X.; Rothmund, L.; He, X.; Yang, Y.; Van Landuyt, K.L.; Kehe, K.; Polydorou, O.; Hickel, R.; Högg, C. Effect of Opalescence® bleaching gels on the elution of bulk-fill composite components. *Dent. Mater.* **2016**, *32*, 127–135. [CrossRef] [PubMed]
33. Schuster, L.; Rothmund, L.; He, X.; Van Landuyt, K.L.; Schweikl, H.; Hellwig, E.; Carell, T.; Hickel, R.; Reichl, F.-X.; Högg, C. Effect of Opalescence® bleaching gels on the elution of dental composite components. *Dent. Mater.* **2015**, *31*, 745–757. [CrossRef] [PubMed]
34. Heintze, S.D. How to qualify and validate wear simulation devices and methods. *Dent. Mater.* **2006**, *22*, 712–734. [CrossRef]
35. Ozkanoglu, S.; Akin, E.G. Evaluation of the effect of various beverages on the color stability and microhardness of restorative materials. *Niger J. Clin. Pract.* **2020**, *23*, 322. [CrossRef] [PubMed]
36. Güler, A.U.; Güler, E.; Yücel, A.Ç.; Ertaş, E. Effects of polishing procedures on color stability of composite resins. *J. Appl Oral Sci* **2009**, *17*, 108–112. [CrossRef]

37. Elwardani, G.; Sharaf, A.A.; Mahmoud, A. Evaluation of colour change and surface roughness of two resin-based composites when exposed to beverages commonly used by children: An in-vitro study. *Eur Arch. Paediatr. Dent.* **2019**, *20*, 267–276. [CrossRef] [PubMed]
38. Dikova, T.; Maximov, J.; Todorov, V.; Georgiev, G.; Panov, V. Optimization of Photopolymerization Process of Dental Composites. *Processes* **2021**, *9*, 779. [CrossRef]
39. Kowalska, A.; Sokolowski, J.; Gozdek, T.; Krasowski, M.; Kopacz, K.; Bociong, K. The Influence of Various Photoinitiators on the Properties of Commercial Dental Composites. *Polymer* **2021**, *13*, 3972. [CrossRef] [PubMed]
40. Szalewski, L.; Wójcik, D.; Bogucki, M.; Szkutnik, J.; Różyło-Kalinowska, I. The Influence of Popular Beverages on Mechanical Properties of Composite Resins. *Materials* **2021**, *14*, 3097. [CrossRef] [PubMed]
41. Szalewski, L.; Wójcik, D.; Sofińska-Chmiel, W.; Kuśmierz, M.; Różyło-Kalinowska, I. How the Duration and Mode of Photopolymerization Affect the Mechanical Properties of a Dental Composite Resin. *Materials* **2023**, *16*, 113. [CrossRef] [PubMed]
42. Dionysopoulos, D.; Tolidis, K.; Gerasimou, P.; Papadopoulos, C. Analyzing the radiopacity of dental composite restoratives. *SPEPRO* **2017**. [CrossRef]
43. Ermis, R.B.; Yildirim, D.; Yildiz, G.; Gormez, O. Radiopacity evaluation of contemporary resin composites by digitization of images. *Eur. J. Dent.* **2014**, *8*, 342–347. [CrossRef]
44. Neves, A.A.; Jaecquesa, S.; Van Ende, A.; Cardoso, M.V.; Coutinho, E.; Lührs, A.K.; Zicari, F.; Van Meerbeek, B. 3D-microleakage assessment of adhesive interfaces: Exploratory findings by μCT. *Dent. Mater.* **2014**, *30*, 799–807. [CrossRef]
45. Jacker-Guhr, S.; Ibarra, G.; Oppermann, L.S.; Lührs, A.K.; Rahman, A.; Geurtsen, W. Evaluation of microleakage in class V composite restorations using dye penetration and micro-CT. *Clin. Oral Invest.* **2016**, *20*, 1709–1718. [CrossRef]
46. Rengo, C.; Goracci, C.; Ametrano, G.; Chieffi, N.; Spagnuolo, G.; Rengo, S.; Ferrari, M. Marginal Leakage of Class V Composite Restorations Assessed Using Microcomputed Tomography and Scanning Electron Microscope. *Oper. Dent.* **2015**, *40*, 440–448. [CrossRef]
47. Tyndall, D.A.; Rathore, S. Cone-Beam CT Diagnostic Applications: Caries, Periodontal Bone Assessment and Endodontic Applications. *Dent. Clin. N. Am.* **2008**, *52*, 825–841. [CrossRef] [PubMed]
48. Labuneț, A.; Objelean, A.; Almășan, O.; Kui, A.; Buduru, S.; Sava, S. Bruxism's Implications on Fixed Orthodontic Retainer Adhesion. *Dent. J.* **2022**, *10*, 141. [CrossRef] [PubMed]

Disclaimer/Publisher's Note: The statements, opinions and data contained in all publications are solely those of the individual author(s) and contributor(s) and not of MDPI and/or the editor(s). MDPI and/or the editor(s) disclaim responsibility for any injury to people or property resulting from any ideas, methods, instructions or products referred to in the content.

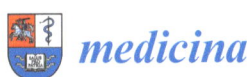

Case Report

Full-Mouth Rehabilitation of a Patient with Gummy Smile—Multidisciplinary Approach: Case Report

Kinga Mária Jánosi [1], Diana Cerghizan [1,*], Florentin Daniel Berneanu [1,†], Alpár Kovács [2], Andrea Szász [2], Izabella Mureșan [1], Liana Georgiana Hănțoiu [1] and Aurița Ioana Albu [1]

1. Faculty of Dental Medicine, George Emil Palade University of Medicine, Pharmacy, Science, and Technology of Targu Mures, 38 Gh. Marinescu Str., 540142 Targu Mures, Romania
2. Private Practice, SC Maxdent Office SRL, 540501 Targu Mures, Romania
* Correspondence: diana.cerghizan@umfst.ro; Tel.: +40-740-076-876
† Authors with equal contribution as the first author.

Abstract: The impairment of aesthetic function leads to a decreased quality of life. An unaesthetic smile due to excessive gingival exposure demands, most of the time, a complex treatment in which the objective is the vertical reduction of the amount of exposed fixed gingiva by obtaining a complete exposure of the anatomical crown of the teeth and restoring the ideal dimensions of the biological width. This paper presents a case of a 48-year-old female patient who was unsatisfied with her aesthetics and had disturbed masticatory function due to the absence of some posterior teeth. The cone beam computed tomography was performed to evaluate the facial and dental morphology. The treatment plan included diode laser and piezo-surgery utilization for the frontal area of the upper arch and implants to restore the distal area of the lower and upper arch. Zirconia ceramic was used for the final restorations. This complex and multidisciplinary full-mouth rehabilitation lasted for two years, and the patient was pleased with the result. This case showed that a well-established treatment plan is necessary to obtain long-lasting results. The use of adequate procedures and equipment ensures a predictable result.

Keywords: oral rehabilitation; laser-assisted crown-lengthening; piezo-surgery; implants; zirconia ceramics

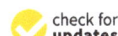

Citation: Jánosi, K.M.; Cerghizan, D.; Berneanu, F.D.; Kovács, A.; Szász, A.; Mureșan, I.; Hănțoiu, L.G.; Albu, A.I. Full-Mouth Rehabilitation of a Patient with Gummy Smile—Multidisciplinary Approach: Case Report. *Medicina* 2023, 59, 197. https://doi.org/10.3390/medicina59020197

Academic Editor: Gaetano Isola

Received: 9 December 2022
Revised: 5 January 2023
Accepted: 16 January 2023
Published: 19 January 2023

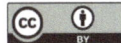

Copyright: © 2023 by the authors. Licensee MDPI, Basel, Switzerland. This article is an open access article distributed under the terms and conditions of the Creative Commons Attribution (CC BY) license (https://creativecommons.org/licenses/by/4.0/).

1. Introduction

Inadequate facial aesthetics due to an unaesthetic smile, especially in the case of a gummy smile, with a high smile line, can harm patients' quality of life, even leading to psychical problems in some cases [1]. The American Academy of Periodontology (AAP) defines the gummy smile as a deformity and mucogingival condition that affects the area around the teeth [2]. The excessive gingival display is characterized by overexposure of the maxillary gingiva during smiling or speaking [3]. According to Allen, gum exposure of less than 2–3 mm can be considered attractive. An overexposure of more than three mm is known as the gummy smile [4] and is generally considered an aesthetic problem [5]. In some European countries, a gingival display up to 4 mm or more is acceptable [4]. Etiological factors related to a gummy smile can be gingival (passive eruption), skeletal (vertical maxillary excess), and muscular (upper lip hyperfunction) [6]. The high smile line and excessive gingival exposure must be considered during the treatment plan [6] because sometimes corrections are needed during full-mouth rehabilitation.

The treatment procedure depends on the diagnosis and the etiological factors.

Aesthetic crown lengthening is one of the most common surgical treatments for a gummy smile. The objective of this procedure is the vertical reduction of the amount of exposed fixed gingiva by obtaining a complete exposure of the anatomical crown of the teeth and restoring the ideal dimensions of the biological width [7]. Following crown-lengthening surgery, the biological width is restored to a minimum of 2 mm, with the epithelial attachment of 0.97 mm and connective tissue of 1.07 mm width [8].

During the development of the treatment plan, tridimensional imagistic investigations are necessary. Cone beam computed tomography (CBCT) can provide accurate information about the alveolar bone and the periodontal status of the teeth. Measurements can be performed to define the length of the anatomical crown and root, which is necessary to realize the surgery correctly [9].

The greatest desire during the surgery is good visibility, without bleeding in the working area. The diode laser's most significant advantages are the non-bleeding operative field, tissue evaporation ability, adequate sterilization of the interventional area and minimal postoperative pain and edema [10].

Piezo-surgery offers a promising alternative to bone resection with significant benefits compared to traditional methods. It reduces the bleeding rate by 25–30% because it does not damage the soft tissues or blood vessels, ensuring a clean operating field during the intervention [11]. Its combination with the minimal flap technique significantly reduces postoperative pain and edema [12].

The gingival phenotype and the suture technique influence the evolution of the healing process after the surgery [13].

Dental implants have been considered one of the most important discoveries in dentistry in the past decades. In modern dentistry, the implant-prosthetic approach allows the treatment of partially edentulous spaces with fixed restorations, considerably improving the patient's quality of life [14]. The implant therapy, combined with zirconia ceramic restorations, allows the rehabilitation of function and aesthetics [15].

2. Case Report

This case report is a full-mouth rehabilitation of a 48-year-old female patient. She wanted to improve her aesthetics, disturbed by the shape and orientation of the upper frontal teeth and the excessive visibility of the gingiva. The patient also reports difficulties in mastication due to the absence of numerous posterior teeth in the lower arch. To establish the preliminary diagnosis, intraoral examinations (Figure 1a) and a panoramic X-ray (Figure 1b) were performed.

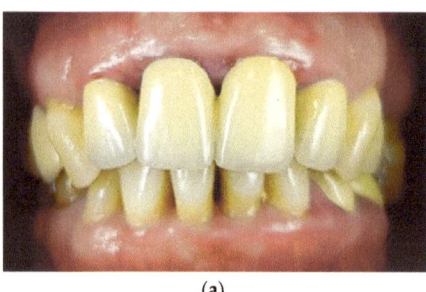
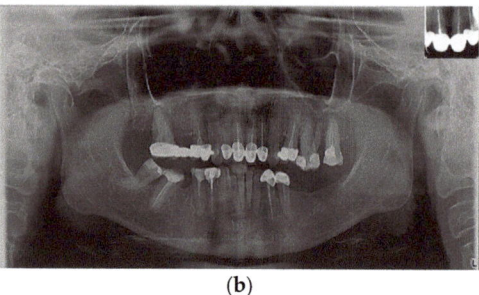

(a) (b)

Figure 1. Initial situation of the patient: (**a**) Unaesthetic metal-ceramic crowns with chronic inflammation of the gingival margins and oblique interincisal line; (**b**) Initial panoramic X-ray.

The clinical examination revealed the presence of inadequate metal-ceramic restorations, teeth with unsatisfactory periodontal status (grade I mobility), aesthetical and functional problems. A full-mouth CBCT scan was performed for the final diagnosis and to establish the treatment plan. The treatment objective was to perform full-mouth rehabilitation and improve the smile's aesthetics by reducing the excessive gingival displacement.

A crown-lengthening surgery was planned before the prosthodontic rehabilitation. The long-term success of future restorations is conditioned by accurately reestablishing the vertical dimension and the occlusal plane. The functional rehabilitation of the jaws needed an implant-prosthodontic approach. The treatment plan was established following the patient's agreement, considering the principles of the Declaration of Helsinki involving humans as revised in 2013. Informed consent was obtained from the patient regarding the treatment, and written informed consent has been obtained to publish this paper.

The full-mouth rehabilitation of this case was performed for two years.

Based on the CBCT measurements, the postoperative maxillary crown/root ratio was defined (Figure 2). The right central incisor presented a short root length to support future exposure during the crown-lengthening procedure. Therefore, it was decided to extract this tooth. The extraction of periodontally compromised 17 and 15 teeth was recommended with implant-prosthodontic rehabilitation of the right posterior area.

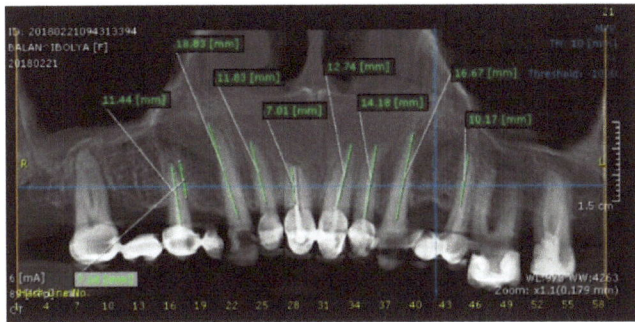

Figure 2. Evaluation of the periodontal status and root length of the maxillary teeth on CBCT.

The surgical pre-prosthetic treatment protocol combines laser therapy with the piezo-surgery to achieve a minimally invasive intervention with reduced postoperative symptomatology. Intraoral mock-ups were created to simulate and individualize future results and to guide the surgery (Figure 3).

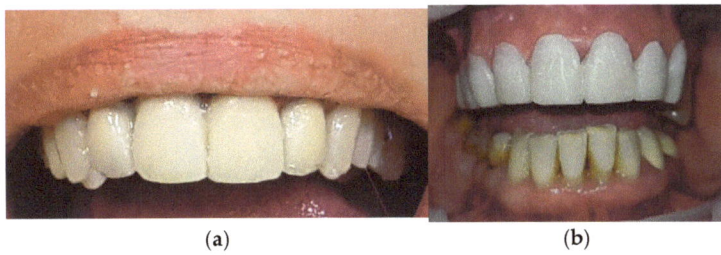

(a) (b)

Figure 3. Planning the surgical treatment outcomes: (a) Initial mock-up; (b) Surgical guide.

The old restorations were removed. The surgical guide was realized after the preliminary preparation of the abutments with the vertical preparation technique. During the surgical interventions, the Optragate (Ivoclar Vivadent AG, Schaan, Principality of Liechtenstein) retractor was used, which ensured good visibility and adequate access to the working area. The Lasotronix Smart M Pro diode laser (Lasotronix Sp. z o.o., Piaseczno, Poland) was used for the guiding incisions at the gingival margin, following the cervical line of the mock-up. No elongation was performed at the right central incisor because this tooth needed to be extracted at the end of the surgery. The alveolar bone margins were removed using the Ultrasurgery US-III LED piezo-surgery device (Guilin Woodpecker Medical Instrument Co., Ltd, Guangxi, P. R. China) (Figure 4).

To obtain long-lasting results, the placement of the margins of the future restorations must be at a minimum distance of 5 mm from the alveolar bone. Therefore, this desirability was considered during the surgery (Figure 5).

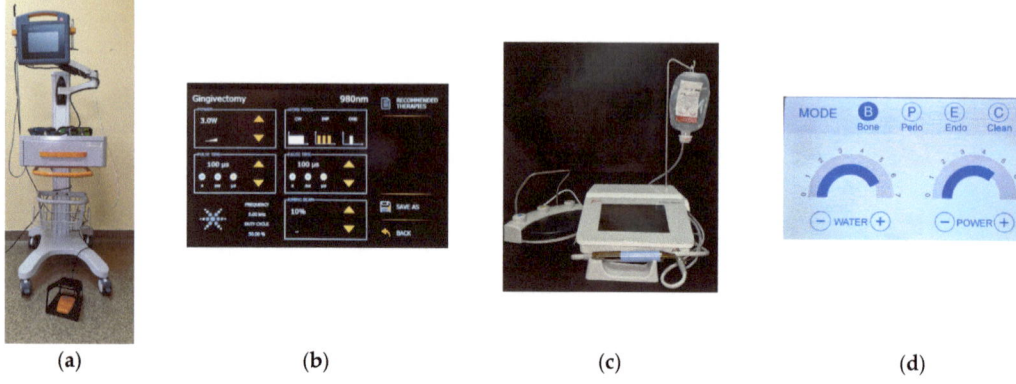

(a) (b) (c) (d)

Figure 4. The used devices and the settings: (**a**) Lasotronix Smart M Pro laser; (**b**) The setting of the laser device for the gingivectomy; (**c**) Ultrasurgery III LED piezo-surgery device; (**d**) The setting of the piezo-surgery device.

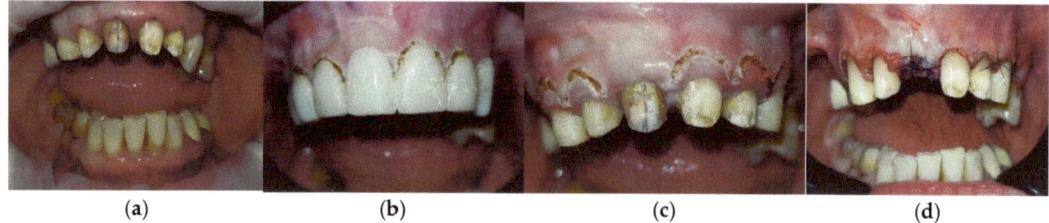

(a) (b) (c) (d)

Figure 5. The steps of the crown-lengthening surgery: (**a**) The abutments after the removal of the old restorations and a preliminary preparation before the surgery; (**b**) Predefinition of the gingival margins using the surgical guide and the Lasotronix Smart M Pro laser; (**c**) The limits of the new gingival margins after the removal of the surgical guide; (**d**) The aspect of the prosthodontic field after the piezo and laser surgery.

After performing the surgery and extracting the right central incisor, socket preservation and bone augmentation were done to maintain the alveolar bone dimensions. Provisional restoration was made to restore the aesthetics and function temporarily. Complete healing was achieved after six months. As expected, the results obtained were stable. The gingival contour was exposed but symmetrical and satisfactory during the smile. The final preparation of the abutments was performed with a heavy chamfer finish line, and zirconia ceramic restorations were used for the prosthodontic rehabilitation (Figure 6). The bite template was used to reestablish the vertical dimension. The color of the restorations was B1 (Vita Classical shade guide).

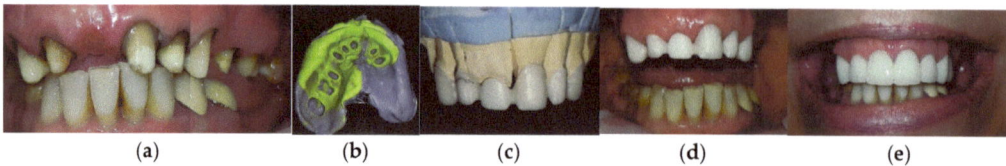

(a) (b) (c) (d) (e)

Figure 6. The steps of the prosthodontic rehabilitation: (**a**) Final aspect of the abutment after the healing period; (**b**) One-step impression with A silicone—Variotime Heavy Tray and Medium Flow (Zhermack); (**c**) The zirconia frame on the master cast; (**d**) The try-in of the zirconia frame; (**e**) The final restoration after cementation.

After the extraction of teeth 15 and 17, two implants were inserted. The osseointegration of the implants can be seen in the panoramic X-ray after six months (Figure 7).

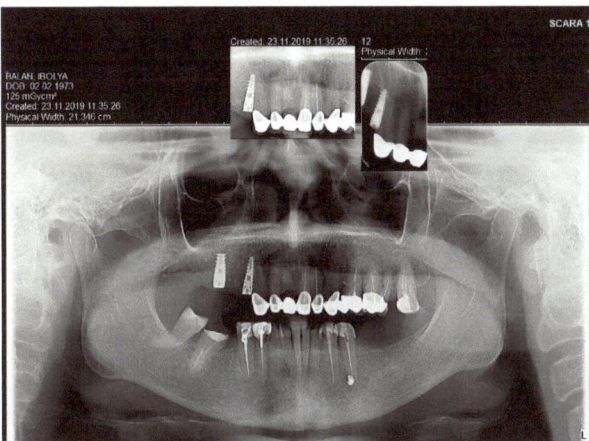

Figure 7. Panoramic X-ray with the osseointegrated implants and the maxillary prosthodontic rehabilitation on the natural teeth.

Pre-prosthetic treatments were performed on the lower arch during the upper arch healing period. The endodontic retreatments of the lower premolars were successful. The preparation of the teeth was carried out with a subgingivally placed heavy chamfer finish line. Single crown zirconia ceramic restorations and a bridge were realized, preserving tooth vitality in all abutments (Figure 8).

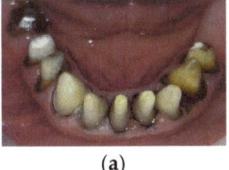 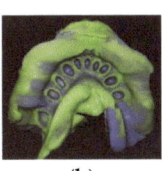 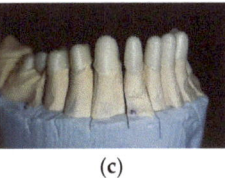 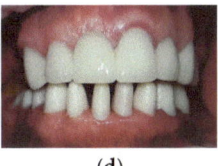 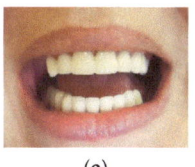

(a) (b) (c) (d) (e)

Figure 8. The steps of the prosthodontic rehabilitation: (**a**) The prepared abutments with the first impression cord; (**b**) One step impression with A silicone; (**c**) The zirconia frame on the master cast; (**d**) The try-in of the zirconia frame; (**e**) The final restoration after cementation.

For the restoration of the edentulous space on the lower arch, implant therapy was applied. Two implants were inserted.

In the case of the upper arch, a screw-retained titanium-based zirconia ceramic bridge was realized after the osseointegration period. The closed impression tray technique was used (Figure 9).

A panoramic X-ray was taken to verify the osseointegration of the lower implants (after six months) (Figure 10).

Due to the lack of parallelism of the implant bodies, a cemented zirconia ceramic bridge was realized to re-establish the function on the lower arch. In this case, the open-tray technique was used for the impression (Figure 11).

The final aspect of the complex, multidisciplinary full-mouth rehabilitation is presented in Figure 12.

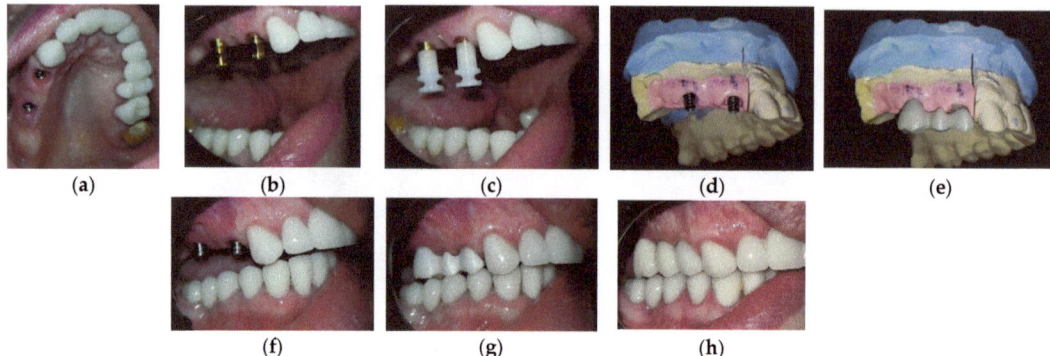

Figure 9. The sequences of the implant-prosthodontic therapy in the maxilla: (**a**) The emergence profile after the removal of the healing caps; (**b**) The impression copings in the mouth; (**c**) The transfer caps applied on the impression copings; (**d**) The master cast with the artificial gingiva and titanium abutments; (**e**) The zirconia frame on the master cast; (**f**) The intraoral try-in of the titanium abutments; (**g**) The intraoral try-in of the zirconia frame; (**h**) The final restoration after the intraoral fixation.

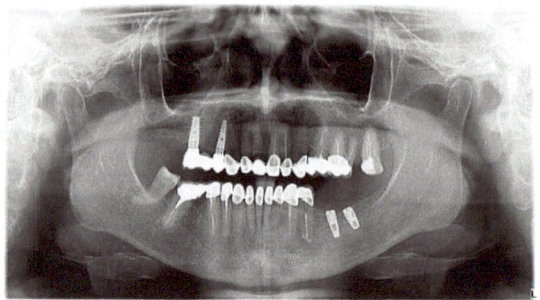

Figure 10. Panoramic X-ray with the osseointegrated implants on the lower arch and the good marginal adaptation of all the restorations.

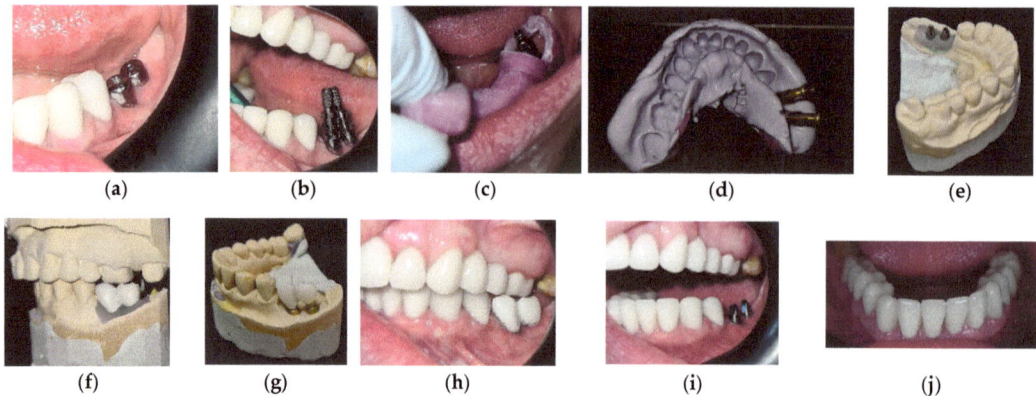

Figure 11. The sequences of the implant-prosthodontic therapy in the mandible: (**a**) The healing caps; (**b**) The impression copings in the mouth; (**c**) The try-in of the open tray; (**d**) The impression with the technical analogs (**e**) The prepared abutments and the artificial gingiva on the master cast; (**f**) The zirconia framework on the cast.; (**g**) The final restoration on the cast; (**h**) The try-in of the zirconia frame; (**i**) Closing the hole on the abutments; (**j**) The final restoration after the cementation.

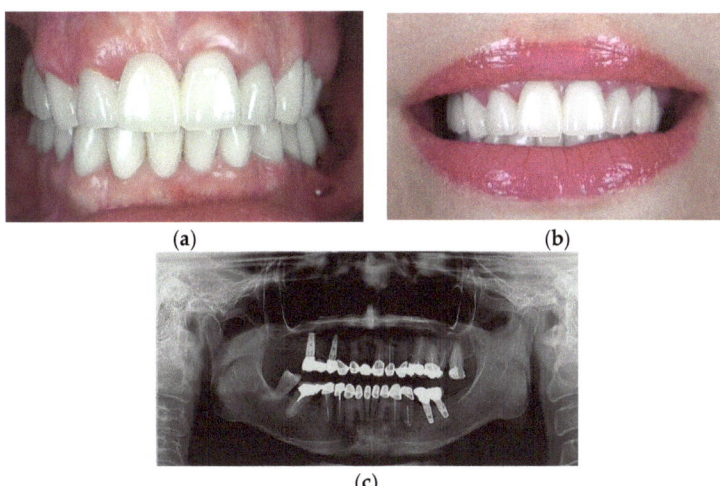

Figure 12. The final result of the full-mouth rehabilitation: (**a**) Intraoral aspect of the restorations; (**b**) The improved smile with minimal gingival display; (**c**) Panoramic X-ray after one year.

3. Discussion

Several studies have demonstrated the need for these surgical interventions to obtain an aesthetic smile, predominantly in the case of female patients [16], as in the presented case. The patient's initial problem was the gingival smile with the visibility of unaesthetic metal-ceramic prosthetic works. In this situation, resolving the patient's primary problems was possible only by performing full-mouth rehabilitation.

The surgical correction of the upper clinical crown:root ratio and gingival displacement was necessary before the prosthodontic approach.

According to Narayan et al., the pretreatment planning included a complex clinical evaluation regarding:

- The patient's systemic health and her expectations;
- The evaluation of the face and smile line;
- The lip thickness and size;
- The size and shape of the teeth;
- The gingival biotype and the width of keratinized gingiva;
- The thickness and contour of the alveolar bone [17].

CBCT evaluation was performed by measuring the existent and the future crown: root ratio and the crestal bone relation to the cementoenamel junction to decide the surgery type.

In the presented case a, mock-up guided crown lengthening procedure was performed based on the diagnostic wax-up, similar to the technique described by Jurado et al. [18] in their case report. Using a precise 3D-printed surgical guide for crown lengthening can help to prevent or reduce the chance of under or over-contouring hard and soft tissues during the procedure [19].

The crown-lengthening surgery combined two modern, minimally invasive techniques (laser therapy for soft tissue remodeling and piezo-surgery for bone resection) and the conventional technique to obtain long-lasting results with minor post-interventional symptoms and reduced healing time. The methods reduced surgical chair time and operative trauma, accelerating the healing process and making the patient more comfortable. The flapless surgery was undesirable because it did not allow direct visualization of the operative field and can be challenging regarding soft tissue damage [20]. Performing a reduced flap without vertical incisions was beneficial.

The thick gingival phenotype of the patient facilitated the healing process. Three months post-operatively, stabile results were obtained, probably due to minimally invasive techniques and the favorable gingival phenotype. The recovery period, a controversial topic in the literature, can differ individually. After soft tissue remodeling, the final rehabilitation can be done after a healing period of three months [21,22]. According to Herrero et al., in the case of bone remodeling with biological width modification, the healing period must be about six months before the prosthodontic rehabilitation [23], and it is essential to define a proper distance between the finish line and the bone margin during post-surgical prosthodontic treatment [24]. In our case, the healing period was six months.

After this period, the re-preparation of the teeth was carried out with a subgingivally-placed heavy chamfer finish line at a greater distance from the bone margin than 5 mm. Zirconia ceramic single crown restorations and bridges were used for aesthetic and functional rehabilitation. Several studies have been carried out regarding the marginal adaptation of these restorations, which are superior to conventional metal-ceramics [25,26]. Proper teeth preparation and a good impression technique are essential to achieve the best results [27,28]. In the case of digital workflow during the zirconia frame's design, the cementation space can influence the quality of the marginal adaptation. Defining the dimensions of this space must be done with caution [29]. Dittmer et al. [30] and Kohorst et al. [31] demonstrated in their studies that the successive application and firing of ceramic layers on the zirconia frame could cause marginal discrepancies, contradictory to Vigolo et al. findings [32]. The zirconia framework presents a lower occurrence of discrepancies than metal-ceramics [33]; this can contribute to obtaining long-lasting aesthetical results. The perfect marginal fit of the restorations is essential in maintaining periodontal health and ensuring the restorations' natural appearance, especially in the frontal area.

In the literature, different recommendations can be found for the cementation of zirconia ceramic restorations on teeth and implants. Some studies recommend the adhesive cementation technique in case of poor retention of the abutments [34,35]. Other studies have shown the importance of treating the inner surfaces of zirconia restorations to achieve good adhesion after cementation [36,37]. In the presented case, the zirconia restoration internal surface was sandblasted and treated with Ivoclean (Ivoclar). The vitality of the teeth influenced our choice of adhesive material. The adhesive cementation was abandoned to avoid pulpal irritation related to etching. Resin-modified glass ionomer cement was used for the final cementation of the restorations in the case of natural teeth.

In the case of implants, the fixation method (screw or cement retained) of the restorations might not directly influence their survival rate. However, it can lead to certain complications (mainly periimplantitis) [38]. Each retention method has its indication with advantages and disadvantages [39]. According to de Brandao et al., there is no evidence of differences in the marginal bone loss around the cement and screw-retained restorations [40]. Several studies demonstrated a higher success rate of screw-retained restorations versus classically cemented ones [38,41]. Park et al. recommend choosing the appropriate fixation method depending on the implants' parallelism and considering the occlusal relations. It is crucial in the case of the upper premolar region the possibility to place the access hole of the screw on the central fossa [42], as it was in our case.

The patient was satisfied with the obtained results, even though she still had a moderate gummy smile. The lip-repositioning surgery represents future possibilities for better aesthetical results [43], as does the injection of botulinum toxin A [44].

The patient chose a less invasive way to improve the final aesthetics in the future by using hyaluronic acid filler to make the lips look fuller and more youthful.

The limitations during the follow-up:

- Lack of periodical CBCT evaluation (at three months, six months, and one year)
- Lack of periodical periodontal evaluation using periodontal probing.

Digital planning and using a 3D-printed surgical guide can improve the expected results. A good collaboration between a multidisciplinary dental team and a facial plastic surgeon can result in even better aesthetics.

4. Conclusions

The crown-lengthening surgery is an efficient method to improve aesthetics in the case of a gingival smile. Laser therapy and piezo-surgery are modern methods that allow minimally invasive and efficient interventions with fast postoperative recovery. The zirconia ceramic restorations can be used to restore aesthetics and function with good results. Screw-retained restorations have a better long-term prognosis compared to cemented ones, demonstrated by the one-year follow-up Panoramic X-ray.

Author Contributions: Conceptualization: K.M.J.; methodology: K.M.J. and F.D.B.; formal analysis: A.S. and A.K.; investigation: I.M.; resources: L.G.H.; data curation: A.I.A.; writing—original draft preparation: K.M.J., F.D.B. and A.I.A.; writing—review and editing: K.M.J.; visualization: D.C.; supervision: D.C. All authors have read and agreed to the published version of the manuscript.

Funding: This research received no external funding.

Institutional Review Board Statement: The case report was conducted according to the guidelines of the Declaration of Helsinki on experimentation involving human subjects, as revised in 2013. Ethical review and approval were waived due to the design of the present case report. Our Institutional policy does not require the Ethical Committee approval in this case as the patient signed the informed consent requested for the publication of the present case report. Ethical approval was not sought for the present case report also because no experimental procedures were performed during the patient's treatment, and none of the materials or equipment used were prototypes. All of them are available on the market in their current form, and they were used according to the manufacturer's instructions without requiring off-label protocols.

Informed Consent Statement: Informed consent was obtained from the patient. Written informed consent has been obtained from the patient to publish this paper.

Data Availability Statement: The dataset analyzed during this case report are available from the first author on request.

Acknowledgments: The authors declare no financial affiliation or involvement with any commercial organization with a direct financial interest in the materials discussed in this manuscript.

Conflicts of Interest: The authors declare no conflict of interest.

References

1. Izraelewicz-Djebali, E.; Chabre, C. Gummy smile: Orthodontic or surgical treatment? *J. Dentofac. Anom. Orthod.* **2015**, *8*, 102. [CrossRef]
2. Armitage, G.C. Development of a Classification System for Periodontal Diseases and Conditions. *Ann. Periodontol.* **1999**, *4*, 1–6. [CrossRef] [PubMed]
3. Panduric, D.G.; Blašković, M.; Brozović, J.; Sušić, M. Surgical Treatment of Excessive Gingival Display Using Lip Repositioning Technique and Laser Gingivectomy as an Alternative to Orthognathic Surgery. *J. Oral. Maxillofac. Surg.* **2014**, *72*, 404.e1–404.e11. [CrossRef] [PubMed]
4. Allen, E.P. Use of mucogingival surgical procedures to enhance esthetics. *Dent. Clin. North Am.* **1988**, *32*, 307–330. [CrossRef] [PubMed]
5. Abou-Arraj, R.V.; Souccar, N.M. Periodontal treatment of excessive gingival display. *Semin. Orthod.* **2013**, *19*, 267–278. [CrossRef]
6. Tjan, A.H.; Miller, G.D.; The, J.G. Some esthetic factors in a smile. *J. Prosthet. Dent.* **1984**, *51*, 24–28. [CrossRef]
7. Hempton, T.J.; Dominici, J.T. Contemporary crown-lengthening therapy: A review. *J. Am. Dent. Assoc.* **2010**, *141*, 647–655. [CrossRef]
8. Lee, E.A. Aesthetic Crown Lengthening: Contemporary Guidelines for Achieving Ideal Gingival Architecture and Stability. *Curr. Oral. Health Rep.* **2017**, *4*, 105–111. [CrossRef]
9. Batista, E.L., Jr.; Moreira, C.C.; Batista, F.C.; de Oliveira, R.R.; Pereira, K.K. Altered passive eruption diagnosis and treatment: A cone beam computed tomography-based reappraisal of the condition. *J. Clin. Periodontal.* **2012**, *39*, 1089–1096. [CrossRef]
10. Arora, S.A.; Chhina, S.; Kazimm, J.; Goel, A.; Mishra, S.; Nidhi, S. Clinical Crown Lengthening using soft tissue diode laser: A case series. *Int. J. Oral. Health Med. Res.* **2015**, *2*, 81–83.
11. Hennet, P. Piezoelectric Bone Surgery: A Review of the Literature and Potential Applications in Veterinary Oromaxillofacial Surgery. *Front. Veter-Sci.* **2015**, *2*, 8. [CrossRef] [PubMed]
12. Kirmani, M.; Trivedi, H.; Bey, A.; Sharma, V.K. Postoperative Complications of Periodontal Surgery. *Int. J. Contemp. Med. Res.* **2016**, *3*, 1285–1286.

13. Paolantoni, G.; Marenzi, G.; Mignogna, J.; Wang, H.L.; Blasi, A.; Sammartino, G. Comparison of three different crown-lengthening procedures in the maxillary anterior aesthetic regions. *Quintessence Int.* **2016**, *47*, 407–416.
14. Mitrea, M.; Niculescu, S.; Dmor, A.; Al Hage, W.E.; Florea, C.; Săveanu, I.C.; Balcos, C.; Forna, N.C. Esthetic rehabilitation with implants-supported fixed dentures after periodontitis. *Rom. J. Oral Rehabil.* **2021**, *13*, 102–113.
15. Sorrentino, R.; Ruggiero, G.; Toska, E.; Leone, R.; Zarone, F. Clinical Evaluation of Cement-Retained Implant-Supported CAD/CAM Monolithic Zirconia Single Crowns in Posterior Areas: Results of a 6-Year Prospective Clinical Study. *Prosthesis* **2022**, *4*, 383–393. [CrossRef]
16. Moura, D.; Lima, E.; Lins, R.; Souza, R.; Martins, A.; Gurgel, B. The treatment of gummy smile: Integrative review of literature. *Rev. Clin. Periodontia. Implantol. Oral Rehabil.* **2017**, *10*, 26–28. [CrossRef]
17. Narayan, S.; Narayan, T.V.; Jacob, P.C. Correction of gummy smile: A report of two cases. *J. Indian Soc. Periodontol.* **2011**, *15*, 421–424. [CrossRef]
18. Jurado, C.A.; Parachuru, V.; Tinoco, J.V.; Guzman-Perez, G.; Tsujimoto, A.; Javvadi, R.; Afrashtehfar, K.I. Diagnostic Mock-Up as a Surgical Reduction Guide for Crown Lengthening: Technique Description and Case Report. *Medicina* **2022**, *58*, 1360. [CrossRef]
19. Alhumaidan, A.; Alqahtani, A.; Al-Qarni, F. 3D-Printed Surgical Guide for Crown Lengthening Based on Cone Beam Computed Tomography Measurements: A Clinical Report with 6 Months Follow Up. *Appl. Sci.* **2020**, *10*, 5697. [CrossRef]
20. Clear, A.G. Guidelines for flapless surgery. *J. Oral. Maxillofac. Surg.* **2007**, *65*, 20–32.
21. Fletcher, P. Biologic rationale of aesthetic crown lengthening using innovative proportion gauges. *Int. J. Periodontics Restor. Dent.* **2011**, *31*, 523–532.
22. Robert, L.; McGuire, M. The diagnosis and treatment of the gummy smile. *Compend. Contin. Educ. Dent.* **1997**, *18*, 757–762+764; quiz 766.
23. Herrero, F.; Scott, J.B.; Maropis, P.; Yukna, R.A. Clinical comparison of desired versus actual amount of surgical crown lengthening. *J. Periodontal.* **1995**, *66*, 568–571. [CrossRef] [PubMed]
24. Kois, J.C. The restorative-periodontal interface: Biological parameters. *Periodontology* **1996**, *11*, 29–38. [CrossRef] [PubMed]
25. Bindl, A.; Mörmann, W.H. Marginal and internal fit of all-ceramic CAD/CAM crown-copings on chamfer preparations. *J. Oral Rehabil.* **2005**, *32*, 441–447. [CrossRef] [PubMed]
26. Beuer, F.; Aggstaller, H.; Richter, J.; Edelhoff, D.; Gernet, W. Influence of preparation angle on marginal and internal fit of CAD/CAM-fabricated zirconia crown copings. *Quintessence Int.* **2009**, *40*, 243–250.
27. Komine, F.; Iwai, T.; Kobayashi, K.; Matsumura, H. Marginal and Internal Adaptation of Zirconium Dioxide Ceramic Copings and Crowns with Different Finish Line Designs. *Dent. Mater. J.* **2007**, *26*, 659–664. [CrossRef]
28. Comlekoglu, M.; Dundar, M.; Ozcan, M.; Gungor, M.; Gokce, B.; Artunc, C. Influence of cervical finish line type on the marginal adaptation of zirconia ceramic crowns. *Oper. Dent.* **2009**, *34*, 586–592. [CrossRef]
29. Iwai, T.; Komine, F.; Kobayashi, K.; Saito, A.; Matsumura, H. Influence of convergence angle and cement space on adaptation of zirconium dioxide ceramic copings. *Acta Odontol. Scand.* **2008**, *66*, 214–218. [CrossRef]
30. Dittmer, M.P.; Borchers, L.; Stiesch, M.; Kohorst, P. Stresses and distortions within zirconia-fixed dental prostheses due to the veneering process. *Acta Biomater.* **2009**, *5*, 3231–3239. [CrossRef]
31. Kohorst, P.; Brinkmann, H.; Dittmer, M.P.; Borchers, L.; Stiesch, M. Influence of the veneering process on the marginal fit of zirconia fixed dental prostheses. *J. Oral Rehabil.* **2010**, *37*, 283–291. [CrossRef] [PubMed]
32. Vigolo, P.; Fonzi, F. An In Vitro Evaluation of Fit of Zirconium-Oxide-Based Ceramic Four-Unit Fixed Partial Dentures, Generated with Three Different CAD/CAM Systems, before and after Porcelain Firing Cycles and after Glaze Cycles. *J. Prosthodont.* **2008**, *17*, 621–626. [CrossRef] [PubMed]
33. Gonzalo, E.; Suárez, M.J.; Serrano, B.; Lozano, J.F. A comparison of the marginal vertical discrepancies of zirconium and metal ceramic posterior fixed dental prostheses before and after cementation. *J. Prosthet. Dent.* **2009**, *102*, 378–384. [CrossRef] [PubMed]
34. Tinschert, J.; Natt, G.; Mautsch, W.; Augthun, M.; Spiekermann, H. Fracture resistance of lithium disilicate-, alumina-, and zirconia-based three-unit fixed partial dentures: A laboratory study. *Int. J. Prosthodont.* **2001**, *14*, 231–238.
35. Rosentritt, M.; Behr, M.; Thaller, C.; Rudolph, H.; Feilzer, A. Fracture performance of computer-aided manufactured zirconia and alloy crowns. *Quintessence Int.* **2009**, *40*, 655–662.
36. Derand, T.; Molin, M.; Kvam, K. Bond strength of composite luting cement to zirconia ceramic surfaces. *Dent. Mater.* **2005**, *21*, 1158–1162. [CrossRef]
37. Kitayama, S.; Nikaido, T.; Ikeda, M.; Alireza, S.; Miura, H.; Tagami, J. Internal coating of zirconia restoration with silica-based ceramic improves bonding of resin cement to dental zirconia ceramic. *Bio-Medical Mater. Eng.* **2010**, *20*, 77–87. [CrossRef]
38. Wittneben, J.G.; Joda, T.; Weber, H.P.; Brägger, U. Screw retained vs. cement retained implant-supported fixed dental prosthesis. *Periodontology* **2017**, *73*, 141–151. [CrossRef]
39. Shadid, R.; Sadaqa, N. A Comparison Between Screw- and Cement-Retained Implant Prostheses. *A Lit. Review. J. Oral Implant.* **2012**, *38*, 298–307. [CrossRef]
40. de Brandão, M.L.; Vettore, M.V.; Vidigal Júnior, G.M. Peri-implant bone loss in cement- and screw-retained prostheses: Systematic review and meta-analysis. *J. Clin. Periodontol.* **2013**, *40*, 287–295. [CrossRef]
41. Rosenstiel, S.F.; Land, M.F.; Fujimoto, J. *Contemporary Fixed Prosthodontics*, 5th ed.; Elsevier Inc.: St Louis, MO, USA, 2016; pp. 334+358–361.

42. Park, D.U.; Kim, J.Y.; Lee, J.R.; Kim, H.S.; Sim, H.Y.; Lee, H.; Han, Y.S. Screw-and-cement-retained prosthesis versus cement-retained prosthesis: Which is more appropriate for the upper premolar area? *J. Dent. Sci.* **2022**, *17*, 1553–1558. [CrossRef] [PubMed]
43. Dym, H.; Pierre, R. Diagnosis and Treatment Approaches to a "Gummy Smile". *Dent. Clin. North Am.* **2020**, *64*, 341–349. [CrossRef] [PubMed]
44. Nasr, M.W.; Jabbour, S.F.; Sidaoui, J.A.; Haber, R.N.; Kechichian, E.G. Botulinum Toxin for the Treatment of Excessive Gingival Display: A Systematic Review. *Aesthetic Surg. J.* **2015**, *36*, 82–88. [CrossRef] [PubMed]

Disclaimer/Publisher's Note: The statements, opinions and data contained in all publications are solely those of the individual author(s) and contributor(s) and not of MDPI and/or the editor(s). MDPI and/or the editor(s) disclaim responsibility for any injury to people or property resulting from any ideas, methods, instructions or products referred to in the content.

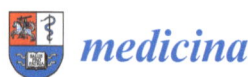 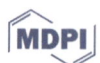

Article

Modular Digital and 3D-Printed Dental Models with Applicability in Dental Education

Alexandru Eugen Petre [1], Mihaela Pantea [1,*], Sergiu Drafta [1,*], Marina Imre [1], Ana Maria Cristina Țâncu [1], Eduard M. Liciu [2], Andreea Cristiana Didilescu [3] and Silviu Mirel Pițuru [4]

1 Department of Prosthodontics, Faculty of Dentistry, "Carol Davila" University of Medicine and Pharmacy, 17–23 Calea Plevnei, 010221 Bucharest, Romania
2 Coordinator of the 3D Printing Department, Center for Innovation and e-Health (CieH), "Carol Davila" University of Medicine and Pharmacy, 20 Pitar Mos Str., 010454 Bucharest, Romania
3 Department of Embryology, Faculty of Dentistry, "Carol Davila" University of Medicine and Pharmacy, 8 Eroii Sanitari Boulevard, 050474 Bucharest, Romania
4 Department of Professional Organization and Medical Legislation-Malpractice, Faculty of Dentistry, "Carol Davila" University of Medicine and Pharmacy, 020021 Bucharest, Romania
* Correspondence: mihaela.pantea@umfcd.ro (M.P.); sergiu.drafta@umfcd.ro (S.D.); Tel.: +40-722-387-969 (M.P.); +40-722-657-800 (S.D.)

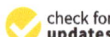

Citation: Petre, A.E.; Pantea, M.; Drafta, S.; Imre, M.; Țâncu, A.M.C.; Liciu, E.M.; Didilescu, A.C.; Pițuru, S.M. Modular Digital and 3D-Printed Dental Models with Applicability in Dental Education. *Medicina* 2023, 59, 116. https://doi.org/10.3390/medicina59010116

Academic Editors: Giuseppe Minervini, Stefania Moccia and Ricardo Faria Ribeiro

Received: 17 November 2022
Revised: 20 December 2022
Accepted: 30 December 2022
Published: 6 January 2023

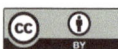

Copyright: © 2023 by the authors. Licensee MDPI, Basel, Switzerland. This article is an open access article distributed under the terms and conditions of the Creative Commons Attribution (CC BY) license (https://creativecommons.org/licenses/by/4.0/).

Abstract: *Background and Objectives*: The ever more complex modern dental education requires permanent adaptation to expanding medical knowledge and new advancements in digital technologies as well as intensification of interdisciplinary collaboration. Our study presents a newly developed computerized method allowing virtual case simulation on modular digital dental models and 3D-printing of the obtained digital models; additionally, undergraduate dental students' opinion on the advanced method is investigated in this paper. *Materials and Methods*: Based on the digitalization of didactic dental models, the proposed method generates modular digital dental models that can be easily converted into different types of partial edentulism scenarios, thus allowing the development of a digital library. Three-dimensionally printed simulated dental models can subsequently be manufactured based on the previously obtained digital models. The opinion of a group of undergraduate dental students (n = 205) on the proposed method was assessed via a questionnaire, administered as a Google form, sent via email. *Results*: The modular digital models allow students to perform repeated virtual simulations of any possible partial edentulism cases, to project 3D virtual treatment plans and to observe the subtle differences between diverse teeth preparations; the resulting 3D-printed models could be used in students' practical training. The proposed method received positive feedback from the undergraduate students. *Conclusions*: The advanced method is adequate for dental students' training, enabling the gradual design of modular digital dental models with partial edentulism, from simple to complex cases, and the hands-on training on corresponding 3D-printed dental models.

Keywords: dental students; digital dental models; digital technology; 3D printing; digital libraries; dental education; digital learning

1. Introduction

The digital revolution has spread across all medical fields, including dentistry [1], and, as expected, it has also touched the under- and postgraduate medical education. In dentistry, we are witnessing extraordinary progress generated by digital technology, such as clinical and technical procedures related to intraoral or extraoral scanning [1–5], 3D printing [6,7], guided dental implantology, complex maxillo-facial guided surgery or orthodontic digital planning [8], design and production of diverse prosthetic restorations using subtractive or additive methods [9–12], computerized validation of diverse fixed or mobile prostheses and computerized patient monitoring [1]. The importance of these beneficial elements constantly increases due to the encouraging perspectives in the development of digital dentistry. Today's top trending elements in dentistry digitalization and in influencing the directions of scientific research in this field are considered to be the following: rapid prototyping (RP); augmented and virtual reality (AR/VR), artificial intelligence (AI) and machine learning (ML); personalized and precision medicine; and tele-medicine [13–17].

Dental students' training holds a special place in this technological universe and, as a consequence, it must adapt to the characteristic rhythm of development of the actual digital era [18–20]. Thus, the concept of "virtual teaching and learning" ("e-teaching and e-learning"), which includes the use of digital dental didactic models, has been proposed and successfully applied in university education, facilitating students' understanding of theoretical and practical aspects [21–23]; these methods ensure students' efficient transition from a preclinical to a clinical context, thus proving their high educational value [21–23]. Haptic models employing virtual reality techniques represent an alternative to the standard models used in the preclinical training of students [24–26]. The famous Simodont (Nissin Dental Products Europe BV, Nieuw-Vennep, The Netherlands) was the first simulator that offered the possibility of learning proprioceptive abilities. The results of certain studies demonstrate that a clinically relevant qualitative feedback can be provided via a VR dental simulator [27,28]. While the cost of virtual simulation equipment is, unfortunately, still high, Nassar [29] pointed out in a relatively recent review that "none can deny the benefits of using these simulations strategies especially in saving faculty time as well as allowing the students to perform repeated attempts to achieve mastery at their own pace and after hours".

On the other hand, digital applications are not intended to completely replace the traditional, conventional methods of teaching and learning [18,30], which have proved their efficiency and have already been validated. In this respect, the training on mechanical patient simulators ("phantom heads") using standard dental models undisputedly remains an important stage in the preclinical training of dental students. Practical exercises performed on standard dental didactic models aim to form and, subsequently, to enhance the practical abilities of under- and postgraduate dental students, so that, in contact with real patients, they can demonstrate appropriate precision, correctness and expeditiousness in performing practical daily dentistry [31–33]. The dental models obtained with 3D printing have been used in dental education for some time. Deployment of 3D scanners, of CBCT and of 3D printers has enabled the precise replication of real anatomical structures, achieving simulated dental models having a real clinical correspondent, which can be successfully used in dental education [34,35] The combination of traditional simulation techniques with digital simulation broadens the educational possibilities towards decision-making training and deliberate practice, which are less possible in traditional settings.

Given the previously presented context, this paper has two major objectives: (Objective 1) to advance a new computerized method that allows the simulation of different virtual partial edentulism cases on modular digital dental models and the 3D printing of the obtained digital models; (Objective 2) to assess the opinion of a group of undergraduate dental students (n = 205) on the use of the proposed method in university dental education.

2. Materials and Methods

As previously mentioned, our study includes two distinct sections: the first one addresses a computerized method for obtaining modular digital and 3D-printed dental models and the second one presents undergraduate dental students' opinion on the advanced method.

2.1. Obtaining the Modular Digital and 3D-Printed Dental Models

The construction of the simulation models is based on CAD/CAM technology and consist of the following phases:

Section 2.1.1: scanning of standard dental models (with intact anatomic teeth), and separate scanning of intact artificial teeth and of prepared artificial teeth for different types of fixed prosthetic restorations;

Section 2.1.2: based on the acquired data, simulated modular dental models are developed using CAD software;

Section 2.1.3: based on the previously obtained digital models, 3D-printed simulated dental models can be manufactured.

2.1.1. Digital Data Acquisition

The proposed method for creating and accessing modular digital dental models is as follows. As a first step, digital dental models were achieved by digitalizing a maxillary and a mandibular standard dental model, their artificial teeth having intact anatomic dental crowns (Frasaco AN3, Frasaco GmbH, Tettnang, Germany). Subsequently, the upper and lower digital dental models were positioned in maximum intercuspation and scanned accordingly. All digital data corresponding to the dental arches, alveolar processes and maximum intercuspation position were obtained as .stl files (Standard Tessellation Language) using a Trios 3 intraoral scanner (3Shape, Copenhagen, Denmark). Successively, two groups of teeth were scanned separately, as follows: group A: represented by 32 artificial unprepared teeth, with intact anatomic dental crowns and their radicular extensions, corresponding to the full upper and lower dental arches, as produced by the manufacturer (Frasaco GmbH, Tettnang, Germany); group B: represented by 69 artificial teeth prepared for various types of fixed prosthetic restorations for total or partial coverage (Frasaco GmbH, Tettnang, Germany). These two groups were formed so that each unprepared artificial tooth, with an intact dental crown (from group A), corresponds to at least two prepared artificial teeth from Group B.

2.1.2. Design of the Modular Dental Models

The digital models of the two dental arches were uploaded in a prosthetic restorations design application (CAD) (Ceramill Mind, Amann Girrbach AG, Koblach, Austria) and, observing anthropometric criteria, were mounted in the virtual articulator (Figure 1).

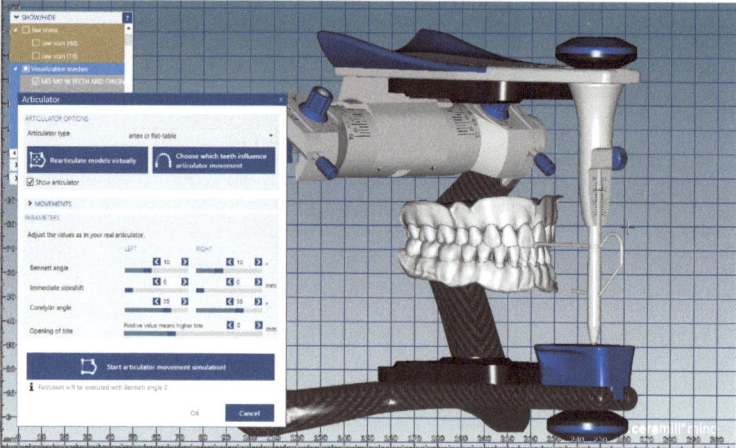

Figure 1. Image of digital dental model mounted in the virtual articulator in maximum intercuspation position.

The .stl files corresponding to the intact (unprepared) artificial teeth that were separately scanned (group A) were uploaded one by one, in the same order, in the form of "Generic Visualization Mesh", by indexing them with the intact dental models. The scanned images were indexed by reference to the corresponding surfaces of the dental crowns (Figure 2). The same procedure was applied for all the teeth of the two dental arches. Each artificial tooth scanned image (from Group A) was exported as a standard .stl file, maintaining the reference system.

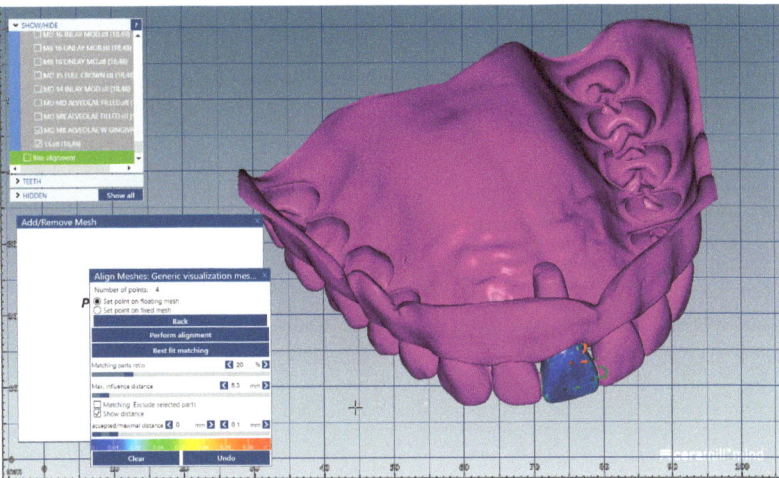

Figure 2. Image representing the .stl file obtained after separate scanning of the unprepared tooth # 1.1 (crown and radicular extension) indexed by reference to the corresponding surfaces of the digital dental model.

The scanned images of the prepared artificial teeth belonging to group B were uploaded one at a time, also in the form of "Generic Visualization Mesh", by indexation in relation with intact teeth models, using as reference the corresponding surfaces of the radicular extensions (Figure 3). The same procedure was applied for all prepared teeth from group B. Each prepared scanned image was exported as a standard .stl file, observing the reference system. The areas of the digital dental model corresponding to alveolar processes were isolated using the "Edit Mesh" tool (teeth are separated and their corresponding alveolar spaces are "closed") (Figure 4). The two dental alveolar processes, corresponding to upper and lower dental arches, were exported as .stl files, observing the reference system.

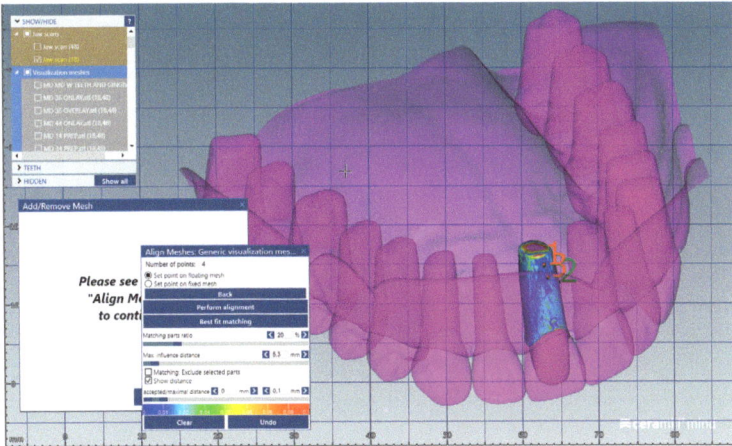

Figure 3. Image representing the indexation of the prepared tooth #1.1, by reference to the corresponding surfaces of the radicular extension.

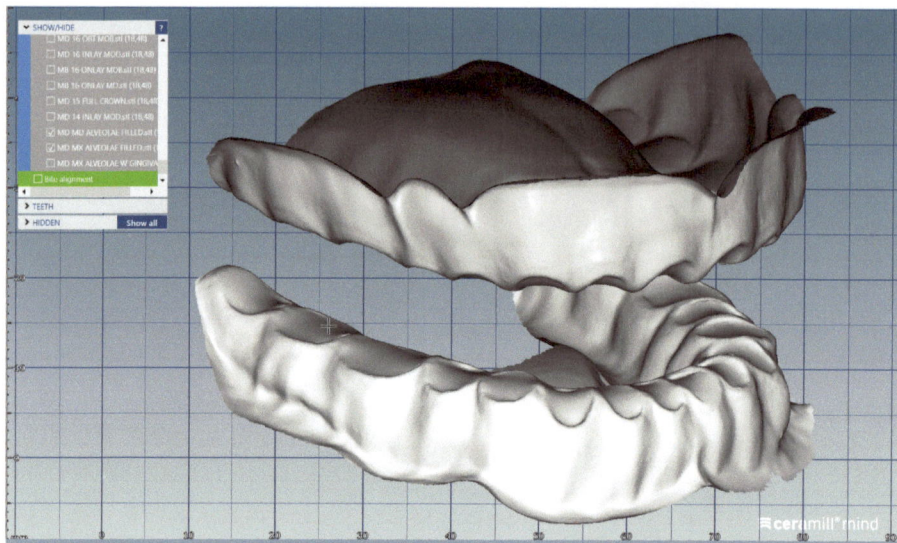

Figure 4. Image of the upper and lower dental alveolar processes obtained using the "Edit Mesh" tool.

Following the steps previously presented, the system of modular didactic digital dental models was created. This system is formed of: 1. edentulous ridge models; 2. unprepared teeth models (group A); 3. prepared teeth models (group B). It is important that all models should observe the same reference system so that, when combined, they will be placed in the correct position in relation to both their adjacent teeth and their antagonists. The resulting modular digital models allow students to perform repeated virtual simulation of any possible partial edentulism scenario. In order to generate a didactic modular digital dental model corresponding to a certain configuration, a new order is created in the CAD (Computer Aided Design) program. The two dental alveolar processes are uploaded as a digital wax-up, to which Boolean additions of prepared or unprepared teeth are performed.

We present a clinical situation corresponding to the absence of tooth #2.6/first upper left molar (edentation of 2.6), where the teeth next to the edentation (the abutment teeth) are prepared for complete fixed prosthetic coverage, with a circular cervical shoulder. At the lower arch, we generate a digital dental model corresponding to the edentation of all molars. In order to obtain the complete system of the modular didactic digital dental model, the following steps are to be followed: the .stl files corresponding to the two alveolar processes, respectively "MX GINGIVA FILLED.stl" (maxillary alveolar process) and "MD GINGIVA FILLED.stl" (mandibular alveolar process) are uploaded as digital wax-ups; the .stl files of the unprepared teeth from #1.8 to #2.4 and tooth #2.8 (Figure 5), and the respective files of the prepared teeth #25 and #27—the abutments—(Figure 6) are added to the "MX GINGIVA FILLED.stl" file as Boolean addition; the .stl files of the unprepared teeth from #3.5 to #4.5 are added to the file "MD GINGIVA FILLED.stl" (Figure 7). The areas corresponding to edentulous ridges can be edited in order to simulate bone resorption (Figure 8).

Moreover, this method can also use a dental model generated from a real patient. In this case, the following steps are required: 1. obtain digital intraoral impression; 2. generate models with removable dies/abutments; 3. print the removable dies/abutments; 4. prepare the abutments from the previous point (3) for different types of crowns; 5. re-scan the printed model with intact teeth and prepared teeth (abutments). A digital library is thus created, as in the case of the commercial didactic model.

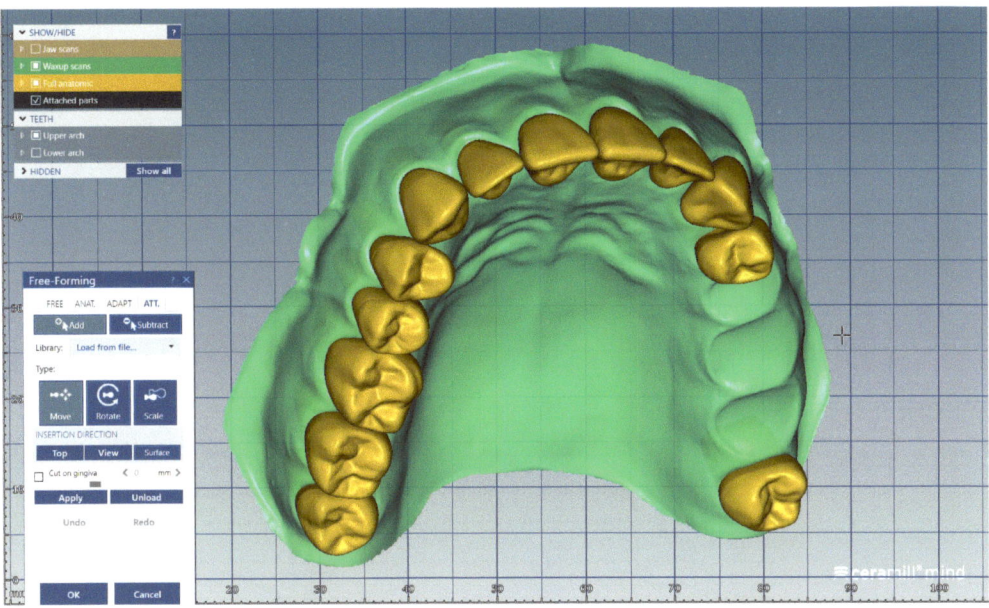

Figure 5. Image representing the .stl files of the unprepared teeth from #1.8 to #2.4 and tooth #2.8 that are added to the .stl file of the maxillary alveolar process ("MX GINGIVA FILLED.stl" file) as Boolean additions.

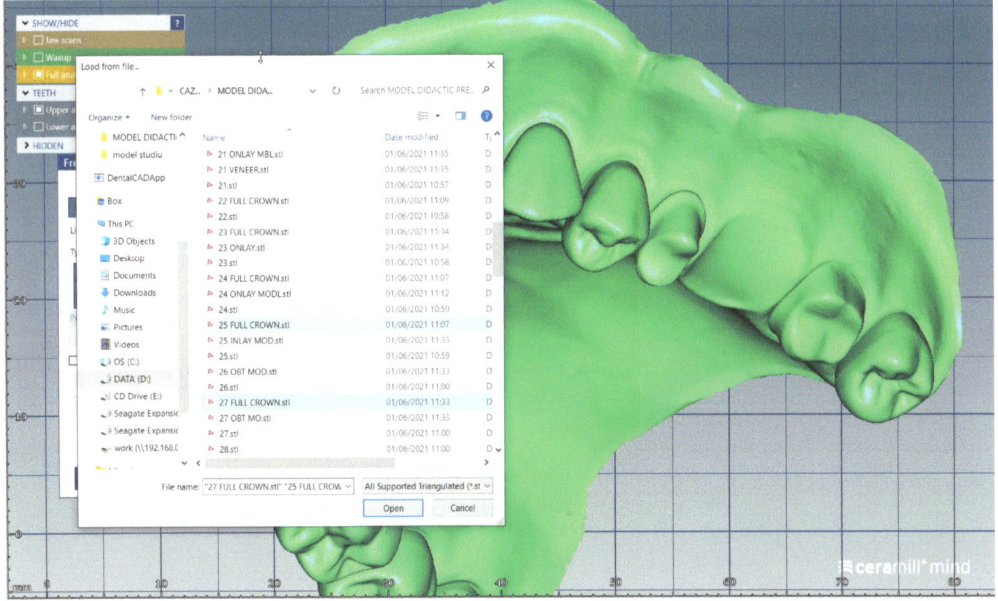

Figure 6. Image representing the .stl files of the prepared teeth #25 and #27 that are added to the .stl file of the maxillary alveolar process ("MX GINGIVA FILLED.stl" file) as Boolean additions.

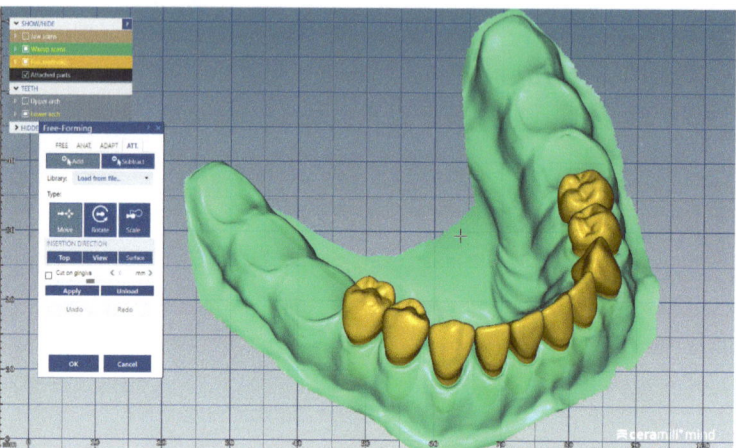

Figure 7. Image representing the .stl files of the unprepared teeth from #3.5 to #4.5 that are added to the .stl file of the mandibular alveolar process ("MD GINGIVA FILLED.stl" file) as Boolean additions.

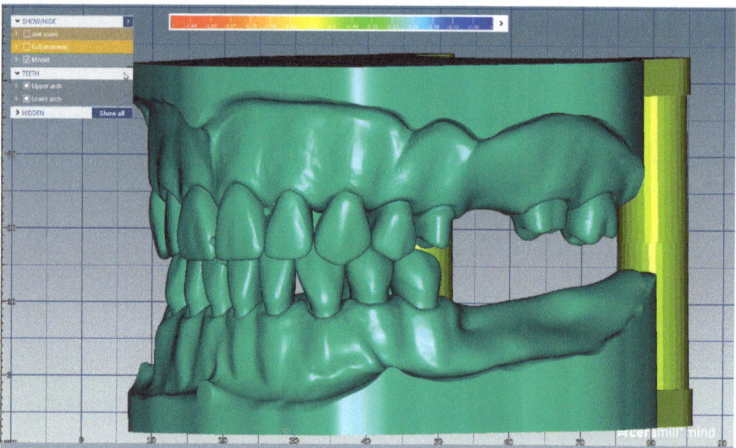

Figure 8. The obtained modular didactic dental model; the areas corresponding to edentulous ridges can be edited to simulate bone resorption.

All procedures in this scientific study were conducted in accordance with the manufacturers' recommendations. It should also be noted that the software's license is currently available.

2.1.3. Additive Manufacturing of the Dental Models

The obtained digital dental models (corresponding to standard models or to real patients) can be 3D printed. The STL files were generated and exported to an SLA (Stereolithography) 3D printer (Form 3B+, Formlabs Inc., Somerville, MA, USA) in order to fabricate the printed resin models using their proprietary resin (White Resin, Formlabs Inc., Somerville, MA, USA). Printing tests were performed at a layer height of 0.050 mm, 0.100 mm and 0.020 mm; a layer height of 0.050 mm was chosen to be used in printing, combining both a reduced printing time and a proper level of detail. The resulting plates designated for printing consisted of 7 models, placed in a vertical position, to maximize the available space. Printing was carried out at a layer height of 0.050 mm, 4.5 s layer exposure time, at 60% UV power. The printing time of 7 h and 38 min allowed for multiple plates to be printed per day, significantly reducing the total production time. When the printing program had finished, the printed models were removed from the platform and first cleaned (washed) for ten minutes in 98% Isopropyl Alcohol (Anycubic Wash & Cure Plus Machine, Hongkong Anycubic Technology Co., Kowloon, Hong Kong, China) to remove any excess resin. After cleaning and drying, the printed models rested for at least 10 min to make sure that they were dry and free of ethanol residue. The printed parts were placed for 6 min for curing under UV light (Formlabs Cure Station, Formlabs Inc., Somerville, MA, USA) at ambient temperature, for final, optimal polymerization. The support structures were removed and the obtained 3D-printed dental models did not require any further finishing or polishing. In case of the modular dental model, this can be printed with or without mobile dies/abutments. It is worth noting that the dental models' bases were designed and 3D printed so that they can be mounted (using a magnetic metal plate) in the dental patient simulators (Dental Patient Simulator (DPS) "Adam" TM, KaVo Dental GmbH, 88400 Biberach/Riß, Germany) which the faculty makes available to students.

2.2. Evaluation of Undergraduate Students' Opinion on the Use of Modular Digital and 3D-Printed Dental Models in University Dental Education

2.2.1. Survey Methodology and Ethical Approval

This survey was approved by the Scientific Research Ethics Committee of "Carol Davila" University of Medicine and Pharmacy, Bucharest, Romania (Project identification Code: PO-35-F-03; Protocol number:15596; date: 8 June 2022). The students' opinion on the use of modular digital dental models and 3D-printed simulated dental models in university dental education was assessed via a questionnaire, administered as a Google form sent via email. The study was conducted in accordance with the Declaration of Helsinki of 1975, revised in 2013. Subjects selected to participate in the study were invited to fill in the questionnaire and were informed about the survey in accordance with the World Medical Association Declaration of Helsinki and the current European privacy law, highlighting, in an introduction section of the questionnaire, the scientific aim of the study, that the questionnaire was anonymous and that they had the right to interrupt the completion of the form at any moment in case of withdrawal. Subjects who were invited to participate in this study received an e-mail containing written information about the study and the informed consent. All subjects gave their informed consent for inclusion before they participated in the study. All subjects that agreed to participate in the study expressed their consent by completing the survey; informed consent was obtained from the subjects involved in the study to publish this paper. No personal data were collected through the form and, as an anonymous web survey, no sensitive data were collected. The questionnaire was secured so as to be completed only once by every participant.

2.2.2. Selection of Participants

This study was designed to be a pilot study and was conducted among third- and fourth-year dental students undergoing theoretical and practical training in Prosthodontics, Faculty of Dentistry, "Carol Davila" University of Medicine and Pharmacy, Bucharest, Romania. The inclusion criteria for the participants were: third- and fourth-year dental students; students that completed the theoretical and practical training in Fixed Prosthodontics and Occlusology, for an entire semester; students that used the modular digital and 3D-printed dental models in their training activities, during an entire semester (14 weeks), at least once per week; females or males aged >18 years. The exclusion criteria were: students not willing to participate in the study; students that have not completed their training in Fixed Prosthodontics and Occlusology for an entire semester. These students' opinions on the use of modular digital dental models and 3D-printed simulated dental models in university dental education was assessed via a questionnaire, administered as a Google form sent via email. The request to participate in the survey was applied to 240 students, of which 205 voluntarily agreed to participate, which means a percentage of acceptance of participation of 85.42%.

2.2.3. Survey Questionnaire

The questionnaire used for the assessment (as presented in Table 1) was formed of 20 items represented by both multiple or single-choice questions, referring to the following main aspects: (1) socio-demographic data (age, gender, year of study—first three questions of the questionnaire); (2) participants' perception of the proposed computerized method allowing virtual case simulation on modular digital dental models (questions 4 to 10); (3) participants' perception of the practical training on 3D-printed dental models (questions 11 to 17); (4) participants' perception of certain particularities of the proposed methods and on their further use in university dental education (questions 18 to 20). Items 4 to 7 and 11 to 14 were represented by multiple-choice questions; the other items were represented by single-choice questions. The estimated time needed to fill in the questionnaire was a maximum of 5 min.

Table 1. The questionnaire used to assess the opinions of dental students on the use of modular digital and 3D-printed dental models in university dental education; the questionnaire was administered as a Google form and sent via email.

Investigated Aspects	Questions (Q) and Possible Answers
(1) Socio-demo-graphic data	Q1. Please enter your age
	Q2. Please enter your gender
	Q3. Please enter your study year
(2) Modular digital dental models	Q4. Modular digital dental models allow the following:
	a. realistic simulation of various classes of partial edentulism
	b. easy identification of various classes of partial edentulism
	c. realistic simulation of the alveolar ridges resorption of various degrees
	d. realistic simulation of malpositioned teeth and the destruction of dental crowns, of various degrees
	e. easy elaboration of various treatment plans
	Q5. The three main advantages of using modular digital dental models in my university training are as follows:
	a. it allows a 3D visualization of details, in contrast to 2D images
	b. it allows repeated virtual simulations (reiteration of virtual simulations)
	c. it is an accessible and flexible method of learning
	d. it is a quick way to learn
	e. it is a comfortable way of learning
	Q6. The three main advantages of using modular digital models as a method of e-learning in university dental education are as follows:
	a. it allows easy access from various locations
	b. it allows virtual interaction (synchronous and asynchronous) between students and teachers
	c. it allows fast virtual feedback to students from teachers
	d. it allows the storage of digital data for a long time
	e. it allows the evaluation of the program's effectiveness (number of registered downloads)

Table 1. Cont.

Investigated Aspects	Questions (Q) and Possible Answers
	Q7. The three main disadvantages of using modular digital models as a method of e-learning in university dental education are as follows:
	a. it requires technological resources (dedicated electronic devices: computer, laptop etc.)
	b. it requires (minimum) experience in the field of computers/(minimum) digital skills
	c. limitation of direct interaction with teachers (face-to-face contact)
	d. limitation of direct interaction with patients
	e. dependence on internet connection
	Q8. Using the proposed virtual simulation method makes me feel better prepared for my clinical activity:
	a. Yes
	b. No
	Q9. The proposed virtual simulation method fits my way of learning:
	a. Yes
	b. No.
	Q10. I am interested in further use of the proposed virtual simulation method in my university training:
	a. Yes
	b. No
(3) 3D-printed dental models	**Q11.** Practical training on 3D-printed dental models allows me the following:
	a. to improve my practical skills
	b. to learn diverse practical procedures risk-free
	c. hands-on training under the supervision of teachers
	d. to better understand the performed procedures (dental preparations, impressions, wax-up procedures, interim restorations)
	e. good visualization of teeth (position, destruction) and edentulous areas
	Q12. The three main advantages of using 3D-printed dental models in my university training are as follows:
	a. it allows a real/3D visualization of the details, in contrast to the 2D images
	b. it allows repeated attempts of various practical procedures
	c. it is an accessible, flexible method of learning
	d. it is a quick way to learn
	e. it is a comfortable way of learning
	Q13. The three main advantages of using 3D-printed dental models in university dental education are as follows:
	a. 3D-printing of models is facilitated by the university
	b. it allows direct interaction between students and teachers
	c. it allows direct feedback to students from teachers
	d. 3D-printed models can be scanned and archived as digital models which allow virtual evaluation
	e. 3D-printed models can be used for practical training in various dental specialties in different years of study

Table 1. Cont.

Investigated Aspects	Questions (Q) and Possible Answers
	Q14. The three main disadvantages of using 3D-printed dental models in my university dental training are as follows:
	a. the colour of the printed material is different from that of natural teeth
	b. the hardness of the printed material is different from that of natural teeth
	c. the lightness of the printed material is different from that of natural teeth
	d. the absence of a gingival mask
	e. the 3D-printed models are brittle
	Q15. Practicing on 3D-printed dental models makes me feel better prepared for my clinical activity:
	a. Yes
	b. No
	Q16. The practical training on 3D-printed dental models fits my way of learning:
	a. Yes
	b. No
	Q17. I am interested in further use of 3D-printed dental models in my university training:
	a. Yes
	b. No
(4) Aspects common to both modular digital and 3D-printed dental models	**Q18.** I believe that obtaining virtual and 3D-printed dental models from real clinical cases through the proposed methods is an advantage:
	a. Yes
	b. No
	Q19. I believe that the use of the proposed methods in my university training can help me to improve my own professional skills in digital technology and 3D-printing:
	a. Yes
	b. No
	Q20. I think that the development of these teaching / learning methods (virtual and 3D-printed dental models) would be of interest to future generations of students:
	a. Yes
	b. No

2.2.4. Data Analysis

All the data from the study were analyzed using IBM SPSS Statistics 25 and illustrated using Microsoft Office Excel/Word 2021. Quantitative variables were tested for normal distribution using the Shapiro–Wilk Test and were summarized as averages with standard deviations or medians with interquartile ranges. Qualitative variables were reported as counts or percentages and differences between groups were tested using Fisher's Exact tests. Quantitative independent variables with non-parametric distributions were tested between groups using Mann–Whitney U. Correlations between quantitative variables with non-parametric distributions were measured using Spearman's rho correlation coefficients.

3. Results

3.1. Modular Digital and 3D-Printed Dental Models

Theoretical and hands-on courses on the use of modular digital dental models and of 3D-printed simulated dental models were organized weekly by experienced specialists in prosthodontics (university teaching staff) for the third- and fourth-year dental students, and the students used these models in their training activities during an entire semester (14 weeks) at least once per week. The modular digital models were used by the dental students under the supervision of the teaching staff. The students could perform repeated virtual simulation of any possible partial edentulism scenario, the virtual identification of classes of partial edentulism requiring prosthetic treatment, the digital analysis of diverse partial edentulous cases, occlusal examination (i.e., malpositioned teeth, occlusal plane) and the selection of the proper dental preparation and of fixed dental prostheses for different virtual clinical situations.

In Figures 9–13 certain sequences from the development of a modular digital dental model are presented; this specific model was classified by our teaching staff as a "training digital dental model". The "training digital dental model" was designed to be relevant to undergraduate students in fixed prosthodontics, as it presented different edentulous areas, migrated teeth and bone resorptions. Based on this "digital training dental model", "3D-printed training dental models" were subsequently manufactured. The previously mentioned 3D-printed models were made available to both third-year and fourth-year dental students, who performed hands-on practice on these models throughout an entire semester. Students' practical training on these 3D-printed models included procedures related to fixed prosthodontics, such as teeth preparations, wax-ups, fabrication of interim restorations, partial and full-arch impressions, evaluation and provisional cementation of interim fixed prosthetic restorations. Additionally, 3D-printed dental models that presented diverse ideal teeth preparations for prosthetic restorations were made available to students; students could check their own dental preparations using these models as reference. During the respective semester, the students succeeded in combining virtual training on modular digital dental models with practical training on their corresponding 3D-printed models.

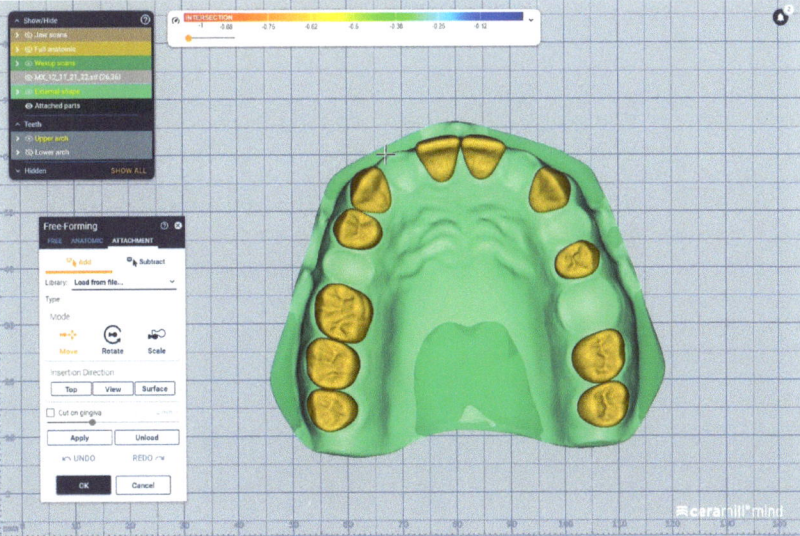

Figure 9. Sequence for obtaining the "training digital dental model": the .stl files of the unprepared teeth are added to the .stl file of the maxillary alveolar process ("MX GINGIVA FILLED.stl" file) as Boolean additions.

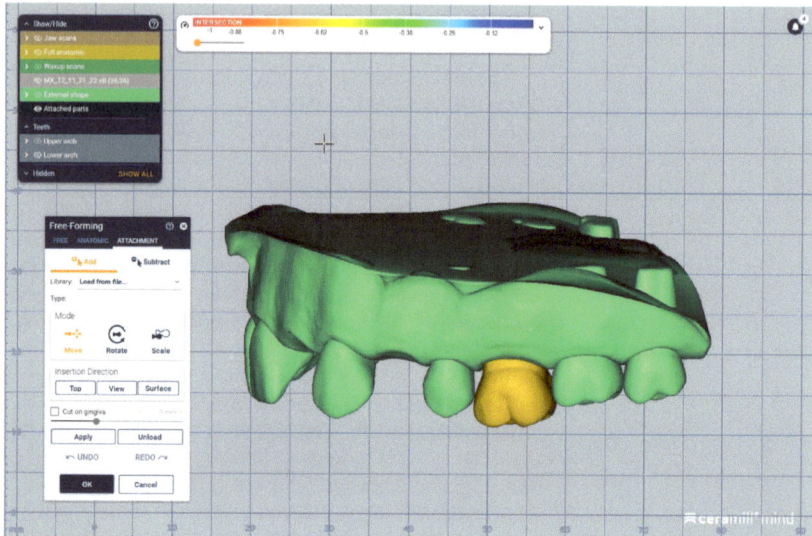

Figure 10. Sequence for obtaining the "training digital dental model": the migrated tooth (#2.6) is separately added.

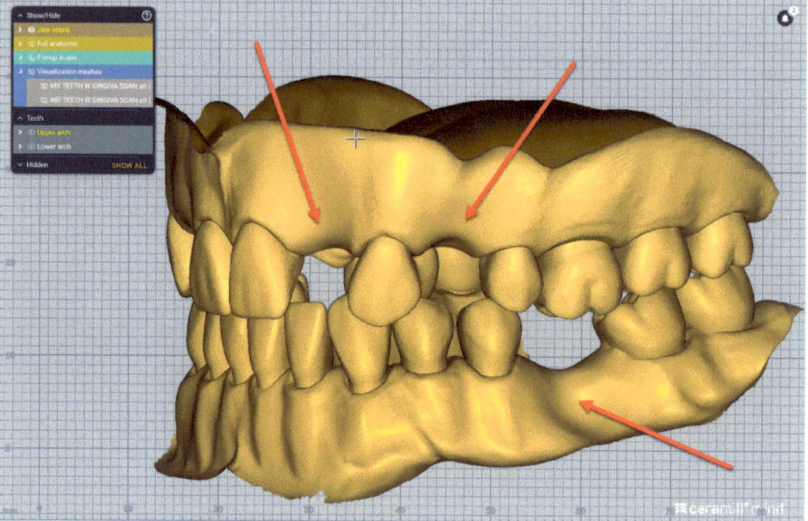

Figure 11. Sequence for obtaining the "training digital dental model": the areas corresponding to edentulous ridges are edited to simulate bone resorption (indicated by red arrows).

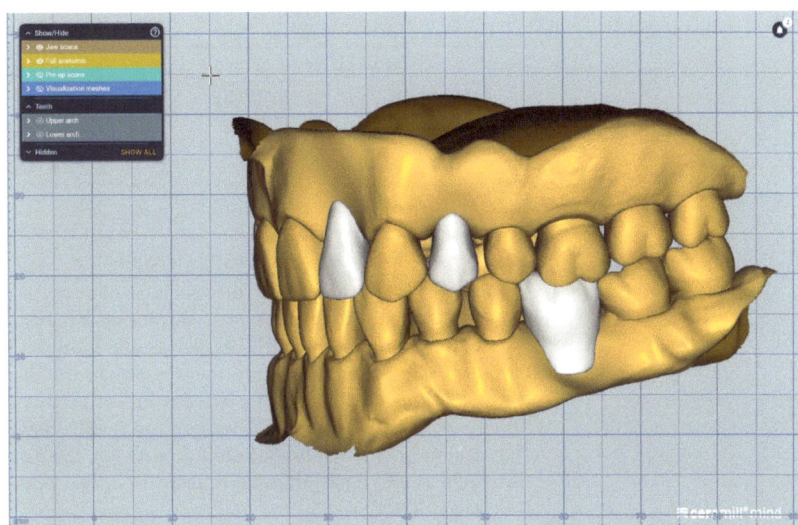

Figure 12. Sequence for obtaining the "training digital dental model": As an additional option, the absent teeth can be added in order to observe certain aesthetic and functional challenges.

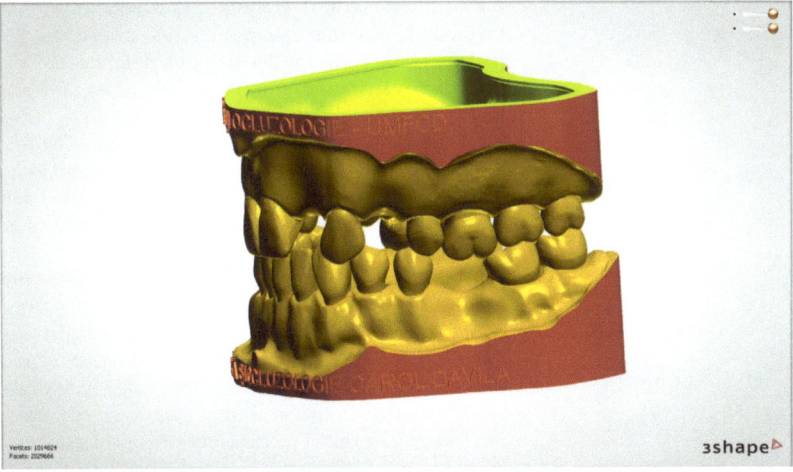

Figure 13. The corresponding printable digital model is obtained.

3.2. Students' Opinion on the Use of Modular Digital and 3D-Printed Dental Models in University Dental Education

The statistical analysis of the results obtained from the applied survey revealed the following presented aspects. Data in Table 2 show the demographic characteristics of the analyzed students. Mean age was 22.31 ± 1.74, with a median of 22 years. Most of the students were women (74.6%). A 58% proportion of the students were in their fourth academic year and 42% of the students were in their third academic year.

Table 2. Demographic characteristics of the analyzed students.

Parameter	Value
Age (Mean ± SD, Median (IQR)	22.31 ± 1.74, 22 (21–23)
Gender (No., %)	153 (74.6%) Female, 52 (25.4%) Male
Year of study (No., %)	86 (42%) Third year, 119 (58%) Fourth year

Data in Table 3 show the distribution of the students according to their answers in the survey. The results show the following elements:

- the most-selected answer for the functions of modular digital dental models (question 4) was the realistic simulation of various classes of partial edentulism (81%); corresponding to functions of 3D-printed dental models (question 11), the most-selected answer was option A (improvement of practical skills) (78.5%);
- the most-selected answer for advantages of modular digital dental models in university training (question 5) was option A (3D visualization of details) (85.9%); in the same line, the most-selected answer for the advantages of 3D-printed dental models in university training (question 12) was option A (real/3D visualization of details) (82.9%);
- the most-selected answer for advantages of modular digital dental models as a method of e-learning (question 6) was option A (easy access from various locations) (86.8%); in the case of 3D-printed dental models, the most-selected advantage was that the use of these 3D-printed models allows direct feedback to students from teachers (77.1%);
- the most-selected answer for the disadvantages of modular digital dental models as a method of e-learning (question 7) was option D (limitation of direct interaction with patients) (69.3%); as for the 3D-printed dental models, the most-selected answer for their disadvantages was option B (hardness of the printed material is different from that of natural teeth) (91.7%);
- most responses were affirmative to questions 8 (76.6%), 9 (82.9%) and 10 (91.7%), which are related to the virtual simulation method, and to questions 15 (84.9%), 16 (90.2%), and 17 (92.7%), which are related to the 3D-printed dental models. The students were asked if they feel better-prepared for their clinical activity by using the proposed methods (question 8 and 15), if the methods fits their way of learning (question 9 and 16) and if they are interested in further use of the proposed methods in university training (question 10 and 17). It can be noted that the questions related to 3D-printed dental models registered a slightly higher affirmative response percentage than the questions related to the virtual simulation method (modular digital models);
- most of the students responded affirmatively to question 18 (obtaining virtual/3D-printed models from real clinical cases is an advantage) (96.6%), question 19 (usage of virtual/3D-printed models improves professional skills in digital technology and 3D-printing) (92.7%), and question 20 (development of virtual/3D-printed dental models would be of interest to future generations of students) (96.6%).

Data from Table 4 show the comparison of ages between different question item answers. The distribution of age between groups was non-parametric according to the Shapiro–Wilk test ($p < 0.001$). According to the Mann–Whitney U test, students who selected item 5D (modular digital dental models are a quick way to learn) had a significantly lower age (median = 22 years, IQR = 21–23) than students who did not select 5D (median = 22 years, IQR = 22–23) ($p = 0.034$).

Table 3. Distribution of the students according to the answers from the survey.

Question	Selected/Affirmative Answer (No., %)
Q4	4A-81%, 4B-79.5%, 4C-59.5%, 4D-70.2%, 4E-78%
Q5	5A-85.9%, 5B-68.3%, 5C-66.3%, 5D-35.6%, 5E-43.9%
Q6	6A-86.8%, 6B-76.6%, 6C-56.6%, 6D-64.4%, 6E-15.6%
Q7	7A-62.4%, 7B-55.6%, 7C-57.6%, 7D-69.3%, 7E-55.1%
Q8	48 (23.4%) Negative, 157 (76.6%) Affirmative
Q9	35 (17.1%) Negative, 170 (82.9%) Affirmative
Q10	17 (8.3%) Negative, 188 (91.7%) Affirmative
Q11	11A-78.5%, 11B-75.6%, 11C-54.6%, 11D-78%, 11E-62.9%
Q12	12A-82.9%, 12B-70.2%, 12C-35.6%, 12D-35.6%, 12E-42.9%
Q13	13A-53.2%, 13B-51.7%, 13C-77.1%, 13D-52.7%, 13E-64.9%
Q14	14A-61.5%, 14B-91.7%, 14C-58%, 14D-42.4%, 14E-44.4%
Q15	31 (15.1%) Negative, 174 (84.9%) Affirmative
Q16	20 (9.8%) Negative, 185 (90.2%) Affirmative
Q17	15 (7.3%) Negative, 190 (92.7%) Affirmative
Q18	7 (3.4%) Negative, 198 (96.6%) Affirmative
Q19	15 (7.3%) Negative, 190 (92.7%) Affirmative
Q20	7 (3.4%) Negative, 198 (96.6%) Affirmative

Table 4. Comparison of ages between different question item answers.

	Age/Item	Q5-D	Q5-E	Q6-E	Q13-B
	Average ± SD	22.48 ± 1.98	22.18 ± 1.78	22.22 ± 1.75	22.01 ± 1.07
	Median (IQR)	22 (22–23)	22 (21–23)	22 (21–23)	22 (21–23)
	Mean Rank	109.22	96.12	98.49	93.64
Selected	Average ± SD	21.99 ± 1.15	22.47 ± 1.69	22.78 ± 1.66	22.58 ± 2.16
	Median (IQR)	22 (21–23)	22 (22–23)	23 (22–23)	22 (22–23)
	Mean Rank	91.75	111.79	127.41	111.75
	p *	0.034	0.048	0.008	0.022

* Mann–Whitney U Test.

Also, students who selected item 5E (modular digital dental models are a comfortable way of learning) (median = 22 years, IQR = 22–23 vs. median = 22 years, IQR = 21–23, p = 0.048), 6E (modular digital dental models allow the evaluation of the program's effectiveness) (median = 23 years, IQR = 22–23 vs. median = 22 years, IQR = 21–23, p = 0.008) or 13B (3D-printed dental models allow direct interaction between students and teachers) (median = 22 years, IQR = 22–23 vs. median = 22 years, IQR = 21–23, p = 0.022) had a significantly higher age than students who did not select these items.

Data from Table 5 show the distribution of the students according to academic year of study and item answers. The results show the following:

- Students who selected option 4A (modular digital dental models allow realistic simulation of various classes of partial edentulism) were more frequently in their fourth academic year (85.7% vs. 74.4%) (p = 0.048);
- Students who selected option 4C (modular digital dental models allow realistic simulation of alveolar ridge resorption) were more frequently in their fourth academic year (65.5% vs. 51.2%) (p = 0.044);

- Students who selected option 4D (modular digital dental models allow realistic simulation of malpositioned teeth and destruction of dental crowns) were more frequently in their fourth academic year (76.5% vs. 61.6%) ($p = 0.030$);
- Students who selected option 5D (modular digital dental models are a quick way to learn) were more frequently in their third academic year (46.5% vs. 27.7%) ($p = 0.008$);
- Students who selected option 7C (modular digital dental models are limited in terms of direct interaction with teachers) were more frequently in their fourth academic year (64.7% vs. 47.7%) ($p = 0.022$);
- Students who answered that modular digital dental models fit their way of learning (question 9) were more frequently in their third academic year (89.5% vs. 78.2%) ($p = 0.039$);
- Students who selected option 12D (3D-printed dental models are a quick way to learn) were more frequently in their third academic year (45.3% vs. 28.6%) ($p = 0.018$);
- Students who selected option 13B (3D-printed dental models allow direct interaction between students and teachers) were more frequently in their fourth academic year (59.7% vs. 40.7%) ($p = 0.011$);
- Students who answered that virtual/3D-printed dental models would be of interest to future generations of students (question 20) were more frequently in their third academic year (100% vs. 94.1%) ($p = 0.043$).

Table 5. Distribution of the students according to academic year of study and item answers.

Selected Item /Year of Study	Third Year (N = 86)		Fourth Year (N = 119)		p *
	No.	%	No.	%	
Q4-A	64	74.4%	102	85.7%	0.048
Q4-C	44	51.2%	78	65.5%	0.044
Q4-D	53	61.6%	91	76.5%	0.030
Q5-D	40	46.5%	33	27.7%	0.008
Q7-C	41	47.7%	77	64.7%	0.022
Q9 (Affirmative)	77	89.5%	93	78.2%	0.039
Q12-D	39	45.3%	34	28.6%	0.018
Q13-B	35	40.7%	71	59.7%	0.011
Q20 (Affirmative)	86	100%	112	94.1%	0.043

* Fisher's Exact Test.

Data from Table 6 show the comparisons of item answers among the analyzed students. Differences between groups that are significant according to Fisher's Exact Tests ($p < 0.05$) show the following:

- Students who selected item 5A (modular digital dental models allow 3D visualization of details) more frequently also selected item 12A (3D-printed dental models allow 3D visualization of details) (90.6% vs. 62.9%) ($p < 0.001$);
- Students who selected item 5B (modular digital dental models allow repeated virtual simulations) more frequently also selected item 12B (3D-printed dental models allow repeated attempts of various practical procedures) (81.9% vs. 36.1%) ($p < 0.001$);
- Students who selected item 5C (modular digital dental models are an accessible and flexible method of learning) more rarely also selected item 12C (3D-printed dental models are an accessible and flexible method of learning) (78.8% vs. 43.8%) ($p < 0.001$);
- Students who selected item 5D (modular digital dental models are a quick way to learn) more frequently also selected item 12D (3D-printed dental models are a quick way to learn) (68.5% vs. 17.4%) ($p < 0.001$);

- Students who selected item 5E (modular digital dental models are a comfortable way of learning) more frequently also selected item 12E (3D-printed dental models are a comfortable way of learning) (67% vs. 26.5%) ($p < 0.001$);
- Students who selected item 6C (modular digital dental models allow fast virtual feedback to students from teachers) more frequently also selected item 13C (3D-printed dental models allow direct feedback to students from teachers) (60.8% vs. 42.6%) ($p = 0.030$);
- Students who answered that modular digital models are a good way to prepare for their clinical activity (question 8) more frequently also answered that 3D-printed dental models are a good way to prepare for their clinical activity (question 15) (83.3% vs. 38.7%) ($p < 0.001$);
- Students who answered that modular digital models fit their way of learning (question 9) more frequently also answered that 3D-printed dental models fit their way of learning (question 16) (87.6% vs. 40%) ($p < 0.001$);
- Students who answered that they are interested in further use of modular digital models (question 10) more frequently also answered that they are interested in further use of 3D-printed dental models (question 17) (95.3% vs. 46.7%) ($p < 0.001$);
- Students who answered that obtaining virtual/3D-printed dental models from real clinical cases is an advantage (question 18) more frequently also answered that virtual/3D-printed dental models can help them improve their professional skills in digital technology and 3D-printing (question 19) (98.9% vs. 66.7%) ($p < 0.001$);
- Students who answered that obtaining virtual/3D-printed dental models from real clinical cases is an advantage (question 18) more frequently also answered that development of virtual/3D-printed dental models would be of interest to future generations of students (question 20) (98.5% vs. 42.9%) ($p < 0.001$);
- Students who answered that virtual/3D-printed dental models can help them improve their professional skills in digital technology and 3D-printing (question 19) more frequently also answered that development of virtual/3D-printed dental models would be of interest to future generations of students (question 20) (94.9% vs. 28.6%) ($p < 0.001$).

Table 6. Comparisons of item answers among analyzed students.

Item Q5-A/Q12-A	12-A-Not Selected		12-A-Selected		p *
	No.	%	No.	%	
5-A-Not selected	13	37.1%	16	9.4%	<0.001
5-A-Selected	22	62.9%	154	90.6%	
Item Q5-B/Q12-B	12-B-Not selected		12-B-Selected		p *
	No.	%	No.	%	
5-B-Not selected	39	63.9%	26	18.1%	<0.001
5-B-Selected	22	36.1%	118	81.9%	
Item Q5-C/Q12-C	12-C-Not Selected		12-C-Selected		p *
	No.	%	No.	%	
5-C-Not selected	28	21.2%	41	56.2%	<0.001
5-C-Selected	104	78.8%	32	43.8%	
Item Q5-D/Q12-D	12-D-Not Selected		12-D-Selected		p *
	No.	%	No.	%	
5-D-Not selected	109	82.6%	23	31.5%	<0.001
5-D-Selected	23	17.4%	50	68.5%	

Table 6. *Cont.*

Item Q5-E/Q12-E	12-E-Not Selected		12-E-Selected		*p* *
	No.	%	No.	%	
5-E-Not selected	86	73.5%	29	33%	<0.001
5-E-Selected	31	26.5%	59	67%	
Item Q6-C/Q13-C	13-C-Not Selected		13-C-Selected		*p* *
	No.	%	No.	%	
6-C-Not selected	27	57.4%	62	39.2%	0.030
6-C-Selected	20	42.6%	96	60.8%	
Item Q8/Q15	15-Negative		15-Affirmative		*p* *
	No.	%	No.	%	
8-Negative	19	61.3%	29	16.7%	<0.001
8-Affirmative	12	38.7%	145	83.3%	
Item Q9/Q16	16-Negative		16-Affirmative		*p* *
	No.	%	No.	%	
9-Negative	12	60%	23	12.4%	<0.001
9-Affirmative	8	40%	162	87.6%	
Item Q10/Q17	17-Negative		17-Affirmative		*p* *
	No.	%	No.	%	
10-Negative	8	53.3%	9	4.7%	<0.001
10-Affirmative	7	46.7%	181	95.3%	
Item Q18/Q19	19-Negative		19-Affirmative		*p* *
	No.	%	No.	%	
18-Negative	5	33.3%	2	1.1%	<0.001
18-Affirmative	10	66.7%	188	98.9%	
Item Q18/Q20	20-Negative		20-Affirmative		*p* *
	No.	%	No.	%	
18-Negative	4	57.1%	3	1.5%	<0.001
18-Affirmative	3	42.9%	195	98.5%	
Item Q19/Q20	20-Negative		20-Affirmative		*p* *
	No.	%	No.	%	
19-Negative	5	71.4%	10	5.1%	<0.001
19-Affirmative	2	28.6%	188	94.9%	

* Fisher's Exact Test.

Based on the numbers of items chosen for question 4 a score was constructed: Score_Q4—number of functions chosen for modular digital dental models. Data from Table 7 and Figure 14 show the comparison of Score_Q4 between academic years of study. Based on the numbers of items chosen for questions 4 and 11 scores were constructed: Score_Q4—number of functions chosen for modular digital dental models, Score_Q11—number of functions chosen for 3D-printed dental models. Distribution of the Score_Q4 between groups was non-parametric according to the Shapiro–Wilk test ($p < 0.001$). According to the Mann–Whitney U test, fourth year students selected significantly more functions for modular digital dental models (median = 4, IQR = 3–5) than third year students (median = 3, IQR = 2–5) ($p = 0.046$).

Table 7. Comparison of Score_Q4 between academic years of study.

Year of Study/ Score_Q4	Average ± SD	Median (IQR)	Mean Rank	p *
Third year	3.42 ± 1.53	3 (2–5)	93.76	0.046
Fourth year	3.87 ± 1.29	4 (3–5)	109.68	

* Mann–Whitney U Test.

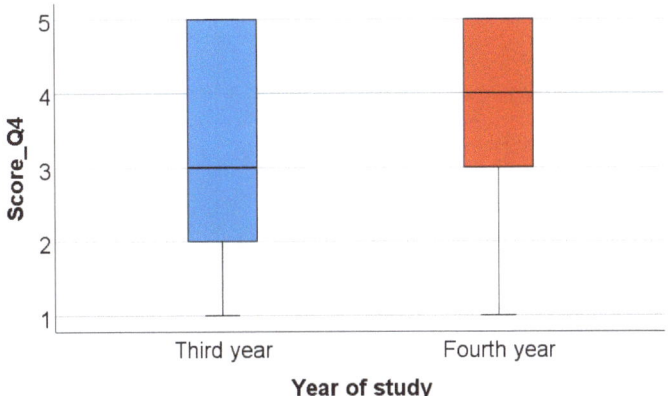

Figure 14. Comparison of Score_Q4 between academic years of study.

Data from Table 8 show the correlation between Score_Q4 and Score_Q11. Both scores have a non-parametric distribution according to the Shapiro–Wilk Test ($p < 0.001$). The correlation observed is statistically significant and positive with a weak power ($p < 0.001$, $R = 0.242$), indicating that students who chose more functions for modular digital dental models also chose more functions for 3D-printed dental models.

Table 8. Correlation between Score_Q4 and Score_Q11.

Correlation	p *
Score_Q4 ($p < 0.001$ **) × Score_Q11 ($p < 0.001$ **)	<0.001, R = 0.242

* Spearman's rho Correlation Coefficient, ** Shapiro–Wilk Test.

4. Discussion

Digital technology is already advanced in the medical domain, and has an extraordinary pace of and potential for development [36,37]. As regards the educational area in dentistry, new digital means for theoretical teaching and practical training have appeared in recent years, as well as various modalities for virtually interacting with students or testing their abilities.

Based on the digitization of standard dental models, of artificial intact teeth, and of artificial prepared teeth for diverse types of prosthetic restorations, the virtual method presented in this paper allows the following: simulation of any possible partial edentulism scenario; digital identification of diverse classes of partial edentulism; occlusal examination; establishment of appropriate prosthetic treatment plans for different virtual clinical situations; and selection of the proper dental preparation and fixed dental prosthesis. In light of the published literature, as other authors have also shown, this type of digital training improves students' 3D visualization skills while enabling them to better understand and assimilate the required didactic information [22,38–40]. The virtual partial edentulism cases that can be designed by this method correspond to clinical situations that a dentist encounters in daily practice. Furthermore, based on the designed modular digital model, dental educators can add details inspired from real clinical cases to their interactive discussions with their students, including anatomical variations or ectopic dental positions. Nevertheless, this method also allows the creation of modular digital models based on real clinical cases. The digital library created by the digitalization of standard dental models and of real clinical cases allows virtual simulations of any possible partial edentulism scenario; in our opinion, this enables us to enrich our faculty's own digital library, which could be of great benefit to our students. The proposed method also allows the 3D printing of dental simulated models, which have already proved their usefulness in undergraduate students' pre-clinical practical training, as other scientific studies have pointed out [18,30–33,41–44]. Certain authors have suggested that 3D-printed dental models represent a "more realistic and cost-efficient alternative to commercial models" in undergraduate dental training [42]. Our presented method is, indeed, software-based and available to all licensed users; however, to our understanding, this method could be regarded as being accessible, convenient and user friendly. Moreover, in our study, the 3D-printed simulated dental models were manufactured in our university, using our own internal resources, which leads to reduced fabrication costs.

Regarding the use of the proposed modular digital dental models, the possibility to constantly and rapidly vary the clinical scenarios but also to return to certain elements of interest at any time could result in the enhancement of students' ability to promptly identify classes of partial edentulism, establish diagnoses and fixed or removable prosthetic treatment plans, and observe the succession of therapeutic stages, as other authors also stated in their studies [22,45]. As a result, students may be stimulated to elaborate several 3D virtual treatment plans for the same clinical situation, previsualize (repeatedly, if needed) these therapeutic alternatives and acknowledge the pros and cons of each possible solution. Other recent studies [46,47], whose observations support the method we put forward in our study, confirm students' appreciation for e-learning or virtual teaching; the authors stated that e-learning offers easy access to the shared materials and feasibility, which help students better understand complex clinical cases or theoretical subjects. Mladenovic et al. [48] also reported that students appreciate the flexibility of a suggested mobile application for the dynamic study of dental traumatology. The digital method proposed in this paper also enables the computerized analysis of the discrete differences between various types of dental preparations: the unique details of each preparation can be 3D- and computer-visualized. Goodacre [40] reports that, thanks to the 3D education in dentistry, students manage to enhance their ability to visualize diverse structures three dimensionally and operate them in their minds ("spatial ability"). Other studies state, in the light of the results obtained, the necessity of virtual instruments for controlling the dental preparations achieved by the students [22,49,50]. As other authors have mentioned, students can assimilate, by means of this digital training, the notions that are important for an adequate presentation of the treatment plan to future patients, and thus improve their communication and relational skills, aspects that other authors refer to as well [21,51].

On the other hand, the idea of combining 3D virtual models with 3D-printed dental models in university dental education is also suggested by other authors [44] in order to ease visual recognition and understanding of teeth preparation. In our study, the possibility to 3D-print the dental models on the basis of the designed digital modular models obtained via the suggested method opens up new directions for applicability in dental education. The obtained 3D-printed simulation models are hence designated for hands-on training (tooth preparation for fixed prosthetic restorations or fillings, impressions, wax-up procedures, provisional restorations, evaluation and cementation of fixed prosthetic restorations) or for exercising other specific practical techniques. We have noticed that the possibility to constantly and rapidly return to certain elements of interest in the digital models allowed our students to manage the procedures they performed on the 3D-printed models. These 3D-printed dental models are also useful for additional analysis of the elements specific to edentulism cases or for establishing treatment plans and the succession of the treatment stages in dental prosthetics, occlusology and in other specialties (implantology, maxillofacial prosthodontics, orthodontics) [11,52–55]. Scientific studies found in the specialized literature reveal the contribution that teaching methods applying 3D-printed models have in dental education, as follows. Lambrecht (2010) [56] achieved 3D-printed training models for implantology surgery, which were fabricated on the basis of real patients' CBCT. Soares (2013) [44] created virtual models and prototypes of teeth with various cavity preparations. Kroger (2017) [57] obtained 3D-printed models by digitally scanning real patients. Hohne (2019) [58,59] created models in which the enamel and dentine can be discerned as well as 3D-printed models with caries (both studies were evaluated and validated using questionnaires filled in by students). Boonsiriphant (2019) [60] printed models with ideal preparations of teeth and reported high advantages in students' achieving practical abilities thanks to real 3D visualization in contrast to 2D images in books or courses. Werz (2018) [61] and Hanish (2020) [62] obtained printed models for exercising surgery techniques (sinus lift, extraction of wisdom teeth, apical resection). Lee (2015) [63] demonstrated that printing technology can also be useful in orthodontics, while Marty (2018) [64] presented a comparison between students' perception on 3D-printed models based on real cases and their perception on standard models, in pedodontics.

Furthermore, the responses collected from the survey of third- and fourth-year dental students in our faculty indicate that the proposed method (the combined use of modular digital and 3D-printed dental models in university dental training) received good feedback from the participants in the survey. The findings of our survey were consistent with those of other studies found in the dental literature [65–70]. However, to our knowledge, few scientific studies have been dedicated to topics related to the influence of students' age or academic year on their perception of the use of digital dentistry and technological advancement such as 3D-printing in dental education. Certain aspects were revealed through the statistical analysis that was performed in our study; for example, the opinion of the students participating in the study is different depending on their age: students who selected the item indicating that "modular digital dental models are considered a quick way to learn" had a significantly lower age than students who did not select this item ($p = 0.034$). When compared to younger students, older students were more interested in academic, teaching aspects, valuing the fact that modular digital dental models allow the evaluation of the method's effectiveness ($p = 0.008$) (number of registered downloads) and that 3D-printed dental models allow direct interaction between students and teachers ($p = 0.022$). Significant differences were registered between the students' responses to the applied questionnaire, depending on their academic year of study. Thus, when comparing the fourth-year students to the third-year students, the latter responded more frequently that modular digital dental models are a quick way to learn ($p = 0.008$) and fit their way of learning ($p = 0.039$), and that the 3D-printed dental models allow them to learn quicker ($p = 0.018$). On the other hand, fourth-year students showed greater concerns towards exploring detailed anatomical elements: fourth-year students selected more frequently the items indicating that modular digital dental models allow realistic simulation of various classes of partial edentulism ($p = 0.048$), of alveolar ridge resorption ($p = 0.044$) and of malpositioned teeth or destruction of dental crowns ($p = 0.030$). Moreover, fourth-year students selected significantly more functions for modular digital dental models than third-year students; students who chose more functions for modular digital dental models also chose more functions for 3D-printed dental models ($p < 0.001$). To our understanding, the older fourth-year students are able to better discern the value of the proposed modular digital and 3D-printed dental models because they have greater practical experience and higher theoretical knowledge. Even though the fourth-year students partake in various clinical training sessions, they have expressed their willingness to continue using the modular digital and 3D-printed dental models in their university education.

Although we registered certain relevant differences in students' perception of the use of the advanced method, depending on their age and academic year of study, it is worth noting that the performed statistical analysis confirms that there is a coherent pattern in students' answers. For example, the questionnaire's items corresponding to the modular digital models were answered similarly to those corresponding to the 3D-printed models; students gave balanced answers to the questions regarding the advantages and the usage of these two types of dental models. We can consequently conclude that the students participating in this study appreciated the value of both modular digital and 3D-printed dental models in a similar manner.

The survey represents an important tool which could contribute to the improvement of students' training activity, especially when modern, recent innovations such as CAD/CAM technology or digital dentistry are introduced in a curriculum. Moreover, we consider that our study lines up with the idea of sustainability in university dental education which has been at the center of recent scientific studies [70–73]. In addition, other studies pointed out that, in the context of the recent COVID-19 pandemic evolution [74–78], hybrid teaching and educational platforms have proved to be very useful; these issues back up our proposed method.

As other authors have already pointed out [65,79] it is debatable whether digital learning methods improve dental students' skills. Despite the noticeable, evident enthusiasm of the undergraduate dental students toward digital technology that was highlighted in this paper, structured self-learning and self-evaluation of students represent important issues for further development of dental curricula, as other authors have indicated [68]. On the other hand, implementation of dental technology in university dental education could face diverse barriers such as limited resources, funds, time and availability of teaching staff [67]. Therefore, as regards the limits of the advanced digital method, it is worth noting that it requires technological resources and certain digital skills for the students. Additionally, the hardness and the color of the printed resin that we used to obtain the 3D-printed dental models is different from that of natural teeth, as the students also noticed; in this context, the properties of different resin materials used in manufacturing the 3D-printed dental models will be a subject of our further research. Another limitation of our paper is the fact that the questionnaire was conducted at a single dental school and in a single department (Prosthodontics); therefore, its results may not be extended to students in other programs or to other dental specialties. Moreover, the results of the applied questionnaires are based on perceived experiences and not on objective evaluations; we thus consider that the development of students' competence, skills and self-assessment should be investigated from more of an objective standpoint in future studies.

Nevertheless, our study, along with other recent ones [18,40,74,80,81], further stimulates interest in developing scientific research in the area of digital dentistry education and also in investing in technological innovations [37,82–84], in order to provide the proper, sustainable education to the next generations of dentists.

5. Conclusions

1. The present paper advances an alternative digital proposal dedicated to dental education of students in the domain of prosthodontics, allowing the creation digital modular dental models corresponding to various clinical situations of partial edentulism and to subsequently obtain 3D-printed dental models that can be used for students' practical training. The suggested method stimulates students to project, create, previsualize and interact with modular didactic digital models and to perform repeated virtual simulation of any possible partial edentulism scenario; on the other hand, the 3D-printed models offer the possibility to enhance students' practical skills.
2. As we registered positive feedback from students participating in the survey, the proposed method could offer students at the pre-clinical stage of their education the opportunity to train and prepare themselves better for their future clinical activities.
3. The proposed method could pave the way for various practical training applications in dental education, fostering its sustainability and encouraging interdisciplinary collaboration.

Author Contributions: Conceptualization, A.E.P. and M.P.; methodology, A.E.P. and S.M.P.; software, A.E.P. and E.M.L.; validation, M.I., A.M.C.Ț., A.C.D. and S.M.P.; formal analysis, S.D.; investigation, S.D. and E.M.L.; resources, A.M.C.Ț. and E.M.L.; data curation, M.I. and A.C.D.; writing—original draft preparation, M.P. and S.D.; writing—review and editing, M.P.; visualization, M.I., A.M.C.Ț. and A.C.D. ; supervision, A.E.P. and S.M.P.; project administration, M.P. All authors have read and agreed to the published version of the manuscript.

Funding: This research received no external funding.

Institutional Review Board Statement: This study was conducted in accordance with the Declaration of Helsinki, and approved by the Scientific Research Ethics Committee of "Carol Davila" University of Medicine and Pharmacy, Bucharest, Romania (Project identification Code: PO-35-F-03; Protocol number:15596; date: 8 June 2022).

Informed Consent Statement: Informed consent was obtained from all subjects involved in the study. Informed consent was also obtained from the subjects involved in the study to publish this paper.

Data Availability Statement: The data that support the findings of this study are available from the corresponding authors upon request.

Acknowledgments: The authors gratefully acknowledge F.M. Medident—Institute for Dental Radiology, Bucharest, Romania; Center for Innovation and e-Health (CieH)—"Carol Davila" University of Medicine and Pharmacy, Bucharest, Romania; Laboratory for Digital Technologies in Dentistry—"Carol Davila" University of Medicine and Pharmacy, Bucharest, Romania; and Alex Pantea and Florina Popescu (who participated in the technical editing of the manuscript) for their support provided during this study.

Conflicts of Interest: The authors declare no conflict of interest.

References

1. Revilla-León, M.; Jiang, P.; Sadeghpour, M.; Piedra-Cascón, W.; Zandinejad, A.; Özcan, M.; Krishnamurthy, V.R. Intraoral digital scans—Part 1: Influence of ambient scanning light conditions on the accuracy (trueness and precision) of different intraoral scanners. *J. Prosthet. Dent.* **2020**, *124*, 372–378. [CrossRef] [PubMed]
2. Bandiaky, O.N.; Le Bars, P.; Gaudin, A.; Hardouin, J.B.; Cheraud-Carpentier, M.; Mbodj, E.B.; Soueidan, A. Comparative assessment of complete-coverage, fixed tooth-supported prostheses fabricated from digital scans or conventional impressions: A systematic review and meta-analysis. *J. Prosthet. Dent.* **2020**, *127*, 71–79. [CrossRef] [PubMed]
3. Winkler, J.; Gkantidis, N. Trueness and precision of intraoral scanners in the maxillary dental arch: An In Vivo analysis. *Sci. Rep.* **2020**, *10*, 1172. [CrossRef] [PubMed]
4. Nedelcu, R.; Olsson, P.; Nyström, I.; Rydén, J.; Thor, A. Accuracy and precision of 3 intraoral scanners and accuracy of conventional impressions: A novel in vivo analysis method. *J. Dent.* **2018**, *69*, 110–118. [CrossRef] [PubMed]
5. Bosniac, P.; Rehmann, P.; Wöstmann, B. Comparison of an indirect impression scanning system and two direct intraoral scanning systems In Vivo. *Clin. Oral. Investig.* **2018**, *23*, 2421–2427. [CrossRef]
6. Javaid, M.; Haleem, A. Current status and applications of additive manufacturing in dentistry: A literature-based review. *J. Oral Biol. Craniofacial Res.* **2019**, *9*, 179–185. [CrossRef] [PubMed]
7. Ligon, S.C.; Liska, R.; Stampfl, J.; Gurr, M.; Mülhaupt, R. Polymers for 3D-printing and Customized Additive Manufacturing. *Chem. Rev.* **2017**, *117*, 10212–10290. [CrossRef]
8. Jockusch, J.; Özcan, M. Additive manufacturing of dental polymers: An overview on processes, materials and applications. *Dent. Mater. J.* **2020**, *39*, 345–354. [CrossRef]
9. Nassani, M.; Ibraheem, S.; Shamsy, E.; Darwish, M.; Faden, A.; Kujan, O. A Survey of Dentists' Perception of Chair-Side CAD/CAM Technology. *Healthcare* **2021**, *9*, 68. [CrossRef]
10. Tahayeri, A.; Morgan, M.; Fugolin, A.P.; Bompolaki, D.; Athirasala, A.; Pfeifer, C.S.; Ferracane, J.L.; Bertassoni, L.E. 3D-printed versus conventionally cured provisional crown and bridge dental materials. *Dent. Mater.* **2018**, *34*, 192–200. [CrossRef]
11. Revilla-León, M.; Meyers, M.J.; Zandinejad, A.; Özcan, M. A review on chemical composition, mechanical properties, and manufacturing work flow of additively manufactured current polymers for interim dental restorations. *J. Esthet. Restor. Dent.* **2019**, *31*, 51–57. [CrossRef] [PubMed]
12. Pituru, S.M.; Greabu, M.; Totan, A.; Imre, M.; Pantea, M.; Spinu, T.; Tancu, A.M.C.; Popoviciu, N.O.; Stanescu, I.-I.; Ionescu, E. A Review on the Biocompatibility of PMMA-Based Dental Materials for Interim Prosthetic Restorations with a Glimpse into Their Modern Manufacturing Techniques. *Materials* **2020**, *13*, 2894. [CrossRef] [PubMed]
13. Joda, T.; Bornstein, M.M.; Jung, R.E.; Ferrari, M.; Waltimo, T.; Zitzmann, N.U. Recent trends and future direction of dental research in the digital era. *Int. J. Environ. Res. Public Health* **2020**, *17*, 1987. [CrossRef] [PubMed]
14. Schwendicke, F.; Samek, W.; Krois, J. Artificial intelligence in dentistry: Chances and challenges. *J. Dent. Res.* **2020**, *99*, 769–774. [CrossRef] [PubMed]

15. Ho, D.; Quake, S.R.; McCabe, E.R.; Chng, W.J.; Chow, E.K.; Ding, X.; Gelb, B.D.; Ginsburg, G.S.; Hassenstab, J.; Ho, C.-M.; et al. Enabling Technologies for Personalized and Precision Medicine. *Trends Biotechnol.* **2020**, *38*, 497–518. [CrossRef] [PubMed]
16. Grischke, J.; Johannsmeier, L.; Eich, L.; Griga, L.; Haddadin, S. Dentronics: Towards robotics and artificial intelligence in dentistry. *Dent. Mater.* **2020**, *36*, 765–778. [CrossRef]
17. Neville, P.; van der Zande, M.M. Dentistry, E-health and digitalisation: A critical narrative review of the dental literature on digital technologies with insights from health and technology studies. *Community Dent. Health J.* **2020**, *37*, 51–58. [CrossRef]
18. Barour, S.; Richert, R.; Virard, F.; Wulfman, C.; Iozzino, R.; Elbashti, M.; Naveau, A.; Ducret, M. Immersive 3D Educational Contents: A Technical Note for Dental Educators. *Healthcare* **2021**, *9*, 178. [CrossRef]
19. Wulfman, C.; Bonnet, G.; Carayon, D.; Lance, C.; Fages, M.; Vivard, F.; Daas, M.; Rignon-Bret, C.; Naveau, A.; Millet, C.; et al. Digital removable complete denture: A narrative review. *Fr. J. Dent. Med.* **2020**, *10*, 1–9.
20. Rekow, E.D. Digital Dentistry: The New State of the Art—Is It Disruptive or Destructive? *Dent. Mater.* **2020**, *36*, 9–24. [CrossRef]
21. Kato, A.; Ziegler, A.; Utsumi, M.; Ohno, K.; Takeichi, T. Three-dimensional imaging of internal tooth structures: Applications in dental education. *J. Oral Biosci.* **2016**, *58*, 100–111. [CrossRef]
22. Schepke, U.; Palthe, M.E.V.W.; Meisberger, E.W.; Kerdijk, W.; Cune, M.S.; Blok, B. Digital assessment of a retentive full crown preparation—An evaluation of prepCheck in an undergraduate pre-clinical teaching environment. *Eur. J. Dent. Educ.* **2020**, *24*, 407–424. [CrossRef] [PubMed]
23. Bonnet, G.; Lance, C.; Bessadet, M.; Tamini, F.; Veyrune, J.-L.; Francois, O.; Nicolas, E. Teaching removable partial denture design: 'METACIEL', a novel digital procedure. *Int. J. Med. Educ.* **2018**, *9*, 24–25. [CrossRef] [PubMed]
24. De Boer, I.R.; Wesselink, P.R.; Vervoorn, J.M. The creation of virtual teeth with and without tooth pathology for a virtual learning environment in dental education. *Eur. J. Dent. Educ.* **2013**, *17*, 191–197. [CrossRef] [PubMed]
25. De Boer, I.R.; Wesselink, P.R.; Vervoorn, J.M. Student performance and appreciation using 3D vs. 2D vision in a virtual learning environment. *Eur. J. Dent. Educ.* **2015**, *20*, 142–147. [CrossRef] [PubMed]
26. Güth, J.F.; Ponn, A.; Mast, G.; Gernet, W.; Edelhoff, D. Description and evaluation of a new approach on pre-clinical implant dentistry education based on an innovative simulation model. *Eur. J. Dent. Educ.* **2010**, *14*, 221–226. [CrossRef] [PubMed]
27. Dixon, J.; Towers, A.; Martin, N.; Field, J. Re-defining the virtual reality dental simulator: Demonstrating concurrent validity of clinically relevant assessment and feedback. *Eur. J. Dent. Educ.* **2021**, *25*, 108–116. [CrossRef]
28. Towers, A.; Field, J.; Stokes, C.; Maddock, S.; Martin, N. A scoping review of the use and application of virtual reality in pre-clinical dental education. *Br. Dent. J.* **2019**, *226*, 358–366. [CrossRef]
29. Nassar, H.M.; Tekian, A. Computer simulation and virtual reality in undergraduate operative and restorative dental education: A critical review. *J. Dent. Educ.* **2020**, *84*, 812–829. [CrossRef]
30. Sajdłowski, D.; Świątkowski, W.; Rahnama, M. Dental Education in COVID-19 Pandemic. *World J. Surg. Res.* **2021**, *4*, 1283.
31. Jalali, P.; Glickman, G.N.; Umorin, M. Do didactics improve clinical skills: A retrospective educational study. *Saudi Endod. J.* **2021**, *11*, 31.
32. Sjöström, M.; Brundin, M. The Effect of Extra Educational Elements on the Confidence of Undergraduate Dental Students Learning to Administer Local Anaesthesia. *Dent. J.* **2021**, *9*, 77. [CrossRef]
33. McGleenon, E.L.; Morison, S. Preparing dental students for independent practice: A scoping review of methods and trends in undergraduate clinical skills teaching in the UK and Ireland. *Br. Dent. J.* **2021**, *230*, 39–45. [CrossRef] [PubMed]
34. Savoldi, F.; Yeung, A.W.K.; Tanaka, R.; Zadeh, L.S.M.; Montalvao, C.; Bornstein, M.M.; Tsoi, J.K.H. Dry skulls and cone beam computed tomography (CBCT) for teaching orofacial bone anatomy to undergraduate dental students. *Anat. Sci. Educ.* **2021**, *14*, 62–70. [CrossRef] [PubMed]
35. Shaikh, S.; Nahar, P.; Shaikh, S.; Sayed, A.J.; Habibullah, M.A. Current perspectives of 3D-printing in dental applications. *Braz. Dent. Sci.* **2021**, *24*, 2481. [CrossRef]
36. Coro-Montanet, G.; Monedero, M.J.P.; Ituarte, J.S.; Calvo, A.d.l.H. Train Strategies for Haptic and 3D Simulators to Improve the Learning Process in Dentistry Students. *Int. J. Environ. Res. Public Health* **2022**, *19*, 4081. [CrossRef]
37. Murbay, S.; Neelakantan, P.; Chang, J.W.W.; Yeung, S. Evaluation of the introduction of a dental virtual simulator on the performance of undergraduate dental students in the pre-clinical operative dentistry course. *Eur. J. Dent. Educ.* **2020**, *24*, 5–16. [CrossRef]
38. Zitzmann, N.U.; Matthisson, L.; Ohla, H.; Joda, T. Digital undergraduate education in dentistry: A systematic review. *Int. J. Environ. Res. Public Health* **2020**, *17*, 3269. [CrossRef]
39. Mahrous, A.; Schneider, G.B.; Holloway, J.A.; Dawson, D.V. Enhancing student learning in removable partial denture design by using virtual three-dimensional models versus traditional two-dimensional drawings: A comparative study. *J. Prosthodont.* **2019**, *28*, 927–933. [CrossRef]
40. Goodacre, C.J. Digital Learning Resources for Prosthodontic Education: The Perspectives of a Long-Term Dental Educator Regarding 4 Key Factors. *J. Prosthodont.* **2018**, *27*, 791–797. [CrossRef]
41. Ferro, A.S.; Nicholson, K.; Koka, S. Innovative Trends in Implant Dentistry Training and Education: A Narrative Review. *J. Clin. Med.* **2019**, *8*, 1618. [CrossRef] [PubMed]
42. Richter, M.; Peter, T.; Rüttermann, S.; Sader, R.; Seifert, L.B. 3D printed versus commercial models in undergraduate conservative dentistry training. *Eur. J. Dent. Educ.* **2022**, *26*, 643–651. [CrossRef] [PubMed]

43. Zaharia, C.; Gabor, A.G.; Gavrilovici, A.; Stan, A.T.; Idorasi, L.; Sinescu, C.; Negruțiu, M.L. Digital dentistry-3D printing applications. *J. Interdiscip. Med.* **2017**, *2*, 50–53. [CrossRef]
44. Soares, P.V.; Milito, G.d.A.; Pereira, F.A.; Reis, B.R.; Soares, C.; Menezes, M.D.S.; Santos-Filho, P.C.D.F. Rapid prototyping and 3D-virtual models for operative dentistry education in Brazil. *J. Dent. Educ.* **2013**, *77*, 358–363. [CrossRef]
45. Terry, A.; Liu, D.; Divnic-Resnik, T. The impact of an electronic guide on students' self-directed learning in simulation clinic. *Eur. J. Dent. Educ.* **2021**, *25*, 86–99. [CrossRef] [PubMed]
46. Schlenz, M.A.; Schmidt, A.; Wöstmann, B.; Krämer, N.; Schulz-Weidner, N. Students' and lecturers' perspective on the implementation of online learning in dental education due to SARS-CoV-2 (COVID-19): A cross-sectional study. *BMC Med. Educ.* **2020**, *20*, 354. [CrossRef]
47. Shrivastava, K.J.; Nahar, R.; Parlani, S.; Murthy, V.J. A cross-sectional virtual survey to evaluate the outcome of online dental education system among undergraduate dental students across India amid COVID-19 pandemic. *Eur. J. Dent. Educ.* **2021**, *26*, 123–130. [CrossRef]
48. Mladenovic, R.; Bukumiric, Z.; Mladenovic, K. Influence of a dedicated mobile application on studying traumatic dental injuries during student isolation. *J. Dent. Educ.* **2020**, *85*, 1131–1133. [CrossRef]
49. Tang, L.; Cao, Y.; Liu, Z.; Qian, K.; Liu, Y.; Liu, Y.; Zhou, Y. Improving the quality of preclinical simulation training for dental students using a new digital real-time evaluation system. *Eur. J. Dent. Educ.* **2021**, *25*, 100–107. [CrossRef]
50. Mino, T.; Kurosaki, Y.; Tokumoto, K.; Higuchi, T.; Nakanoda, S.; Numoto, K.; Tosa, I.; Kimura-Ono, A.; Maekawa, K.; Kim, T.H.; et al. Rating criteria to evaluate student performance in digital wax-up training using multi-purpose software. *J. Adv. Prosthodont.* **2022**, *14*, 203–211. [CrossRef]
51. Lee, B.; Kim, J.; Shin, S.; Kim, J.; Park, J.; Kim, K.; Kim, S.; Shim, J. Dental students' perceptions on a simulated practice using patient-based customised typodonts during the transition from preclinical to clinical education. *Eur. J. Dent. Educ.* **2022**, *26*, 55–65. [CrossRef] [PubMed]
52. Garcia, J.; Yang, Z.; Mongrain, R.; Leask, R.L.; Lachapelle, K. 3D-printing materials and their use in medical education: A review of current technology and trends for the future. *BMJ Simul. Technol. Enhanc. Learn.* **2018**, *4*, 27–40. [CrossRef]
53. Wang, Y.; Xu, Z.; Wu, D.; Bai, J. Current status and prospects of polymer powder 3D-printing technologies. *Materials* **2020**, *13*, 2406. [CrossRef] [PubMed]
54. Revilla-León, M.; Sadeghpour, M.; Özcan, M. An update on applications of 3D-printing technologies used for processing polymers used in implant dentistry. *Odontology* **2020**, *108*, 331–338. [CrossRef] [PubMed]
55. Özcan, M.; Hotza, D.; Fredel, M.; Cruz, A.; Volpato, C. Materials and Manufacturing Techniques for Polymeric and Ceramic Scaffolds Used in Implant Dentistry. *J. Compos. Sci.* **2021**, *5*, 78. [CrossRef]
56. Lambrecht, J.; Berndt, D.; Christensen, A.; Zehnder, M. Haptic model fabrication for undergraduate and postgraduate teaching. *Int. J. Oral. Maxillofac. Surg.* **2010**, *39*, 1226–1229. [CrossRef]
57. Kröger, E.; Dekiff, M.; Dirksen, D. 3D-printed simulation models based on real patient situations for hands-on practice. *Eur. J. Dent. Educ.* **2017**, *21*, e119–e125. [CrossRef] [PubMed]
58. Höhne, C.; Schwarzbauer, R.; Schmitter, M. 3D-printed teeth with enamel and dentin layer for educating dental students in crown preparation. *J. Dent. Educ* **2019**, *83*, 1457–1463. [CrossRef] [PubMed]
59. Höhne, C.; Schmitter, M. 3D-printed Teeth for the Preclinical Education of Dental Students. *J. Dent. Educ.* **2019**, *83*, 1100–1106. [CrossRef]
60. Boonsiriphant, P.; Al-Salihi, Z.; Holloway, J.A.; Schneider, G.B. The use of 3D-printed tooth preparation to assist in teaching and learning in preclinical fixed prosthodontics courses. *J. Prosthod.* **2019**, *28*, e545–e547. [CrossRef]
61. Werz, S.M.; Zeichner, S.J.; Berg, B.-I.; Zeilhofer, H.-F.; Thieringer, F. 3D-printed surgical simulation models as educational tool by maxillofacial surgeons. *Eur. J. Dent. Educ.* **2018**, *22*, e500–e505. [CrossRef] [PubMed]
62. Hanisch, M.; Kroeger, E.; Dekiff, M.; Timme, M.; Kleinheinz, J.; Dirksen, D. 3D-printed Surgical Training Model Based on Real Patient Situations for Dental Education. *Int. J. Environ. Res. Public Health* **2020**, *17*, 2901. [CrossRef] [PubMed]
63. Lee, K.-Y.; Cho, J.-W.; Chang, N.-Y.; Chae, J.-M.; Kang, K.-H.; Kim, S.-C.; Cho, J.-H. Accuracy of three-dimensional printing for manufacturing replica teeth. *Korean J. Orthod.* **2015**, *45*, 217–225. [CrossRef] [PubMed]
64. Marty, M.; Broutin, A.; Vergnes, J.-N.; Vaysse, F. Comparison of student's perceptions between 3D-printed models versus series models in paediatric dentistry hands-on session. *Eur. J. Dent. Educ.* **2019**, *23*, 68–72. [CrossRef] [PubMed]
65. Schlenz, M.A.; Michel, K.; Wegner, K.; Schmidt, A.; Rehmann, P.; Wostmann, B. Undergraduate dental students' perspective on the implementation of digital dentistry in the preclinical curriculum: A questionnaire survey. *BMC Oral. Health* **2020**, *20*, 78. [CrossRef] [PubMed]
66. Kim, Y.; Kim, J.; Jeong, Y.; Yun, M.; Lee, H. Comparison of digital and conventional assessment methods for a single tooth preparation and educational satisfaction. *Eur. J. Dent. Educ.* **2022**, 1–9. [CrossRef]
67. Ishida, Y.; Kuwajima, Y.; Kobayashi, T.; Yonezawa, Y.; Asack, D.; Nagai, M.; Kondo, H.; Ishikawa-Nagai, S.; Da Silva, J.; Lee, S.J. Current Implementation of Digital Dentistry for Removable Prosthodontics in US Dental Schools. *Int. J. Dent.* **2022**, *2022*, 7331185. [CrossRef] [PubMed]
68. Sharab, L.; Adel, M.; Abualsoud, R.; Hall, B.; Albaree, S.; de Leeuw, R.; Kutkut, A. Perception, awareness, and attitude toward digital dentistry among pre-dental students: An observational survey. *Bull. Natl. Res. Cent.* **2022**, *46*, 246. [CrossRef]

69. Zotti, F.; Cominziolli, A.; Pappalardo, D.; Rosolin, L.; Bertossi, D.; Zerman, N. Proposal for Introducing a Digital Aesthetic Dentistry Course in Undergraduate Program: Contents and Ways of Administration. *Educ. Sci.* **2022**, *12*, 441. [CrossRef]
70. Turkyilmaz, I.; Hariri, N.H.; Jahangiri, L. Student's perception of the impact of e-learning on dental education. *J. Contemp. Dent. Pract.* **2019**, *20*, 616–621. [CrossRef]
71. Duane, B.; Dixon, J.; Ambibola, G.; Aldana, C.; Couglan, J.; Henao, D.; Daniela, T.; Veiga, N.; Martin, N.; Darragh, J.; et al. Embedding environmental sustainability within the modern dental curriculum—Exploring current practice and developing a shared understanding. *Eur. J. Dent. Educ.* **2021**, *25*, 541–549. [CrossRef]
72. Cocârță, D.; Prodana, M.; Demetrescu, I.; Lungu, P.; Didilescu, A. Indoor Air Pollution with Fine Particles and Implications for Workers' Health in Dental Offices: A Brief Review. *Sustainability* **2021**, *13*, 599. [CrossRef]
73. Joury, E.; Lee, J.; Parchure, A.; Mortimer, F.; Park, S.; Pine, C.; Ramasubbu, D.; Hillman, L. Exploring environmental sustainability in UK and US dental curricula and related barriers and enablers: A cross-sectional survey in two dental schools. *Br. Dent. J.* **2021**, *230*, 605–610. [CrossRef]
74. Varvara, G.; Bernardi, S.; Bianchi, S.; Sinjari, B.; Piattelli, M. Dental education challenges during the COVID-19 pandemic period in Italy: Undergraduate student feedback, future perspectives, and the needs of teaching strategies for professional development. *Healthcare* **2021**, *9*, 454. [CrossRef] [PubMed]
75. Chang, T.-Y.; Hong, G.; Paganelli, C.; Phantumvanit, P.; Chang, W.-J.; Shieh, Y.-S.; Hsu, M.-L. Innovation of dental education during COVID-19 pandemic. *J. Dent. Sci.* **2021**, *16*, 15–20. [CrossRef] [PubMed]
76. Kui, A.; Jiglau, A.L.; Chisnoiu, A.; Negucioiu, M.; Balhuc, S.; Constantiniuc, M.; Buduru, S. A survey on dental students' perception regarding online learning during COVID-19 pandemic. *Med. Pharm. Rep.* **2022**, *95*, 203–208. [CrossRef]
77. Poudevigne, M.; Armstrong, E.S.; Mickey, M.; Nelson, M.A.; Obi, C.N.; Scott, A.; Thomas, N.; Thompson, T.N. What's in Your Culture? Embracing Stability and the New Digital Age in Moving Colleges of Health Professions Virtually during the COVID-19 Pandemic: An Experiential Narrative Review. *Educ. Sci.* **2022**, *12*, 137. [CrossRef]
78. Antoniadou, M.; Rahiotis, C.; Kakaboura, A. Sustainable Distance Online Educational Process for Dental Students during COVID-19 Pandemic. *Int. J. Environ. Res. Public Health* **2022**, *19*, 9470. [CrossRef] [PubMed]
79. Wolgin, M.; Grabowski, S.; Elhadad, S.; Frank, W.; Kielbassa, A.M. Comparison of a prepCheck-supported self-assessment concept with conventional faculty supervision in a pre-clinical simulation environment. *Eur. J. Dent. Educ.* **2018**, *22*, e522–e529. [CrossRef]
80. Iozzino, R.; Champin, P.-A.; Richert, R.; Bui, R.; Palombi, O.; Charlin, B.; Tamimi, F.; Ducret, M. Assessing decision-making in education of restorative and prosthetic dentistry: A pilot study. *Int. J. Prosthodont.* **2020**, *34*, 585–590. [CrossRef]
81. Höhne, C.; Jentzsch, A.; Schmitter, M. The "Painting by Numbers Method" for education of students in crown preparation. *Eur. J. Dent. Educ.* **2020**, *25*, 261–270. [CrossRef] [PubMed]
82. Monterubbianesi, R.; Tosco, V.; Vitiello, F.; Orilisi, G.; Fraccastoro, F.; Putignano, A.; Orsini, G. Augmented, Virtual and Mixed Reality in Dentistry: A Narrative Review on the Existing Platforms and Future Challenges. *Appl. Sci.* **2022**, *12*, 877. [CrossRef]
83. Moussa, R.; Alghazaly, A.; Althagafi, N.; Eshky, R.; Borzangy, S. Effectiveness of virtual reality and interactive simulators on dental education outcomes: Systematic review. *Eur. J. Dent.* **2022**, *16*, 14–31. [CrossRef]
84. Imran, E.; Adanir, N.; Khurshid, Z. Significance of Haptic and Virtual Reality Simulation (VRS) in the Dental Education: A Review of Literature. *Appl. Sci.* **2021**, *11*, 10196. [CrossRef]

Disclaimer/Publisher's Note: The statements, opinions and data contained in all publications are solely those of the individual author(s) and contributor(s) and not of MDPI and/or the editor(s). MDPI and/or the editor(s) disclaim responsibility for any injury to people or property resulting from any ideas, methods, instructions or products referred to in the content.

Article

Evaluation of the Sensitivity of Selected *Candida* Strains to Ozonated Water—An In Vitro Study

Anna Kuśka-Kiełbratowska [1,*], Rafał Wiench [1], Anna Mertas [2], Elżbieta Bobela [2], Maksymilian Kiełbratowski [3], Monika Lukomska-Szymanska [4], Marta Tanasiewicz [5] and Dariusz Skaba [1]

[1] Department of Periodontal Diseases and Oral Mucosa Diseases, Faculty of Medical Sciences in Zabrze, Medical University of Silesia, 40-055 Katowice, Poland
[2] Chair and Department of Microbiology and Immunology, Faculty of Medical Sciences in Zabrze, Medical University of Silesia, 40-055 Katowice, Poland
[3] Conservative Dentistry and Endodontics Clinic, General Dentistry Clinic, Academic Centre of Dentistry, 41-902 Bytom, Poland
[4] Department of General Dentistry, Medical University of Lodz, 251 Pomorska St., 92-213 Lodz, Poland
[5] Chair and Department of Conservative Dentistry with Endodontics, Faculty of Medical Sciences in Zabrze, Medical University of Silesia, 40-055 Katowice, Poland
* Correspondence: anna.kuska@hotmail.com; Tel.: +48-663073488

Abstract: (1) *Background and Objectives:* Oral candidiasis has increased significantly in recent years. Increasingly, we encounter treatment difficulties related to drug resistance. Therefore, it is necessary to search for other therapies such as ozone therapy, which has antimicrobial activity. The aim of this study was to determine the sensitivity of selected *Candida* strains to ozonated water based on concentration and contact time (2) *Methods:* The sensitivity of *Candida* strains to ozonated water with a concentration of 5 µg/mL, 30 µg/mL, and 50 µg/mL was assessed using Mosmann's Tetrazolium Toxicity (MTT) assay. Statistical differences were assessed by the analysis of variance (ANOVA) and the Newman-Keuls post-hoc test. A *p*-value of ≤0.05 was considered to indicate a statistically significant difference. (3) *Results:* In all the strains and research trials, the number of viable cells was reduced by ozonated water. The reduction depended on the exposure time and concentration of ozonated water. The highest percentage reduction (34.98%) for the tested samples was obtained for the *C. albicans* strain after 120 s of exposure at the highest concentration-50 µg/mL. (4) *Conclusions:* The selected strains of *Candida* spp. were sensitive to ozonated water at all tested concentrations (5 µg/mL, 30 µg/mL, and 50 µg/mL). The sensitivity of strains to ozonated water increased with concentration and application time. Moreover, the sensitivity of *Candida* strains to ozonated water is comparable to that of 0.2% chlorhexidine gluconate.

Keywords: oral surgery; oral candidiasis; ozonated water; MTT; DMSO

1. Introduction

Candida fungi are part of the physiological saprophytic flora of the human oral cavity and are found in up to 25–65% of patients [1,2]. However, under certain conditions, namely disturbances of the balance and homeostasis of the organism or the incompetence of the host immune system, opportunistic infections and the development of candidiasis may occur. Due to the numerous and mutually overlapping risk factors for infection occurrence, the number of infections with *Candida* fungi has dramatically increased recently [3]. In clinical practice, doctors encounter increasingly huge difficulties in choosing the right pharmacological treatment because of reduced drug sensitivity or even complete resistance to fungi. Such a situation urged the search for new methods and substances with antifungal properties in order to supplement or even replace conventional therapy [4,5]. Alternative methods include essential oils (oregano, lemongrass, tea tree) [6–10], nano-metal colloidal solutions (silver, copper, gold) [11–13], antimicrobial photodynamic therapy (aPDT) (a type of light therapy that causes irreversible damage to target cells) [14–16], and ozone therapy (in various gaseous forms, water solutions, or ozonated oils) [17–20].

There are two forms of oxygen naturally occurring in the Earth's atmosphere: molecular oxygen (O_2), consisting of two oxygen atoms, and the allotropic form found in the stratosphere, ozone (O_3), consisting of three oxygen atoms. O_3 is a pale blue gas with a pungent, characteristic smell. It is heavier than air; therefore, as it moves from the higher layers of the atmosphere, it naturally cleans the air of pollutants. The solubility of ozone in water is 10-fold greater than that of diatomic oxygen, which decreases with increasing water temperature. The half-life of ozone in distilled water at room temperature is assumed to be approximately 30 min. It decomposes into a diatomic oxygen (O_2) and an active singlet oxygen ($^1O_2$) molecule, whose strong oxidizing properties (resulting from a high redox potential) make ozone one of the strongest oxidants among substances with a disinfecting effect; its redox potential is respectively 2.07 V for ozone, 1.76 V for hydrogen peroxide, and 1.45 V for chloric acid (I) [21,22]. As a result, ozone has a wide therapeutic window, and therefore gram-positive bacteria, gram-negative bacteria, viruses, fungi, and vegetative cells are susceptible to its effects [23,24]. Its antimicrobial action is based on damaging the cell wall and subsequent destruction of the lipids in the cell membrane, causing an increase in its permeability and breakdown. Oxidized radicals act on fungi of the genus *Candida* by destabilizing the cell membrane and damaging cytoplasmic organelles. They also interact with purine and pyrimidine bases, damaging the genetic material, disrupting enzyme systems, and leading to the destruction of the cell [24].

It is worth emphasizing that ozone has many applications in dentistry. For example, ozone can be used to disinfect carious cavities and the root canal system before the final filling, and due tits deep penetration into the dentinal tubules, ozone enables more thorough decontamination. Additionally, ozone can be applied to treat dentine hypersensitivity by opening dentinal tubules and enhancing the penetration of calcium or fluorine ions, ensuring their long-term retention [23,25]. Regular application of low doses of ozone, alone or in combination with conventional therapy, improves the treatment effectiveness of mucosal diseases (aphthous erosions, cold sores, oral mycosis, lichen planus, and angular cheilitis). Tissue microscopic studies have shown that ozone therapy reduces inflammation and swelling and is useful in wound healing in soft tissues [26–28]. Additionally, a similar mechanism of action can be expected in the course of treatment of oral candidiasis [29].

A common form of antiseptic or medication used in the oral cavity are rinses. Mouth rinsing is most often recommended in the time range from 30 s to 2 min.

This study took these rinse requirements into account.

Therefore, the aim of the present study was to assess the sensitivity of selected *Candida* strains to ozonated water based on concentration and contact time.

The null hypothesis to be tested is that the contact time and concentration of ozonated water do not influence the sensitivity of selected *Candida* strains.

2. Materials and Methods

2.1. Organisms and Growth Conditions

This research was carried out on reference strains of *Candida* fungi from the American Type Culture Collection (ATCC, Manassas, VA, USA): *Candida albicans* ATCC 10,231, *Candida glabrata* ATCC 2001, and *Candida krusei* ATCC 34,135. These represent the most common strains causing oral candidiasis [30]. These strains were selected due to their high frequency of occurrence in patients treated for oral mycosis. However, they often show great difficulties in treatment due to reduced sensitivity to antifungal drugs. The approval of the bioethics committee was not required due to the use of reference strains from the ATCC collection.

Cultures of each strain were placed separately onto Sabouraud dextrose agar plates from bioMerieux (Marcy-l'Étoile, France), which contain peptone (10.0 g/L) and agar (8.0 g/L), and incubated in atmospheric air at 37 °C. After 24 h of incubation, a sample of colonies was removed from the surface of the plate and suspended in sterile physiological solution (0.9% NaCl). The number of viable cells in used suspension was counted in a Densi-La-Meter II densitometer (ERBA LACHEMA, Prague, Czech Republic) using the optical density of McFarland = 5.0.

2.2. Ozone Water

Ozonated water in a concentration of 5 µg/mL, 30 µg/mL, and 50 µg/mL was used, obtained with the use of an ATO-3 ozone therapy device (Metrum CryoFlex, Blizne Łaszczyńskiego, Warsaw, Poland). Distilled water (400 mL) was ozonated for 7 min. according to the manufacturer's instructions. In order to preserve the properties of ozonated water, a new portion was prepared before each stage (due to the short half-life).

2.3. Chlorhexidine Digluconate

The 0.2% working solution was prepared immediately before the test by diluting a 2% aqueous solution of chlorhexidine digluconate (Cerkamed, Stalowa Wola, Poland) in water of pharmacopoeial purity. The choice of this substance is supported by studies showing its effectiveness against *Candida* spp. [26,31,32].

2.4. MTT Assay Protocol

The fungal cell viability was assessed using the MTT test. This is a quantitative study to determine the end product, formazan, which is formed by adding [3-(4,5-dimethyl-2-yl)-2,5-diphenyltetrazole] bromide (MTT reagent) from Sigma Chemical Company (St. Louis, MO, USA) to a fungus suspension previously treated with ozonated water. The MTT test assesses the activity of mitochondrial dehydrogenase, which is active only in living fungus cells. The amount of insoluble formazan formed is directly proportional to the number of viable cells. In order to dissolve the formazan crystals accumulating in the cells, it was necessary to use a solution of dimethylsulfoxide (DMSO) (Merck, Darmstadt, Germany). The concentration of the released dye was quantified in a universal microplate spectrophotometer at a wavelength of $\lambda = 550$ nm, comparing the values in the test samples to the control samples [33].

2.5. Experimental Groups and Inactivation of Candida spp. In Vitro

A total of 192 tests were prepared, 64 for each tested *Candida* strain. They were divided into the following groups: O_3, the experimental groups in which the working yeast suspensions were treated with ozonated water (5 µg/mL, 30 µg/mL, and 50 µg/mL), and two control groups. In the positive control, the yeast working suspensions were treated with 0.2% chlorhexidine digluconate (CHX), while in the negative one (K) the working suspensions were exposed neither to ozonated water nor chlorhexidine solution. The experiments were performed under uniform experimental conditions in 8 independent replications (n = 8). In each of the experimental and control groups, the effects of different ozonated water concentrations and their exposure times on the reduction of viable cells were assessed as follows: 200 µL of yeast working suspensions were added to the wells of a 96-well plate. The plates were then centrifuged (at 2000 rpm per 5 min, in Jouan, France) to separate the microbial pellet from the supernatant, which was then drained. A volume of 200 µL of ozonated water was added to the test wells with a sterile pipette for a duration of 30, 60, and 120 s, respectively. A positive control (CHX) was carried out according to the above-described scheme, replacing ozonated water with freshly prepared 0.2% chlorhexidine digluconate. In the case of the control group (K), ozonated water was replaced with liquid Sabouraud medium (Marcy-l'Étoile, France). After the specified time, ozonated water, chlorhexidine, and Sabouraud's liquid medium were removed, and 180 µL of bioMerieux Sabouraud liquid medium and 20 µL of MTT reagent were added to the wells. The plates with cells prepared in this way were incubated under aerobic conditions for 4 days at 37 °C. After this time, the samples were centrifuged (at 2000 rpm per 5 min, in Jouan, France), the supernatant was drained, and 200 µL of DMSO was added to the test cultures to extract insoluble formazan from the fungal cells. Then, 150 µL of the solution were collected and the absorbance was determined using an EonTM universal microplate spectrophotometer (BioTek Instruments, Winooski, USA) at a wavelength of $\lambda = 550$ nm. The color intensity of the test solution is proportional to the amount of formazan formed. Values of mitochondrial dehydrogenase activity determining the percentage of viable cells for the tested suspensions were calculated based on the following formula: cell viability = [AB/AK] × 100% (AB-absorbance of the experimental sample, AK-absorbance of the control sample).

2.6. Statistical Analysis

The results were presented in histograms as the mean of the cell viability ± standard deviation. Statistical analysis was performed with the use of Excel 2013 by Microsoft and Statistica v. 7.1 PL by StatSoft Poland (Poland, Cracow). The convergence of the results with the normal distribution was assessed with the Shapiro-Wilk test. Statistical differences were assessed by the analysis of variance (ANOVA) and the Newman-Keuls post-hoc test. A *p*-value of ≤0.05 was considered to indicate a statistically significant difference (Figure 1).

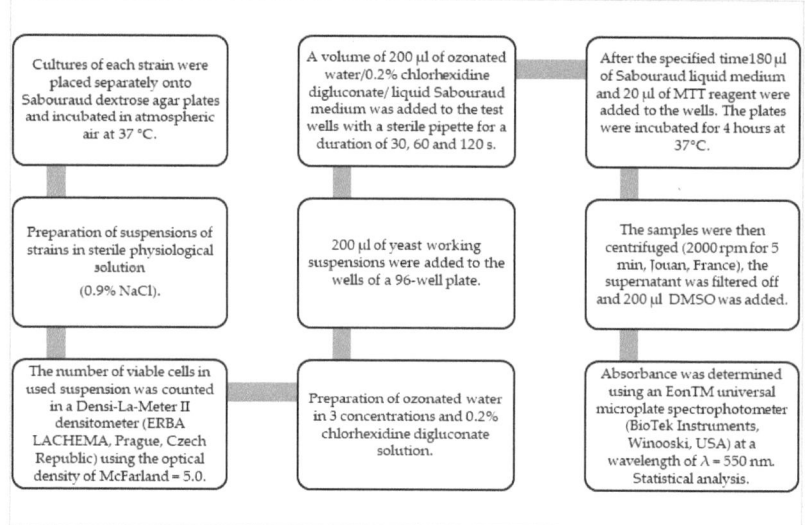

Figure 1. The study design.

3. Results

In the present study, the inhibitory effect of ozonated water at three concentrations (5 µg/mL, 30 µg/mL, and 50 µg/mL) on the viability of *Candida* spp. cells was assessed after 30, 60, and 120 s of incubation in experimental and control groups.

Figures 2–4 show the mean number of viable cells in percent and the standard deviation (M SD). In all strains, both in the test and the control groups (CHX), the number of live cells was reduced after exposure to ozonated water. The percentage reduction depended on the concentration of ozonated water and the time of exposure. The lowest viability for the test samples (50 µg/mL O_3) was observed for the strain *C. albicans* ATCC 10,231 and amounted to 34.98% (Figure 2). Subsequently, for *C. glabrata* ATCC 2001, it was 40.85% (Figure 3), and for *C. krusei* ATCC 34,135 it was 55,79% (Figure 4). The lowest viability for all strains was found for the longest exposure time in ozonated water in the highest concentration. In the entire experiment, the lowest cell viability was obtained for *C. albicans* ATCC 10,231, as a result of the action of 0.2% chlorhexidine, and was 28.07% (Figure 2). Figure 5 shows the influence of different exposure times for ozonated water at three concentrations on the cell viability of the investigated strains. The study used a *p*-value where * $p < 0.05$, ** $p < 0.01$, and *** $p < 0.001$. The lowest concentration of ozonated water was the most effective against the *C. glabrata* ATCC 2001 strain, after 60 s of exposure; the viability of the strain amounted to 69.92%. However, statistically significant differences for this concentration and different exposure times have not been demonstrated. The greatest reduction in cell viability in the shortest time of ozonated water application was demonstrated for the *C. glabrata* ATCC 2001 strain; the cell viability of this strain amounted up to 49.25%. For this time, differences between individual concentrations of ozonated water for the described strain were statistically significant in each comparison ($p < 0.001$). On the other hand, for the longest exposure time to ozonated water- 50 µg/mL O_3, the highest sensitivity was demonstrated for the strain *C. albicans* 10,231, where the cell viability was only 34.98%. The comparison between individual exposure times within this concentration of ozone water (50 µg/mL O_3) showed a positive correlation between contact time with the active substance and the survival rate of *C. albicans* cells. Differences in this concentration of ozonated water for the described strain between individual exposure times were statistically significant in each comparison ($p < 0.001$) In 0.2% aqueous chlorhexidine digluconate the lowest cell viability at 30, 60 and 120 s was recorded for *C. albicans* ATCC 10,231 strain. It amounted to 57.36% for the shortest time and 28.07% for the longest application time (Figure 6).

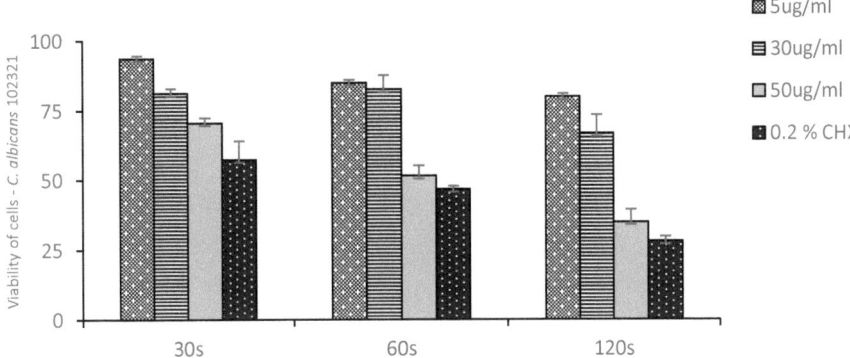

Figure 2. Viability of cells of *Candida albicans* ATCC 10,231 to ozonated water and chlorhexidine after three exposure times. n = 8 where n is the number of independent replications.

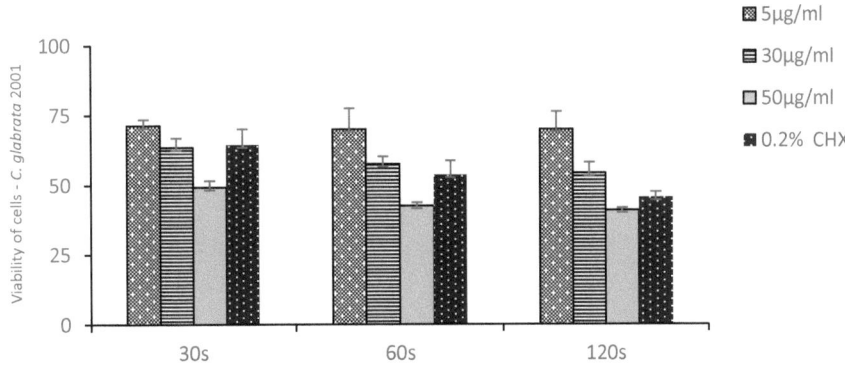

Figure 3. Viability of cells of *Candida glabrata* ATCC 2001 to ozonated water and chlorhexidine in three exposure times. n = 8.

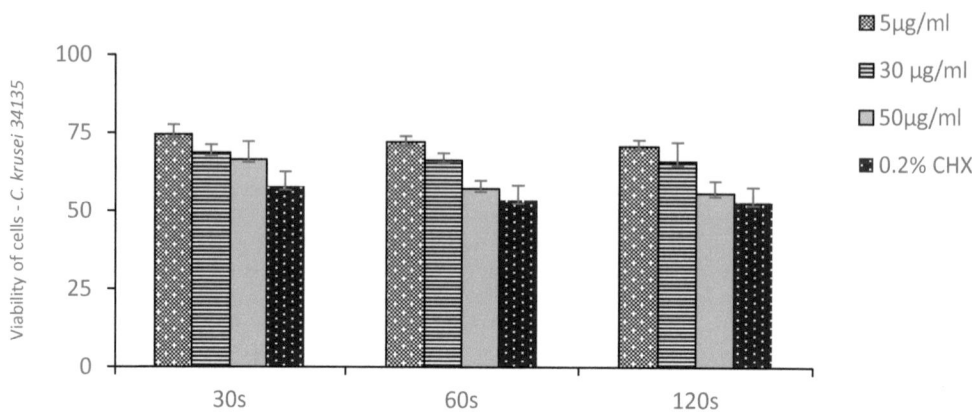

Figure 4. Viability of cells of *Candida krusei* ATCC 34,135 to ozonated water and chlorhexidine at three exposure times. n = 8.

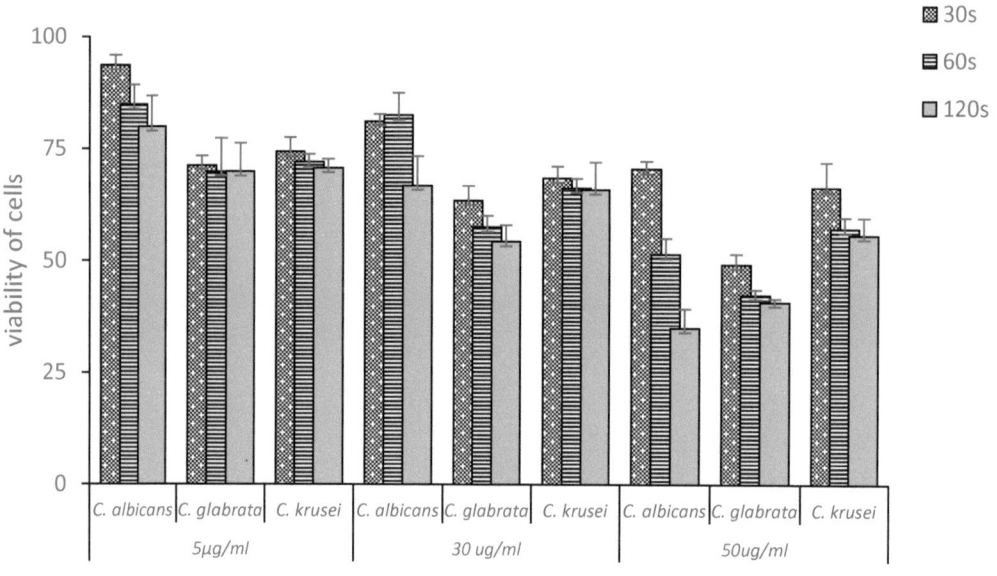

Figure 5. The effect of different exposure times (30 s–120 s) of ozonated water at three concentrations (5 µg/mL, 30 µg/mL, and 50 µg/mL) on cell viability (percentage of viability). Comparison between fungal strains *C. albicans* ATCC 10,231, *C. glabrata* ATCC 2001, and *C. krusei* ATCC 34,135.

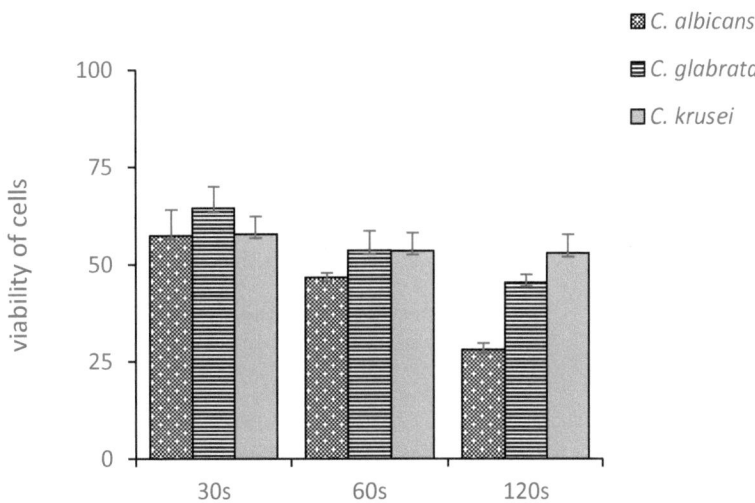

Figure 6. Effect of different exposure times on 0.2% chlorhexidine digluconate (30 s–120 s) on the number of viable cells (percentage of viability). Comparison between fungal strains *C. albicans* ATCC 10,231, *C. glabrata* ATCC 2001, and *C. krusei* ATCC 34,135.

4. Discussion

Ozone therapy is a method that uses ozone in various forms and its properties. It has been successfully applied in medicine and dentistry for years [21].

The present results showed that the strain *C. albicans* ATCC 10,231 had the highest sensitivity during the longest exposure to ozonated water for 120 s. The cell viability of this strain was 34.98%, while the viability of the *C. krusei* ATCC 34,135 strain, in the same conditions, amounted to 55.79%. The viability of cells after a 120-s exposure to 0.2% chlorhexidine digluconate was found to be similar. It was 28.07% for *C. albicans* and 52.93% for the *C. krusei* strain. Additionally, the *C. albicans* strain is more sensitive to commonly used antiseptics, such as 0.2% chlorhexidine digluconate and ozonated water, than other tested strains. Accordingly, the null hypothesis tested in this study could be rejected. Similar results were obtained by Monzillo V. et al. [34], who analyzed the antifungal efficacy (*C. albicans*, *C. parapsilosis*, *C. glabrata*, and *C. tropicalis*) of GeliO$_3$ ozonated oil compared to 0.2% chlorhexidine digluconate (Plakgel ®). Both products demonstrated antifungal activity against all *Candida* species tested. All species exhibited equal sensitivity to chlorhexidine. In the case of GeliO$_3$, differences in sensitivity were found. The greatest ones were observed for *C. glabrata* and *C. albicans*, and the lowest for *C. parapsilosis* and *C. tropicalis* [34].

Other researchers confirmed the current study's finding, demonstrating that the longer ozone application time, the more effective it is. De Faria et al. [35] assessed and compared the sensitivity to ozonated water of standard strains of *C. albicans* ATCC 18,804 and isolates collected from healthy students. The reduction in the number of strains progressed with increasing exposure time; however, complete reduction of colonies of the reference *C. albicans* strain occurred only after 5 min of exposure to ozone at a concentration of 3.3 mg/L. Moreover, freshly isolated strains of *C. albicans* showed higher resistance to ozone than the reference strains [35].

It is worth emphasizing that in the oral cavity there are pre-existing mixed bacterial and fungal biofilms. Moreover, fungi most often adhere to the surfaces occupied by bacteria. This phenomenon can be observed in the environments occupied by commensal flora, such as the oral cavity, and on the surfaces of dental materials, both in healthy and diseased individuals [36]. *Candida* spp. fungi can co-aggregate with other microorganisms living in the oral cavity, such as bacteria of the genera *Streptococcus, Staphylococcus, Actinomyces* and *Fusobacterium*, thus creating a species-diverse biofilm. Such interactions facilitate the survival and proliferation of fungi in the diverse microflora of the oral cavity. Currently, there are no studies available that would determine the sensitivity of microorganisms in mixed biofilms to ozonated water. However, based on the results for individual microorganisms, it can be presumed that it would also be effective against such a structure [20,22,25,36]. The use of an antifungal substance as medicine is often associated with many side effects and, in the case of the oral cavity, often with adverse effects on the surrounding tissues. In addition, the effects of water and ozonated oil were shown to be less toxic compared to other commonly used antiseptics [37]. The toxicity of ozone in various forms was evaluated for individual cells. Colombo M. et al. [37] proved the lack of cytotoxicity (MTT test) of ozonated olive oil and moderate to severe cytotoxicity of chlorhexidine digluconate (0.5% and 1%) against gingival fibroblasts (HGFs). Due to the fact that oral candidiasis often coexists with other mucosa pathologies, such as the severe form of lichen planus, it is desirable to have ozone stimulating the metabolic activity of fibroblasts, as well as immunomodulatory and anti-inflammatory effects based on the stimulation of the proliferation of immunocompetent cells and the synthesis of immunoglobulins. It also activates the phagocytic function of macrophages. In addition, it is believed that the effect of eliminating pain and inflammation is associated with the improvement in microcirculation and oxygenation of cells and tissues, as well as with the reduced production of pro-inflammatory cytokines and elimination of pain mediators [27,28].

The present results confirmed earlier reports that showed high activity of ozonated water against yeasts of the genus *Candida* [35]. It is well known that *non-albicans* strains are less sensitive to ozone [34]. The effectiveness of the therapy seems to be dependent on the concentration of the ozone solution used and the exposure time. Single laboratory tests also show low toxicity to epithelial cells and fibroblasts [37]. All this points to the potential possibility of using ozone (in the form of water or oil solutions) in local therapy not only on the oral mucosa but also on the mucosa in other parts of the body, and on the skin and its appendages. The ozone activity also shows activity against bacteria, thus the application of ozonated water solutions for mixed bacterial and fungal infections can be considered. However, there are no clinical studies on this subject in the available literature.

For this reason, the laboratory experience gained should be used to plan and conduct further studies and allow for the use of this substance as a supportive therapy or monotherapy.

The great advantage of this research, which contributes to its innovativeness and novelty, is the use of ozone water prepared ex tempore at particularly selected times of its impact. Exposure times were chosen to reflect the effectiveness of antiseptics with proven anti-fungal activity. Such studies using these conditions had not been conducted before.

One of the main goals of this study was to use the shortest possible time of exposure to ozonated water. In clinical terms, ozonated water would be used as a mouthwash. The time range of 30 to 120 s is most often recommended for mouthwash with other antibacterial substances. It is also a real and practical time that can be used by the patient in the dental office and at home. For this reason, our main goal was to test the sensitivity of the assessed strains to ozonated water under these conditions and exposure times.

In our study, we assessed the number of live cells after a single treatment. As with most antifungal substances, a single application is unlikely to be sufficient. In the future, it should be considered to conduct research defining a treatment regimen (number of days and frequency of use) using ozonated water, allowing for complete eradication. The presented study may be a preparation for further studies involving our patients. In the study, we plan to eliminate microorganisms not only from the mucous membrane but also from the denture plate. A limitation of the present study was the fact that only three concentrations were investigated; therefore, future research should include more concentrations of ozonated water. However, it should be acknowledged that it was a limitation of the device used for the study. Moreover, additional antiseptics as a control should be examined. The present study used only three reference strains of *Candida* fungi, thus more fungi strains were needed, including mixtures of several Candida strains and those collected from patients.

5. Conclusions

Within the limitations of this study, it can be concluded that selected strains of *Candida* spp. were sensitive to ozonated water at all tested concentrations (5 µg/mL, 30 µg/mL, and 50 µg/mL). The sensitivity of strains to ozonated water increased with concentration and application time. Moreover, the sensitivity of *Candida* strains to ozonated water is comparable to that of 0.2% chlorhexidine gluconate.

Author Contributions: Conceptualization, A.K.-K., R.W. and D.S.; methodology, A.K.-K., R.W., D.S., A.M. and E.B.; validation, A.K.-K., D.S., R.W., M.T., A.M. and E.B.; formal analysis, A.K.-K., R.W., M.T., A.M., E.B. and M.K.; investigation, A.K.-K., A.M., E.B. and R.W.; data curation, A.K.-K., R.W., D.S. and M.L.-S.; writing—original draft preparation, A.K.-K., R.W., E.B., M.L.-S, M.K. and M.T.; writing—review and editing, A.K.-K., R.W., D.S., M.K. and M.T.; visualization, A.K.-K., M.K., R.W. and E.B.; supervision, D.S., M.L.-S., M.T. and A.M.; project administration, R.W. and A.K.-K. All authors have read and agreed to the published version of the manuscript.

Funding: This research received no external funding.

Institutional Review Board Statement: Not applicable.

Informed Consent Statement: Not applicable.

Data Availability Statement: Not applicable.

Conflicts of Interest: The authors declare no conflict of interest.

References

1. Giacobbe, D.R.; Maraolo, A.E.; Simeon, V.; Magnè, F.; Pace, M.C.; Gentile, I.; Chiodini, P.; Viscoli, C.; Sanguinetti, M.; Mikulska, M.; et al. Changes in the relative prevalence of candidaemia due to non-albicans Candida species in adult in-patients: A systematic review, meta-analysis and meta-regression. *Mycoses* **2020**, *63*, 334–342. [CrossRef] [PubMed]
2. Nobile, C.J.; Johnson, A.D. *Candida albicans* Biofilms and Human Disease. *Annu. Rev. Microbiol.* **2016**, *69*, 71–92. [CrossRef] [PubMed]
3. Vila, T.; Sultan, A.S.; Montelongo-jauregui, D. Oral Candidiasis: A Disease of Opportunity. *J. Fungi* **2020**, *6*, 15. [CrossRef] [PubMed]
4. Rodrigues, C.F.; Rodrigues, M.E.; Henriques, M.C.R. Promising Alternative Therapeutics for Oral Candidiasis. *Curr. Med. Chem.* **2018**, *26*, 2515–2528. [CrossRef]
5. Welk, A.; Zahedani, M.; Beyer, C.; Kramer, A.; Müller, G. Antibacterial and antiplaque efficacy of a commercially available octenidine-containing mouthrinse. *Clin. Oral Investig.* **2016**, *20*, 1469–1476. [CrossRef]
6. Soares, I.H.; Loreto, S.; Rossato, L.; Mario, D.N.; Venturini, T.P.; Baldissera, F.; Santurio, J.M.; Alves, S.H. In vitro activity of essential oils extracted from condiments against fluconazole-resistant and -sensitive Candida glabrata. *J. Mycol. Med.* **2015**, *25*, 213–217. [CrossRef]
7. Srivatstava, A.; Ginjupalli, K.; Perampalli, N.U.; Bhat, N.; Ballal, M. Evaluation of the properties of a tissue conditioner containing origanum oil as an antifungal additive. *J. Prosthet. Dent.* **2013**, *110*, 313–319. [CrossRef]
8. Ninomiya, K.; Hayama, K.; Ishijima, S.A.; Maruyama, N.; Irie, H.; Kurihara, J.; Abe, S. Suppression of inflammatory reactions by terpinen-4-ol, a main constituent of tea tree oil, in a murine model of oral candidiasis and its suppressive activity to cytokine production of macrophages In Vitro. *Biol Pharm Bull.* **2013**, *36*, 838–844. [CrossRef]
9. Szweda, P.; Gucwa, K.; Kurzyk, E.; Romanowska, E.; Dzierżanowska-Fangrat, K.; Zielińska Jurek, A.; Kuś, P.M.; Milewski, S. Essential Oils, Silver Nanoparticles and Propolis as Alternative Agents Against Fluconazole Resistant Candida albicans, Candida glabrata and Candida krusei Clinical Isolates. *Indian J. Microbiol.* **2015**, *55*, 175–183. [CrossRef]
10. Dalwai, S.; Rodrigues, S.J.; Baliga, S.; Shenoy, V.K.; Shetty, T.B.; Pai, U.Y.; Saldanha, S. Comparative evaluation of antifungal action of tea tree oil, chlorhexidine gluconate and fluconazole on heat polymerized acrylic denture base resin—An in vitro study. *Gerodontology* **2016**, *33*, 402–409. [CrossRef]
11. Jebali, A.; Hajjar, F.H.E.; Pourdanesh, F.; Hekmatimoghaddam, S.; Kazemi, B.; Masoudi, A.; Daliri, K.; Sedighi, N. Silver and gold nanostructures: Antifungal property of different shapes of these nanostructures on Candida species. *Med. Mycol.* **2014**, *52*, 65–72. [CrossRef] [PubMed]
12. Ingle, A.P.; Duran, N.; Rai, M. Bioactivity, mechanism of action, and cytotoxicity of copper-based nanoparticles: A review. *Appl. Microbiol. Biotechnol.* **2014**, *98*, 1001–1009. [CrossRef] [PubMed]

13. Nam, K.Y. In vitro antimicrobial effect of the tissue conditioner containing silver nanoparticles. *J. Adv. Prosthodont.* **2011**, *3*, 20–24. [CrossRef]
14. Wiench, R.; Nowicka, J.; Pajaczkowska, M.; Kuropka, P.; Skaba, D.; Kruczek-Kazibudzka, A.; Kuśka-Kiełbratowska, A.; Grzech-Leśniak, K. Influence of incubation time on ortho-toluidine blue mediated antimicrobial photodynamic therapy directed against selected Candida strains—An in vitro study. *Int. J. Mol. Sci.* **2021**, *22*, 10971. [CrossRef]
15. Wiench, R.; Skaba, D.; Matys, J.; Grzech-Leśniak, K. Efficacy of Toluidine Blue—Mediated Antimicrobial Photodynamic on *Candida* spp. A systematic Review. *Antibiotics* **2021**, *10*, 349. [CrossRef] [PubMed]
16. Wiench, R.; Skaba, D.; Stefanik, N.; Kępa, M.; Gilowski, Ł.; Cieślar, G.; Kawczyk-Krupka, A. Assessment of sensitivity of selected Candida strains on antimicrobial photodynamic therapy using diode laser 635 nm and toluidine blue—In vitro research. *Photodiagnosis Photodyn. Ther.* **2019**, *27*, 241–247. [CrossRef] [PubMed]
17. Kumar, T.; Arora, N.; Puri, G.; Aravinda, K.; Dixit, A.; Jatti, D. Efficacy of ozonized olive oil in the management of oral lesions and conditions: A clinical trial. *Contemp. Clin. Dent.* **2016**, *7*, 51. [CrossRef]
18. Khatri, I.; Moge, G.; Kumar, N.A. Evaluation of effect of topical ozone therapy on salivary Candidal carriage in oral candidiasis. *Indian J. Dent. Res.* **2015**, *26*, 158–162.
19. Sechi, L.; Lezcano, I.; Nunez, N.; Espim, M.; Pinna, A.; Molicotti, P.; Dupre, I.; Microbiologia, I. Antibacterial activity of ozonized sunfower oil (Oleozon). *J. Appl. Microbiol.* **2001**, *90*, 279–284. [CrossRef]
20. Lezcano, I.; Nuñez, N.; Espino, M.; Gómez, M. Antibacterial activity of ozonized sunflower oil, oleozon, against *Staphylococcus aureus* and *Staphylococcus epidermidis*. *Ozone Sci. Eng.* **2000**, *22*, 207–214. [CrossRef]
21. Garg, R. Ozone: A new face of dentistry. *Internet J. Dent. Sci.* **2009**, *7*, 1–7. [CrossRef]
22. Tiwari, S.; Avinash, A.; Katiyar, S.; Iyer, A.A. Dental applications of ozone therapy : A review of the literature. *Saudi J. Dent. Res.* **2016**, *8*, 105–111. [CrossRef]
23. Kumar, P.; Tyagi, P.; Bhagawati, S.; Kumar, A. Current interpretations and scientific rationale of the ozone usage in dentistry: A systematic review of literature. *Eur. J. Gen. Dent.* **2014**, *3*, 175. [CrossRef]
24. Zeng, J.; Lu, J. Mechanisms of action involved in ozone-therapy in skin diseases. *Int. Immunopharmacol.* **2018**, *56*, 235–241. [CrossRef] [PubMed]
25. Suh, Y.; Patel, S.; Kaitlyn, R.; Gandhi, J.; Joshi, G.; Smith, N.L.; Khan, S.A. Clinical utility of ozone therapy in dental and oral medicine. *Med. Gas Res.* **2019**, *9*, 163–167. [CrossRef]
26. Gupta, G.; Mansi, B. Ozone therapy in periodontics. *J. Med. Life* **2012**, *5*, 59–67.
27. Naik, S.V.; Kohli, S.; Zohabhasan, S.; Bhatia, S. Ozone—A Biological Therapy in Dentistry-Reality or Myth. *Open Dent. J.* **2016**, *10*, 196–206. [CrossRef]
28. Colombo, M.; Gallo, S.; Garofoli, A.; Poggio, C.; Arciola, C.R.; Scribante, A. Ozone gel in chronic periodontal disease: A randomized clinical trial on the anti-inflammatory effects of ozone application. *Biology* **2021**, *10*, 625. [CrossRef]
29. Cardoso, M.G.; de Oliveira, L.D.; Koga-Ito, C.Y.; Jorge, A.O.C. Effectiveness of ozonated water on Candida albicans, Enterococcus faecalis, and endotoxins in root canals. *Oral Surg. Oral Med. Oral Pathol. Oral Radiol. Endodontol.* **2008**, *105*, 85–91. [CrossRef]
30. Falagas, M.E.; Roussos, N.; Vardakas, K.Z. Relative frequency of albicans and the various non-albicans *Candida* spp among candidemia isolates from inpatients in various parts of the world: A systematic review. *Int. J. Infect. Dis.* **2010**, *14*, e954–e966. [CrossRef]
31. Kolliyavar, B.; Shettar, L.; Thakur, S. Chlorhexidine: The Gold Standard Mouth Wash. *J. Pharm. Biomed. Sci.* **2016**; *6*, 106–109. [CrossRef]
32. Nogales, C.G.; Ferrari, P.H.; Olszewer, K.E. Ozone Therapy in Medicine and Dentistry. *J. Contemp. Dent. Pract.* **2008**, *9*, 75–84. [CrossRef] [PubMed]
33. Kumar, P.; Nagarajan, A.; Uchil, P. Analysis of Cell Viability by the MTT Assay. *Cold Spring Harb. Protoc.* **2018**, *6*, pdb-prot095489. [CrossRef] [PubMed]
34. Monzillo, V.; Lallitto, F.; Russo, A.; Poggio, C.; Scribante, A.; Arciola, C.R.; Bertuccio, F.R.; Colombo, M. Ozonized gel against four Candida species: A pilot study and clinical perspectives. *Materials* **2020**, *13*, 1731. [CrossRef] [PubMed]
35. De Faria, I.D.S.; Ueno, M.; Yumi Koga-Ito, C.; Urrichi Irrazabal, W.; Balducci, I.; Jorge, A.O.C. Effects of ozonated water on Candida albicans oral isolates. *Braz. J. Oral Sci.* **2005**, *4*, 783–786.
36. Lohse, M.B.; Gulati, M.; Johnson, A.D.; Nobile, C.J. Development and regulation of single- and multi-species *Candida albicans* biofilms. *Nat. Publ. Gr.* **2017**, *16*, 19–31. [CrossRef]
37. Colombo, M.; Ceci, M.; Felisa, E.; Poggio, C.; Pietrocola, G. Cytotoxicity evaluation of a new ozonized olive oil. *Eur. J. Dent.* **2018**, *12*, 585–589. [CrossRef]

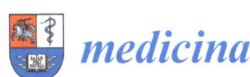

Case Report

The Stability Guided Multidisciplinary Treatment of Skeletal Class III Malocclusion Involving Impacted Canines and Thin Periodontal Biotype: A Case Report with Eight-Year Follow-Up

Juan Li [†], Xiaoyan Feng [†], Yi Lin and Jun Lin *

Department of Stomatology, The First Affiliated Hospital, College of Medicine, Zhejiang University, Hangzhou 310003, China
* Correspondence: linjun2@zju.edu.cn; Tel.: +86-0571-8723-6338
† These authors contributed equally to this work.

Abstract: Skeletal class III malocclusion with severe skeletal disharmonies and arch discrepancies is usually treated via the conventional orthodontic-surgical approach. However, when associated with tooth impaction and periodontal risks, the treatment is more challenging and complex. The esthetic, occlusal, and periodontal stability of the treatment outcome is more difficult to obtain. The 16-year-old female patient in this case was diagnosed with dental and skeletal Class III malocclusion, bilateral impacted maxillary canines, and scalloped thin gingiva. The multidisciplinary management included a segmental arch technique, extracting two premolars, a subepithelial connective tissue graft surgery, and orthognathic surgery. The esthetic facial profile, pleasant smile, appropriate occlusion, and functional treatment results were obtained and maintained in 8-year follow-up.

Keywords: skeletal class III malocclusion; connective tissue graft; orthognathic surgery; impacted maxillary canines

1. Introduction

Skeletal class III malocclusion has a high rate of prevalence in Asian people, and it has a high rate of relapse following orthodontic treatment, which poses a challenge to orthodontists [1]. Combined orthodontic and orthognathic surgery is a conventional option to correct the malocclusion and dentofacial deformities in adults with severe skeletal class III malocclusion.

In this type of patient, hypodevelopment of the maxilla is common, and an insufficient length and width of the maxilla can lead to maxillary teeth impaction, of which canines are the most frequent [2]. Maxillary canine impaction occurs in approximately 2% of the population, while the incidence in the maxilla is more than twice that in the mandible, and only 17% of labially impacted canines have enough space [3]. The various treatment options available are observation, intervention, relocation, and extraction. Orthodontic traction is a widely used and efficient method to reserve and position the canine in its proper location within the arch; however, there are difficulties and considerations since it may cause pulp necrosis, gingival recession, or alveolar-dental ankylosis [4].

In addition, the periodontal condition has a significant impact on the limitation of orthodontic tooth movement, macro and micro aesthetics, and stability [5]. In patients with skeletal class III malocclusion, the gingival thickness in the area is also found to be thinner, with a so-called thin scalloped gingival biotype accompanied by relatively deficient underlying bone and attached gingiva [6]. The teeth in the mandibular anterior area is moved labially on the narrow alveolus in the pre-surgery decompensation period [7]. These all indicate that the risk of gingival recession, fenestrations, and dehiscence is highly elevated. Dealing with the corresponding periodontal risks and maintaining stability are also huge challenges.

The treatment for skeletal class III malocclusion patients with both impacted canines and thin periodontal biotype is more complicated in plan elaborating and retention designing. This clinical report provides an interdisciplinary treatment strategy through a typical case study. In the case, a segmental arch technique, a subepithelial connective tissue graft surgery, and an orthognathic surgery were performed, and favorable esthetic and stable occlusion were obtained and maintained in follow-up period of 8 years.

2. Case Report

2.1. Diagnosis and Etiology

The patient, a 16-year-old female with no significant medical history, presented to the Orthodontic Department seeking to correct occlusion and improve her face aesthetic.

The facial examination displayed a concave profile, a prominent chin, an increased lower third of the face, and an unconfident smile. The upper lip was retruded 4.8 mm in relation to the E plane (Figure 1). The intraoral photographs (Figure 1) and dental casts (Figure 2) showed a bilateral Class III molar relationship and an anterior crossbite with a negative overjet of 2 mm. The width of the maxilla was narrow compared to the mandible, which led to a crossbite in the right posterior region and a compensatory lingual inclination in the left mandibular posterior region. All the mandibular deciduous molars and maxillary deciduous canines were retained with the left permanent maxillary canine erupted labially. Scalloped thin gingiva was evident in the mandibular anterior region with an obvious root shape. Temporomandibular disorder symptoms or bad oral habits were not detected. The mandible cannot retreat to the edge-to-edge occlusion.

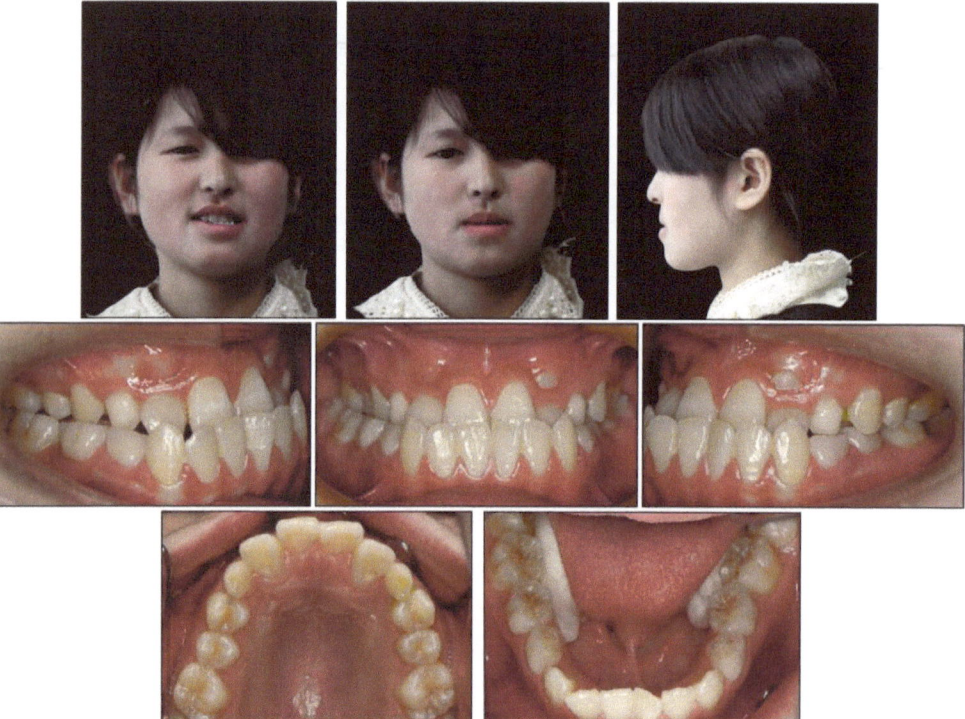

Figure 1. Pretreatment intraoral and facial photographs.

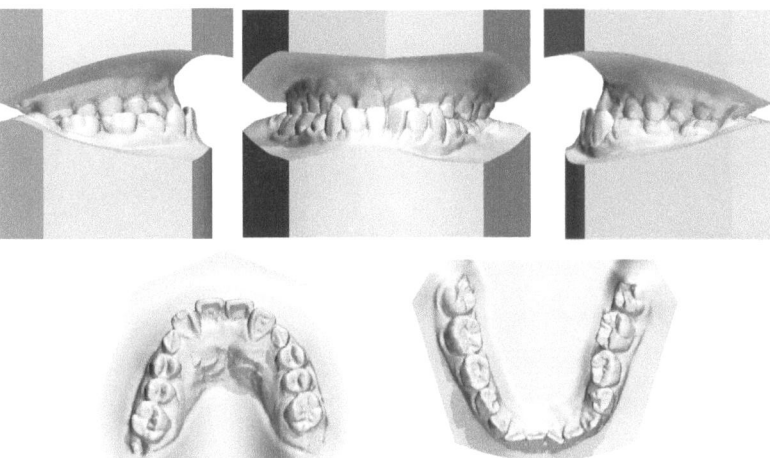

Figure 2. The pretreatment dental cast.

The panoramic radiograph showed that both the maxillary canines and all the third molars were impacted, and no significant periodontal support loss was found. The cephalometric analysis (Figure 3 and Table 1) showed a severe skeletal Class III relationship (ANB, −4.0°) with an insufficient developed maxilla (SNA, 77.2°). The maxillary incisors were relatively well-positioned, while the mandibular incisors were lingually inclined (U1-SN,104°; L1-MP, 86.5°) [8].

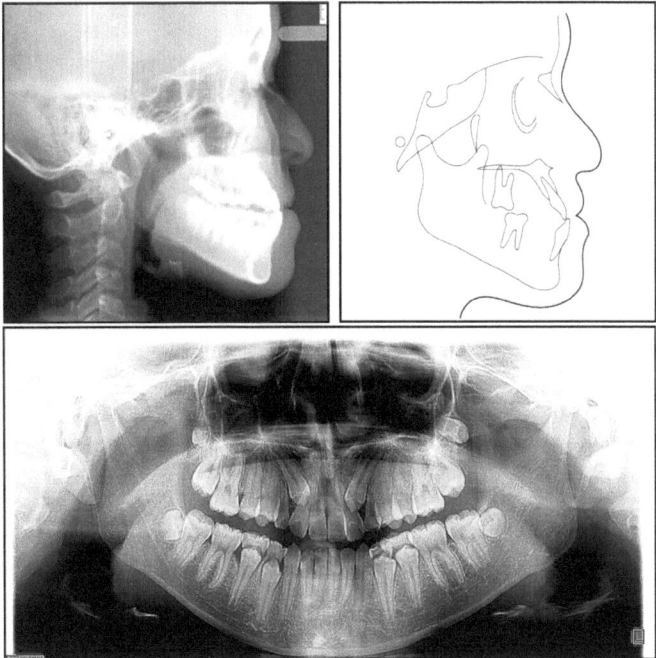

Figure 3. A pretreatment lateral cephalometric radiograph and tracing and a panoramic radiograph.

Table 1. Cephalometric measurements.

Measurement	Norm ± SD	Pretreatment	Posttreatment	8-Year Follow-Up
FMIA (°)	64.8 ± 8.5	67.6	69.0	68.0
FMA (°)	23.9 ± 4.5	26.6	21.5	22.6
SNA (°)	82.0 ± 3.5	77.2	83.0	83.4
SNB (°)	80.9 ± 3.4	81.3	81.6	81.5
ANB (°)	1.6 ± 1.5	−4.0	1.3	1.9
L1-MP (°)	95.0 ± 7.0	86.5	89.6	89.3
Occ-Plane (°)	6.8 ± 5.0	8.1	9.5	10.7
U1-SN (°)	102.8 ± 5.5	104.0	105.6	103.5
Upper Lip-E (mm)	6.0 ± 2.0	−4.8	−4.0	−4.2
Lower Lip-E (mm)	−2.0 ± 2.0	−0.3	−1.5	−1.1
S-Go (mm)	82.5 ± 5.0	67.9	67.8	68.1
Na-Me (mm)	128.5 ± 5.0	111.8	103.7	105.4
S-Go/Na-Me (%)	65.0 ± 4.0	60.7	65.4	64.6

S, sella; N, nasion; MP, mandibular plane; Occ-Plane, occlusion plane; E, aesthetic line; Go, Gonion; Me, Menton.

2.2. Treatment Objectives

The treatment objectives were to: (1) tract the impacted maxillary permanent canines; (2) improve the periodontal phenotype of the lower anterior region and reduce the risk of gingival recession through mucogingival surgery; (3) solve the horizontal and sagittal discrepancy between the mandible and the maxilla to improve the facial profile through two-jaw surgery; and (4) align the dentition to establish function occlusion.

2.3. Treatment Alternatives

Little or no orthopedic maxillary and mandible response could be expected because the female patient was already 16 years old with little growth potential. Therefore, orthognathic surgery could be a proper choice to solve her complaints. Two-jaw surgery includes LeFort I osteotomy for maxilla advancement and bilateral split sagittal osteotomy for mandible setback because the stability of isolated mandibular setback is relatively poor.

As for the dental problem, the first option was the extraction of two impacted maxillary canines to shorten the treatment time and offer the spaces to decompensate and retract the maxillary incisors. However, the maxillary canines were vital in dentition, as they frame the smile and guide occlusion [9]. The second option was the removal of the maxillary first premolars, which would resolve the crowding of the anterior area and regain space for traction. This approach would contribute to an extended course of presurgical treatment. However, according to her age, the timing of orthognathic surgery was not yet appropriate, so the whole treatment course would not be extended. Considering the periodontal conditions described above, mucogingival surgery was arranged to improve the periodontal tissue quality and the treatment outcome [10].

2.4. Treatment Progress

Before the orthodontic treatment, the extraction of all retained deciduous teeth and maxillary first premolars were scheduled. After the extraction, both arches were bonded with preadjusted brackets (0.022-inch slot; 3M Unitek, Monrovia, CA, USA), aligned with initial 0.014-inch nickel titanium arch wires, and changed sequentially to eliminate crowding and provide leveling. Meanwhile, two impacted maxillary permanent canines were tracted through two auxiliary segmental 0.019 × 0.025-inch stainless steel arch wires with vertical helical loops (Figure 4). After 12 months, the canines were basically tracted into the right place. Presurgical decompensation started to increase the magnitude of surgical movement. The unfavorable tooth inclinations were corrected with 0.019 × 0.025-inch stainless steel arch wires through sliding mechanics to increase reverse overjet. A subepithelial connective tissue graft was also performed. Two connective tissue grafts were harvested from the palate and positioned in the prepared recipient site corresponding to the mandibular anterior region. The attached gingiva and keratinized tissue were augmented after the mucogingival surgery (Figure 5). After 34 months, the dentition preparation phase of presurgical treatment was completed in both arches (Figure 6).

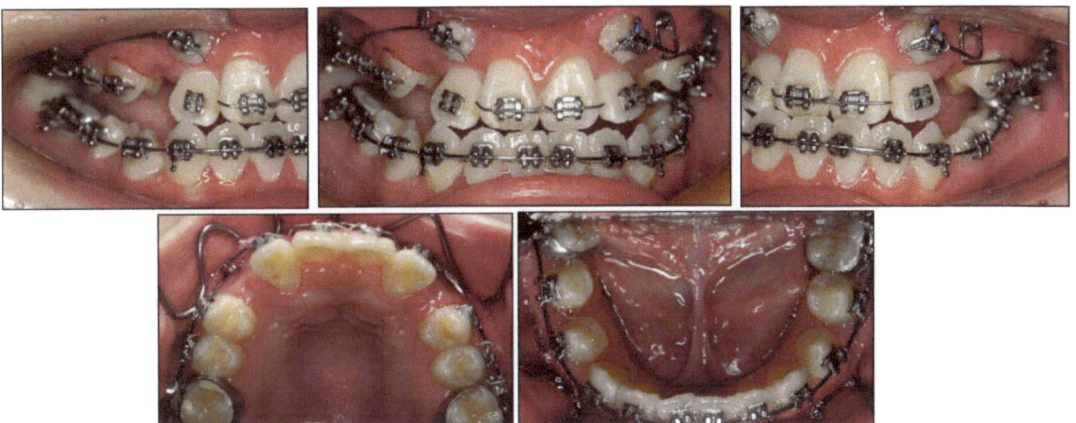

Figure 4. Tracting the impacted maxillary permanent canines with the segmental arch technique.

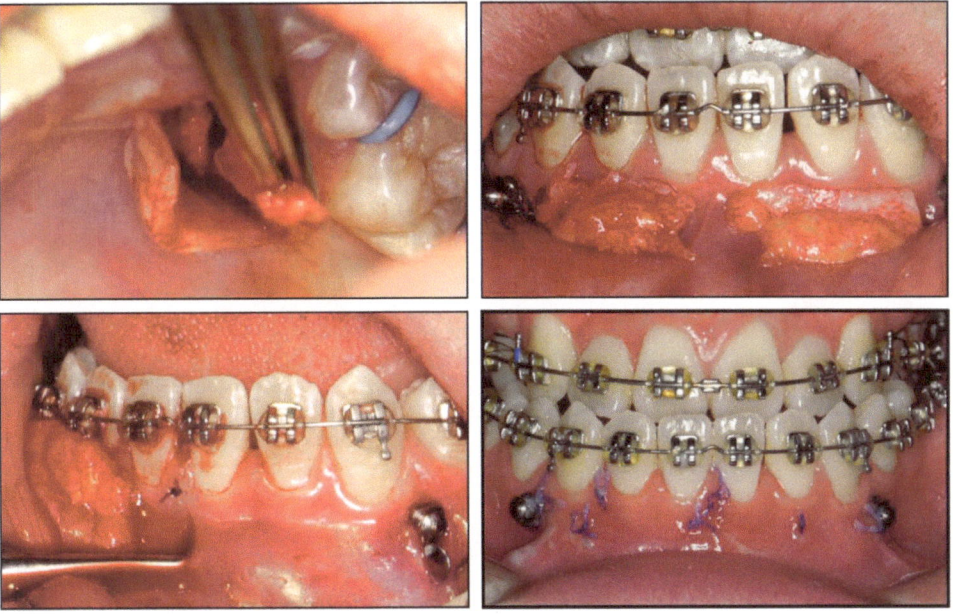

Figure 5. Subepithelial connective tissue transplantation.

Based on the reconstructed data of CBCT(cone-beam computed tomography) and cast surgery, the orthognathic surgery was determined to require a LeFort I maxillary osteotomy to advance the maxillary in 5 mm and the bilateral sagittal split osteotomy to setback the mandible in 3 mm. During the surgery, two splints were subsequently applied to assist in accurately placing and maintaining the jaw's position. Then, the new position was fixed with rigid internal fixation (RIF) and intermaxillary elastics. The patient was monitored closely after the procedure, and she was also taught how to perform opening and lateral movement exercises.

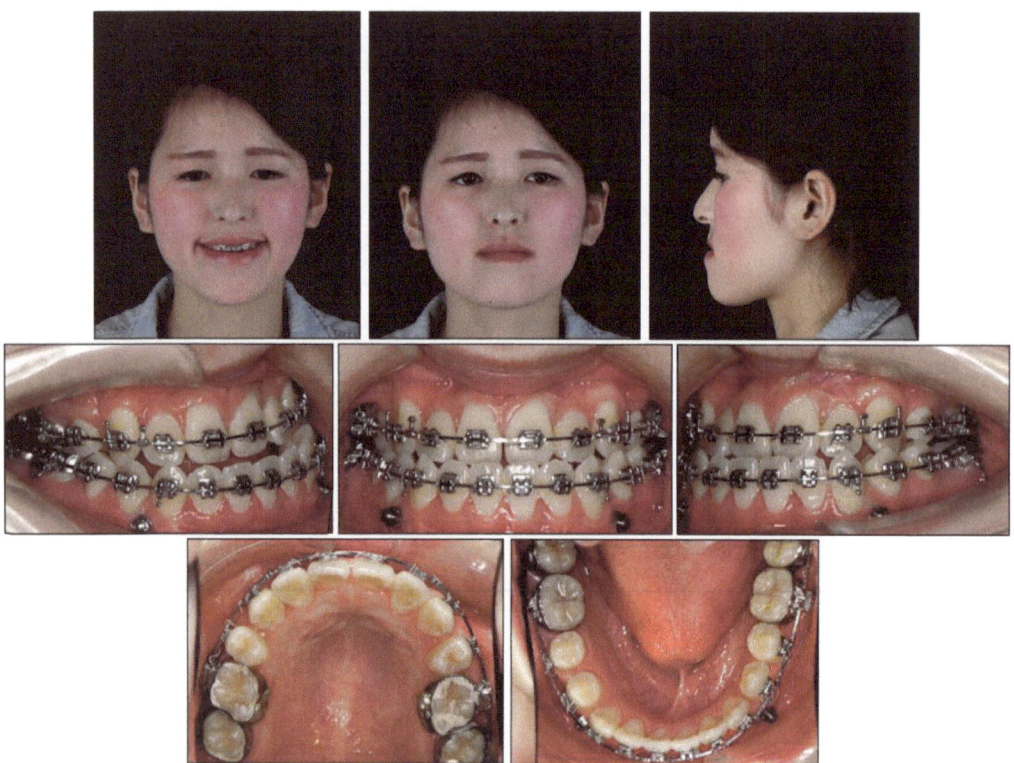

Figure 6. Presurgical facial and intraoral photographs.

One month after the surgery, the spaces in the upper arch were closed with 0.019 × 0.025-inch stainless steel arch wires with a double key loop. At the finishing stage, a fine adjustment of the occlusion was applied to improve the anterior overjet, the overbite, and the canine and molar relationship. After a total treatment of 48 months, the multi-bracket system and all Micro-Implant Anchorages were removed. Lingual bonded retainers from canine to canine and Hawley retainers were placed immediately after removal.

2.5. Treatment Results

All the initial treatment objectives, including occlusion, periodontal health, and facial esthetics, were achieved by a satisfactory multidisciplinary approach, partly due to the cooperation of the patient. The facial photographs showed a pleasant profile and a harmonious smile. The patient was satisfied with the facial improvement, and she became more confident (Figure 7). Posttreatment intraoral photographs and dental casts (Figure 8) showed bilateral Class II molar and Class I canine relationships with an ideal overjet and overbite. The gingiva tissue in the mandibular anterior region was evidently augmented, which indicated lower periodontal risks.

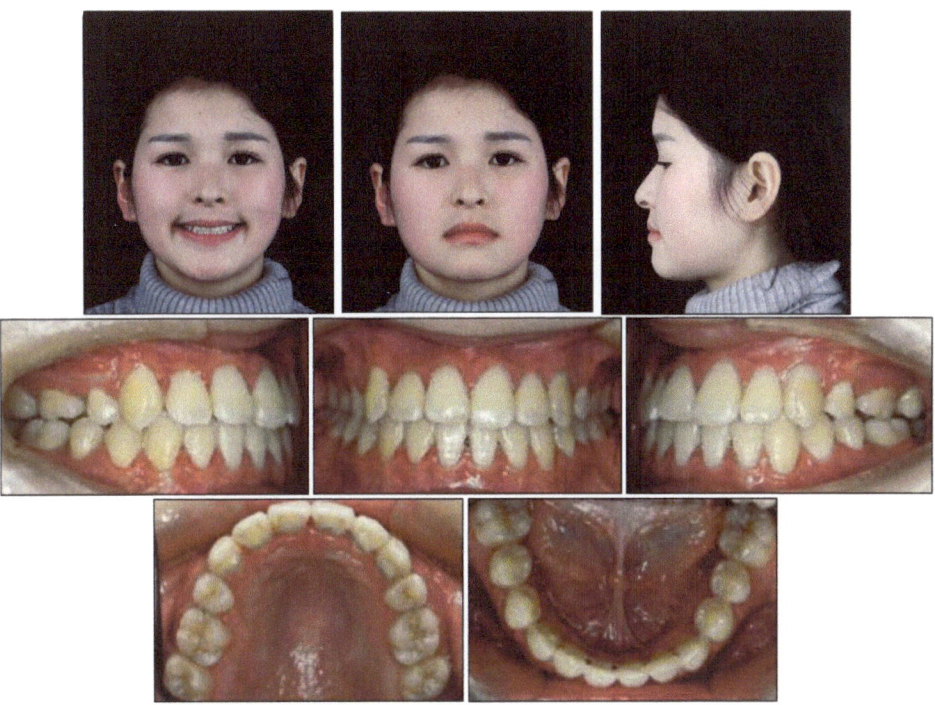

Figure 7. Posttreatment facial and intraoral photographs.

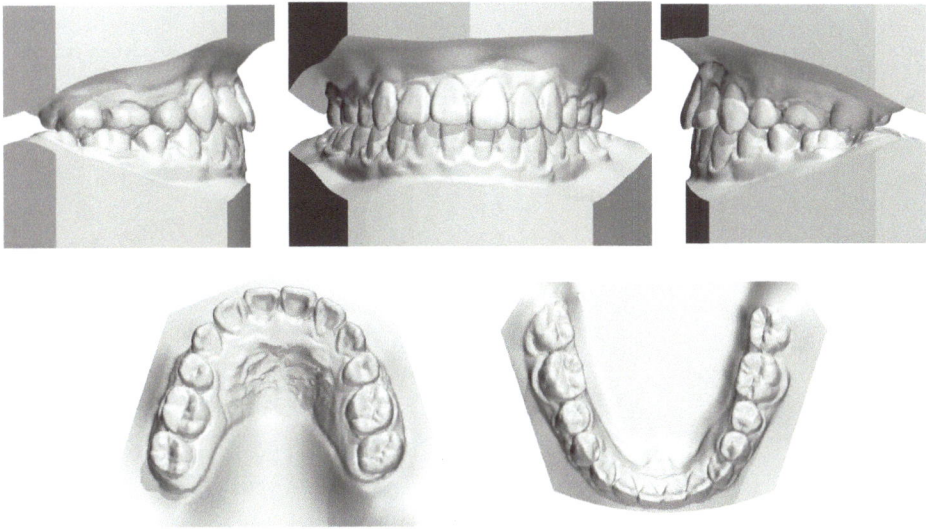

Figure 8. Posttreatment dental casts.

The final panoramic radiograph confirmed parallel roots with no apparent root resorption. Cephalometric analysis (Figure 9 and Table 1) indicated a normal anteroposterior (AP) relationship (ANB, from −4° to 1.3°) and decreased lower third (FMA: from 26.6° to 21.5°;

Na-Me: from 111.8 mm to 103.7 mm). Furthermore, the distance from the upper and lower lips to the E-line were significantly decreased, which helped improve the soft tissue profile.

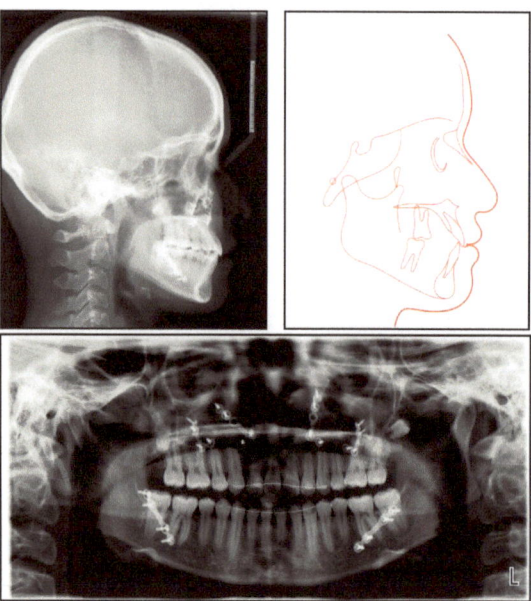

Figure 9. Posttreatment lateral cephalometric radiograph and tracing and a panoramic radiograph.

The 8-year follow-up photographs showed excellent stability of the occlusion and the profile (Figure 10). The pretreatment, posttreatment, and follow-up cephalometric superimposition revealed a significant improvement and stability in the facial profile and the skeletal and dental relationship. Superimposition of the posttreatment and retention digital dental models indicated generally stable results (Figure 11).

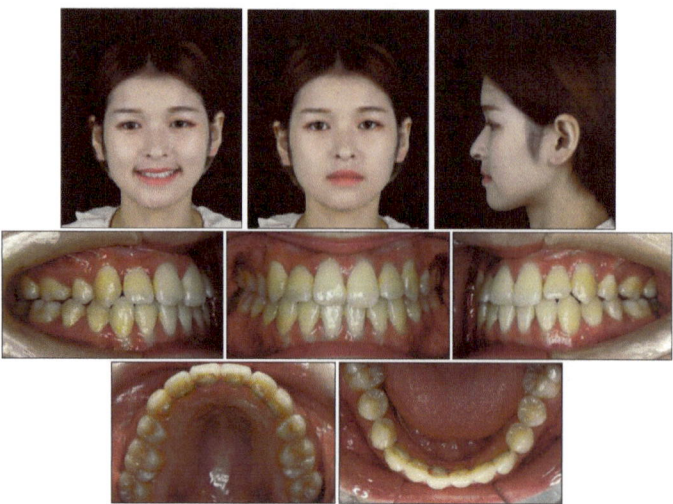

Figure 10. Facial and intraoral photographs after the 8-year follow-up.

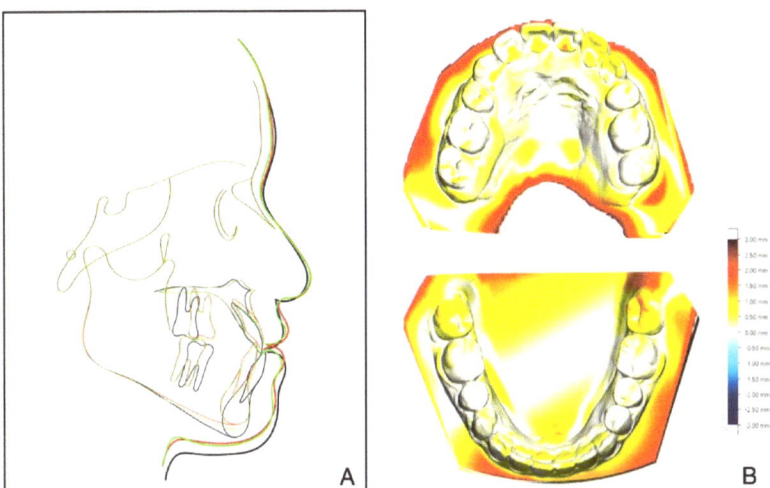

Figure 11. (**A**) Superimposed cephalometric tracings: pretreatment (black), posttreatment (red), and 8-year follow-up (green). (**B**) Superimposition of the posttreatment and retention digital dental models.

3. Discussion

Treatment plans for nongrowing patients with skeletal class III malocclusion are varied, including sole orthodontic treatment for dental camouflage or combined orthodontic-orthognathic treatment, including single or double-jaw surgery and genioplasty [11]. Johnston et al. reported that bimaxillary surgery was 3.4 times more likely to fully correct the ANB angle than mandibular surgery [12]. Previous studies have shown that maxillary advancement was stable, while large mandibular setback was a risk factor for relapse due to its habitual mandibular forward movement and prolonged growth. Double-jaw surgery, including bilateral sagittal split osteotomy and maxillary advancement, is the most effective way to improve stability [13]. Considering the degree of skeletal discrepancy in three dimensions in this case (ANB: −5.2°; Wits appraisal: −11.3 mm; FMA: from 26.6°; Na-Me 111.8 mm), the conventional surgical approach was determined to advance maxilla in 5 mm and setback mandible in 3 mm.

In addition to the maxilla-mandible relationship, the arch and the dentition play an important role in long-term stability. The etiology of the impacted teeth was related to the arch-length deficiency, which occurs in hypo-developed maxilla and may lead to bilateral impacted canines, which happened in this case. A treatment alternative is extraction; however, after extraction, there is a need to figure out an approach to replace the pivotal esthetic and the occlusion function of the missing canines, such as implant-retained crown restoration, conventional bridge, or premolar substitution through orthodontic treatment. The panoramic radiograph showed the canine crown was in the buccal side and distal to the midline of the lateral incisor, which noted a higher rate of successful traction, even up to 91% [3]. However, it takes space to decompensate and tract maxillary anterior teeth, so the extraction project was beneficial to create space [14]. Meanwhile, extraction guided the posterior dental arch to move relatively forward, which was equivalent to increasing the arch of the upper jaw and conducive to the establishment of a normal overjet and overbite of the posterior teeth. All things considered, a removal of the deciduous canines and the first premolars was decided, and then surgical exposure and a segmental arch technique were performed to tract the canines (Figure 12). The pre-surgical planning was mainly to tract the impacted teeth and create enough overjet and overbite for jaw movement, which was established a stable jaw–tooth relationship and improved the profile. The pre-surgical treatment went on for 2 years to achieve the traction of canines and reach the proper timing for the orthognathic surgery, which seemed longer compared to routine cases. Finally, we placed the canines correctly and established an ideal occlusion. Proper overjet and overbite, coordinate width, and close occlusion helped maintain the stable dentition relationship and further ensured the stability of the jaw's position and soft tissue aesthetic.

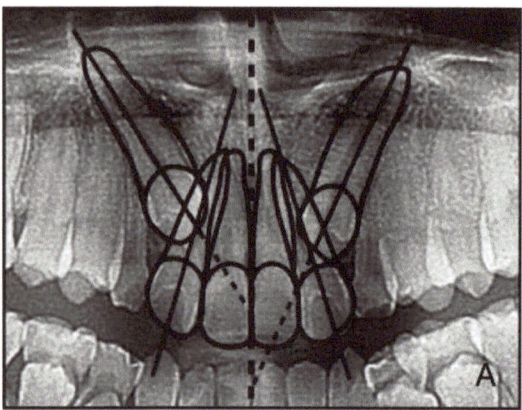 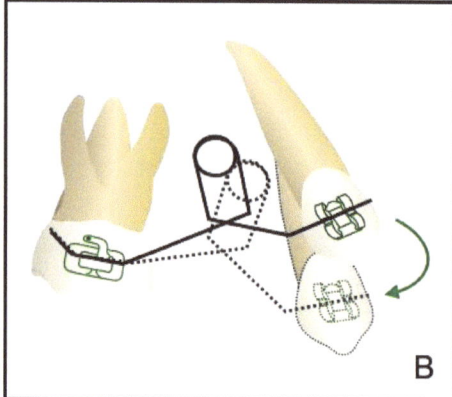

Figure 12. (**A**): The relative position of the canine crown and lateral incisor in a panoramic radiograph. (**B**): Biomechanism of canine traction through segmental arch. The green arrow illustrates the path of canine movement.

Dental decompensation during presurgical orthodontic treatment is aimed to correct the torque of anterior teeth [15]. It is vital to keep an eye on the periodontal condition because mandibular anterior teeth always express crown lingual torque in skeletal class III malocclusion, which enhances the risks of gingival recession, fenestrations, and dehiscence [16]. Mucogingival surgery is a widely used technique to obtain attached gingiva, including free gingival graft, laterally positioned flap, and subepithelial connective tissue graft [17]. According to the thin periodontal biotype, we chose to use a subepithelial connective tissue graft, which was the best way to convert a thin, soft tissue to a thick biotype. Occlusal trauma caused by anterior crossbite was relieved by acquiring proper anterior overjet [18]. The outcome displayed that the keratinized and attached gingiva gained sufficient thickness, which preserved healthy a periodontal state and better represented the pink-white esthetic.

Retention and stability following an orthodontic-surgical approach is an important indicator to judge whether a case is successful. The 8-year follow-up showed a stable effect in hard or soft tissues in this case. We applied a rigid internal fixation to settle the jaws during the active orthodontic period, and then we applied a lingual bonded retainer and a Hawley retainer for both arches during the retention period [19]. In addition, the adaptable finishing occlusion and TMJ position were indispensable factors for long-term stability in our case.

In our treatment, digital technology was applied to visualize and design the treatment plan. Dolphin software was used to simulate the jaw movement and carry out a visual surgical design to clarify the target position (Figure 13). However, digital technology was not applied to design and manufacture the surgery splints. Virtual surgical planning with CAD/CAM technology [20] and artificial intelligence has been gaining popularity in orthognathic surgery. It can provide doctors and patients with more predictive treatment outcomes, and it can also contribute to more accurate surgical processes and more stable results [21].

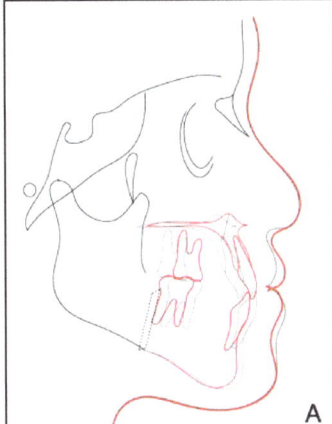
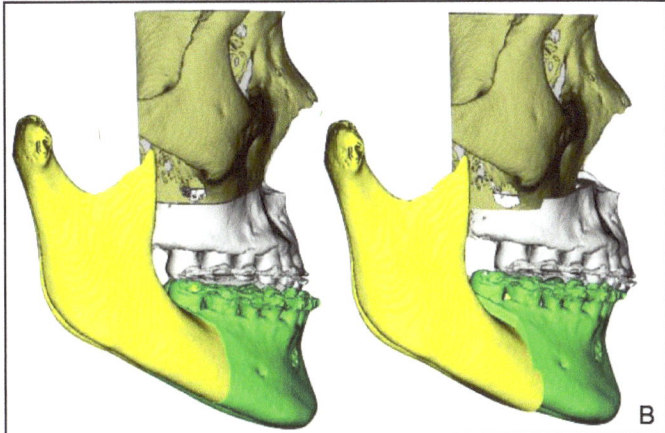

Figure 13. (**A**) VTO (Visual Treatment Objective): The postoperative effects were simulated by lateral radiographs. Pretreatment (black) and post-treatment (red). (**B**) Digital orthognathic surgery design through Dolphin software.

4. Conclusions

Due to the multidisciplinary treatment, including the orthognathic surgery, the orthodontic treatment, and the periodontal procedures, the skeletal and dental class III relationship was corrected, the impacted canines returned to a normal position, and the periodontal condition was in a relatively stable state. Additionally, during the 8-year follow-up, the facial esthetics, functional occlusion, and periodontal health were successfully maintained. A stability-guided, close interdisciplinary approach is critical for successful and stable outcomes in similar cases.

Author Contributions: Conceptualization, J.L. (Jun Lin) and J.L. (Juan Li); methodology, J.L. (Juan Li) and X.F.; software, X.F.; validation, J.L. (Jun Lin), J.L. (Juan Li), and X.F.; formal analysis, X.F. and Y.L.; investigation, X.F. and Y.L.; resources, X.F.; data curation, X.F.; writing—original draft preparation, J.L. (Juan Li) and X.F.; writing—review and editing, Y.L.; visualization, X.F.; supervision, J.L. (Jun Lin); project administration, J.L. (Jun Lin); funding acquisition, J.L. (Jun Lin) and J.L. (Juan Li). All authors have read and agreed to the published version of the manuscript.

Funding: This research was funded by the National Natural Science Foundation of China (No. 81970978) and the Zhejiang Provincial Natural Science Foundation of China (No. LY22H140006).

Institutional Review Board Statement: The study was conducted in accordance with the Declaration of Helsinki and approved by the Institutional Review Board of The First Affiliated Hospital, College of Medicine, Zhejiang University (protocol code: (2019) IIT (1483) with a date of approval 26 November 2019).

Informed Consent Statement: Informed consent was obtained from all subjects involved in the study.

Data Availability Statement: All experimental data supporting the results of this study are available from The First Affiliated Hospital, College of Medicine, Zhejiang University.

Conflicts of Interest: The authors declare no conflict of interest. The funders had no role in the design of the study; in the collection, analyses, or interpretation of data; in the writing of the manuscript; or in the decision to publish the results.

References

1. Park, J.U.; Baik, S.H. Classification of Angle Class III malocclusion and its treatment modalities. *Int. J. Adult Orthod. Orthognath. Surg.* **2001**, *16*, 19–29.
2. Ellis, E., 3rd; McNamara, J.A., Jr. Components of adult Class III malocclusion. *J. Oral Maxillofac. Surg.* **1984**, *42*, 295–305. [CrossRef]

3. Becker, A.; Chaushu, S. Etiology of maxillary canine impaction: A review. *Am. J. Orthod. Dentofac. Orthop.* **2015**, *148*, 557–567. [CrossRef] [PubMed]
4. Ferreira, J.T.L.; Romano, F.L.; Sasso Stuani, M.B.; Assed Carneiro, F.C.; Nakane Matsumoto, M.A. Traction of impacted canines in a skeletal Class III malocclusion: A challenging orthodontic treatment. *Am. J. Orthod. Dentofac. Orthop.* **2017**, *151*, 1159–1168. [CrossRef] [PubMed]
5. Vaden, J.L. Long-term stability—It begins with the treatment plan. *Semin. Orthod.* **2017**, *23*, 149–165. [CrossRef]
6. Park, J.H.; Hong, J.Y.; Ahn, H.W.; Kim, S.J. Correlation between periodontal soft tissue and hard tissue surrounding incisors in skeletal Class III patients. *Angle Orthod.* **2018**, *88*, 91–99. [CrossRef]
7. Kahn, S.; Almeida, R.A.; Dias, A.T.; Rodrigues, W.J.; Barceleiro, M.O.; Taba, M., Jr. Clinical Considerations on the Root Coverage of Gingival Recessions in Thin or Thick Biotype. *Int. J. Periodontics Restor. Dent.* **2016**, *36*, 409–415. [CrossRef]
8. Manhartsberger, C.; Richter, M. Cephalometric analysis of the results of orthopedic and orthodontic treatment in skeletal Angle Class III. *Z. Stomatol.* **1988**, *85*, 27–33.
9. Thiruvenkatachari, B.; Javidi, H.; Griffiths, S.E.; Shah, A.A.; Sandler, J. Extraction of maxillary canines: Esthetic perceptions of patient smiles among dental professionals and laypeople. *Am. J. Orthod. Dentofac. Orthop.* **2017**, *152*, 509–515. [CrossRef]
10. Wennstrom, J.L. Mucogingival considerations in orthodontic treatment. *Semin. Orthod.* **1996**, *2*, 46–54. [CrossRef]
11. Ngan, P.; Moon, W. Evolution of Class III treatment in orthodontics. *Am. J. Orthod. Dentofac. Orthop.* **2015**, *148*, 22–36. [CrossRef] [PubMed]
12. Johnston, C.; Burden, D.; Kennedy, D.; Harradine, N.; Stevenson, M. Class III surgical-orthodontic treatment: A cephalometric study. *Am. J. Orthod. Dentofac. Orthop.* **2006**, *130*, 300–309. [CrossRef] [PubMed]
13. Rizzatto, S.M.D.; Macedo de Menezes, L.; da Cunha Filho, J.J.; Allgayer, S. Conventional surgical-orthodontic approach with double-jaw surgery for a patient with skeletal Class III malocclusion: Stability of results 10 years posttreatment. *Am. J. Orthod. Dentofac. Orthop.* **2018**, *154*, 128–139. [CrossRef] [PubMed]
14. Bellot-Arcis, C.; Garcia-Sanz, V.; Paredes-Gallardo, V. Nonsurgical treatment of an adult with skeletal Class III malocclusion, anterior crossbite, and an impacted canine. *Am. J. Orthod. Dentofac. Orthop.* **2021**, *159*, 522–535. [CrossRef] [PubMed]
15. Choi, Y.J.; Chung, C.J.; Kim, K.H. Periodontal consequences of mandibular incisor proclination during presurgical orthodontic treatment in Class III malocclusion patients. *Angle Orthod.* **2015**, *85*, 427–433. [CrossRef]
16. Jakobsone, G.; Stenvik, A.; Sandvik, L.; Espeland, L. Three-year follow-up of bimaxillary surgery to correct skeletal Class III malocclusion: Stability and risk factors for relapse. *Am. J. Orthod. Dentofac. Orthop.* **2011**, *139*, 80–89. [CrossRef]
17. Rana, T.K.; Phogat, M.; Sharma, T.; Prasad, N.; Singh, S. Management of gingival recession associated with orthodontic treatment: A case report. *J. Clin. Diagn. Res.* **2014**, *8*, ZD05. [CrossRef]
18. Zimmer, B.; Seifi-Shirvandeh, N. Changes in gingival recession related to orthodontic treatment of traumatic deep bites in adults. *J. Orofac. Orthop.* **2007**, *68*, 232–244. [CrossRef]
19. Joss, C.U.; Vassalli, I.M. Stability after bilateral sagittal split osteotomy advancement surgery with rigid internal fixation: A systematic review. *J. Oral Maxillofac. Surg.* **2009**, *67*, 301–313. [CrossRef]
20. Lin, H.H.; Lonic, D.; Lo, L.J. 3D printing in orthognathic surgery—A literature review. *J. Formos Med. Assoc.* **2018**, *117*, 547–558. [CrossRef]
21. Hong, M.; Kim, I.; Cho, J.H.; Kang, K.H.; Kim, M.; Kim, S.J.; Kim, Y.J.; Sung, S.J.; Kim, Y.H.; Lim, S.H.; et al. Accuracy of artificial intelligence-assisted landmark identification in serial lateral cephalograms of Class III patients who underwent orthodontic treatment and two-jaw orthognathic surgery. *Korean J. Orthod.* **2022**, *52*, 287–297. [CrossRef] [PubMed]

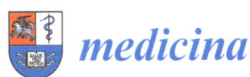

Case Report

Diagnostic Mock-Up as a Surgical Reduction Guide for Crown Lengthening: Technique Description and Case Report

Carlos A. Jurado [1], Venkata Parachuru [1,*], Jose Villalobos Tinoco [2], Gerardo Guzman-Perez [3], Akimasa Tsujimoto [4,5], Ramya Javvadi [6] and Kelvin I. Afrashtehfar [7,8]

[1] Woody L Hunt School of Dental Medicine, Texas Tech University Health Sciences Center El Paso, El Paso, TX 79905, USA
[2] Graduate Program in Periodontics, School of Dentistry, National University of Rosario, Rosario S2000CGK, Argentina
[3] Private Practice, Uriangato, Guanajuato 36260, Mexico
[4] Department of Operative Dentistry, College of Dentistry and Dental Clinics, The University of Iowa, Iowa City, IA 52242, USA
[5] Department of General Dentistry, School of Dentistry, Creighton University, Omaha, NE 68102, USA
[6] Oasis Dental, El Paso, TX 79905, USA
[7] Evidence-Based Practice Unit, Clinical Sciences Department, College of Dentistry, Ajman University, Ajman City P.O. Box 346, United Arab Emirates
[8] Department of Reconstructive Dentistry and Gerodontology, School of Dental Medicine, University of Bern, CH-3010 Berne, Switzerland
* Correspondence: venkata.parachuru@ttuhsc.edu

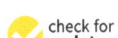

Citation: Jurado, C.A.; Parachuru, V.; Villalobos Tinoco, J.; Guzman-Perez, G.; Tsujimoto, A.; Javvadi, R.; Afrashtehfar, K.I. Diagnostic Mock-Up as a Surgical Reduction Guide for Crown Lengthening: Technique Description and Case Report. *Medicina* 2022, 58, 1360. https://doi.org/10.3390/medicina58101360

Academic Editors: Giuseppe Minervini and Stefania Moccia

Received: 30 August 2022
Accepted: 25 September 2022
Published: 28 September 2022

Publisher's Note: MDPI stays neutral with regard to jurisdictional claims in published maps and institutional affiliations.

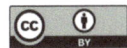

Copyright: © 2022 by the authors. Licensee MDPI, Basel, Switzerland. This article is an open access article distributed under the terms and conditions of the Creative Commons Attribution (CC BY) license (https://creativecommons.org/licenses/by/4.0/).

Abstract: *Background and Objectives:* The report describes a technique using a diagnostic mock-up as a crown-lengthening surgical guide to improve the gingival architecture. *Materials and Methods:* The patient's primary concern was improving her smile due to her "gummy smile" and short clinical crowns. After clinical evaluation, surgical crown lengthening accompanied by maxillary central full-coverage single-unit prostheses and lateral incisor veneers was recommended. The diagnostic mock-up was placed in the patient's maxillary anterior region and used as a soft tissue reduction guide for the gingivectomy. Once the planned gingival architecture was achieved, a flap was reflected to proceed with ostectomy in order to obtain an appropriate alveolar bone crest level using the overlay. After six months, all-ceramic crowns and porcelain veneers were provided as permanent restorations. *Results:* A diagnostic mock-up fabricated with a putty guide directly from the diagnostic wax-up can be an adequate surgical guide for crown-lengthening procedures. The diagnostic wax-up was used to fabricate the diagnostic mock-up. These results suggested that it can be used as a crown-lengthening surgical guide to modify the gingival architecture. Several advantages of the overlay used in the aesthetic complex case include: (1) providing a preview of potential restorative outcomes, (2) allowing for the appropriate positioning of gingival margins and the desired alveolar bone crest level for the crown-lengthening procedure, and (3) serving as a provisional restoration after surgery. *Conclusions:* The use of a diagnostic mock-up, which was based on a diagnostic wax-up, as the surgical guide resulted in successful crown lengthening and provisional restorations. Thus, a diagnostic overlay can be a viable option as a surgical guide for crown lengthening.

Keywords: crowns; aesthetic dentistry; mock-up; wax-up; periodontal plastic surgery

1. Introduction

The gingival architecture surrounding natural teeth or dental implants is an important component of aesthetics in the anterior region [1–3]. When the natural dentition lacks symmetry or has poor gingival architecture, these conditions can markedly alter the harmony of the dentition [4]. In recent years, it has become common for patients to have high aesthetic demands, going beyond a simple desire for a smile makeover [5–8]. Thus, clinicians must aim for an optimal gingival architecture during treatment [9]. Crown lengthening can be used in several clinical situations, such as excessive gingival display or a "gummy smile", teeth with an inadequate amount of tooth structure, or short clinical restorations [10]. In these cases, crown lengthening can re-establish the gingival architecture and enhance the restorative outcome.

Before initiating restorative treatment with crown lengthening, the patient's aesthetic concerns and expectations should be evaluated in detail. A diagnostic wax-up representing the desired outcome can be completed. Then, an intraoral diagnostic overlay can be fabricated to provide the patient and clinician with a tactile evaluation of the proposed treatment [11]. In addition, excellent communication between the surgeon and the restorative dentist is necessary to achieve the desired harmonious gingival architecture, especially in patients with high aesthetic demands [6,12–14]. Based on the diagnostic evaluations made by the restorative dentist, the surgeon can re-establish the soft and hard tissues to relocate the margins and alveolar crest and achieve periodontal health and an aesthetically pleasing gingival architecture.

Generally, a vacuum-formed surgical guide for crown lengthening is made from a duplicated cast from the diagnostic wax-up to establish the desired gingival architecture and alveolar bone crest level [15]. However, very few reports using a diagnostic overlay fabricated using a temporary bis-acrylic resin with a putty guide directly from the wax-up as a surgical guide for crown-lengthening procedures are available in the literature [16]. This case report aims to describe a technique wherein a diagnostic overlay can be used as a crown-lengthening surgical guide to help a surgeon achieve optimal gingival architecture.

2. Materials and Methods

A 30-year-old female patient presented to the clinic with the chief complaint of wanting to improve her smile (Figure 1). The patient had received ceramic restorations made from lithium disilicate on her central incisors two years ago. However, she disliked the results and was looking for a second opinion in an effort to improve her smile. After a detailed clinical evaluation, the patient was diagnosed with an excessive gingival display of Type IB (altered active eruption), non-ideal gingival contours, altered passive eruption of the maxillary central incisors, and incisal wear of teeth #7 and #11. She was offered the following treatment plan: (1) a crown-lengthening procedure to improve the gingival architecture, (2) replacement of the two crowns on the maxillary central incisors, (3) veneers on both lateral incisors, and (4) an incisal resin composite restoration on the left maxillary canine.

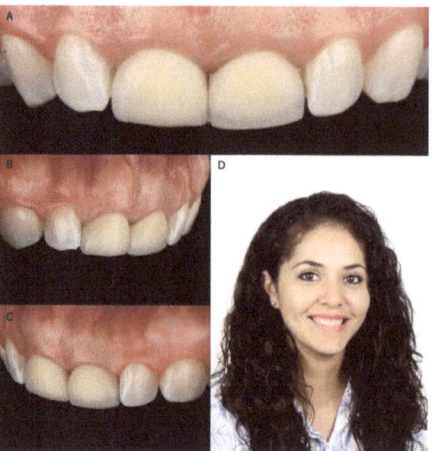

Figure 1. Initial scenario: (**A**) Intraoral frontal view; (**B**) Intraoral right-side view; (**C**) Intraoral left-side view; (**D**) Headshot of face smiling.

Diagnostic casts were made, and a wax-up (Wax GEO Classic, Renfert, Hilzingen, Germany) was fabricated to generate a harmonious smile according to the patient's wishes. After showing the patient the diagnostic wax-up, a diagnostic overlay was made with temporary bis-acrylic resin (Structur Premium, VOCO, Cuxhaven, Germany). The patient consented to the treatment after approving the diagnostic wax-up and overlay. Rubber dam isolation (Nic Tone Dental Dam, MDC Dental, Guadalajara, Mexico) was placed, and the existing ceramic restorations on the central incisors were sectioned with a diamond bur (Conical End 850, Jota AG, Rüthi, Switzerland) and removed (Figure 2).

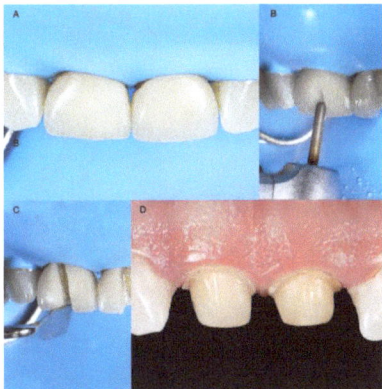

Figure 2. Crown prostheses removal: (**A**) Rubber dam isolation; (**B**) Initial channel in buccal surface; (**C**) Use of hand instrument for wedging; (**D**) Abutment assessment.

The diagnostic overlay was placed over the teeth to guide the desired contour through gingivoplasty with an electrosurgical unit (Sensimatic 700SE Electrosurge, Parkell, Edgewood, NY, USA) (Figures 3 and 4).

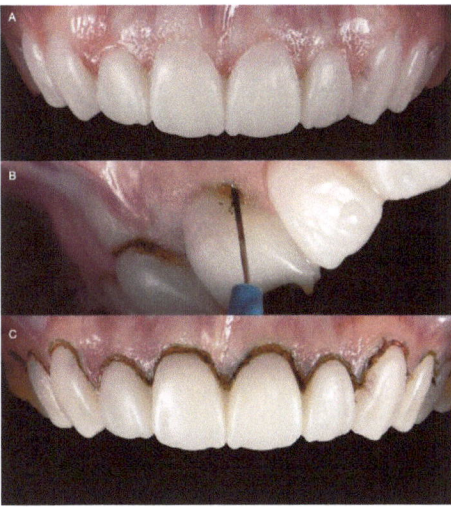

Figure 3. Diagnostic overlay and tissue recontour: (**A**) Placement of the diagnostic overlay intraorally; (**B**) Gingivoplasty with an electrosurgical unit; (**C**) Finishing the contouring with the laser.

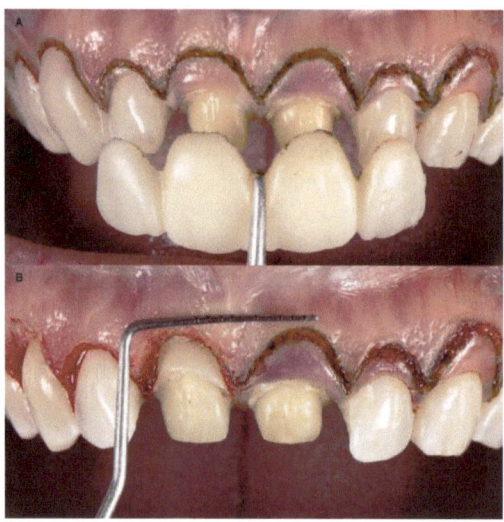

Figure 4. Diagnostic overlay removal and evaluation: (**A**) Removal of the diagnostic overlay; (**B**) Gingival tissue architecture evaluation.

After the new gingival architecture was achieved, buccal flap reflection provided a clear view for the surgeon performing the ostectomy. Flap reflection revealed the proper position of the osseous crest relative to the cemento-enamel junction (CEJ), which, in this case, was at the CEJ (Figure 5). An ostectomy procedure was performed using the diagnostic overlay as a guide to remove the alveolar bone. The crown-lengthening procedure was conducted within the recommended range of the Root/Crown (R/C) ratio: (1) R/C ratio of at least 1/1.5 for an abutment, and (2) R/C ratio of at least 1/1 for a crown.

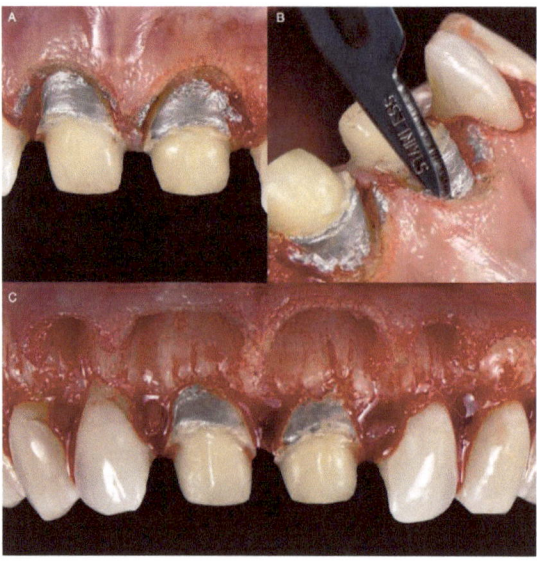

Figure 5. Crown-lengthening procedure: (**A**) Gingivectomy completed; (**B**) Initiation of flap; (**C**) Flap reflation.

The flap was repositioned (Figure 6), crown margins were refined, and provisional restorations (adjusted diagnostic overlay) were placed on the central incisors with temporary resin luting cement.

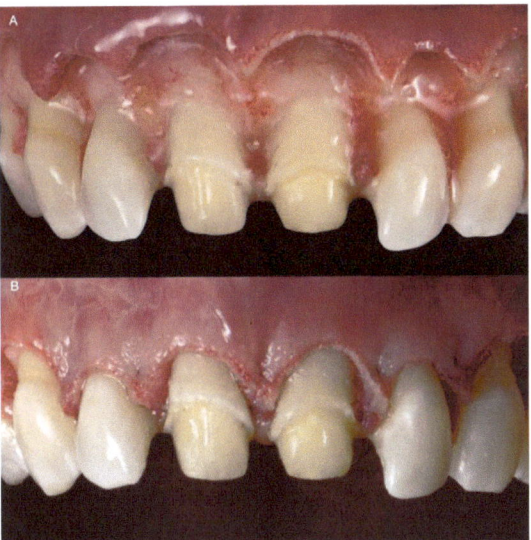

Figure 6. Flap release and reposition: (**A**) Flap release; (**B**) Flap reposition after suturing.

After six months, veneer preparations were performed on lateral incisors to allow for the proper healing of the periodontal complex (Figure 7), and a final impression was made with polyvinyl siloxane impression material (Virtual 380, Ivoclar Vivadent, Schaan, Liechtenstein).

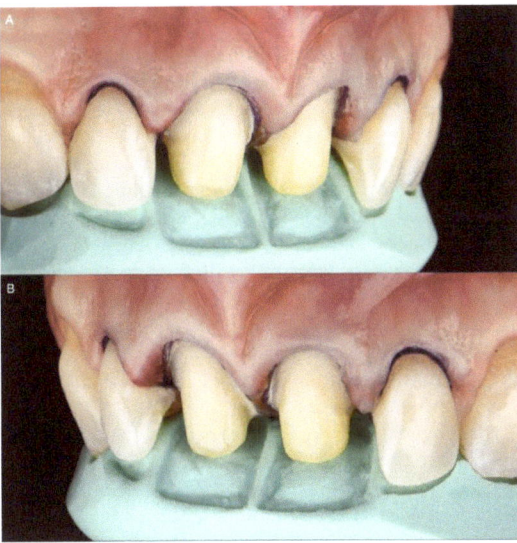

Figure 7. Lateral incisors veneer preparations: (**A**) Right side of the lateral veneer preparation with the reduction guide; (**B**) Left side of the lateral veneer preparation with the reduction guide.

The final master cast was fabricated with type IV stone (Fujirock, GC, Tokyo, Japan). Restorations, fabricated following the contours of the diagnostic wax-up, were made of refractory feldspathic porcelain (Noritake Super Porcelain EX-3, Kuraray Noritake Dental, Tokyo, Japan) for the veneers and full-coverage crowns (Figure 8).

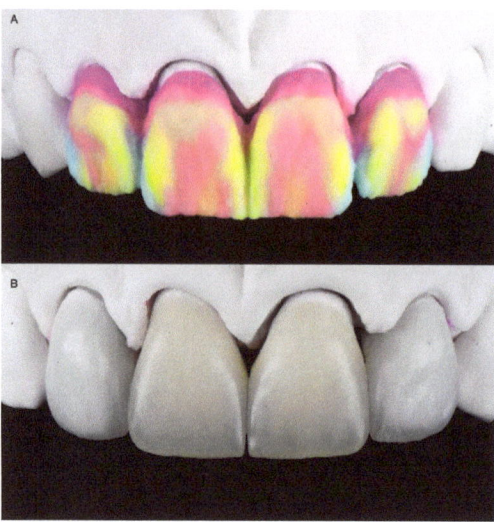

Figure 8. Feldspathic veneers on the master cast: (**A**) Porcelain build-up before baking; (**B**) Definitive restorations.

A try-in of the final ceramic restorations was performed to evaluate the fit and contours, and the patient approved the final appearance. For bonding the ceramic restorations, isolation was provided via rubber dam placement. The teeth were air-abraded with 20-micron aluminum oxide particles (AquaCare Aluminium Oxide Air Abrasion Powder, Velopex, London, UK). The teeth receiving veneers were surface treated with 37% phosphoric acid (Total Etch, Ivoclar Vivadent, Schaan, Liechtenstein) for 15 s and then rinsed with water. A primer (Syntac Primer, Ivoclar Vivadent, Schaan, Liechtenstein) was applied, and any excess was gently removed with air. Adhesive (Syntac Adhesive, Ivoclar Vivadent, Schaan, Liechtenstein) was applied, and any excess was removed with air according to the manufacturer's recommendations. The intaglio surfaces of the ceramic restorations were etched with 5% hydrofluoric acid (IPS Ceramic Etching Gel, Ivoclar Vivadent, Schaan, Liechtenstein) for 60 s, and Monobond Plus (Ivoclar Vivadent, Schaan, Liechtenstein) was applied to the etched surfaces. Light-cure resin luting cement (Variolink Esthetic LC, Ivoclar Vivadent, Schaan, Liechtenstein) was applied to the veneers, and they were seated. Excess cement was removed, and the restorations were cured using an LED light-curing unit (VALO Cordless, Ultradent, South Jordan, UT, USA) on each surface (facial, palatal, mesial, and distal) for 20 s. The crowns were cemented with a dual-cure resin luting cement (Panavia V5, Kuraray Noritake Dental, Tokyo, Japan) and light-cured, followed by applying appropriate pre-treatments to the teeth and ceramic restorations.

After adjusting the occlusion as needed, the restorations were finalized with polishing points (Dialite Feather Lite, Brasseler USA Dental, Savannah, GA, USA) and polishing paste (Dialite Intra-Oral Polishing Paste, Brasseler USA Dental, Savannah, GA, USA). The incisal wear was addressed as follows. The maxillary left canine received 37% phosphoric acid etching gel for 15 s, and an adhesive (Tetric N-Bond Universal, Ivoclar Vivadent, Schaan, Liechtenstein) was applied for 20 s, gently air-thinned, and light-cured for 20 s. A nano-hybrid flowable composite resin (Tetric N-Flow, Shade A1, Ivoclar Vivadent, Schaan, Liechtenstein) was placed on the incisal edge and light-cured for 30 s. The resin composite restoration was re-shaped on the incisal edge with a fine diamond bur (Diamond bur FG 859012, Jota AG, Rüthi, Switzerland). The restoration was final-polished with green and grey composite polishers (Composite Diamond Polisher, Jota AG, Ruthi, Switzerland) using a polishing paste (Diamond Polish Mint, Ultradent, South Jordan, UT, USA) and a polishing brush (Jiffy Composite Polishing Brush, Ultradent, South Jordan, UT, USA). The patient approved of the shape and size of the final restorations, and the treatment fulfilled her aesthetic desire (Figure 9).

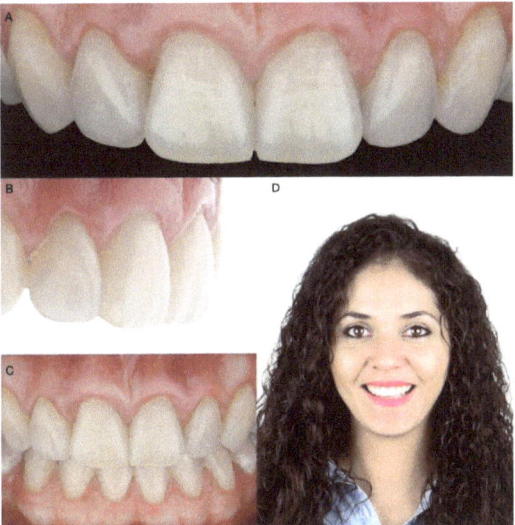

Figure 9. Final restorations: (**A**) Frontal view; (**B**) Lateral view; (**C**) Frontal in occlusion; (**D**) Final smile.

An occlusal night guard was also provided to prevent damage to the final restorations. At the patient's five-year follow-up, she was fascinated with the clinical outcome (Figure 10).

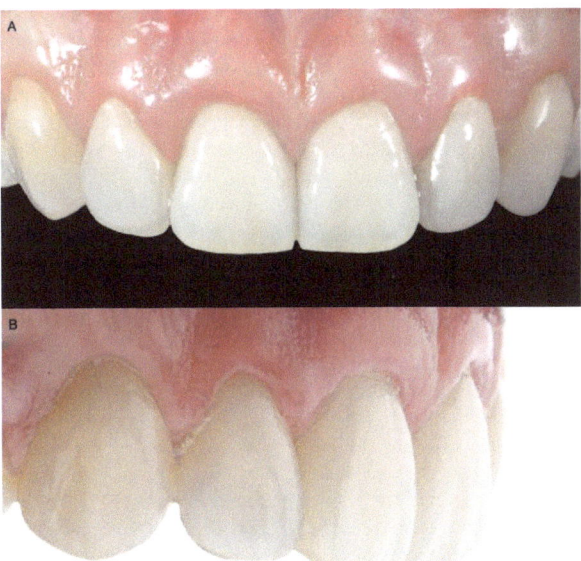

Figure 10. Five-year follow-up: (**A**) Frontal view; (**B**) Lateral view.

3. Discussion

Despite the lack of clinical case reports, evidence from this case suggests that a diagnostic overlay for crown lengthening allows outcomes to be predictable for follow-up periods of at least five years. These findings are essential for the anterior region, where soft tissue changes may compromise treatment outcomes without a vacuum-formed surgical guide. Typically, the restorative process of crown lengthening using a vacuum-formed surgical guide needs both provisional restorations and a surgical guide. However, this clinical case shows that a diagnostic overlay can be used to confirm the proposed treatment plan with the patient and provide a two-for-one surgical guide and provisional restorations, thus reducing costs. Recently, a fully digital workflow for crown lengthening, using a single surgical guide, was reported [17–20]. However, this technique requires an intraoral scanner, 3D printer, and cone beam computed tomography (CBCT) scan, relying on many kinds of expertise in the digital workflow. Most clinicians are still not familiar with digital workflow [21], and the additional time and costs required before surgery are disincentives for its introduction.

In contrast, it is simpler to use conventional methods to prepare the soft and hard tissues based on a diagnostic overlay when it is placed in the mouth if the clinician knows the appropriate distances to the alveolar bone crest level from the gingival margins. Most clinicians know that the distance from the alveolar crest to the gingival margin on the facial and palatal aspects is in the range of 3 mm, while the distance from the alveolar crest to the gingival margin on the interproximal aspect is about 5 mm due to the height of the interproximal papilla [22]. Thus, it appears easier to determine the desired alveolar bone crest level using only a diagnostic overlay. This would be a simplified approach to performing crown lengthening without a traditional surgical guide.

In the present case, the use of a diagnostic overlay, based on the diagnostic wax-up, was an easy and powerful tool for the diagnostic planning of a treatment with high aesthetic demands. Given this outcome, the placement of a diagnostic overlay could be adopted as a routine protocol by clinicians, as it provides a high predictability of outcomes in aesthetically complex cases. Furthermore, the overlay can also be considered as a useful promotional tool for acquiring the patient approval of the treatment plan presented by the dental professional. In this case report, the diagnostic overlay was made based on the patient's requests, and after it was placed in her mouth, the patient immediately indicated that she liked the result and requested the treatment.

Soft tissue crown lengthening is performed with gingivoplasty using a scalpel, an electrosurgical unit, a radiosurgical unit, or a laser [23]. If the new gingival margin position is near the underlying bone, a flap should be reflected for an ostectomy to re-establish an adequate biologic width. In the current case, the diagnostic overlay was placed and guided the use of the electrosurgical unit for the external gingivoplasty. A flap was reflected to recontour hard tissues and re-establish the biologic width of 3 mm. Compared with a traditional scalpel, an electrosurgical unit allows the clinician to cut, ablate, and re-shape soft tissues with no resulting bleeding and no need for suturing. The diagnostic overlay was an excellent guide.

Another consideration when performing crown lengthening is the healing period. The periodontal phenotype is a crucial factor, especially in aesthetic outcomes, because it impacts both the healing and final position of the gingival margin [24]. Research suggests that a thin biotype has a thickness of 1.5 mm or less, and a thick biotype has a thickness of 2.0 mm or more. Patients with a thin biotype may experience more gingival recession than those with a thick one [25]. The patient in this case had a thick biotype; thus, the likelihood of gingival recession was minimal. When considering aesthetic outcomes during this kind of treatment, the ideal healing time ranges from six weeks to six months, and a longer time may be required for patients with a thin biotype [26,27]. In the present case, the clinicians decided to wait six months before finalizing the ceramic restorations. This period provided adequate time for tissue healing and resulted in a stable gingival margin position for a pleasing aesthetic result. The diagnostic overlay was used as the provisional restoration and performed well during this time.

A limitation of this traditional workflow can happen if the diagnostic wax-up is excessive; then, it will create bulky restorations. In order to prevent this, the lip support is evaluated by the clinician and patient during the mock-up. Thus, the diagnostic overlay is necessary to demonstrate the likely outcome to the patient, and, as a provisional restoration during the healing of the hard and soft tissue, it can also be used as the surgical guide while attaining good aesthetic results. This suggests that a separate surgical guide may be unnecessary in many cases, and the assumed additional precision resulting from the use of a dedicated surgical guide may similarly be unnecessary. A simplified procedure using the diagnostic overlay may achieve all treatment goals at a lower cost.

4. Conclusions

The case presented in this clinical report shows that using a diagnostic overlay, which was based on a diagnostic wax-up, as the surgical guide resulted in successful crown lengthening. These results suggest that a diagnostic overlay may be viable for surgically guiding crown lengthening in aesthetically complex cases.

Author Contributions: Conceptualization, C.A.J. and J.V.T.; methodology, V.P.; investigation, G.G.-P.; resources, A.T. and R.J.; data curation, K.I.A.; writing—original draft preparation, C.A.J.; writing—review and editing, A.T. and K.I.A. All authors have read and agreed to the published version of the manuscript.

Funding: This research received no external funding.

Institutional Review Board Statement: The study was conducted in accordance with the Declaration of Helsinki, and approved by the Institutional Review Board of Cenro de Estudios Odontologicos de Queretaro (protocol code XXXDENT/0430121-16 and 11/01/2016)." for studies involving humans.

Informed Consent Statement: Written informed consent has been obtained from the patient to publish this paper.

Data Availability Statement: Not applicable.

Acknowledgments: K. I. Afrashtehfar thanks the Universität Bern for partially supporting the open-access publication of this work.

Conflicts of Interest: The authors declare no conflict of interest.

References

1. Jurado, C.A.; Tinoco, J.V.; Tsujimoto, A.; Barkmeier, W.; Fischer, N.; Markham, M. Clear matrix use for composite resin core fabrication. *Int. J. Esthet. Dent.* **2020**, *15*, 108–117. [PubMed]
2. Afrashtehfar, K.I.; Assery, M.K.A.; Bryant, S.R. Aesthetic Parameters and patient-perspective assessment tools for maxillary anterior single implants. *Int. J. Dent.* **2021**, *2021*, 6684028. [CrossRef] [PubMed]
3. Del Monte, S.; Afrashtehfar, K.I.; Emami, E.; Abi Nader, S.; Tamimi, F. Lay preferences for dentogingival esthetic parameters: A systematic review. *J. Prosthet. Dent.* **2017**, *118*, 717–724. [CrossRef] [PubMed]
4. Miranda, M.E.; Olivieri, K.A.; Rigolin, F.J.; de Vasconcellos, A.A. Esthetic challenges in rehabilitating the anterior maxilla: A case report. *Oper. Dent.* **2016**, *41*, 2–7. [CrossRef] [PubMed]
5. Afrashtehfar, K.I.; Assery, M.K. Five considerations in cosmetic and esthetic dentistry. *J. New Jersey Dent. Assoc.* **2014**, *85*, 14–15.
6. Afrashtehfar, K.I.; Assery, M.K.A.; Bryant, S.R. Patient Satisfaction in Medicine and Dentistry. *Int. J. Dent.* **2020**, *2020*, 6621848. [CrossRef]
7. Alikhasi, M.; Yousefi, P.; Afrashtehfar, K.I. Smile Design: Mechanical Considerations. *Dent. Clin. North Am.* **2022**, *66*, 477–487. [CrossRef]
8. Afrashtehfar, K.I.; Bryant, S.R. Understanding the lived experience of north american dental patients with a single-tooth implant in the upper front region of the mouth: Protocol for a qualitative Study. *JMIR Res. Protoc.* **2021**, *10*, e25767. [CrossRef]
9. Jurado, C.A.; Tsujimoto, A.; Guzman, L.G.; Fischer, N.G.; Markham, M.D.; Barkmeier, W.W.; Latta, M.A. Implant therapy with monolithic translucent zirconia restorations in the esthetic zone. *Gen. Dent.* **2020**, *68*, 46–49.
10. Marzadori, M.; Stefanini, M.; Sangiorgi, M.; Mounssif, I.; Monaco, C.; Zucchelli, G. Crown lengthening and restorative procedures in the esthetic zone. *Periodontol. 2000* **2018**, *77*, 84–92. [CrossRef]
11. Simon, H.; Magne, P. Clinically based diagnostic wax-up for optimal esthetics: The diagnostic mock-up. *J. Calif. Dent. Assoc.* **2008**, *36*, 355–362. [PubMed]

12. Jurado, C.; Watanabe, H.; Tinoco, J.V.; Valenzuela, H.U.; Perez, G.G.; Tsujimoto, A. A conservative approach to ceramic veneers: A case report. *Oper. Dent.* **2020**, *45*, 229–234. [CrossRef] [PubMed]
13. Afrashtehfar, K.I.; Igarashi, K.; Bryant, S.R. Canadian Dental Patients with a Single-Unit Implant-Supported Restoration in the Aesthetic Region of the Mouth: Qualitative and Quantitative Patient-Reported Outcome Measures (PROMs). *Data* **2021**, *6*, 90. [CrossRef]
14. Afrashtehfar, K.I. Conventional free-hand, dynamic navigation and static guided implant surgery produce similar short-term patient-reported outcome measures and experiences. *Evid.-Based Dent.* **2021**, *22*, 143–145. [CrossRef]
15. Longo, E.; Frosecchi, M.; Marradi, L.; Signore, A.; de Angelis, N. Guided periodontal surgery: A novel approach for the treatment of gummy smile. A case report. *Int. J. Esthet. Dent.* **2019**, *14*, 384–392.
16. Gurrea, J.; Bruguera, A. Wax-up and mock-up. A guide for anterior periodontal and restorative treatments. *Int. J. Esthet. Dent.* **2014**, *9*, 146–162. [PubMed]
17. Liu, X.; Yu, J.; Zhou, J.; Tan, J. A digitally guided dual technique for both gingival and bone resection during crown lengthening surgery. *J. Prosthet. Dent.* **2018**, *119*, 345–349. [CrossRef]
18. Kongkiatkamon, S.; Rokaya, D. Full digital workflow in the esthetic dental restoration. *Case Rep Dent.* **2022**, *2022*, 8836068. [CrossRef]
19. Mendoza-Azpur, G.; Cornejo, H.; Villanueva, M.; Alva, R.; Barbisan de Souza, A. Periodontal plastic surgery for esthetic crown lengthening by using data merging and a CAD-CAM surgical guide. *J. Prosthet. Dent.* **2022**, *127*, 556–559. [CrossRef]
20. Jurado, C.A.; Tsujimoto, A.; Watanabe, H.; Villalobos-Tinoco, J.; Garaicoa, J.L.; Markham, M.D.; Barkmeier, W.W.; Latta, M.A. Chair-side CAD/CAM fabrication of a single-retainer resin bonded fixed dental prosthesis: A case report. *Restor. Dent. Endod.* **2020**, *45*, e15. [CrossRef]
21. Alazmi, S.O. Three dimensional digitally designed surgical guides in esthetic crown lengthening: A clinical case report with 12 months follow up. *Clin. Cosmet Investig. Dent.* **2022**, *14*, 55–59. [CrossRef] [PubMed]
22. Takei, H.H.; Bevilacqua, F.; Cooney, J. Surgical crown lengthening of the maxillary anterior dentition: Aesthetic considerations. *Pract. Periodontics Aesthetic Dent.* **1999**, *11*, 639–644.
23. Hempton, T.J.; Dominici, J.T. Contemporary crown-lengthening therapy: A review. *J. Am. Dent. Assoc.* **2010**, *141*, 647–655. [CrossRef] [PubMed]
24. Pontoriero, R.; Carnevale, G. Surgical crown lengthening: A 12-month clinical wound healing study. *J. Periodontol.* **2001**, *72*, 841–848. [CrossRef]
25. Kois, J.C. Altering gingival levels: The restorative connection part I: Biologic variables. *J. Esthet. Restor. Dent.* **1994**, *6*, 3–7. [CrossRef]
26. Deas, D.E.; Moritz, A.J.; McDonnell, H.T.; Powell, C.A.; Mealey, B. Osseous surgery for crown lengthening: A 6-month clinical study. *J. Periodontol.* **2004**, *75*, 1288–1294. [CrossRef] [PubMed]
27. Afrashtehfar, K.I.; Moshaverinia, A. Five things to know about regenerative periodontal therapies in dental medicine. *J. New Jersey Dent. Assoc.* **2015**, *86*, 12–13.

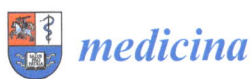

Systematic Review

Misfit of Implant-Supported Zirconia (Y-TZP) CAD-CAM Framework Compared to Non-Zirconia Frameworks: A Systematic Review

Hussain D. Alsayed

Prosthetic Dental Science Department, College of Dentistry, King Saud University, Riyadh 60169, Saudi Arabia; halsayed@ksu.edu.sa; Fax: +966-1467-8639

Abstract: *Objective*: The aim of the study was to systematically review the overall outcomes of studies comparing the misfit of yttria-stabilized zirconia (Y-TZP) CAD-CAM implant-supported frameworks with frameworks fabricated with other materials and techniques. *Methods*: An electronic literature search of English literature was performed using Google Scholar, Scopus, Web of Science, MEDLINE (OVID), EMBASE, and PubMed, using predetermined inclusion criteria. Specific terms were utilized in conducting a search from the inception of the respective database up to May 2022. After the search strategy was applied, the data were extracted and the results were analyzed. The focused question was: Is the misfit of the implant-supported zirconia CAD-CAM framework lower than that of non-Y-TZP implant-supported fixed restorations? *Results*: Eleven articles were included for qualitative assessment and critical appraisal in this review. In the included studies, Y-TZP CAD-CAM implant-supported frameworks were compared to Titanium (Ti), Ni-Cr, Co-Cr, PEEK and high-density polymer, and cast and CAD-CAM frameworks. The studies used scanning electron microscopy, one-screw tests, digital or optical microscopy, 3D virtual assessment, and replica techniques for analyzing the misfit of frameworks. Six studies showed comparable misfits among the Y-TZP CAD-CAM frameworks and the controls. Three studies showed higher misfits for the Y-TZP CAD-CAM frameworks, whereas two studies reported lower misfits for Y-TZP CAD-CAM implant frameworks compared to controls. *Conclusion*: Y-TZP CAD-CAM implant-supported frameworks have comparable misfits to other implant-supported frameworks. However, due to heterogeneity in the methodologies of the included studies, the overall numerical misfit of the frameworks assessed in the reviewed studies is debatable

Keywords: systematic review; misfit; implant frameworks; Zirconium; metal alloys

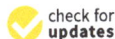

Citation: Alsayed, H.D. Misfit of Implant-Supported Zirconia (Y-TZP) CAD-CAM Framework Compared to Non-Zirconia Frameworks: A Systematic Review. *Medicina* **2022**, *58*, 1347. https://doi.org/10.3390/medicina58101347

Academic Editors: Stefania Moccia and Giuseppe Minervini

Received: 7 September 2022
Accepted: 19 September 2022
Published: 25 September 2022

Publisher's Note: MDPI stays neutral with regard to jurisdictional claims in published maps and institutional affiliations.

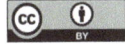

Copyright: © 2022 by the author. Licensee MDPI, Basel, Switzerland. This article is an open access article distributed under the terms and conditions of the Creative Commons Attribution (CC BY) license (https://creativecommons.org/licenses/by/4.0/).

1. Introduction

Dental implants are surgically placed devices that have direct contact with the alveolar bone [1,2]. In addition to supporting single-tooth restorations, they are also used to support and retain prostheses for the restoration of partially or completely edentulous patients [3]. Implant-supported removable and fixed prostheses possess significant advantages over conventional prostheses. In addition to offering superior support [4] and stability [5], implant-supported prostheses preserve residual bone [6] and are esthetically pleasing [7]. It has been estimated that the 5-year success-rate of implant-supported prostheses is as high as 95% [8,9].

Frameworks of implant-supported dentures have conventionally been constructed from cast metals [10]. However, cast implant-supported prostheses have several drawbacks. The clinical phase of these prostheses includes taking impressions which may become easily distorted and damaged during or after the impression-taking process [11]. In addition, the cast metal alloys may undergo distortion during the casting process, resulting in a misfit of up to 450 µm [12,13]. Moreover, the wax pattern of the cast framework may also undergo dimensional changes, resulting in a misfit of the prosthesis [14]. Ideally, a framework should fit passively by not exerting biologically detrimental forces on the supportive teeth, the supportive tissues, and the framework [15]. Furthermore, there should be no gap between the margins of the framework and the supportive tissues and teeth. The misfit is measured by evaluating the distance between the final restoration and the corresponding fitting surfaces. Although the misfit of cast prostheses may be reduced by sectioning and then re-connecting the framework, the mechanical properties of the cast metal may be diminished, which can lead to fractures of the prostheses [16]. Additionally, misfit causes micro-gaps between the implant and the framework. This gap harbors bacteria which may cause infection of the peri-implant tissues [17]. A misfitting framework can also lead to the loosening or even the fracture of prosthetic implant screws [18]. Eventually, long-standing misfit results in the instability of the framework, inducing failure of the dental implants [19].

Over the last few years, prostheses designed and constructed via computer-aided design and computer-aided manufacturing (CAD-CAM) have gained popularity [20]. Briefly, the CAD-CAM process involves three-dimensional (3D) digital scanning of the teeth and related structures in the oral cavity to produce a virtual 3D model. The virtual model is then processed by a computer connected to a milling machine that constructs the prostheses. The milling system produces a prosthesis from a block of homogenous material such as Titanium (Ti) or yttria-stabilized zirconia (Y-TZP) [21]. Studies have indicated that CAD-CAM-constructed prostheses have a significantly lower misfit compared to cast frameworks [22]. There are two types of CAD-CAM systems: additive and subtractive [20]. Additive manufacturing focuses on building appliances and objects layer by layer, while subtractive systems remove material from pre-formed blocks into appliances. Subtractive manufacturing has seen more clinical use than additive manufacturing; however, the latter has gained popularity in the last few years [20]. A recent systematic review of in vitro and clinical studies indicated that CAD-CAM frameworks have significantly better fits compared to cast frameworks [23].

Y-TZP has been a popular material for the construction of CAD-CAM implant-supported frameworks over the last decade, and its market-share is expected to double by 2024 [24]. Indeed, Y-TZP frameworks exhibit exceptional strength and fracture toughness [25]. Clinical studies suggest that Y-TZP frameworks remain stable for more than 5 years post-insertion [26]. Moreover, due to its higher color stability and the biocompatibility and accuracy of CAD-CAM fabrication, Y-TZP presents an attractive alternative to metal alloys from the patients' perspective [27]. Several in vitro studies have compared the fit (or misfit) of metal alloys and Ti and polymer frameworks with that of Y-TZP CAD-CAM frameworks [28–38]. In a study by Abduo et al., the vertical misfits for Y-TZP and Ti CAD-CAM frameworks were comparable [28]. By contrast, in a study by de Rio Silva et al., Ti CAD-CAM frameworks had a lower misfit compared to Y-TZP frameworks [38]. A controversy exists among the studies reporting the misfit of Y-TZP CAD-CAM with other materials and techniques. So, the aim was to systematically review the overall outcomes of studies comparing the misfit of Y-TZP CAD-CAM implant-supported frameworks with frameworks fabricated with other materials and techniques. I hypothesize that, overall, the misfit of Y-TZP CAD-CAM frameworks will be lower compared to that of frameworks fabricated with other materials.

2. Materials and Methods

2.1. Focused Question

Following the Participants, Intervention, Control, and Outcomes principal described in the Preferred Reporting Items in Systematic Reviews and Meta-Analysis (PRISMA) statement [39], the following focused question was constructed: 'Is the misfit of implant-supported Zirconia CAD-CAM frameworks lower than that of non-Y-TZP implant-supported fixed restorations?' (Participants: Patients or study casts; Intervention: Y-TZP CAD-CAM implant-supported dental prostheses; Controls: Non-Y-TZP-supported fixed restorations; Outcomes: Misfit).

2.2. Eligibility Criteria

Before conducting the literature search, eligibility criteria were decided on by the author. Prospective clinical studies, case reports and series, animal studies, and laboratory studies focusing on comparing the fit or misfit of CAD-CAM implant-supported Zirconia fixed restorations with other non-Y-TZP implant-supported restorations were included. Literature from inception to May 2022 was searched. Additionally, only articles in English were included. Studies not in the English language, systematic or literature reviews, and letters to the editor were excluded.

2.3. Literature Search

An electronic search using the keywords ((Zirconia) OR (Y-TZP) AND (Restoration or bridge or framework) AND ((computer-aided design OR CAD)) or (computer-aided manufacture) OR CAM)) AND (full arch OR partial OR complete) AND (control OR titanium OR resin OR cobalt chromium) AND (misfit OR gap OR adaptation) AND (implant)) was conducted on the following databases: PubMED/MEDLINE, ISI Web of Science/Knowledge, Scopus, Embase, and Google Scholar, including studies up to May 2022. Following the exclusion of the non-relevant articles on the basis of titles and abstracts, the full texts of studies appearing to meet the inclusion criteria were downloaded. Additionally, the reference lists of the full-text documents were scanned manually to look for relevant articles. Furthermore, a similar search was repeated using the same keywords on the clinical trial registers CONTROL and clinicaltrials.gov. The literature search was conducted by author (HA) interpedently, and any disagreements were solved by discussion with a statistician.

2.4. Data Extraction

Using predetermined items, the data from each study were extracted to construct tables. Briefly, the materials used to construct the dentures in the test and control groups (if any), the method of denture fabrication, the type of misfit (or fit) assessment employed, measurements of any other variables, and the qualitative outcomes of the studies were summarized in the first table. Summarized information on the implant or abutment system, the dimensions and positions of the dental implants, the type of implant-supported prostheses (fixed or removable, along with the number of units), the CAD-CAM fabrication system, and the numerical values of the misfit or fit was also prepared.

2.5. Quality Assessment

The overall quality of the studies and any bias present in the studies were assessed using a modified version of the 'Guidelines For Reporting Pre-Clinical In Vitro Studies On Dental Materials' developed by Mariano [40]. Briefly, in each study, the following items were assessed: an adequate abstract, introduction (background and objects), and methodology (replicability, reporting of adequate outcomes, a predetermined sample size, and details of any randomization, blinding, or concealment employed), adequate statistics, a mention of any limitations in the discussion, funding details, and, if any, the protocol of the study was accessible. A 15-point checklist was used to grade each study. Each study was assigned an overall quality of low (score: 0–5), medium (score: 6–10), or high (score: 11–15).

3. Results

3.1. Results of the Literature Search

The primary literature search resulted in 105 articles. 25 articles were eliminated on the basis of titles. Of the 80 articles, 66 articles were further excluded after the review of the abstracts and on the basis of relevance. Therefore, the full texts of 14 articles were downloaded to assess their eligibility for inclusion in this review. Three full-text articles were excluded because two of them were systematic reviews [41,42] and one did not include any controls to which to compare the misfit of the Y-TZP prosthesis [43]. Hence, 11 articles were included for qualitative assessment and critical appraisal in this review [28–38]. The study methodology is presented in Figure 1. The overall Kappa (intra-examiner reliability) score was calculated as 0.87.

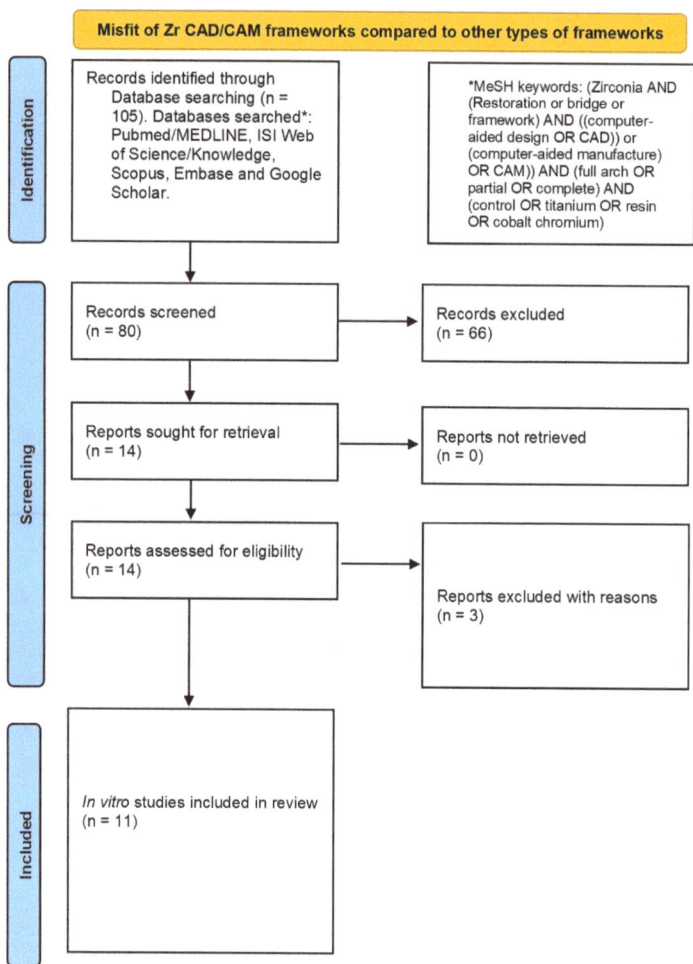

Figure 1. PRISMA flow diagram employed for the literature search.

3.2. General Characteristics

All studies included in this review were in vitro laboratory studies that compared the fit or misfit of Y-TZP CAD-CAM implant-supported frameworks with other materials or fabrication methods [28–38] (Table 1). In six studies, Ti CAD-CAM frameworks were included in the comparison groups [28,31,36–38]. In one study, cast Ni-Cr frameworks were included as a comparison [29], and Cast Co-Cr frameworks were compared with CAD-CAM Y-TZP in four studies [30–32,38]. In two studies, CAD-CAM was also used to construct Co-Cr frameworks as comparison groups [30,32], and in one study, mechanically scanned CAD-CAM Y-TZP frameworks were also tested [31]. CAD-CAM Y-TZP frameworks were compared with frameworks constructed from CAD-CAM polyetheretherketone (PEEK) and CAD-CAM resin composites in one study [33]. In one study, the effect of porcelain veneering on the misfit of Y-TZP and Ti CAD-CAM frameworks was assessed [34], and in another study, a CAD-CAM high-density polymer (HDP) framework was tested against CAD-CAM Y-TZP [35]. Copy-milled Y-TZP frameworks were constructed in three studies [29,38]. In addition to marginal or vertical misfit, four studies also compared cyclic fatigue [29], retention [33], loosening torque [37,38], and stress [38] between different frameworks.

Table 1. General characteristics and the overall outcomes of the studies included.

No.	Study	Groups (n = Number of Frameworks Constructed)		Method of Fabrication	Misfit Assessment	Other Assessed Variables	Overall Outcomes
		Test	Control				
1	Abduo et al. 2012 [28]	Y-TZP CAD-CAM (n = 5)	Ti CAD-CAM (n = 5)	Copy milling (subtractive)	Optical microscopy; Vertical passive fit	Strain	Vertical misfits for Y-TZP and Ti CAD-CAM groups were comparable. Passive misfit for Y-TZP CAD-CAM was significantly lower than that of Ti CAD-CAM. No significant difference in strain among both groups.
2	Zaghloul & Younis et al. 2013 [29]	Y-TZP CAD-CAM (n = 10) Y-TZP Copy Milling (n = 10)	Ni-Cr Cast (n = 10)	CAD-CAM Copy milling (subtractive)	Digital microscopy; Vertical marginal fit	Cyclic fatigue	Y-TZP CAD-CAM had the highest marginal misfit. No significant difference between Y-TZP copy milling and N-Cr cast frameworks.
3	de França et al. 2014 [30]	Y-TZP CAD-CAM (n = 4)	Co-Cr Cast (n = 8) Co-Cr CAD-CAM (n = 4)	CAD-CAM (milled/subtractive)	SEM; Vertical fit	None	All CAD-CAM frameworks had comparable misfits. CAD-CAM frameworks had significantly lower misfits than cast frameworks.
4	Katsoulis et al. 2014 [31]	Y-TZP CAD-CAM (n = 5)	Co-Cr Cast (n = 5) Y-TZP-M CAD-CAM (n = 5) Ti CAD/AM (n = 6)	CAD-CAM (subtractive/milling) Co-Cr cast	One-screw test, SEM; Vertical passive fit	None	No significant difference was observed for vertical misfit between Y-TZP and CAD-CAM, but both were significantly better than Co-Cr.
5	de Araújo et al. 2015 [32]	Group 1: Y-TZP CAD-CAM (n = 4)	Co-Cr cast (n = 4) Group 2: Co-Cr CAD-CAM (n = 4)	CAD-CAM, Cast (milled/subtractive)	SEM; Vertical passive fit	None	Co-Cr CAD-CAM had a significantly lower misfit than the Y-TZP CAD-CAM and Co-Cr Cast specimens. Y-TZP CAD-CAM had a better fit than the cast frameworks.
6	Ghodsi et al. 2018 [33]	Y-TZP CAD-CAM	PEEK CAD-CAM RC CAD-CAM	CAD-CAM (milled/subtractive)	Replica technique; Internal adaptation	Retention force	Y-TZP CAD-CAM had a significantly lower misfit than PEEK and RC. No difference between PEEK and RC misfits.
7	Yilmaz et al. 2018 [34]	Y-TZP CAD-CAM Before and after veneering	Ti CAD-CAM Before and after veneering	CAD-CAM (milled/subtractive)	3D fit (virtual assessment)	None	Y-TZP and Ti CAD-CAM frameworks before and after veneering were comparable. Significant effect of porcelain veneering on Y-TZP frameworks.
8	Yilmaz et al. 2018 [35]	Y-TZP CAD-CAM	HDP CAD-CAM Ti CAD-CAM	CAD-CAM (milled/subtractive)	Marginal misfit; One-screw test	None	HDP had a significantly lower misfit than the Y-TZP and Ti CAD-CAM specimens. No difference between Y-TZP and Ti misfits.
9	Al-Meraïkhi et al. 2018 [36]	Y-TZP CAD-CAM (n = 5)	Ti CAD-CAM (n = 5)	CAD-CAM (milled/subtractive)	Marginal misfit; One-screw test, CT scanning; Color mapping	None	No significant difference between the fits of the Y-TZP and Ti frameworks was observed.
10	da Cunha Fontoura et al. 2018 [37]	Y-TZP CAD-CAM (n = 5)	Ti CAD-CAM (n = 5)	CAD-CAM (milled/subtractrive)	Vertical misfit; SEM	Torque	No significant difference between the misfits of the Y-TZP and Ti frameworks.
11	Del Rio Silva et al. 2020 [38]	Y-TZP Copy-Milling (n = 5)	Ti CAD-CAM (n = 5) Co-Cr Cast (n = 5)	Co-Cr cast (milled/subtractive)	Marginal fit; One screw test	Stress, loosening torque	Ti had a lower misfit than Y-TZP. Ti and Y-TZP both had lower misfits than Co-Cr. Veneering improved the fit in all groups.

CNC, computer numerical-controlled milling; CAD-CAM, computer-aided design/computer-aided manufacture; HDP, high-density polymer; Ti, titanium; Y-TZP, zirconia; Y-TZP-M, mechanically scanned Zirconia CAD-CAM; Y-TZP-L, laser-scanned zirconia CAD/CM; Ti-L, laser-scanned titanium CAD-CAM; Co-Cr, cobalt-chromium; SEM, scanning electron microscopy; LMC, left maxillary canine; RMC, right maxillary canine; RMFM, right maxillary first molar; PEEK, polyetheretherketone.

In six studies, vertical misfit or fit was analyzed [28–32,35–38]. In one study, the internal misfit was assessed [33], and in another study, the three-dimensional (3D) misfit of the frameworks was assessed [34]. In four studies, scanning electron microscopy (SEM) was used to analyze the misfit [30–32,37]. In four studies, the one-screw test was used to analyze the misfit [31,35,36,38], and in two studies, digital or optical microscopy was used for fit analysis [28,29]. 3D virtual assessment was used to determine the misfit in one study [34], and the 'replica technique' was used to determine the internal misfit in one study [33].

In the studies reviewed, the following implant systems or brands were used: Nobel Biocare Active RP (three studies [30,34,35]), Mk III TiUnite by Nobel Biocare [28], Friatz by Dentsply [29], Replace Select™ Tapered RP by Nobel Biocare [31], Titamax Cortical Ti by Neodent [32], an unspecified brand by Nobel Biocare [36], ITI Straumann [37], and Easy

Grip Porous EH [38]. In one study, the implant system was not specified [33]. The length of the implants ranged from 9 mm to 13 mm and from 3.75 mm to 4.3 mm [28–38] (Table 2).

Table 2. Implant-related characteristics and misfit values in the included studies.

No.	Author	Implant/Abutment System	Implant Dimensions/Location	Implant-Supported Restoration	Fabrication System	Misfit (μm)
1	Abduo et al. 2012 [28]	Mk III TiUnite; Nobel Biocare AB; External hex.	Length: 11.5 mm; diameter: 4.0 mm. First Premolar and second molar on each side	All-on-four full arch fixed denture	Forte, Nobel Biocare, AB (CAD); Fabrication by CAD manufacturer.	Vertical misfit: Y-TZP CAD-CAM: 3.7 μm T CAD-CAM: 3.6 μm Passive misfit: Y-TZP CAD-CAM: 5.5 μm Ti: 13.6 μm
2	Zaghloul & Younis et al. 2013 [29]	Friatiz, Dentsply	Length: 11 mm,; diameter: 4–5 mm Second premolar and second molar	Three-unit FPD	Cerec 3 CAD-CAM (Y-TZP); Y-TZP Copy Milling; Ni-Cr Conventional casting	Y-TZP CAD-CAM: 84.58 ± 3.767 μm Y-TZP copy milling: 50.33 ± 3.415 μm Ni-Cr cast: 42.27 ± 3.766 μm
3	de França et al. 2014 [30]	Tapered RP; Nobel Biocare; Internal hex	Titamax Cortical Ti; Neodent Diameter: 4.1 mm; length: 9 mm. Second premolar and second molar	Three-unit FPD	Not specified	Y-TZP CAD-CAM: 5.9 ± 3.6 μm Co-Cr CAD-CAM: 1.2 ± 2.2 μm Co-Cr Cast: Castable abutment: 12.9 ± 11.0 μm Machined abutment: 11.8 ± 9.8 μm
4	Katsoulis et al. 2014 [31]	Replace Select™ Tapered RP; Nobel Biocare	Diameter: 4.3 mm. RMSPM, RMC, RMCI, LMCI, LMC, LMSPM	Ten-unit fixed denture on six implants	CAD: Nobel Biocare (Nobel Procera™); Nobel Biocare CAM: Nobel Procera Production Facility; Nobel Biocare	Y-TZP-L: Median 14 μm 95% CI: 10–26 μm Y-TZP-M: Median 18 μm 95% CI: 12–27 μm Ti-L: Median 15 μm 95% CI: 6–18 μm Co-Cr Cast: Median 236 μm 95% CI: 181–301 μm
5	de Araújo et al. 2015 [32]	Titamax Cortical Ti; Neodent	Diameter: 3.75 mm; length: 9 mm. Three individual implants (second premolar, first molar, second molar)	Three-unit FPD	Not specified	Y-TZP CAD-CAM: 103.81 ± 43.15 μm Co-Cr CAD-CAM: 48.76 ± 13.45 μm Co-Cr Cast: 187.55 ± 103.63 μm
6	Ghodsi et al. 2018 [33]	Not specified	Not described	12 implants (denture details not stated)	CAD: 3Shape; CAM: 3Shape D810 CAD	Y-TZP CAD-CAM: 74.80 μm PEEK CAD-CAM: 181.39 μm RC: 174.89 μm
7	Yılmaz et al. 2018 [34]	Nobel Biocare Active RP	Length: 13 mm; diameter: 4.3 mm. Two straight in the anterior and two distally tilted internal-hexagon dental implants; canine and molar regions	All-on-four fixed denture	CAD: S600 ARTI; Zirkonzahn CAM: M1 Wet Heavy Metal Milling Unit	Before veneering: Y-TZP CAD-CAM: 89 μm T CAD-CAM μm: 88 After veneering: Y-TZP: 175 Ti: 175
8	Yılmaz et al. 2018 [35]	Nobel Biocare Active RP	Length: 13 mm; diameter: 4.3 mm Perpendicular in RMC and LMC; 30-degree distally inclined in RMFM	All-on-four fixed denture	CAD: Zirkonzahn Software; Zirkonzahn CAM: M1 Wet Heavy Metal Milling Unit	RMC HDP: 60 μm Y-TZP CAD-CAM: 83 μm Ti CAD-CAM: 74 μm LMC Not detectable RMFM HDP: 55 μm Y-TZP CAD-CAM: 74 μm Ti CAD-CAM: 102 μm
9	Al-Meraikhi et al. 2018 [36]	Nobel Bioactive	Implants: 4.3 mm × 13 mm Internal Hex	All-on-four fixed denture. Two implants at canine and two implants at first molar positions	CAD: S600 ARTI Zirkonzahn CAM Milling Unit M1 Heavy; Zirkonzahn	LMC-Ti: 8.2 ± 2.6 μm RMC-Ti: 74 ± 15 μm RMC-Y-TZP: 84.4 ± 12.1 μm RMFM-Ti: 102 ±26.7 μm RMFM-Y-TZP: 93.8 ± 30 μm
10	da Cunha Fontoura et al. 2018 [37]	ITI Straumann	Diameter 4.1; length: Not available. Location: mandibular-2 at central incisors and 2 at canines	All-on-four. First premolar to first premolar	CAD: Zirkozahn Modellier; Zirkonzahn CAM: Milling Unit M5 Heavy; Zirkonzahn	Ti CAD-CAM: 6.011 ± 0.750 μm Y-TZP CAD-CAM: 9.055 ± 3.692 μm
11	Del Rio Silva et al. 2020 [38]	Easy Grip Porous EH	Implants: 4.1 mm × 11.5 mm (premolar region), 4.1 mm × 11.5 mm (incisor region), 5 mm × 7 mm (molar region)	Fixed complete denture supported by six implants	Ceramill Map 400+; Amann Girrbach/Ceramill Motion 2; Amann Girrbach (Y-TZP) and CNC D15W; Yenadent (Co-Cr & Ti)	Mean values not provided. Ti CAD-CAM had the highest fit before veneering. No difference in fit after veneering.

CAD, computer-assisted design; CAM: computer-assisted manufacture; Y-TZP, zirconia; Ti, titanium; Co-Cr, cobalt-chromium; Ni-Cr, nickel-chromium; RMSPM, right maxillary second premolar; RMC, right maxillary canine; RMCI, right maxillary central incisor; LMCI, left maxillary central incisor; LMC, left maxillary canine; LMSPM, left maxillary second premolar; PEEK, polyetheretherketone.

In three studies, three-unit fixed partial dentures (FDP) were constructed [29,30,32], and in five studies, full arch fixed dentures on four implants (all-on-four) were constructed [28,34–37]. In one study, a ten-unit fixed prosthesis supported by six implants was constructed [31], and in one study, six implants supported a fixed prosthesis [38]. In the included studies, the following CAD systems were used: Zirkozahn (four studies [34–37]), Nobel Biocare [28,31], Cerec 3 [29], 3Shape [33], and Ceramill Map [38]. The CAM systems were: M1 Milling Unit (three studies [34–36]), M5 Milling Unit [37], 3Shape [33], and Ceramill Motion [38]. In two studies, the CAD-CAM system was not specified [30,32].

3.3. Outcomes of Included Studies

In five studies, the misfits of the Y-TZP CAD-CAM frameworks were comparable to that of Ti CAD-CAM [28,31,35–37]. In one study, Ti CAD-CAM had a significantly lower misfit compared to Y-TZP CAD-CAM [38]. Compared to Co-Cr CAD-CAM, in one study, Y-TZP CAD-CAM exhibited a comparable fit [30], and in another one, Co-Cr CAD-CAM had a significantly better fit [32]. When compared to copy-milled Y-TZP and Ni-Cr CAD-CAM frameworks, Y-TZP CAD-CAM had a lower misfit in one study [29]. When compared with PEEK and resin composites, Y-TZP CAD-CAM prosthesis had a better fit [33]. On the other hand, in one study, CAD-CAM frameworks constructed from high-density polymer (HDP) had lower misfits than Y-TZP CAD-CAM frameworks [35].

3.4. Results of the Quality Assessment

Eight studies received an overall quality grade of 'Medium' [28–30,32,34–37], one study was graded as 'Low' [33], and only two studies were graded as 'High' [31,38] (Table 3). All studies contained an adequate abstract and described the statistical tests conducted [28–38]. All but one study contained an adequate introduction [28–32,34–38]. Although all studies contained an introduction [28–38], in one study, the objectives and the background were not adequately stated [33]. One study did not describe the reproducibility and the measurements of the outcomes adequately [33]. Additionally, the same study did not present the numerical mean values of the fit or misfit of dentures [33], and only a qualitative summary of the outcomes was described. A pre-determined sample size was used in only two studies [31,32]. Randomization was employed in only one study [33], but the same study did not describe the randomization process and the personnel involved in its implementation. The investigators and the technicians were blinded in only study [31]. Seven studies described their limitations in the discussion section [28,30,32,34–36,38]. On the other hand, two studies did not highlight any limitations of the experiments [33,37], and in two studies, it was not clear if the limitations had been described [29,31]. Three studies did not provide any funding information [29,30,32], and none of the studies provided access to the protocol of the study [28–38] (Table 3).

Table 3. Results of the quality assessment conducted on the studies included in this review.

Assessment Item	Abduo et al. 2012 [28]	Zaghloul & Younis et al. 2013 [29]	de França et al. 2014 [30]	Katsoulis et al. 2014 [32]	de Araújo et al. 2015 [32]	Ghodsi et al. 2018 [33]	Yilmaz et al. 2018 [34]	Yilmaz et al. 2018b [35]	Al-Meraikhi et al. 2018 [36]	Diego et al. 2018 [37]	Silva et al. 2020 [38]
1. Adequate abstract	Yes	Yes	Yes	Yes	Yes	Yes	Yes	Yes	Yes	Yes	Yes
(2a) Introduction (Background)	Yes	Yes	Yes	Yes	Yes	Not clear	Yes	Yes	Yes	Yes	Yes
(2b) Introduction (Objectives)	Yes	Yes	Yes	Yes	Yes	Not clear	Yes	Yes	Yes	Yes	Yes
Methods											
3. Replicable methods	Yes	Yes	Yes	Yes	Yes	Not clear	Yes	Yes	Yes	Yes	Yes
4. Adequate outcomes	Yes	Yes	Yes	Yes	Yes	Not clear	Yes	Yes	Yes	Yes	Yes
5. Pre-determined sample size	No	No	No	Yes	Yes	No	No	No	No	Yes	Yes
6. Allocation of samples											
(a) Randomization	No	No	No	No	No	Yes	No	No	No	No	No
(b) Allocation concealment	No	No	No	No	No	No	No	No	No	No	No
(c) Implementation	No	No	No	No	No	No	No	No	No	No	No
7. Blinding	No	No	No	Yes	No	No	No	No	No	No	No
8. Statistics	Yes	Yes	Yes	Yes	Yes	Yes	Yes	Yes	Yes	Yes	Yes
9. Adequate outcomes & estimation	Yes	Yes	Yes	Yes	Yes	Yes	Yes	Yes	Yes	Yes	Yes
10. Discussion: Limitations	Yes	Not clear	Yes	Not clear	Yes	No	Yes	Yes	Yes	No	Yes
11. Funding	Yes	No	No	Yes	No	Yes	Yes	Yes	Yes	Yes	Yes
12. Accessible protocol	No	No	No	No	No	No	No	No	No	No	No
Overall quality	Medium	Medium	Medium	High	Medium	Low	Medium	Medium	Medium	Medium	High

4. Discussion

CAD-CAM prostheses provide a significant advantage over conventional cast prostheses in terms of the number of patient visits, appointment duration, and accuracy [21]. Additionally, with the application of intraoral scanning and CAD-CAM, there is no need for impression taking and study or cast model construction, making cross infection easier. The aim of this study was to critically appraise and summarize the current evidence comparing the fit of implant-supported Y-TZP CAD-CAM frameworks to that of other metal and non-metal implant frameworks. The majority of the studies included in this review concluded that implant-supported Y-TZP CAD-CAM frameworks have a better or comparable fit to that of cast and CAD-CAM frameworks constructed from Ti, Co-Cr, resin, and PEEK [28,29,31,35–37].

The overall outcome of this systematic review suggests an acceptable fit accuracy of Y-TZP CAD-CAM frameworks, but this should be interpreted with caution due to the heterogeneity in the methodology and outcomes of the studies. Several different CAD-CAM systems were used to construct the frameworks [28–38], making the standardization and comparison of the results difficult. In eight studies, conventional CAD-CAM was used to fabricate frameworks; however, in three studies, copy-milling was employed [28,29,38]. As opposed to conventional CAD-CAM, copy-milling involves the digital scanning of a manually constructed wax or resin pattern of the prostheses. Dimensional changes in the constructed pattern may contribute to discrepancies in the misfit of prostheses constructed with this method. However, to date, no comparative studies have been conducted to assess the misfit of copy-milled Y-TZP frameworks to that of CAD-CAM frameworks. Furthermore, the types of implant abutments used to support the CAD-CAM Y-TZP frameworks [28–38] differed in the reviewed studies, which makes it difficult to prescribe guidelines for constructing CAD-CAM frameworks with an optimal fit or minimal misfit. Another limitation of the studies was that all of them were in vitro laboratory studies [28–38]. Indeed, it is difficult to measure the misfit of prostheses in vivo [44] because there are several factors that affect not only the misfit of implant-supported prostheses but also the overall lifespan of the prostheses. These factors included masticatory forces, parafunctional habits, the age of the patient, systemic health, and the osseointegration of dental implants [45–48]. Hence, future studies should attempt to simulate the effects of these factors on the misfit of Y-TZP CAD-CAM frameworks.

The differences among the methods used for the assessment of the misfit make it difficult to reach a definite conclusion regarding the misfit of Y-TZP CAD-CAM frameworks to other materials. The 'one-screw' test involves the placement of a single screw at the terminal implant abutment, and the opposing abutment is evaluated for movement radiographically or clinically. This test was used in four studies in this review [31,35,36,38]; however, its major limitation is its primary reliance on manual measurements with the naked eye, making the assessments unreliable in many cases. Indeed, this inconsistency is reflected by the results of the four studies that have compared the misfit of Y-TZP CAD-CAM to that of Ti CAD-CAM: in three studies, Y-TZP exhibited either a lower or comparable misfit [31,34,36], and in one study, Ti frameworks possessed a lower misfit [38]. Only two studies made use of CT scanning or virtual scanning to assess the misfit [34,36]. Indeed, the relatively large range of the misfit of the Y-TZP CAD-CAM frameworks (3.7 µm to 103.71 µm) is most likely due to the non-standardization of misfit assessments, so future studies should focus on reproducible and standardized techniques to compare the misfit of frameworks. Nevertheless, due to variations in the fabrication techniques, material phase, and equipment type used, attaining ideal standardization among the Y-TZP misfit studies may not be pragmatic. It is also important to note that CAD-CAM Y-TZP crowns have an approximate success rate of 70% after 24 months, and the most likely reason for this is fatigue-failure [49]. Therefore, more studies focusing on the reasons for CAD-CAM framework misfit and the resultant failures should be conducted. Nevertheless, a recent retrospective clinical study on implant-supported CAD-CAM Y-TZP denture frameworks provided to 50 patients found no long-term failures after 2 years, which makes the long-term viability of Y-TZP

CAD-CAM frameworks promising [50]. Nevertheless, for the adequate functionality and survival of implant-supported prostheses, optimal oral hygiene is vital, and patients should be educated about this during and after treatment [51].

In addition to the above concerns, there were multiple sources of bias found in the studies. A pre-determined sample size was used in only two studies [31,32], and the sample sizes in the remaining studies may have not been sufficient to produce reliable results. Furthermore, no study mentioned any attempt in blinding the investigators or technicians during the experiments. Although it is difficult to blind the investigators from the materials due to their difference in appearance, it may be possible to blind the experimental groups corresponding to the measurements of the misfit assessments in future studies. In the majority of the studies, randomization was not attempted, which may have contributed to selection bias within the studies. A major limitation of this systematic review itself was that it was not possible to conduct a meta-analysis because of the heterogeneity of the studies included. Thus, it was not possible to deduce an overall misfit effect of the results. Therefore, to achieve a certain level of standardization among the misfit evaluation investigations, further studies should incorporate blinding, randomization, similar misfit evaluation methods, and analyzed sample sizes.

In addition to CAD-CAM Zirconia frameworks, the 3D printing of such denture frameworks may provide an additional advantage of additive manufacturing leading to the reduced wastage of material and reduced costs [52]. Nevertheless, a lack of clinical trials or other prospective studies to assess the misfit of the Y-TZP CAD-CAM means that, to date, it is difficult to ascertain whether the misfit of these frameworks is lower or comparable to other types of frameworks. Consequently, large-scale clinical studies and standardized in vitro studies with minimal bias are necessary to make a more definite conclusion.

5. Conclusions

Within the limitations of this review and the included studies, it may be concluded that Y-TZP CAD-CAM implant-supported frameworks have a comparable misfit to other CAD-CAM implant-supported frameworks. However, due to the heterogeneity in the methodologies of the included studies, the overall numerical misfit of the frameworks tested in the studies is debatable. Better-designed in vitro and long-term clinical studies are required to reach a more definite conclusion.

Funding: The research did not receive any funding.

Institutional Review Board Statement: Not applicable (Review study).

Informed Consent Statement: Informed consent was not needed, as it is a review study.

Data Availability Statement: The data are available upon request from the author.

Acknowledgments: I would like to acknowledge the statistician (M.M.) who assisted me in the analysis of data in the review.

Conflicts of Interest: The author declares no conflict of interest.

References

1. Zhang, Y.; Gulati, K.; Li, Z.; Di, P.; Liu, Y. Dental implant nano-engineering: Advances, limitations and future directions. *Nanomaterials* **2021**, *11*, 2489. [CrossRef] [PubMed]
2. Liu, Y.; Rath, B.; Tingart, M.; Eschweiler, J. Role of implants surface modification in osseointegration: A systematic review. *J. Biomed. Mat. Res. Part A* **2020**, *108*, 470–484. [CrossRef] [PubMed]
3. Bagegni, A.; Abou-Ayash, S.; Rücker, G.; Algarny, A.; Att, W. The influence of prosthetic material on implant and prosthetic survival of implant-supported fixed complete dentures: A systematic review and meta-analysis. *J. Prosthodont. Res.* **2019**, *63*, 251–265. [CrossRef] [PubMed]
4. Duong, H.Y.; Roccuzzo, A.; Stähli, A.; Salvi, G.E.; Lang, N.P.; Sculean, A. Oral health-related quality of life of patients rehabilitated with fixed and removable implant-supported dental prostheses. *Periodontology* **2022**, *88*, 201–237. [CrossRef]

5. Varghese, K.G.; Gandhi, N.; Kurian, N.; Daniel, A.Y.; Dhawan, K.; Joseph, M.; Varghese, M.G. Rehabilitation of the severely resorbed maxilla by using quad zygomatic implant-supported prostheses: A systematic review and meta-analysis. *J. Prosthet. Dent.* 2021; in press. [CrossRef]
6. Oh, W.-S.; Saglik, B.; Bak, S.-Y. Bone loss in the posterior edentulous mandible with implant-supported overdentures vs complete dentures: A systematic review and meta-analysis. *Int. J. Prosthodont.* 2020, *33*, 184–191. [CrossRef]
7. Topçu, A.O.; Yamalik, N.; Güncü, G.N.; Tözüm, T.F.; El, H.; Uysal, S.; Hersek, N. Implant-site related and patient-based factors with the potential to impact patients' satisfaction, quality of life measures and perceptions toward dental implant treatment. *Implant Dent.* 2017, *26*, 581–591. [CrossRef]
8. Doundoulakis, J.H.; Eckert, S.E.; Lindquist, C.C.; Jeffcoat, M.K. The implant-supported overdenture as an alternative to the complete mandibular denture. *J. Am. Dent. Assoc.* 2003, *134*, 1455–1458. [CrossRef]
9. Kreissl, M.E.; Gerds, T.; Muche, R.; Heydecke, G.; Strub, J.R. Technical complications of implant-supported fixed partial dentures in partially edentulous cases after an average observation period of 5 years. *Clin. Oral Implants Res.* 2007, *18*, 720–726. [CrossRef]
10. McLaughlin, J.B.; Ramos, V., Jr.; Dickinson, D.P. Comparison of Fit of Dentures Fabricated by Traditional Techniques Versus CAD-CAM Technology. *J. Prosthodont.* 2019, *28*, 428–435. [CrossRef]
11. Yun, M.-J.; Jeon, Y.-C.; Jeong, C.-M.; Huh, J.-B. Comparison of the fit of cast gold crowns fabricated from the digital and the conventional impression techniques. *J. Adv. Prosthodont.* 2017, *9*, 1–13. [CrossRef]
12. Mitha, T.; Owen, C.P.; Howes, D.G. The three-dimensional casting distortion of five implant-supported frameworks. *Int. J. Prosthodont.* 2009, *22*, 248–250. [CrossRef]
13. de Torres, E.M.; Rodrigues, R.C.S.; de Mattos, M.d.G.C.; Ribeiro, R.F. The effect of commercially pure titanium and alternative dental alloys on the marginal fit of one-piece cast implant frameworks. *J. Dent.* 2007, *35*, 800–805. [CrossRef] [PubMed]
14. Diwan, R.; Talic, Y.; Omar, N.; Sadiq, W. The effect of storage time of removable partial denture wax pattern on the accuracy of fit of the cast framework. *J. Prosthet. Dent.* 1997, *77*, 375–381. [CrossRef]
15. Tischler, M.; Patch, C.; Bidra, A.S. Rehabilitation of edentulous jaws with zirconia complete-arch fixed implant-supported prostheses: An up to 4-year retrospective clinical study. *J. Prosthet. Dent.* 2018, *120*, 204–209. [CrossRef] [PubMed]
16. Henriques, G.E.P.; Consani, S.; de Almeida Rollo, J.M.D.; e Silva, F.A. Soldering and remelting influence on fatigue strength of cobalt-chromium alloys. *J. Prosthet. Dent.* 1997, *78*, 146–152. [CrossRef]
17. Lauritano, D.; Moreo, G.; Lucchese, A.; Viganoni, C.; Limongelli, L.; Carinci, F. The impact of implant–abutment connection on clinical outcomes and microbial colonization: A narrative review. *Materials* 2020, *13*, 1131. [CrossRef] [PubMed]
18. Yannikakis, S.; Prombonas, A. Improving the fit of implant prosthetics: An in vitro study. *Int. J. Oral Maxillofac. Implants* 2013, *28*, 126–134. [CrossRef]
19. Pan, Y.; Tsoi, J.K.H.; Lam, W.Y.H.; Pow, E.H.N. Implant framework misfit: A systematic review on assessment methods and clinical complications. *Clin. Implant Dent. Relat. Res.* 2021, *23*, 244–258. [CrossRef]
20. Baba, N.Z.; AlRumaih, H.S.; Goodacre, B.J.; Goodacre, C.J. Current techniques in CAD-CAM denture fabrication. *Gen. Dent.* 2016, *64*, 23–28.
21. Baba, N.Z.; Goodacre, B.J.; Goodacre, C.J.; Müller, F.; Wagner, S. CAD-CAM complete denture systems and physical properties: A review of the literature. *J. Prosthodont.* 2021, *30*, 113–124. [CrossRef]
22. Steinmassl, O.; Dumfahrt, H.; Grunert, I.; Steinmassl, P.A. CAD/CAM produces dentures with improved fit. *Clin. Oral Investig.* 2018, *22*, 2829–2835. [CrossRef] [PubMed]
23. Pereira, A.L.C.; de Medeiros, A.K.B.; de Sousa Santos, K.; de Almeida, É.O.; Barbosa, G.A.S.; Carreiro, A.D.F.P. Accuracy of CAD-CAM systems for removable partial denture framework fabrication: A systematic review. *J. Prosthet. Dent.* 2021, *125*, 241–248. [CrossRef] [PubMed]
24. Share & Trends Analysis Report By Product (Titanium Implants, Zirconium Implants), By Region (North America, Europe, Asia Pacific, Latin America, MEA), And Segment Forecasts, 2018–2024. Personalized Medicine Market Analysis By Product And Segment Forecasts To 2018. 2022. Available online: https://www.marketresearch.com/Grang-View-Research-v4060/Dental-implant-size-share-trends-14163164/Chapter5 (accessed on 10 July 2022).
25. Shetty, R.; Shoukath, S.; Shetty, N.H.G.; Shetty, S.K.; Dandekeri, S.; Ragher, M. A novel design modification to improve flexural strength of zirconia framework: A comparative experimental in vitro study. *J. Pharm. Bioallied Sci.* 2020, *12* (Suppl. 1), S495–S503. [CrossRef] [PubMed]
26. Pott, P.C.; Eisenburger, M.; Stiesch, M. Survival rate of modern all-ceramic FPDs during an observation period from 2011 to 2016. *J. Adv. Prosthodont.* 2018, *10*, 18–24. [CrossRef] [PubMed]
27. Agustín-Panadero, R.; Serra-Pastor, B.; Fons-Font, A.; Solá-Ruíz, M.F. Prospective clinical study of zirconia full-coverage restorations on teeth prepared with biologically oriented preparation technique on gingival health: Results after two-year follow-up. *Oper. Dent.* 2018, *43*, 482–487. [CrossRef] [PubMed]
28. Abduo, J.; Lyons, K.; Waddell, N.; Bennani, V.; Swain, M. A comparison of fit of CNC-milled titanium and zirconia frameworks to implants. *Clin. Implant Dent. Relat. Res.* 2012, *14* (Suppl. 1), e20–e29. [CrossRef] [PubMed]
29. Zaghloul, H.H.; Younis, J.F. Marginal fit of implant-supported all-ceramic zirconia frameworks. *J. Oral Implantol.* 2013, *39*, 417–424. [CrossRef]
30. de França, D.G.; Morais, M.H.; das Neves, F.D.; Barbosa, G.A. Influence of CAD-CAM on the fit accuracy of implant-supported zirconia and cobalt-chromium fixed dental prostheses. *J. Prosthet. Dent.* 2015, *113*, 22–28. [CrossRef]

31. Katsoulis, J.; Mericske-Stern, R.; Rotkina, L.; Zbären, C.; Enkling, N.; Blatz, M.B. Precision of fit of implant-supported screw-retained 10-unit computer-aided-designed and computer-aided-manufactured frameworks made from zirconium dioxide and titanium: An in vitro study. *Clin. Oral Implants Res.* 2014, 25, 165–174. [CrossRef]
32. de Araújo, G.M.; de França, D.G.; Silva Neto, J.P.; Barbosa, G.A. Passivity of conventional and CAD-CAM fabricated implant frameworks. *Braz. Dent. J.* 2015, 26, 277–283. [CrossRef]
33. Ghodsi, S.; Zeighami, S.; Meisami Azad, M. Comparing retention and internal adaptation of different implant-supported, metal-free frameworks. *Int. J. Prosthodont.* 2018, 31, 475–477. [CrossRef] [PubMed]
34. Yilmaz, B.; Alshahrani, F.A.; Kale, E.; Johnston, W.M. Effect of feldspathic porcelain layering on the marginal fit of zirconia and titanium complete-arch fixed implant-supported frameworks. *J. Prosthet. Dent.* 2018, 120, 71–78. [CrossRef] [PubMed]
35. Yilmaz, B.; Kale, E.; Johnston, W.M. Marginal discrepancy of CAD-CAM complete-arch fixed implant-supported frameworks. *J. Prosthet. Dent.* 2018, 120, 65–70. [CrossRef] [PubMed]
36. Al-Meraikhi, H.; Yilmaz, B.; McGlumphy, E.; Brantley, W.; Johnston, W.M. In vitro fit of CAD-CAM complete arch screw-retained titanium and zirconia implant prostheses fabricated on 4 implants. *J. Prosthet. Dent.* 2018, 119, 409–416. [CrossRef] [PubMed]
37. da Cunha Fontoura, D.; de Magalhães Barros, V.; de Magalhães, C.S.; Vaz, R.R.; Moreira, A.N. Evaluation of Vertical Misfit of CAD-CAM Implant-Supported Titanium and Zirconia Frameworks. *Int. J. Oral Maxillofac. Implants* 2018, 33, 1027–1032. [CrossRef] [PubMed]
38. Del Rio Silva, L.; Velôso, D.V.; Barbin, T.; Borges, G.A.; Presotto, A.G.C.; Mesquita, M.F. Can ceramic veneer spark erosion and mechanical cycling affect the accuracy of milled complete-arch frameworks supported by 6 implants? *J. Prosthet. Dent.* 2020, 126, 772–778. [CrossRef] [PubMed]
39. Jadad, A.R.; Moore, R.A.; Carroll, D.; Jenkinson, C.; Reynolds, D.J.; Gavaghan, D.J.; McQuay, H.J. Assessing the quality of reports of randomized clinical trials: Is blinding necessary? *Control. Clin. Trials* 1996, 17, 1–12. [CrossRef]
40. Faggion, C.M., Jr. Guidelines for reporting pre-clinical in vitro studies on dental materials. *J. Evid. Based Dent. Pract.* 2012, 12, 182–189. [CrossRef]
41. Abduo, J.; Lyons, K.; Swain, M. Fit of zirconia fixed partial denture: A systematic review. *J. Oral Rehabil.* 2010, 37, 866–876. [CrossRef]
42. Bousnaki, M.; Chatziparaskeva, M.; Bakopoulou, A.; Pissiotis, A.; Koidis, P. Variables affecting the fit of zirconia fixed partial dentures: A systematic review. *J. Prosthet. Dent.* 2020, 123, 686–692. [CrossRef]
43. Svanborg, P.; Norström Saarva, V.; Stenport, V.; Eliasson, A. Fit of 3Y-TZP complete-arch implant-supported fixed dental prostheses before and after porcelain veneering. *J. Prosthet. Dent.* 2019, 122, 137–141. [CrossRef] [PubMed]
44. Liedke, G.S.; Spin-Neto, R.; da Silveira, H.E.D.; Wenzel, A. Radiographic diagnosis of dental restoration misfit: A systematic review. *J. Oral Rehabil.* 2014, 41, 957–967. [CrossRef] [PubMed]
45. Farina, A.P.; Spazzin, A.O.; Pantoja, J.M.; Consani, R.L.X.; Mesquita, M.F. An in vitro comparison of joint stability of implant-supported fixed prosthetic suprastructures retained with different prosthetic screws and levels of fit under masticatory simulation conditions. *Int. J. Oral Maxillofac. Implants* 2012, 27, 833–838.
46. Farina, A.P.; Spazzin, A.O.; Consani, R.L.; Mesquita, M.F. Screw joint stability after the application of retorque in implant-supported dentures under simulated masticatory conditions. *J. Prosthet. Dent.* 2014, 111, 499–504. [CrossRef] [PubMed]
47. Denardi, R.J.; da Silva, R.D.; Thomé, G.; Andrighetto, A.R.; de Freitas, R.M.; Shimizu, R.H.; Shimizu, I.A.; Melo, A.C. Bone response after immediate placement of implants in the anterior maxilla: A systematic review. *Oral Maxillofac. Surg.* 2019, 23, 13–25. [CrossRef] [PubMed]
48. Zhou, Y.; Gao, J.; Luo, L.; Wang, Y. Does Bruxism Contribute to Dental Implant Failure? A Systematic Review and Meta-Analysis. *Clin. Implant Dent. Relat. Res.* 2016, 18, 410–420. [CrossRef]
49. Gherlone, E.; Mandelli, F.; Capparè, P.; Pantaleo, G.; Traini, T.; Ferrini, F. A 3 years retrospective study of survival for zirconia-based single crowns fabricated from intraoral digital impressions. *J. Dent.* 2014, 42, 1151–1155. [CrossRef]
50. Cappare, P.; Ferrini, F.; Mariani, G.; Nagni, M.; Cattoni, F. Implant rehabilitation of edentulous jaws with predominantly monolithic zirconia compared to metal-acrylic prostheses: A 2-year retrospective clinical study. *J. Biol. Regul. Homeost. Agents* 2021, 35 (Suppl. 1), 99–112.
51. Cattoni, F.; Tetè, G.; D'orto, B.; Bergamaschi, A.; Polizzi, E.; Gastaldi, G. Comparison of hygiene levels in metal-ceramic and stratified zirconia in prosthetic rehabilitation on teeth and implants: A retrospective clinical study of a three-year follow-up. *J. Biol. Regul. Homeost. Agents* 2021, 35 (Suppl. 1), 41–49.
52. Gungor-Ozkerim, P.S.; Inci, I.; Zhang, Y.S.; Khademhosseini, A.; Dokmeci, M.R. Bioinks for 3D bioprinting: An overview. *Biomater. Sci.* 2018, 6, 915–946. [CrossRef]

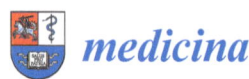

Review

Neural Basis of Etiopathogenesis and Treatment of Cervicogenic Orofacial Pain

Jiří Šedý [1,2,3], Mariano Rocabado [4], Leonardo Enrique Olate [5], Marek Vlna [2] and Radovan Žižka [2,*]

1. 3DK Clinic, U Zdravotniho Ustavu 2213/8, 10000 Prague, Czech Republic
2. Institute of Dentistry and Oral Sciences, Faculty of Medicine, Palacký University, Palackého 12, 77200 Olomouc, Czech Republic
3. Institute of Anatomy, Second Faculty of Medicine, Charles University, V Uvalu 84, 15006 Prague, Czech Republic
4. Facultad de Ciencias de la Rehabilitación, Universidad Andres Bello, República 239, Santiago 8370035, Chile
5. Rocabado Institute, Camino El Alba 8760, Las Condes, Región Metropolitana de Santiago, Santiago 87608760, Chile
* Correspondence: loupaczech@gmail.com

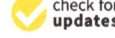

Citation: Šedý, J.; Rocabado, M.; Olate, L.E.; Vlna, M.; Žižka, R. Neural Basis of Etiopathogenesis and Treatment of Cervicogenic Orofacial Pain. *Medicina* 2022, *58*, 1324. https://doi.org/10.3390/medicina58101324

Academic Editors: Giuseppe Minervini and Stefania Moccia

Received: 15 August 2022
Accepted: 19 September 2022
Published: 21 September 2022

Publisher's Note: MDPI stays neutral with regard to jurisdictional claims in published maps and institutional affiliations.

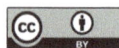

Copyright: © 2022 by the authors. Licensee MDPI, Basel, Switzerland. This article is an open access article distributed under the terms and conditions of the Creative Commons Attribution (CC BY) license (https://creativecommons.org/licenses/by/4.0/).

Abstract: (1) *Background and Objectives*: The aim of this narrative review was to analyze the neuroanatomical and neurophysiological basis of cervicogenic pain in cervico-cranial pain syndromes, focusing particularly on cervico-orofacial syndromes as a background for the proper diagnosis and non-surgical treatment. Relevant literature on the topic from past 120 years has been surveyed. (2) *Material and Methods*: We surveyed all original papers, reviews, or short communications published in the English, Spanish, Czech or Slovak languages from 1900 to 2020 in major journals. (3) *Results*: The cervicogenic headache originates from the spinal trigeminal nucleus where axons from the C_1–C_3 cervical spinal nerves and three branches of the trigeminal nerve converge (trigeminocervical convergence) at the interneurons that mediate cranio-cervical nociceptive interactions. The role of the temporomandibular joint in the broad clinical picture is also important. Despite abundant available experimental and clinical data, cervicogenic orofacial pain may be challenging to diagnose and treat. Crucial non-surgical therapeutic approach is the orthopedic manual therapy focused on correction of body posture, proper alignment of cervical vertebra and restoration of normal function of temporomandibular joint and occlusion. In addition, two novel concepts for the functional synthesis of cervico-cranial interactions are the tricentric concept of mouth sensorimotor control and the concept of a cervicogenic origin of bruxism. (4) *Conclusions*: Understanding the basis of neuroanatomical and neurophysiological neuromuscular relations enables an effective therapeutic approach based principally on orthopedic manual and dental occlusal treatment.

Keywords: cervicogenic; pain; temporomandibular joint; posture; physiotherapy

1. Introduction

Cervicogenic headache, or more broadly, cervicogenic orofacial pain (COP), represents an important clinical entity defined as a secondary, lateralized non-throbbing headache caused by nociceptive sources in the cervical spine [1]. Its negative impact on quality of life is substantial and may be comparable to those of migraines and episodic tension-type headaches [2,3]. Cervicogenic orofacial syndrome is characterized by pain that begins in the neck or occipital region and progresses to adjacent regions of the face and head [4,5]. The anatomical basis for this clinical pattern likely relates to a convergence of the upper cervical and trigeminal nociceptive afferents within the trigeminocervical neural complex [6].

Regarding basic neuroscience, COP is probably one of the best-understood categories of common headaches. Its etiopathogenetic mechanisms are largely known, based mainly on the convergence on afferent nerve fibers from first three cervical nerves and trigeminal branches on the interneurons of the spinal trigeminal nucleus, as a source of referred pain from cervical region to trigeminal area [4–6]. The pain can be induced experimentally in healthy volunteers. It is diagnostically helpful that in some patients, COP can be temporarily relieved by blocking the cervical joints or nerves with local anesthetics [5].

The Cervicogenic Headache International Study Group formally identified the clinical syndrome as a separate entity in 1998. Consequently, it was included in the second and third edition of the International Headache Society classification of Headache in 2004 [7,8] (Table 1). The Study Group classified cervicogenic headache as a side-locked orofacial pain (OP) worsened by diverse stimuli such as neck movements, sustained improper neck positioning, restricted range of cervical spine motion, or ipsilateral shoulder and arm pain [9]. Despite this relatively strict definition, COP may be challenging to diagnose clinically. For example, a sharp pain in the occipital region may reflect neuralgia of the occipital nerve that can mimic COP [10]. Signs and symptoms associated with migraine headaches or other symptoms of vascular headaches, including neck pain, nausea, vomiting, photophobia, and phonophobia can imitate COP [9,11,12]. Despite abundantly available experimental and clinical data, therapeutic modalities based on specific etiopathogenic mechanisms of COP have not been comprehensively elucidated and are the subject of this review. Further text is based elaborating the non-surgical treatment modalities, mainly based on orthopedic manual therapy, based on the author's own concepts, such as Rocabado's tricentric concept of mouth sensorimotor control, the importance of posture, proper alignment of cervical vertebrae and the role of concomitant conservative temporomandibular joint therapy. Moreover, the author's own concept of bruxism etiopathogenesis pathway is presented as well.

Table 1. The International Classification of Headache Disorders (ICHD-3) diagnostic criteria for cervicogenic headache according to the Headache Classification Committee of the International Headache Society (2018).

A. Any headache fulfilling criterion C.
B. Clinical and/or imaging evidence of a disorder or lesion within the cervical spine or soft tissues of the neck, known to be able to cause headache.
C. Evidence of causation demonstrated by at least two of the following: 1. headache has developed in temporal relation to the onset of the cervical disorder or appearance of the lesion; 2. headache has significantly improved or resolved in parallel with improvement in or resolution of the cervical disorder or lesion; 3. cervical range of motion is reduced and headache is made significantly worse by provocative maneuvers; 4. headache is abolished following diagnostic blockade of a cervical structure or its nerve supply.
D. Not better accounted for by another ICHD-3 diagnosis.

2. Data Collection and Analysis

We surveyed all original papers, reviews, or short communications published in the English, Spanish, Czech or Slovak languages from 1900 to 2020 in major journals. Studies were included when they dealt with COP experimentally or clinically based on Medline, Web of Science, OVID, and Google Scholar searches. The parameters studied were mainly neuroanatomy, neurophysiology, etiology, pathogenesis, clinical appearance, and therapeutic modalities. We particularly focused on COP syndromes with more emphasis on cervico-orofacial syndromes.

3. Epidemiology

The prevalence of COP is between 1–4.1% in the general population but could be as high as 17.5% among patients with severe headaches [9,12–14]. The highest prevalence is in the patients with whiplash injury where it could be as high as 53% [15].

4. Clinical Anatomy of Cervico-Cranial Junction

The cervico-cranial complex represents a crucial part of the axial (postural) system. It is involved in many functions including the primary movements of the head, and participating in remote secondary functions such as positioning of the head in accordance with visual and vestibulocochlear inputs, movements of the mandible at the temporomandibular joint, pharyngeal and laryngeal functions, and others. Clinically, the cranio-mandibulo-cervical complex includes the first three vertebrae, skull, mandible, and hyoid bone, together with the muscles, ligaments, fasciae, and other structures involved in their movement [16].

Among the first three cervical vertebrae, only the third represents a typical cervical vertebra with a distinct body, vertebral arch, and typical processes. The C_1 vertebra (*atlas*) lacks a typical vertebral body, being composed of anterior and posterior arches only together with paired lateral masses. The C_2 vertebra (*axis*) serves as an axis for rotation of the *atlas* and head around its strong odontoid process (*dens*), projecting cranially from the superior surface of the body. It is retained in position by the strong transverse ligament of the *atlas*. Further, the tip of the *atlas* is connected to the occipital bone with paired alar ligaments, approximately 11 mm long, and thick collagenous cords. The *atlas* is connected to the occipital bone by two atlanto-occipital joints, developed between occipital condyles and articular surfaces on the superior aspects of the lateral masses of the *atlas*. In this joint, the main movements are flexion and extension (range 16–21°), with limited lateral flexion (range 3°) and rotation (range 6°) [17]. The connection of the *atlas* and *axis* is in the abovementioned, unpaired, median atlanto-axial joint between the *dens axis* and posterior surface of the anterior arch of the *atlas* and paired lateral atlanto-axial zygapophyseal joints. The main movement of this joint is rotation with a normal range of approximately 41° [17]. Atlanto-axial rotation is limited by clinically very important alar ligaments, the left becoming taut on rotation to the right and vice versa. The slightly upward movement of the C_2 vertebra during rotation facilitates a wide range of movement by reducing the tension in the alar ligaments, as it also does in the capsules and accessory ligaments of the lateral atlanto-axial joints [18]. Between the second and third cervical vertebrae, typical intervertebral disc together with paired, lateral, zygapophyseal joints are developed. Together with the four other cervical vertebrae, these structures form a typical convexity directed forward, called cervical lordosis. Moreover, the first two thoracic vertebrae are involved; thus, typical physiological cervical lordosis extends from the *atlas* to the Th_2 vertebra, with its maximum bending being between the C_4 and C_5 vertebrae.

4.1. Spinal Nerves

The cervical vertebrae form the cranial part of the vertebral canal, which encloses the spinal cord giving rise to the spinal nerves, which form by a fusion of motor ventral and sensory dorsal spinal roots to pass as one nerve bundle through the intervertebral foramina. The first cervical spinal nerve (C_1) passes between the occipital bone and C_1 vertebra. The last cervical spinal nerve (C_8) passes between the last cervical vertebra and the first thoracic vertebra—the reason why humans have eight cervical spinal nerves but only seven cervical vertebrae. After passing through the intervertebral foramen (or corresponding space) the spinal nerves emerge laterally and give rise to anterior and posterior nerve branches (*rami*). Importantly, the peripheral branches of the cervical spinal nerves supply neck muscles, which are functionally related to movements of the cervical spine, head, and mandible.

4.2. Spinal System and Trigeminocervical Convergence

The trigeminal nerve is the thickest cranial nerve, and it contains approximately 180,000 nerve fibers. It is a very huge somatosensory part (*radix sensoria, portio major*) that innervates the skin of the face, all teeth, oral, nasal, and paranasal mucosa, anterior two-thirds of the tongue, orbit, part of nasopharynx, mucosa of the Eustachian tube, temporomandibular joint (TMJ), majority of the dura mater, lateral part of the tympanic membrane, external auditory meatus, and small part of the auricle [18–20]. The most intense pain stimuli in this large innervating area are provided by free nerve endings from the dental pulp and cornea. The borders of the innervating areas of particular branches (ophthalmic, maxillary, and mandibular) are *rima palpebrarum* and *rima oris*. Posteriorly, the margin remains the line vertex—external auditory meatus—chin. The importance of the trigeminal sensory innervation is very high—approximately 50% of the cortical representation of all sensory inputs from the body comes from the trigeminal system [21]. Trigeminal primary afferents are dendrites of pseudounipolar neurons in trigeminal (semilunar, Gasserian) ganglion and mesencephalic nucleus [22]. The motor part (*radix motoria, portio minor*) innervates all chewing muscles (masseter, temporalis, and medial and lateral pterygoids) as well as mylohyoid, anterior belly of digastric, tensor tympani, and tensor veli palatini. In the periphery, the trigeminal nerve system is entered by sympathetic, parasympathetic, and gustatory fibers from other origins.

The trigeminal nerve has three sensory nuclei (trigeminal sensory complex) and one motor nucleus.

4.2.1. Trigeminocervical Nucleus

Trigeminocervical nucleus (*nucleus spinalis nervi trigemini*) is an elongated structure, located from the bottom of the pons to upper segments of cervical spinal cord. It has three main parts: (1a) **Subnucleus oralis** (*pars rostralis*) contains afferent fibers from facial region close to the midline, mainly from the oral cavity and nose. (1b) **Subnucleus interpolaris**—contains afferent fibers from the ventrolateral parts of the face, mainly from the cheeks and orbit. (1c) **Subnucleus caudalis**—contains afferent fibers from the lateral parts of the face. Lateral to *subnucleus caudalis*, a bundle of fibers called *tractus spinalis nervi trigemini* is located. This bundle is entered by A-delta and C-type trigeminal fibers leading to pain and thermal stimuli. These fibers are somatotopically organized—most anteriorly, are fibers from the ophthalmic nerve, in the middle, are fibers from the maxillary nerve and dorsally, are fibers from the mandibular nerve. Step by step, these fibers turn medially and enter the trigeminocervical nucleus. To understand COP, it is extremely important to know that the axons of the trigeminocervical nucleus are densely connected with axons of spinal ganglia of C_1–C_3 spinal nerves, via interneurons of the trigeminocervical nucleus [5,23]. This pattern is known as **trigeminocervical functional convergence** [24] (Figure 1). Moreover, the referral of sensations is bi-directional [25]. Thus, there is a possibility of referred pain transfer between the C_1–C_3 and trigeminal innervation areas [4,5]. Pain originating from the teeth, jaws, or TMJ could thus project into the cervical area, and vice versa. Pain from the C_1–C_3 innervation area (e.g., due to improper posture, C_1/C_2 vertebra rotation, cervical trauma) could project to the orofacial region, mainly to the forehead, orbit, cheek, TMJ, and ear, causing problems in differential diagnosis with a high risk of misdiagnosis [5,26]. This relation represents the fundamental neuroanatomical basis of COP [5]. Importantly, no relation has been observed between the trigeminal nerve and spinal nerve C_4 or nerves at lower segments [5].

Posterior to the trigeminocervical nucleus, a fine bundle of somatosensory afferent fibers from facial, glossopharyngeal, and vagus cranial nerves are located, known as the **spinal nerve tract** (*tractus spinalis nervi trigemini*). These fibers also end in the trigeminocervical nucleus—this connection has been confirmed both experimentally and clinically [26–28]. This connection is highly clinically relevant, because it explains the pathogenic background of referred pain between the orofacial area innervated by the facial, glossopharyngeal, and vagus cranial nerves on one side and the spinal C_1–C_3 innervation area on the other side [26]. The knowledge of the organization of nerve fibers in the spinal nerve tract is important for surgical therapy of trigeminal neuralgia—trigeminal tractotomy, employing the destruction of superficially located nerve fibers (for review, see Cetas et al., 2008 [29]). Efferent fibers from the trigeminocervical nucleus run as a ventral trigeminothalamic tract (*tractus trigeminothalamicus ventralis*), together with fibers from the ventrolateral part of the pontine trigeminal nucleus (see below) to the thalamus, from which it runs to the primary sensory cortical area.

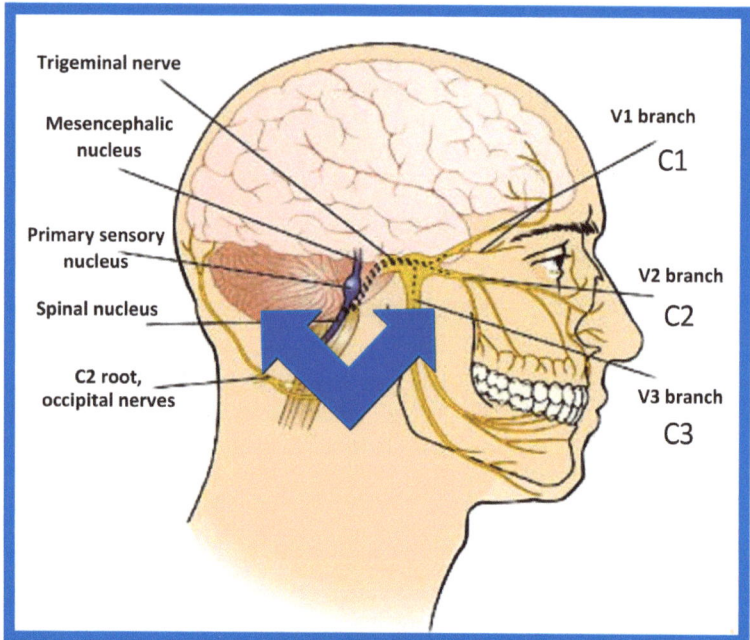

Figure 1. Trigeminocervical convergence. Source: Rocabado Institute, Chile. The convergence of cervical and trigeminal afferents on second-order neurons in the trigeminocervical nucleus may refer to pain from the upper cervical spine into the head and face. Furthermore, bi-directional interactions between the trigeminal and upper cervical afferents may also explain the cervical symptoms of trigeminal origin.

4.2.2. Pontine Trigeminal Nucleus

Pontine trigeminal nucleus (*nucleus pontinus*), also called **principal trigeminal nucleus** (*nucleus principalis nervi trigemini*) is the main somatosensory trigeminal nucleus, located in pons Varoli. Strong A-alpha and A-beta myelinated fibers, leading signals from low-threshold mechanoreceptors of the scalp, end in this nucleus. It has two main parts: (1) The **Dorsomedial part** receives signals from the oral cavity and forms the posterior trigeminothalamic tract (*tractus trigeminothalamicus dorsalis*), which leads ipsilaterally into the thalamus. (2) The **Ventrolateral part** receives signals from all areas innervated by the trigeminal nerve and after crossing the midline, it forms (together with axons of the trigeminocervical nucleus—see above) the ventral trigeminothalamic tract (*tractus trigeminothalamicus ventralis*). This nucleus is functionally related to the gracilis and cuneate nuclei and serves to analyze touch, discrimination, and vibration sensations. It also contains small amounts of proprioceptive fibers, mainly from oculomotor muscles [22]. Efferent fibers from the pontine trigeminal nucleus form a distinct bundle, trigeminal lemniscus (*lemniscus trigeminalis*), which runs into the thalamus and from here to primary sensory cortical areas.

4.2.3. Mesencephalic Nucleus

Mesencephalic nucleus (*nucleus mesencephalicus nervi trigemini*) is an elongated mass of gray matter, located close to the *substantia grisea centralis*. It is unique among central nervous system (CNS) nuclei because it is formed by pseudounipolar neurons [18,22]. Thus, it is considered to be the only intraneuraxial ganglion in the human body [30]. It was originally postulated that these large, glutamatergic pseudounipolar neurons entered the *mesencephalon* from the neural crest during the development; however, recent findings have revealed that they originate primarily from the same material as the future *mesencephalon* [31]. The mesencephalic nucleus is, thereby, the only centrally located nucleus comprising first-order neurons, i.e., they receive impulses directly from receptors, without interpolation. Summarily, 80–90% of dendrites receive proprioceptive signals from the muscle spindles (stretch receptors) of the muscles of mastication, and 10–20% of dendrites receive signals from mechanoreceptors of periodontal tissues, mainly from those at the region of the root apex [32]. Although neurons leading signaling from the masticatory muscles are spread diffusely within the nucleus, i.e., without evident somatotopic organization, neurons registering signals from the periodontal tissues are only localized in the caudal segment of the mesencephalic nucleus [22]. Some anatomical textbooks state that the mesencephalic nucleus also contains signaling from oculomotor muscles and receptors from TMJ [18]; however, this theory has been repeatedly falsified as these pseudounipolar neurons are demonstrably located in the trigeminal ganglion, not in the mesencephalic nucleus [33–35]. The axons of these cells end mainly in the brainstem reticular formation (parvocellular part), in the trigeminal motor nucleus (glutamatergic signals), in the supratrigeminal nucleus and orexinergic hypothalamic nuclei [30,36]. Noteworthy is its projection to the trigeminocervical nucleus and from there, to motor centers of cervical muscles, beside other functions, important for mastication, typically for activation of suprahyoid and infrahyoid muscles during caudal movement (depression) of the mandible [36]. Lateral to the mesencephalic nucleus, are afferent and efferent fibers from the mesencephalic trigeminal tract (*tractus mesencephalicus nervi trigemini*). The mesencephalic nucleus is important for jaw-jerk (masseteric) reflex, as shown by experimental [37] or human studies [38]. However, the role of this nucleus in mastication is not completely elucidated; most likely, it provides the feedback for the masticatory apparatus (stomatognathic system), based on information from proprioceptors of masticatory muscles and mechanoreceptors from the periodontium. If the mesencephalic nucleus is lesioned unilaterally, thus removing all feedback from ipsilateral muscle spindles and important parts of the periodontal mechanoreceptors, experimental animals tend to chew on the contralateral side (they "feel" the food on this side); if the lesion is bilateral, they chew normally on both sides [37]. It remains an interesting result, which reveals that chewing is technically possible without proprioceptive signaling from masticatory muscles [37,39]. In this context, the finding that proprioceptive input does not play a major role in the differentiation of bite force is also important [40]. It was confirmed with findings in patients with lost afferents to mesencephalic nucleus [38]. It shows that proprioceptive signaling is important mainly for teaching of masticatory cycle; moreover, once established, it temporarily becomes less important—until the moment, when a new situation appears and establishment of a new masticatory pattern is necessary, such as after the increase in the vertical dimension of occlusion or loss of the so-called "supporting zones of Eichner" [39,41]. Conversely, experimental work showed that for the regulation of jaw elevation force, the mechanoreceptive signaling from periodontal tissues is necessary [40]. This mechanism protects the teeth against damage (infraction, fracture), as numerous clinical experiences with dental implants (having no periodontal mechanoreceptors) have repeatedly shown [42]. Moreover, the mesencephalic nucleus remains a crucial neural structure in parafunctional orofacial clinical entities such as bruxism (for review, see article by Giovanni and Giorgia [30]).

4.2.4. Motor Trigeminal Nucleus

Motor trigeminal nucleus (*nucleus motorius nervi trigemini*) is a somatomotor nucleus located under the rostral third of the rhomboid fossa. Its fibers form the motor part of the trigeminal nerve, located in the mandibular nerve. It innervates all masticatory muscles (masseter, temporalis, medial and lateral pterygoid) as well as mylohyoid, anterior belly of digastric, tensor tympani, and tensor veli palatini. Cortical projections to the motor trigeminal nucleus are crossed as well as uncrossed; thus, unilateral lesion of this nucleus does not cause significant impairment of the masticatory cycle [18].

4.3. Temporomandibular Joint

TMJ is a compound, paired (bicondylar), and pivoting hinge joint developed between the mandibular (glenoid) fossa and the articular eminence (*tuberculum articulare*) of the temporal bone and mandibular condyle. Between the joint, the articulating disc (*discus articularis*) is inserted. This special and unique biconcave fibrous cartilage divides the joint cavity into the superior discotemporal and inferior discomandibular parts. The articular disc works as a shock absorber as well as a tensile force absorber, forming the basis of convex-concave contact of articular facets [16,26]. Its main parts in the ventrodorsal direction are: (1) anterior attachment of the superior head of the lateral pterygoid muscle, (2) anterior band (anterior rim, anterior dense portion of the disc), (3) biconcave intermediate zone, (4) posterior band (posterior rim, posterior dense portion of the disc), and (5) bilaminar zone, composed of the superior and inferior retrodiscal laminae, which enclose the Zenker's retroarticular fat pad. The main axis of the load of the disc runs through the midpart of its biconcave intermediate zone, where the ventrocranial part of the condyle and dorsocaudal part of the articular eminence are in contact—both parts are convex; hence, the biconcave disk remains the crucial structure for the transfer of convex-convex surfaces to two convex-concave surfaces [16,26].

Temporomandibular Function

Movement of TMJ is limited by many ligaments. Intraarticular (intracapsular) ligaments, which develop in the joint cavity include the anterior, medial, and lateral discal ligaments together with discotemporal ("Tanaka's") and discomalleoar ("Pinto's") ligaments. Ipsiarticular ("collateral") ligaments, formed in proximity to the articular capsule, include the temporomandibular (lateral) and medial ligaments. Extraarticular ligaments, formed at a distance from the articular capsule include sphenomandibular, stylomandibular, pterygomandibular ligaments, and *tractus angularis*. Of particular clinical interest are discomalleoar (Pinto's) and malleomandibular ligaments (part of the sphenomandibular ligament), which connect the structures of the middle ear and the mandibular condyle or articulating disc, thus forming a morphological background for the development of tinnitus in patients with functional problems of TMJ, in particular those of the cervicocranio-mandibular system [43,44].

Importantly, the position of the patient's head is identical to that of the mandibular fossae of TMJ [45]. Thus, any change in alignment of the cervical vertebrae immediately affects the alignment of TMJ structures and their function. For example, if the C_2 vertebra is rotated to the left, the head (together with the mandibular fossae) rotates to the right around the ventrodorsal axis passing through the *glabella* [46]. Accordingly, the bipupilar line (transverse line connecting pupillae of both eyes) is inclined to the right; thus, the right eye (and the right mandibular fossa) is positioned slightly downwards than the left eye (and the left mandibular fossa). A patient may not be aware of this change because the central visual cortex and visual connectomes "re-count" the information such as the head would be in a perfectly horizontal position (for review see Wei, 2018 [47]). This vertebro-cranio-mandibular relation has been repeatedly verified both in experimental animals [48,49] and human patients [50–54]. Elegant experimental study has been provided by D'Attilio et al. [48], who investigated the impact of occlusal interference on the spine of rats creating composite interferences on the right molar of each rat in the experimental group, observing that all such rats developed scoliotic curvature. After creating a composite interference on the opposite side as well (rebalancing of the occlusion), 83% of the rats in the experimental group had their vertebral curvature restored [48]. Moreover, in experimental animals with unilateral occlusal interference, condylar bone resorption of the contralateral side has been observed 1 week later [49]. This finding has been directly and indirectly verified in human patients [50,51,55–60] and the amount of scientific evidence of this phenomenon is rapidly increasing. Of note, when such conditions occur, a change in the occlusal (axilla-mandibular) relationship often leads to misalignment of teeth (malocclusion). The more slowly the cranio-cervical relationship change develops, the greater is the natural tendency to align the teeth (dentoalveolar compensatory mechanism), provided by efficient remodeling capacity of complex periodontal structures. This mechanism is significantly more efficient in growing children than in adults [61]. If this mechanism, and increased attrition/abrasion of the teeth is insufficient, particular teeth (or dental work such as crowns or bridges) are overloaded (traumatic articulation/occlusal trauma) and can suffer from periodontal breakdown and fractures. Moreover, if this malocclusion is fixed, such as in a case of functional unilateral posterior crossbite, it increases the discrepancy of maximum intercuspation and temporomandibular centric relation to pathologic level, which, if not treated properly, can affect further growth and development of the jaws and occlusion, leading to significant skeletal asymmetry, which may require surgical correction [50,51,62]. Moreover, concomitant abnormal mandibular movements may lead to adverse effects both on TMJ and other structures of the stomatognathic system, causing pain and various symptoms [50,51,63,64].

5. Integrative Function of the Cervico-Cranial Complex

The basic control of jaw-opening and jaw-closing is provided by a set of jaw reflexes (trigemino-trigeminal reflexes). The jaw-closers (masseter, temporalis, and pterygoid muscles) serve to close the jaw (mandibular elevation) under normal circumstances and to open it (mandibular depression) when they undergo inhibition. The jaw-closers are excited by A-alpha muscle spindle input and strongly inhibited by A-beta encapsulated mechanoreceptors and possibly A-delta free nerve endings [65]. Uniquely, among the primary sensory neurons, these afferents have their cell bodies in the CNS, in the mesencephalic trigeminal nucleus (see above), rather than in the ganglion, as is typical for other afferents. Moreover, short collaterals connect monosynaptically with synergistic jaw-closing motoneurons in the pontine trigeminal motor nucleus; however, no collaterals cross the midline [65]. Importantly, the excitability of jaw reflex interneurons and primary afferent terminals is controlled during mastication in a way that the sensory detection threshold rises during movement, with a significant change in the perception of oral stimuli during mastication [32].

The rhythmic orofacial movements produced during mastication require the coordination of several jaw, facial, hyoid, and tongue muscles. The basic pattern of rhythmic jaw movements produced during mastication is generated by a neuronal network located in the brainstem and referred to as the masticatory **central pattern generator**. This network, which is composed of neurons mostly associated to the trigeminal system, is found between the rostral borders of the trigeminal motor and facial nuclei [66]. It is capable of the production of rhythmic network activity both and/or without rhythmic inputs from descending or sensory afferents. However, sensory feedback, particularly that from intraoral mechanoreceptors, modifies the basic pattern and is particularly important for the proper coordination of the tongue, lips, and jaws [32]. The central pattern of mastication is generated in two stages: the rhythm, provided by neurons in the midline reticular formation, and the bursts, provided by premotor neurons near the brainstem motor nuclei. The burst generators excite the mandibular opener alpha-motoneurons and inhibit the mandibular closers during the opening phase; however, during closing, the opener motoneurons are not inhibited. Two types of gamma-motoneurons are also involved: dynamic gamma-motoneurons are tonically active during mastication, while static gamma-motoneurons are excited during mandibular closure [32]. The adult masticatory pattern is established at different ages; it varies considerably among individuals [66]. Although mastication is often considered to be stereotyped, there is much variability from cycle to cycle. An older, although important, study of Dellow and Lund showed that the basic pattern could be generated by the brainstem alone in a decerebrated, paralyzed animal [67]. However, the central pattern generator is affected (feedbacked) by many other centers, such as the cortex (including kinesiotopic representation in cortical masticatory area in the most inferior part of the precentral gyrus; via ipsilateral and mainly contralateral corticobulbar tracts), amygdala, hypothalamus, anterior pretectal nucleus, red nucleus, periaqueductal gray, brainstem reticular formation (lesioning of the medial reticular nuclei abolishes mastication), cerebellum or various parts of basal nuclei (for review see Morquette et al., 2012; Lund, 1991 [32,66]). Moreover, inputs from these areas have primarily modulatory functions and are not required to generate the basic masticatory movements that are produced by activation of the masticatory central pattern generator, as shown on decerebrate animals and other models [32,66,68]. However, they are essential for the adaptation of the mandibular movement to the hardness of the food, to compensate for unexpected perturbations and many other delicate masticatory and mastication-related functions [32,66,69]. The central pattern generator also modulates primary afferents and interneurons to suppress unwanted reflexes and favor those that enhance motor performance [32]. More detailed information on the central pattern generator function is available in the literature [32,65,68], but it extends beyond the focus of this review.

The masseter, temporalis, and both medial and lateral pterygoid muscles are often termed the masticatory muscles (muscles of mastication). However, other muscles are also involved in mastication, and are not less important. Due to their position, i.e., attachment from the inferior of the mandible, these muscles can be called **inframandibular masticatory muscles**. Muscles directly attached to the mandible include the anterior belly of the digastric and the mylohyoid. Indirectly attached muscles include platysma, all infrahyoid muscles (sternothyroid, sternohyoid, thyrohyoid, omohyoid), stylohyoid, posterior belly of digastric, pharyngeal constrictors, buccinator, and orbicularis oris. From these, the infrahyoid muscles, innervated by the deep cervical ansa (cervical spinal nerves C_1–C_3), are of particular importance for COP, due to their activation caused by C_1–C_3 spinal nerve irritation. The temporomandibular symptoms including OP appear because inframandibular muscles hold the position of the mandible in perfect midline, but the fossae are positioned incorrectly; thus, the alignment of particular structures of TMJ is incorrect [45,70,71]. Importantly, a significant number of muscle spindles have been found in mandibular elevators, but not in mandibular depressors [32,66]. Thus, the tendency to correct the mandibular position comes mainly from mandibular elevators, thus increasing the possibility of tooth gnashing, grinding, clenching, bracing, thrusting, tapping, and bruxing, together forming a wide range of symptoms of bruxism (for review, see article by Giovanni and Giorgia [30]). Moreover, muscle spindle afferents show various patterns of activity during mastication, ranging from excitation only during mandibular opening to their strong fire during slow closure, thus responding to fusimotor drive [32,37]. Increasing number of data show that the CNS receives several types of feedback signals enabling it to control muscles of mastication in particular movements, both gross and very fine [32,66]. During mastication, trigeminal ganglion neurons provide positive feedback to jaw-closing motoneurons, because heavy pressures generated during the jaw-closing phase of mastication cause the jaw-closing phase to lengthen and jaw-closing motoneurons to fire at higher frequencies [66], leading to a vicious cycle.

Importantly, muscle chains are developed among the particular bony structures. For example, the cervical spine (and occipital bone via pharyngeal raphe attachment) is connected with the anterior mandible (chin) via a muscle chain composed of the superior pharyngeal constrictor muscle, pterygomandibular raphe, buccinator muscle, and inferior part of the orbicularis oris muscle. Dorsally, this muscle chain is connected with the anterior periosteum of the cervical vertebrae via small, but firm pharyngovertebral ligaments. Anteriorly, the orbicularis oris is attached to the periosteum of the anterior mandible. Spasm or any other functional impairment in this muscle chain involves the growth (in children) and movements of the mandible (in all patients), and mandibular protrusion in particular. The involvement of these muscle chains must be considered in differential diagnosis as well as during treatment.

Neurologically, the impairment/loss of occlusal harmony and the development of occlusal interferences significantly impair the execution of jaw reflexes, as well as the function of masticatory central pattern generator in the brain, thus impairing mastication, vital for the preparation of food for digestion by breaking it down into pieces that can be swallowed [66].

6. Novel Concepts of Functional Synthesis of Cervico-Cranial Interactions

Based on scientific evidence and our clinical experience, we recently developed two concepts of OP etiopathogenesis and management, which we present for the first time in this review.

6.1. Rocabado Tricentric Concept of Mouth Sensorimotor Control

Rocabado tricentric concept incorporates (1) craniovertebral, (2) cranio-mandibular, and (3) centric occlusion at rest, all mutually coordinated to allow proper masticatory function and mouth sensory and motor control (Figures 2 and 3). The automatic and dynamic interactions of the three interconnected systems allow for a stable and lasting relation of the mandibular condyle joint facets, functional masticatory system, and physiology of the mouth motor and sensory control. This automatic dynamic mechanism allows for a stable, fossa-condyle, long-lasting, congruent joint-surface relation.

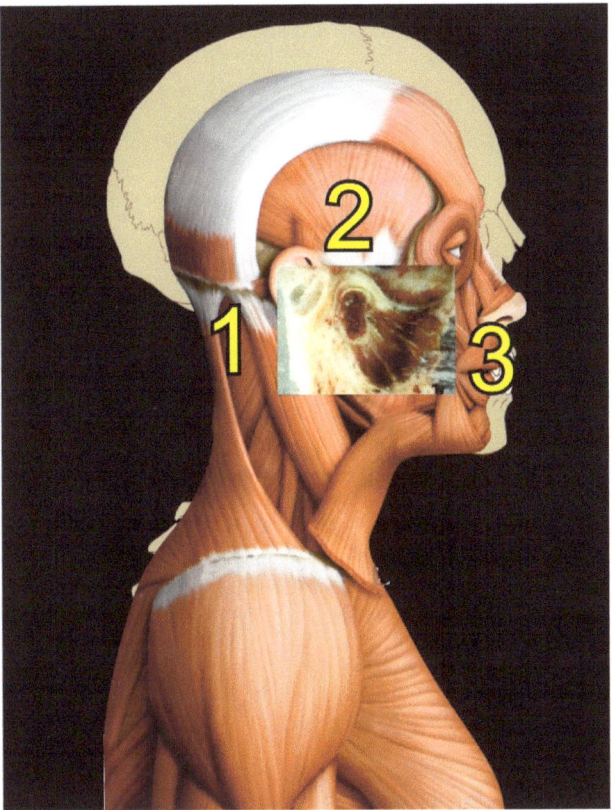

Figure 2. Rocabado tricentric concept. Source: Rocabado Institute, Chile. Craniovertebral, craniomandibular, and centric occlusion at rest are all coordinated to allow functional masticatory system and physiology of the mouth motor and sensory control. This automatic, dynamic mechanism will facilitate a stable fossa-condyle long-lasting congruent joint surface relation.

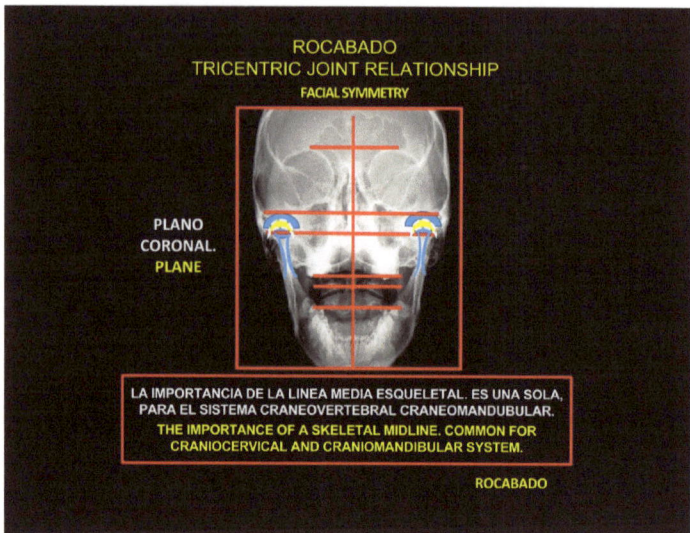

Figure 3. Rocabado tricentric concept.

The Importance of the Skeletal Midline

Physiologically, the mechanism of COP is analogous to the pain felt in the shoulders, chest wall, buttocks, or lower limbs, which is referred from proximal spinal sources; hence its familiarity with pain specialists [5]. The trigeminocervical convergence allows for pain arising from the upper cervical nerves to be referred to regions of the head innervated by trigeminal afferents, such as the orbital, frontal, and parietal regions [4,5,23,72]. Such referral patterns have been elicited in healthy volunteers by experimental noxious stimulation of cervical structures targeting suboccipital and posterior cervical muscles [73,74]. Noxious stimulation of more rostral structures in the cervical spine elicited referred pain in the occipital region, as well as more distant frontal and orbital regions. Conversely, the stimulation of more caudal spine structures elicited pain in the neck radiating to the occipital regions, although not to the anterior regions of the head. It was subsequently shown that noxious stimulation of the atlanto-occipital and lateral atlanto-axial joints, C_2–C_3 zygapophysial joint, and C_2–C_3 intervertebral disc can produce pain in the occipital region [5,75–78].

COP must demonstrate a temporal relationship with the cervical disorder to support causality [10]. Cervical range of motion may be reduced, and headache can worsen with particular movements and/or provocation maneuvers of the neck. The demonstration of a cervical disorder on imaging may be supportive of a diagnosis of cervicogenic pain but does not establish firm evidence of causation. Thus, causation should be considered in the context of the clinical presentation and suspected underlying disorder. Tumors, fractures, infections, cervical spondylosis, osteochondritis, and rheumatoid arthritis of the spine have not been formally validated as causes for OP, but may support causation for COP in certain individual cases. Due to the convergence of cervical and trigeminal nociception, upper cervical myelopathy (C_1, C_2, C_3) may be causal for OP [10,12,79].

Misalignment at the cranio-cervical junction may also play a pathogenic role (Figure 4). Complementary studies have mapped the distribution of referred pain related to the atlanto-axial and zygapophysial (facet) joints of the upper cervical spine [10]. Patients with pain from a particular joint do not experience exactly the same distribution of pain, but there are similarities in the distribution [5]. Misalignment of the first cervical segment can cause impingement of the first two cervical nerve roots (C_1, C_2) as they exit the spine. Stimulation at the C_1 level experimentally evoked occipital or cervical pain in those without migraine, although it was more likely to evoke periorbital and frontal pain in patients with a history of migraine [80]. Moreover, C_2 and C_3 stimulation refers pain to the occipital or cervical region [81]. Although studies have not supported middle- or lower-cervical lesions (below C_4) as being contributory to OP, anastomosis between the spino-cervico-thalamic tract and trigemini-cervical complex may support this possibility [81]. These data show that the structures capable of producing referred pain to the head are those innervated by the C_1, C_2, and C_3 spinal nerves. No experimental studies have shown that structures innervated by lower cervical nerves are capable of directly causing headaches [5]. However, intermediate mechanisms, such as muscle tension and secondary kinematic abnormalities that affect the upper cervical joints may be involved [5,82].

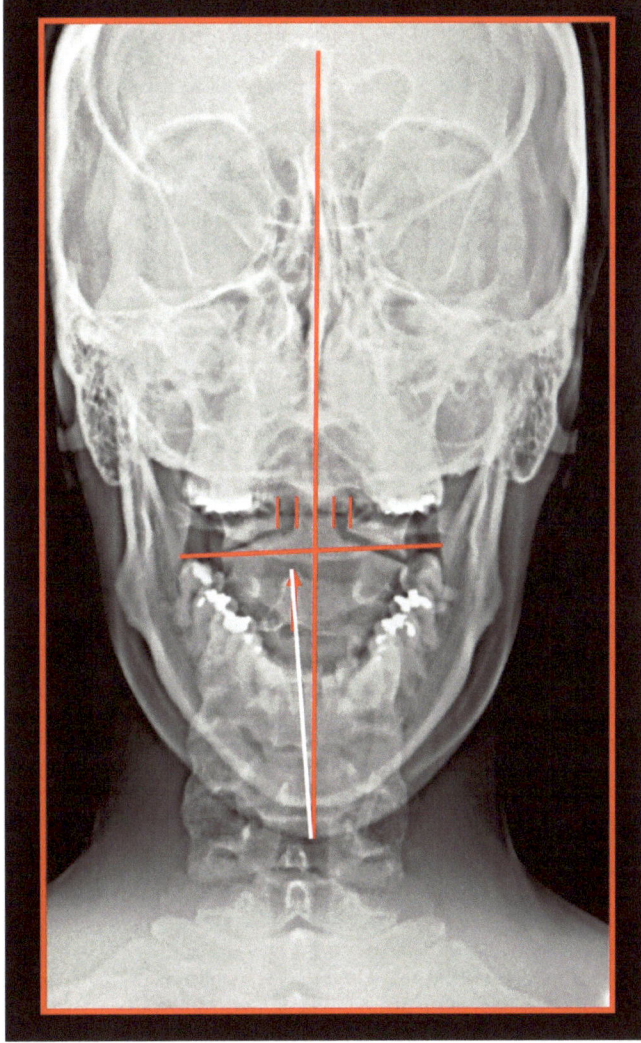

Figure 4. Transoral *atlas-axis* X-ray. Skeletal midline—*dens axis*—spinous process of C_2 should be in one single line. In this patient, spinous process of *axis* is deviated to the right; hence, the *axis* is rotated to the left. The position of the *atlas* is measured from the lateral mass of the *atlas* to the *dens axis*. The space is increased on the right; hence, the *atlas* is rotated to the right. The mandibular occlusal plane is inclined. The cranium is rotated to the left; the left eye pupil is lower than the right.

The relationship to body posture is critical. Many studies have provided evidence of a direct connection between body posture and vertebro-cranio-mandibular system [50,51,55–60]. For example, in children with unilateral crossbite, increased occurrence of postural problems such as oblique shoulder, scoliosis, oblique pelvis, and functional leg length differences have been observed [55].

Faulty body posture and head positioning may result in structural muscle-tissue changes. The deep cervical flexors may undergo a reduction in the number of type I fibers due to muscle inhibition from chronic upper cervical posterior rotation. This, in turn, may help explain the deficits in endurance of the deep cervical flexors observed in patients with COP. According to Watson and Trott, the upper cervical flexors provide a "holding mechanism" for balance and stability of the head [83]. Consequently, the upper or deep cervical flexors have a higher proportion of type I (slow-twitch) versus type II (fast-twitch) fibers, which renders these muscles more resistant to fatigue under normal circumstances. Thus, the importance of posture will be stressed in the following text, as well.

6.2. Concept of Cervical Origin of Bruxism

Bruxism represents a complex of severe clinical symptoms, defined by the American Academy of Orofacial pain as "total parafunctional daily or nightly activity that includes grinding, gnashing, or clenching of the teeth". It occurs in the absence of subjective consciousness, and it can be diagnosed by the presence of tooth-wear facets that have not resulted from the chewing function [84]. There are numerous articles and even comprehensive books focused on bruxism (e.g., Paesani, 2010 [85]). Interestingly, only a few studies and reviews focus on muscles, although they undoubtedly represent a very important factor in the etiopathogenesis of bruxism—simply and concisely, "without muscles, there is no bruxism". Conversely, majority of studies focus on the teeth, where the consequences (but not the etiopathogenesis) are identifiable. Moreover, in the picture of the above mentioned cranio-orofacial, neuro-orthopedic connections, nervous system involvement should be suspected in aspects other than only psychologico-psychiatric facet, as often made by experimenters and clinicians. Furthermore, studies reveal not causation, but a correlation of psychologico-psychiatric aspects and bruxism, indicating they represents mainly secondary, not primary etiological factor in bruxism [86–88]. From our clinical experience, a patient with OP suffering from a primary psychiatric disorder is extremely rare; however, most of these patients have secondary psychological impairments (Šedý, Rocabado, unpublished observation). The crucial factor is time—the proper diagnosis of such patients is often difficult, demanding and time-consuming; contrarily—immediate referring such patients for psychological/psychiatric examination is the opposite. Psychological and psychiatric problems, among the most important seem to be anxiety and depression, thus rather reveal and/or further increase the severity of present bruxism, caused primarily by other (primary) etiopathogenic factors [86–89].

Our concept proposes a chronic irritation of the C_1–C_3 spinal nerves by the improper alignment of the cervical vertebrae and/or degenerative changes in particular vertebrae in close relation to the intervertebral foramina, causing repeated activation of the infrahyoid muscles via branches of the deep cervical ansa (*ansa cervicalis profunda*). These repeated contractions of infrahyoid muscles cause the repetitive minute depression of the hyoid bone as well as the mandible (via the suprahyoid muscles). In the opposite direction, the supramandibular chewing muscles, mainly the mandibular elevators (masseter, temporalis, medial pterygoid) function to reestablish the so-called rest position of the mandible (resting position of the mandible, clinical rest position, rest vertical dimension, mandibular postural position, physiologic rest position, mandibular rest position, vertical dimension of rest) via central pattern generator in the CNS (see above), thus causing sustained muscle contraction leading to bruxism symptomatology, which becomes progressively severe with time.

7. Clinical Syndromes in Cervicogenic Orofacial Pain

Many clinical syndromes have been described in COP. In this review, we describe the ones most important for clinical use in daily practice.

7.1. Cervical Spondylosis

Cervical spondylosis as a primary source of referred OP has been considered important and clinically relevant for decades. Franks in 1968 analyzed 951 patients referred to TMJ specialists during a 5-year period, finding that the problems in 23 were primarily caused by cervical spondylosis [90]. Since then, many studies have identified a cervical origin of orofacial/temporomandibular pain and other symptoms, as detailed in other parts of this review.

7.2. Occipital Neuralgia

The incidence of occipital neuralgia was reported to be 1.8% of headaches [91]. It is caused by irritation of the greater or lesser occipital nerve, characterized by paroxysmal shooting or stabbing pain over the posterior scalp, in the distribution of the occipital nerve. Due to interneural connections in the trigeminal spinal nuclei through the trigeminocervical complex, pain from occipital neuralgia may be referred to the ipsilateral temporal, frontal, or orbital areas [10].

Pain from occipital neuralgia typically irradiates from the suboccipital region towards the vertex and is unilateral in 85% of patients [10]. The pain may be severe, and paroxysmal attacks may last from seconds to minutes. Between paroxysms, there may be a persistent dull ache over the occipital nerve territory, as well as corresponding dysesthesia or allodynia. Continuous occipital pain in the absence of any associated dysesthesia or allodynia should raise suspicion for possible referral of pain from the cervical structures. There is typically tenderness over the affected nerve branches and there may be trigger-point tenderness at the emergence of the greater occipital nerve or in the C_2 distribution. Tingling may also be evoked by light pressure or percussion over the nerve, known as Tinel's sign. Pain with hyperextension or rotation of the neck when patients are in bed may also be a feature, known as the pillow sign [10,92]. Occipital neuralgia must be carefully differentiated from pain in the occiput referred from the atlanto-axial or upper zygapophyseal joints, which should be more appropriately diagnosed as cervicogenic pain (for review, see Barmherzig and Kingston, 2019 [10]).

Importantly, Bogduk and Govind recognized occipital neuralgia as an outdated diagnosis, used before the concept of somatic referred pain was widely understood, when physicians believed that any pain in a particular region was due to some affliction of the nerve that ran through that region. They argued that the proposition that the greater occipital nerve could be compressed between the posterior arch of the *atlas* and the lamina of the *axis* was incompatible with the anatomy and biomechanics of those vertebrae, and that deep aching occipital pain was more likely to be somatic referred pain from an upper cervical joint [5].

7.3. Ponticulus Posticus Syndrome

Any shift/misalignment of the *atlas* can cause a direct impingement of the vertebral artery as it passes through the transverse sulcus or foramen, thus plausibly compromising blood flow to the vertebrobasilar system. One of the most common sources of vertebrobasilar insufficiency, which can also impair the first spinal nerve, is *ponticulus posticus* (Kimmerle anomaly), an artificial bony emergence, crossing the vertebral sulcus of the *atlas*. Through this region, the V_3 part of the vertebral artery is running, together with the abovementioned first cervical nerve and sympathetic as well as venous vertebral plexus [93]. After the calcification of the ligament crossing the vertebral sulcus, an artificial arcuate foramen is formed. It is not a novel finding; although it was first described by W. Allen in 1879 [94], it has not been recognized as a source of COP and/or vertebrobasilar insufficiency until recently. If symptomatic, it represents a morphological basis of tunnel syndrome. A meta-analytic study of 55,985 cases published between 1885–2015 found incomplete *ponticulus posticus* in 13.6% of the population and complete *ponticulus posticus* in 9.1% [95]. In 53.1% of cases, it was bilateral, complete in 59%, and incomplete in the remaining 41% [95]. It occurred more often in North Americans (11.3%) and Europeans (11.2%), and less often in Chinese (4.4%) [95]. Complete *ponticulus posticus* was more frequent in men (10.4%), whereas the incomplete occurred more frequently in women (18.5%) [95]. It more frequently occurs in patients with Gorlin-Gotz syndrome [96]. Morphometric analysis reveals that its mean horizontal diameter (width) is 5.65 mm (range 5.29–5.83 mm) and its mean vertical diameter (height) is 5.16 mm (range 4.86–5.46 mm) [95]. The manifestations of this tunnel syndrome include vertigo, migraine, and Barré-Lieou syndrome, among others. Vertigo is caused by compression of the vertebral artery during head movements, i.e., the movements of the atlanto-occipital joint [95,97,98]. Migraines correspond to COP caused by trigeminocervical convergence, due to irritation of the first cervical spinal nerve [95]. However, the compression of the vertebral artery may also be etiopatogenically involved [98]. Moreover, we must consider that spinal nerves are supplied by branches of the vertebral artery [18]. The Barré-Lieou syndrome represents a combination of headache, nausea, retro-orbital pain, problems with phonation, and visual problems and is clearly associated with *ponticulus posticus* [95,97]. Complete *ponticulus posticus* is 5–11 times more likely to compress the vertebral artery than incomplete *ponticulus posticus* [95]. Regarding diagnosis, computed tomography (CT) has a 20% higher success in uncovering its presence than lateral radiography of the cervical spine [95]. Importantly, the presence of *ponticulus posticus* remains the morphological limitation of conservative treatment; in case of conservative treatment failure, it may be necessary to indicate its surgical removal [95,97,98].

7.4. Triggered Pain

Chronic or persistent pain conditions represent one of the most common causes of disability worldwide. Trigger points are specific sites in muscles, located within taut bands, which are discrete bands of contracture muscle fibers that can be palpated and visualized by particular imaging methods (for review, see Travell and Simons, 2013 [99]. They have greater than normal degree of stiffness than that of normal muscle tissue [100]. They develop most often due to muscle overload, i.e., when an applied load exceeds the capability of the muscle to respond adequately, particularly following unusual or excessive eccentric or concentric loading [101]. Myofascial trigger points in the muscles of the neck can refer pain to the face and head, and vice versa, although less often. Travell and Simons have stated that myofascial trigger points may develop from structural inadequacies, postural stress, and constriction of muscles. At the cranio-cervical junction, the structural inadequacy may be represented by a chronic *atlas* (C_1 vertebra) misalignment that generates mechanical stress, which then leads to the formation of trigger points [99].

7.5. Atypical Facial (Oro-Facial) Pain

Atypical facial pain (AFP), or persistent idiopathic facial pain is a well-recognized syndrome, where the depression or psychosomatic causes are mostly suspected as primary etiological factors. It is a chronic and diffuse distribution of facial pain along the distribution of the trigeminal nerve. This condition occurs in the absence of any neurologic deficit or known etiology. It presents mostly with neck-muscle tension and OP. Despite the limitations of evidence-based literature, tricyclic antidepressants such as amitriptyline or nortriptyline have proven effective and are considered the treatment of choice for AFP [102,103]. However, AFP is one of the most challenging conditions to diagnose due to the lack of clear diagnostic criteria, as well as specific, evidence-based guidelines for management. This condition is diagnosed mostly by the exclusion of other known etiologies. Specific disease modalities cannot be targeted, resulting in a deficiency of a clear treatment protocol. Thus, this diagnostic category is often questioned [103,104]. Based on our empirical clinical experience, we strongly suspect that the diagnosis of AFP is often, but not always, used for patients with unrecognized COP (Šedý, Rocabado, unpublished data).

7.6. Pain Due to Iatrogenic Causes

COP can be caused by iatrogenic factors. Typically, it occurs when the vertical dimension of occlusion drastically increases, typically due to a massive occlusal splint. Such splints are sometimes fabricated for conservative treatment of obstructive sleep apnea, to open upper airways during sleep (for review see Marklund et al., 2019 [105]). However, this extreme posteriorotation of the mandible leads to compensatory posteriorotation of the head, leading to enhancement of cervical lordosis ("hyperlordosis") causing the compression of C_1–C_3 spinal nerves, leading to COP.

8. Diagnosis of Cervicogenic Orofacial Pain

Proper diagnosis of COP remains a crucial part of clinical protocol. Although it can be time-consuming, demanding, and complex, it presents a fundamental take-off step for successful curative treatment of COP.

8.1. Diagnostic Criteria

Antonaci et al. proposed seven criteria for cervicogenic headache: (1) Unilateral headache without side-shift, (2) symptoms and signs of neck involvement: pain triggered by neck movement or sustained awkward posture and/or external pressure of the posterior neck or occipital region; ipsilateral neck, shoulder, and arm pain; reduced range of motion, (3) pain episodes of varying duration or fluctuating continuous pain, (4) Moderate, non-excruciating pain, usually of a non-throbbing nature, (5) pain starting in the neck, spreading to oculo-fronto-temporal areas, (6) anesthetic blockades abolish the pain transiently provided complete anesthesia is obtained, or occurrence of sustained neck trauma shortly before onset [106]. Satisfying criteria 1 and 5 qualify for a diagnosis of possible cervicogenic headache. Satisfying any additional three criteria advances the diagnosis to a probable cervicogenic headache [106].

8.2. Importance of Prompt and Accurate Diagosis

Undiagnosed and unaddressed pain can be refractory, leading to disability, and reduction of quality of life [10]. When deep knowledge and clinical experience of the medical specialist is set aside, the most important factor for a proper diagnosis is the time spent with the patient. Patience is important for obtaining a detailed and valid and reliable medical history of the patient (anamnesis). For COP, the most reliable features are previous neck trauma, pain that starts in the neck and radiates to the fronto-temporal region, pain that radiates to the ipsilateral shoulder and arm, and provocation of pain by neck movement [106–108].

These patients are often frustrated from previous "improper examination/treatment failure" vicious cycles. Although they are highly motivated for treatment, their confidence in medical authorities and proposed treatment methods may be low. In addition, most psychological signs are not primary (i.e., primary psychiatric diseases such as schizophrenia or endogenic depression) but secondary, caused by severe impairment of their psychosocial aspects of life caused by long-term debilitating pain and other orofacial disabilities [109,110]. The following detailed clinical examination is also necessary. Additional maneuvers on physical examination should include movement tests of the cervical spine, such as passive flexion, extension, and rotation; segmental palpation of the cervical facet joints, and; it should also include the assessment for palpation tenderness over the greater-occipital nerve, lesser-occipital nerve and upper-cervical muscle groups [10,16,111] (Figure 5).

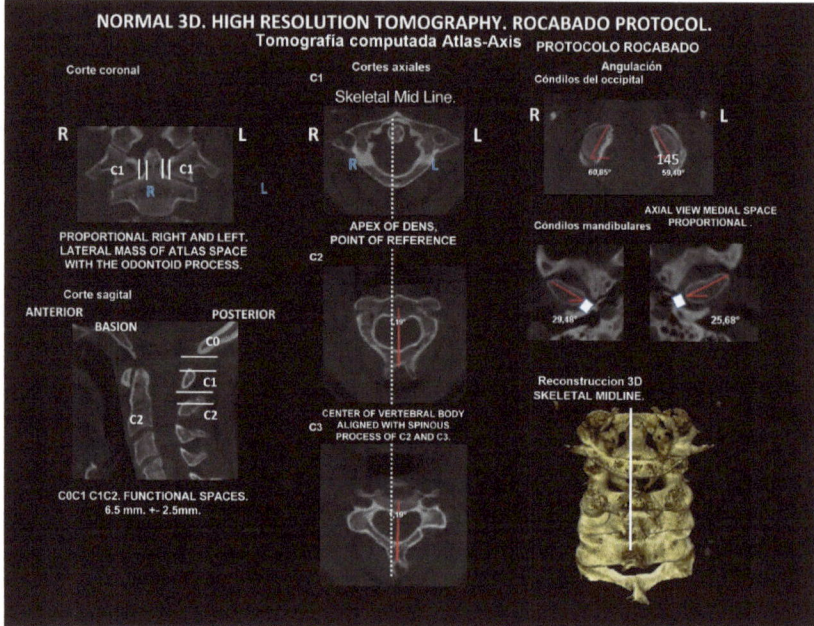

Figure 5. Rocabado diagnostic protocol for cervical spine.

8.3. Local Anesthetic Blockade as a Diagnostic Tool

COP may respond to local anesthetic blockade of the occipital nerves (greater, lesser, or both). While this intervention is sensitive, it is not specific. Many primary headache disorders including migraine, tension-type headache, and cluster headache may also demonstrate a similar response. Clinically, there may be a significant overlap in the clinical appearance between COP, occipital neuralgia, migraine, and tension-type headache with pericranial tenderness [10,79].

Neck pain can be a predominant feature in up to 68% of patients with migraine and tension-type headaches [79]. In the case of migraine, neck pain may occur as a prodromal symptom, intra-attack, or as a postdrome symptom [112]. Due to connections with the vestibulocochlear, glossopharyngeal, and vagus nerves, symptoms such as tinnitus, dizziness, and nausea may be features of both occipital neuralgia and COP [113]. However, these features are less prominent in COP as well as in occipital neuralgia than in migraine.

9. Differential Diagnosis

COP can mimic several diseases, the most clinically important of which are presented here.

9.1. Dissecting Aneurysms

Dissecting aneurysms of the vertebral or internal carotid arteries can present with neck pain and headache. They are indicated by the onset of cerebrovascular features, which typically emerge within 1–3 weeks. If this differential diagnosis is not considered, there is a risk of patients being treated with cervical manipulation, with fatal consequences due to aggravation of the aneurysm [5,114–116].

9.2. Lesions of the Posterior Cranial Fossa

They are also important, as the dura mater and vessels of the posterior fossa are innervated by the upper cervical nerves. These lesions are distinguished by the onset of neurological features or systemic illness, such as meningitis of the upper cervical spine or herpes zoster. Moreover, the tiny, but clinically, extremely important muscles of the suboccipital triangle have an anatomically defined connection of their epimysia with cervical- and lower-cranial dura mater [117]. Importantly, the activity of these muscles is directly connected with the change in the head position [118,119].

9.3. Migraine

While migraine tends to have unilateral shifting, both COP and occipital neuralgia tend to be side-locked, and COP is often triggered by head movement (irritation of C_1–C_3 spinal nerves) (Figure 6). Pain radiation in COP tends to have a postero-anterior direction. However, in migraine, the pain tends to be more anterior, and radiation tends to be anterior-posterior. COP should also be differentiated from other secondary disorders such as headache attributed to cervical dystonia, Chiari malformation, cervical or vertebral artery dissection, whiplash injury, congenital malformations, space-occupying or destructive lesions, or infection [10,79,112,113,120].

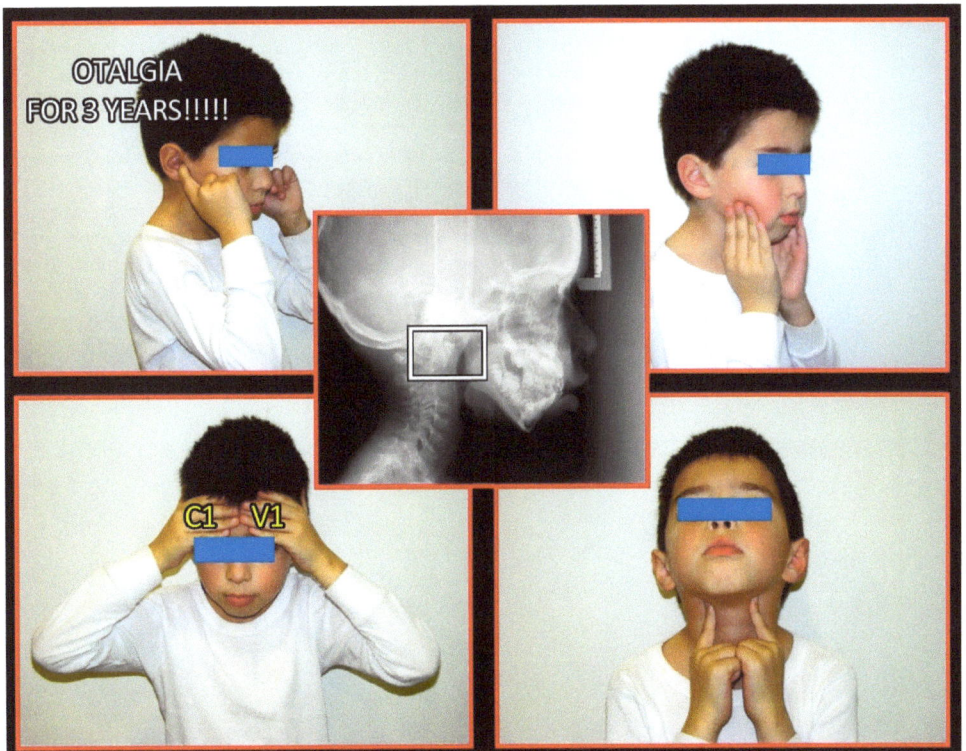

Figure 6. Pediatric patient with otalgia, headache, and pain of the occiput. Source: Rocabado Institute, Chile. *Atlas-axis* syndrome previously not diagnosed. The importance of the neurological connection between the cervical spine and the craniofacial and craniomandibular system. Patient showing sites of pain.

9.4. Neck-Tongue Syndrome

Bogduk and Govind stressed that neck–tongue syndrome and C_2 neuralgia can be confused with COP, because the C_2 spinal nerve runs behind the lateral atlanto-axial joint and is accompanied by its dural sleeve and a substantial plexus of veins. Neck–tongue syndrome occurs when rapid turning of the head subluxates the lateral atlanto-axial joint posteriorly. Tension in the joint capsule causes ipsilateral occipital pain, while compression of the C_2 spinal nerve produces numbness of the tongue [5,121,122].

9.5. Miscellaneous

Moreover, C_2 compression/neuralgia can be caused by various disorders. Inflammatory disorders or injuries of the lateral atlanto-axial joint can result in the adjacent nerve becoming incorporated into the fibrotic changes of chronic inflammation [123,124]. The C_2 spinal nerve can be compromised by a meningioma, neurinoma, anomalous vertebral arteries, and several other vascular anomalies [123–128]. Nerves affected by vascular abnormalities have several features indicative of neuropathy, such as myelin breakdown, chronic hemorrhage, axon degeneration and regeneration, and increased endoneurial and pericapsular connective tissue [125]. Unlike the dull, aching pain of COP, the features of C_2 neuralgia are intermittent, lancinating pain in the occipital region associated with lacrimation and ciliary injection [5,123,125,128].

10. Diagnostic Use of Imaging Techniques

Several imaging methods have been proposed for the diagnosis of COP. However, in their indication, risk-benefit ratio needs to be evaluated in every case, to prevent their overindication (overtreatment). Moreover, analysis of previous medical specialist consultations (ear-nose-throat [ENT], neurological, dental, etc.) and results of previous examination methods (radiography, CT, magnetic resonance imaging [MRI], sonography, etc.) is also necessary. Imaging methods permit clinicians to objectively observe and confirm at least the seven most frequent positional faults among the occiput, *atlas*, *axis*, and C_3 vertebra (Figures 7–9). These positional faults induce craniovertebral intra-joint irritation, as well as capsular connective tissue, ligament soft tissue damage, tears, inflammation, bleeding, and muscle disorders such as shortening, tightness, spasm, adhesions with local or referred patterns of pain. These pathologies need to be addressed prior to reaching any definite therapeutical decision of occlusal contact changes during the process of oral rehabilitation. All dysfunctions are related to the trigeminal-cervical nucleus, affecting the occipito-atlanto-axial joints and synovial TMJ with a broad syndrome of head neck and facial pain with or without synovial TMJ disc pathology.

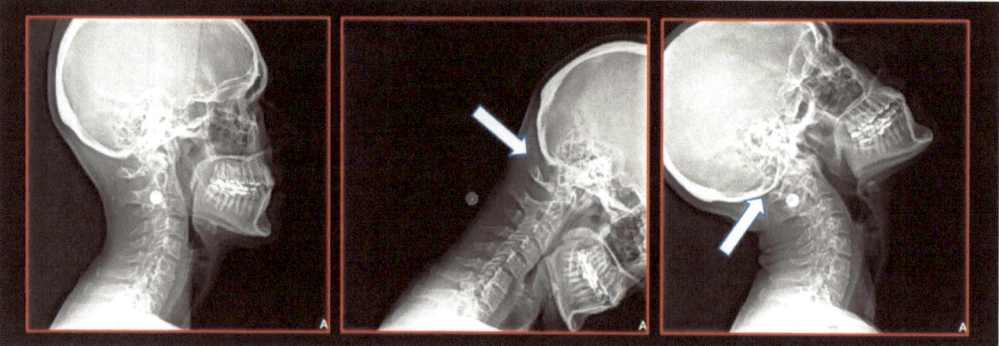

Figure 7. Normal lateral (sagittal) dynamic cephalometric analysis.

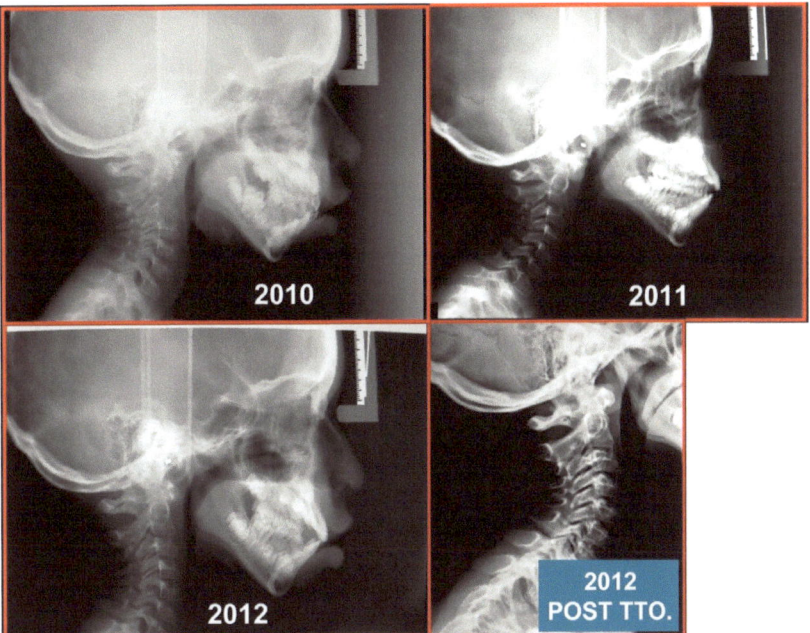

Figure 8. Pediatric patient with otalgia, headache, and facial pain of the occiput. *Atlas-axis* syndrome previously not diagnosed. A series of lateral cephalograms showing the treatment progress. There is the importance of the neurological connection between the cervical spine and craniofacial and craniomandibular systems.

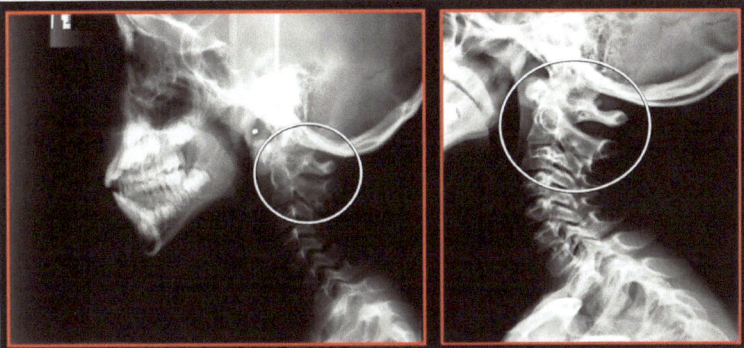

Figure 9. Rotation of the *atlas* on a lateral cephalometric radiograph. **Left:** Pre-treatment. Double ring of the *atlas* showing its rotation. Decreased functional spaces. **Right:** After orthopedic manual therapy. Only one posterior arch of the *atlas* showing the normalization of its rotation. Normalized functional spaces.

10.1. Neck X-ray

The gold standard and most important basic imaging method for the evaluation of COP source is neck X-ray, i.e., frontal X-ray of the upper cervical vertebrae (dorso-ventral image of head with mouth open to maximum) and lateral head and neck image. From these images, the following information can be obtained: general alignment of the cervical spine and head, presence, position (rotation, shift—spondylolisthesis), and morphology of particular vertebrae, changes suggestive of arthritis or cranio-cervical instability, the presence of ponticulus posticus, the position of the hyoid bone, jaw and teeth relationship, and other important changes (Figures 10–14). In addition, particular distances and angle measurements can be easily obtained. These images can be taken by classical medical X-ray, available in most hospitals, or from cephalographs, available in orthodontic or maxillofacial surgical departments. Thus, almost every medical specialist, including a dentist, can obtain this examination quickly and cheaply.

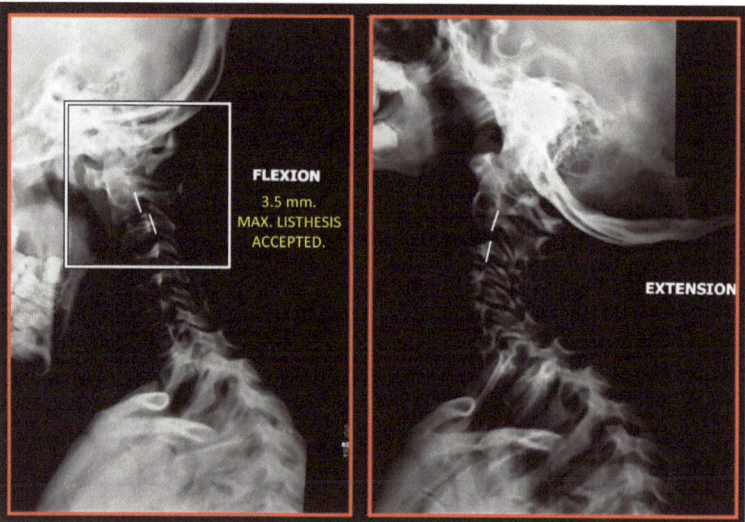

Figure 10. Static *atlas* on the occiput in flexion and extension. Additionally, notice the double ring of posterior arch of the *atlas* showing that it is also rotated and static. A 3.5-mm anterior listhesis of the *axis* on C3 during flexion. Lateral cephalometric study.

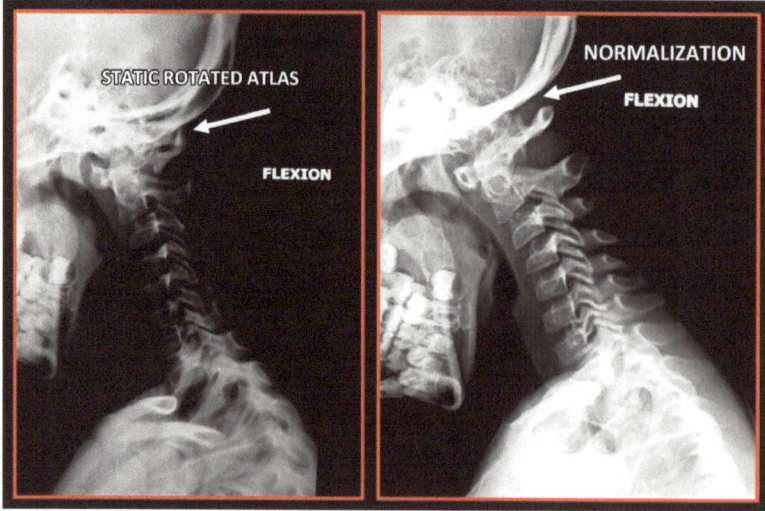

Figure 11. Rotation of the *atlas* on lateral cephalometric radiograph. **Left:** Pre-treatment. Double ring of the *atlas* showing its rotation. Decreased functional spaces. **Right:** After orthopedic manual therapy. Only one posterior arch of *atlas* showing normalization of *atlas* rotation. Normalized functional spaces.

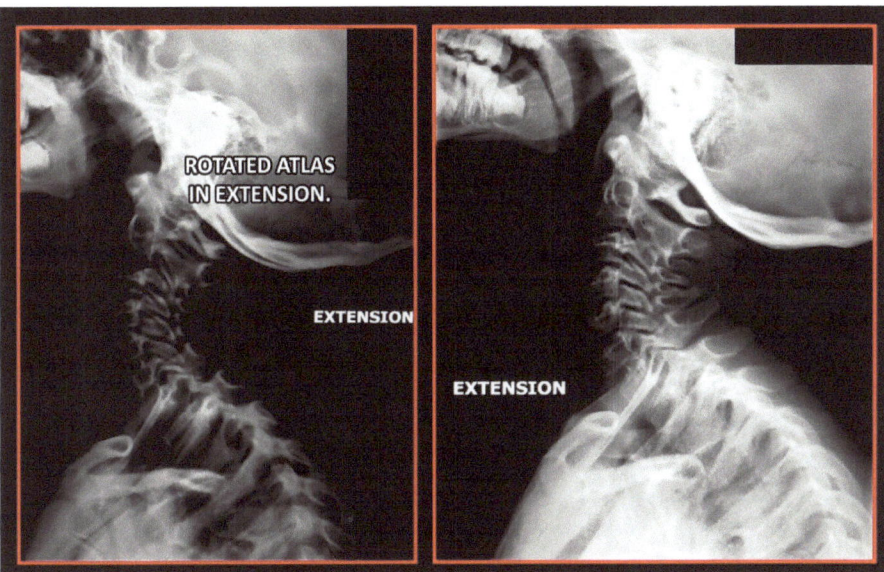

Figure 12. Rotation of the *atlas* on lateral cephalometric radiograph. **Left:** Pre-treatment. Double ring of the *atlas* showing its rotation. Decreased functional spaces. **Right:** After orthopedic manual therapy. Only one posterior arch of the *atlas* showing the normalization of *atlas* rotation. Normalized functional spaces.

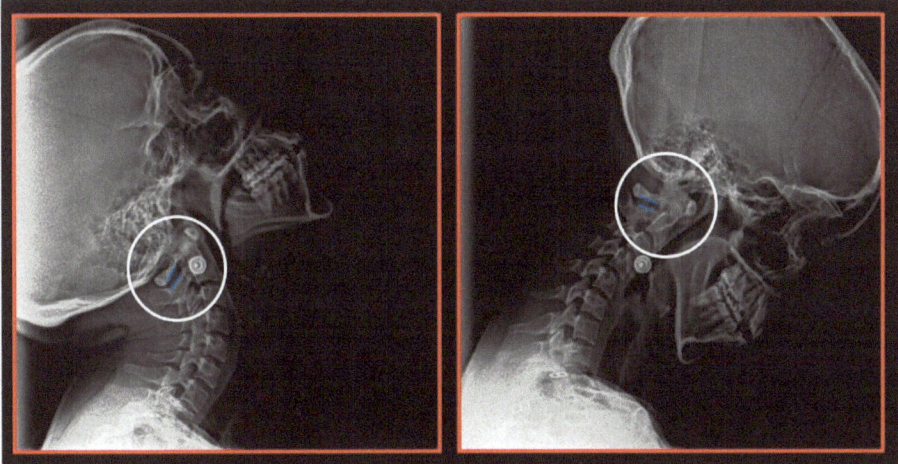

Figure 13. Decreased space between the posterior arch of the *atlas* and spinous process of C_2 in maximal flexion and extension of the cervical spine. Dynamic lateral cephalometric study.

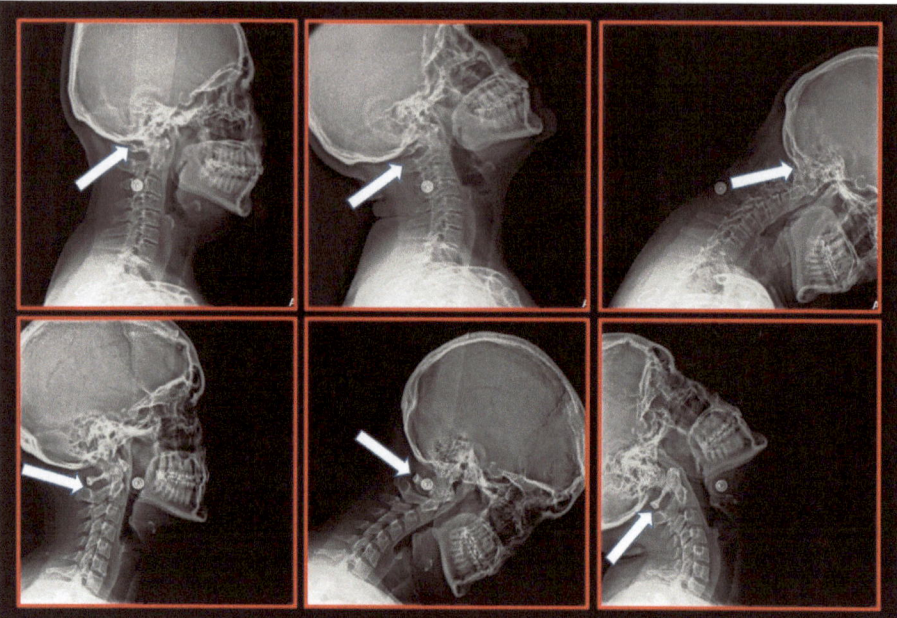

Figure 14. Relations among the occiput, C_1 and C_2 vertebrae. **Upper row:** Static *atlas* on the occiput causing mechanical compression and irritation of the C_1 nerve root, causing occipital supraorbital pain. **Lower row:** Static *atlas* on the *axis* causing additional complaints at the level of the C_2 nerve root, including unilateral craniofacial pain.

10.2. Computed Tomography of Cervical Spine

CT, particularly three-dimensional (3D), high-resolution tomography, should be considered when there is a high index of suspicion for an osseous pathology and/or rotation or suspected malposition of a vertebra (Figures 15–17). It should be noted that osteoarthritic changes are common with advancing age, and the presence of these findings alone on imaging is not diagnostic for COP. Barmherzig and Kingston report from their experience that over-investigating a patient with a clinical history consistent with a primary headache disorder such as migraine carries the risk of discovering these incidental changes [10]. This has the potential for harm in creating patient doubt around the initial primary headache diagnosis. Therefore, there should be a reasonable clinical suspicion of COP prior to initiating these investigations [10]. Moreover, it should be performed in case of significant intervertebral misalignment [70,71]. Although, we can perform CT with classical medical CT scan, it might be better to perform cone-beam CT (CBCT), to minimize the radiation dose [128]. Moreover, CBCT offers the acquisition of an image with high accuracy, reducing the evaluation (measurement) bias and improving the reliability, including the evaluation of data from scientific studies [50,51,129]. To date, CBCT is available in an increasing number of ambulatory offices, becoming the standard examination modality in ENT, dentistry, and cranio-maxillofacial surgery [129].

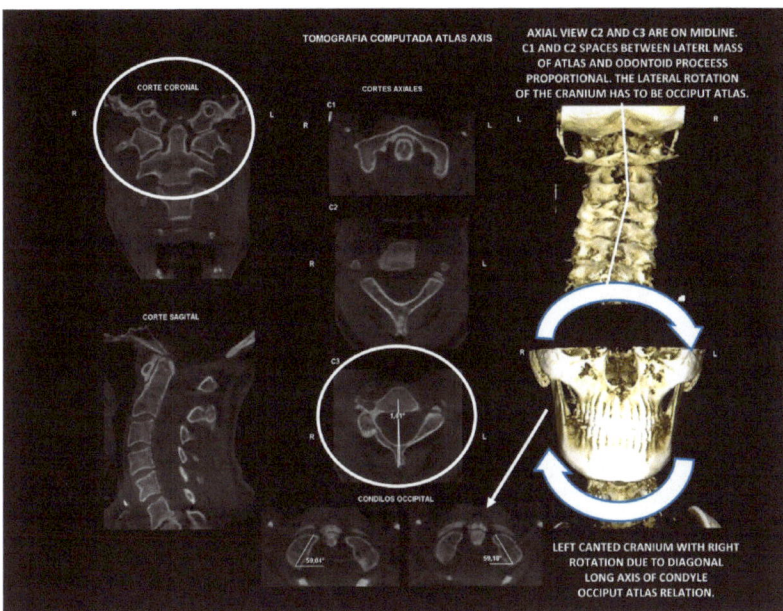

Figure 15. Diagnosis. *Atlas-axis* three-dimensional high-resolution tomography. The cranium is canted with lower cervical spine compensation. It is an occiput-*atlas* lateral or coronal plane disorder. Diagnosed as normal axial and coronal *atlas-axis* relation. Habitually, it is not diagnosed or diagnosed as normal craniovertebral relation.

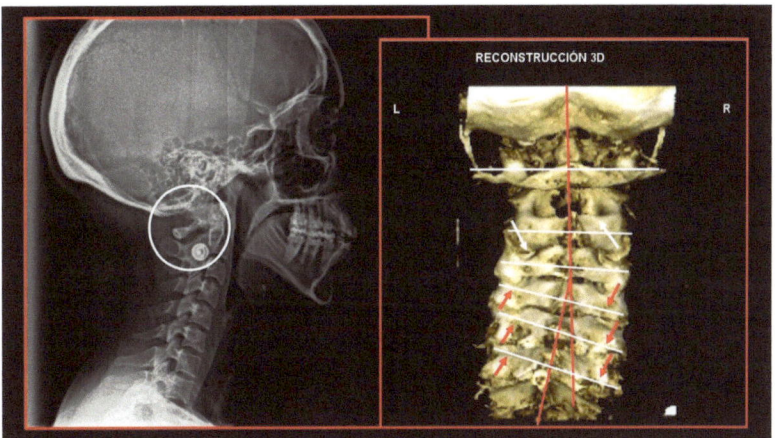

Figure 16. Decreased functional space between posterior arch of the *atlas* and spinous process of C2. Static *atlas* on the *axis*. Loss of cervical lordosis. Scoliosis. **Left:** lateral cephalometric radiography. **Right:** three-dimensional computed tomography reconstruction.

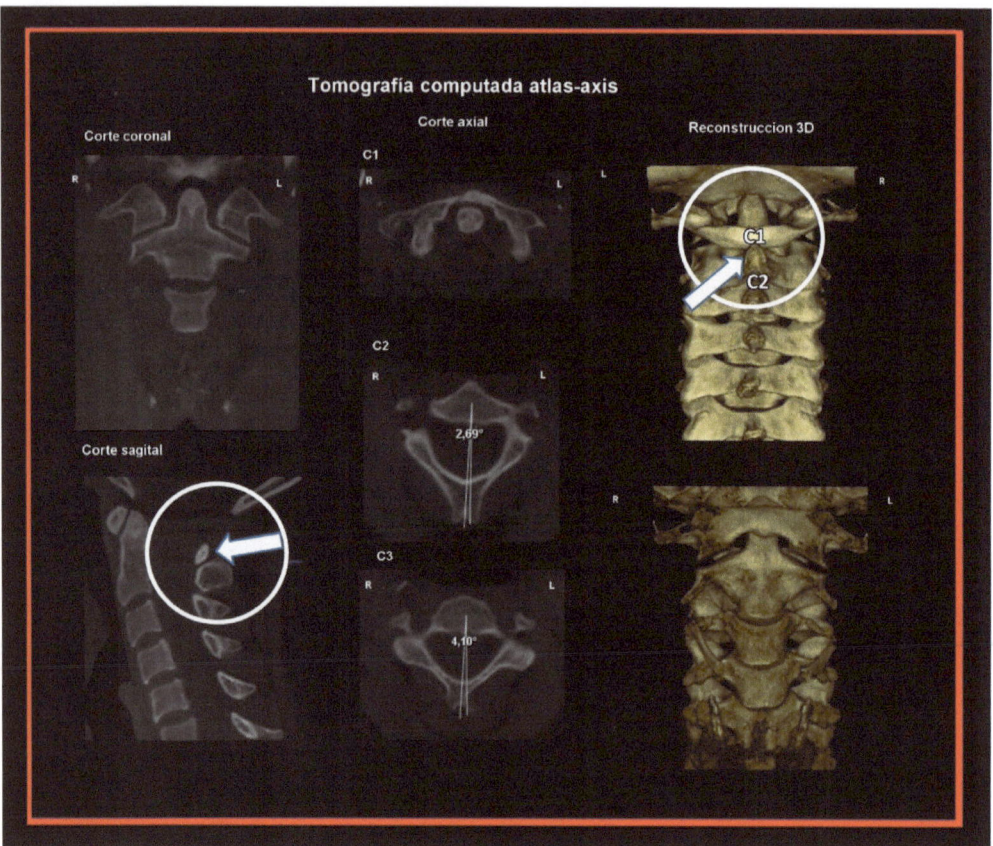

Figure 17. C_2-C_3 segment. The angle of the spinous process of the *axis* determines the degree of *axis* rotation.

10.3. Magnetic Resonance Imaging of Cervical Spine

MRI remains the imaging modality of choice, as it allows for high-quality visualization of both the cervical spine as well as the surrounding occipital and cervical soft tissues (Figures 18–20). The main benefit is the zero radiation dose. Its main disadvantage is the high cost and discomfort in claustrophobic patients.

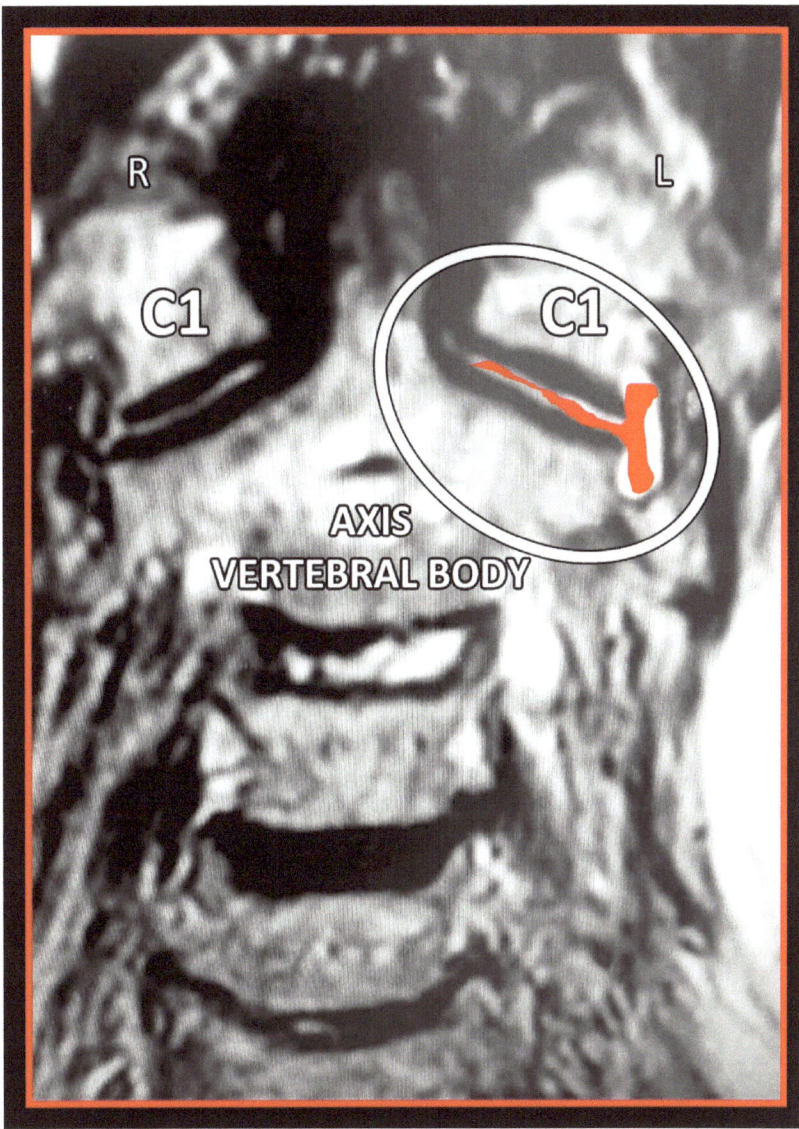

Figure 18. *Atlas-axis* synovitis. Magnetic resonance imaging showing the left lateral effusion of *atlas-axis* intra-joint passive congestion, with increased pain during active axial rotation of the *atlas* on *axis* to either side. C_2 nerve root involvement with unilateral hemicranial pain.

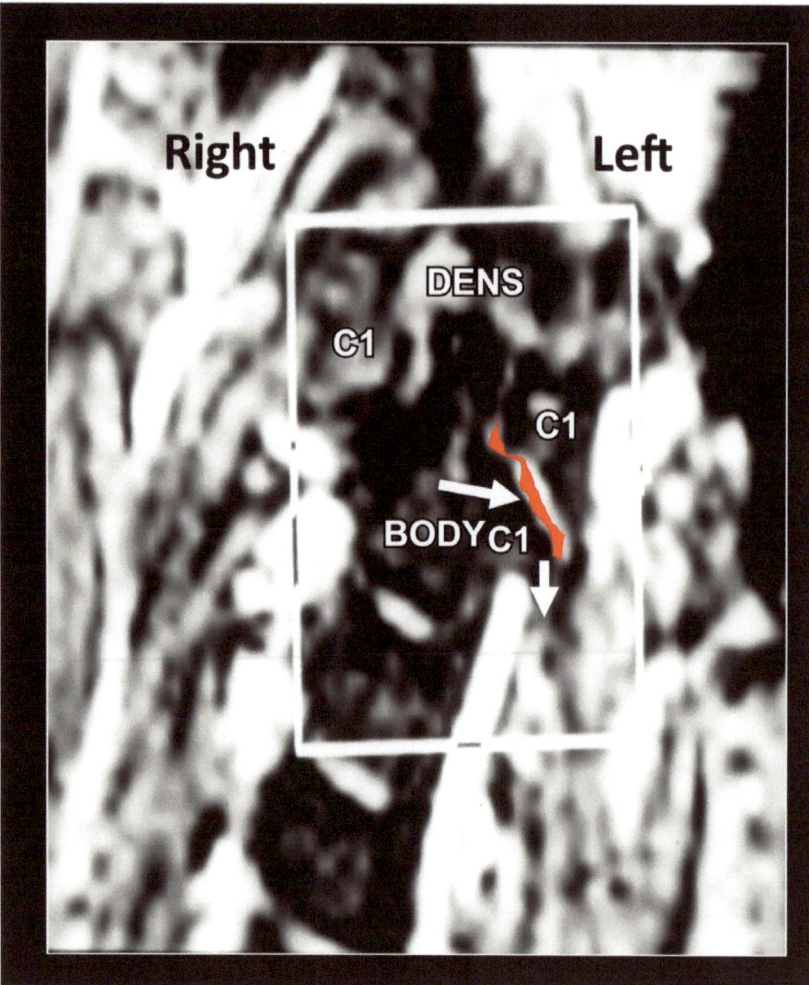

Figure 19. *Atlas-axis* gapping. Left coronal, dynamic magnetic resonance imaging (MRI), showing the lateral gapping of the left facet joint between the *atlas* and *axis*, during lateral cranial rotation (side bending) restriction. The lack of rotational component of the *axis* during lateral rotation of the cranium to the same side induces a dysfunctional pattern of cranial rotation. When the *axis* attempts to rotate towards one side, the superior lateral facet joint of *axis* drops down on the same side of the lateral rotation of the cranium, opening the gap between the lateral mass of the *axis* below the *atlas*. The lateral evaluation of the *axis* is painful on the restricted side of the lateral movement. The *axis* cannot rotate to that side and descends below the *atlas* causing capsular distension of the atlanto-axial joint. The MRI facilitates the understanding of the dysfunction to plan the treatment process and left rotation of the *axis* on the C3 vertebra. During treatment, it is important to maintain proportional rotational patterns of movement between *atlas* and *axis*.

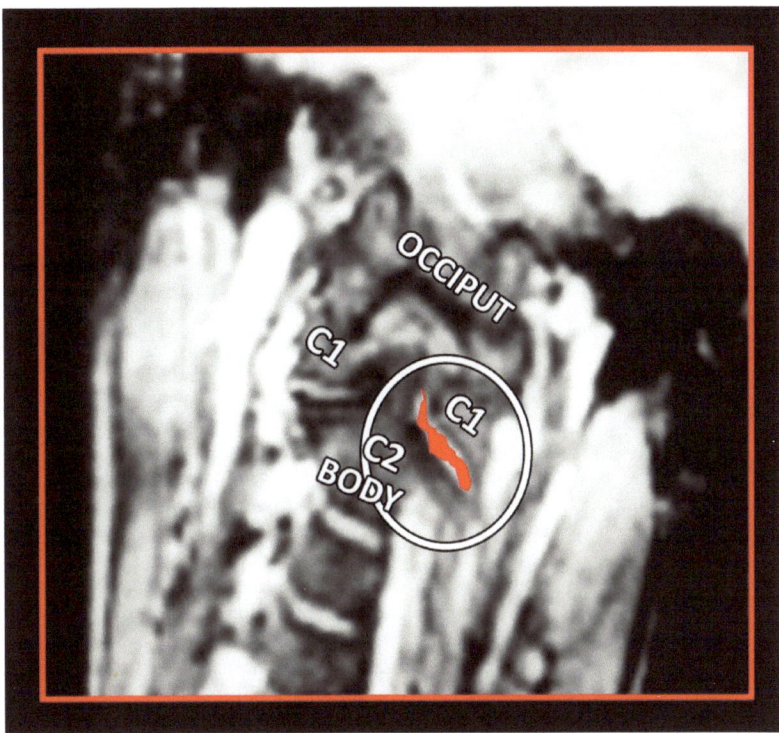

Figure 20. Dynamic coronal magnetic resonance imaging study. Lateral instability of *atlas-axis* segments. The study facilitates the understanding of the dysfunction to plan the treatment process and restore left rotation of the *axis* on the C3. Maintain proportional rotational patterns of movement between the *atlas* and *axis*.

10.4. Sonography of Cervical Area

It may be a useful technique to evaluate the course of the occipital nerve from its origin at the C_2 nerve root until it becomes subcutaneous at the trapezius aponeurosis. This may identify a site of entrapment in occipital neuralgia, corresponding with an enlarged, and swollen nerve appearance. The main benefit of ultrasound is its relatively low cost and zero radiation risk for the patient. However, evaluation with ultrasound relies on expertise in performing the test and interpreting results, which may render it a less valuable diagnostic modality for most clinicians [10]. Moreover, ultrasound does not provide any information about bones and joints, often necessary for the diagnosis of COP. Thus, it remains a rare modality for COP diagnosis.

11. Treatment

Successful treatment requires creating a therapeutic partnership with the patient, to empower the patient to take an active role in the treatment plan. Without the patient's significant investment of time and effort, the treatment cannot be successful. Any underlying or contributory pathology should be appropriately addressed and managed. Interestingly, with the spread of COVID-19 disease during the recent pandemic, teledentistry has been introduced in the management of patients with temporomandibular disorders [130].

11.1. Conservative Treatment

Conservative and non-pharmacologic therapy should be preferred to pharmacologic approaches. Among these approaches, orthopedic manual therapy (targeted physiotherapy) should be the first choice. A randomized-control trial looking at spinal manipulation therapy in a cohort of highly selected patients with COP, in the absence of contraindications to spinal manipulation therapy, suggested a linear dose-response relationship between spinal manipulation therapy therapeutic sessions and days with COP, with a reduction in headache days sustained to 52 weeks after the start of therapy [131]. Another study showed that treatment with manual therapy, specific exercises, or manual therapy plus exercises was significantly more effective at reducing headache frequency and intensity than generalized care by a general practitioner [132]. Approximately 76% of patients achieved a more than 50% decrease in headache frequency and 35% achieved complete relief at the 7-week follow-up. At 12 months, 72% had a more than 50% decrease in headache frequency [132].

11.2. Orthopedic Manual Therapy

Orthopedic manual therapy comprises effective differential diagnosis and treatment approach of both functional disturbances and effectiveness of motor activity in any synovial joint of the body, its connective tissue that holds the joint together and abnormal muscle function (Figures 21–28), including the shortening, weakening, and muscle imbalance and, most important, the loss of muscle chain disconnections altering rest position. This leads to the dysfunction of time direction and load of the joint surfaces and progression to joint wear, tear, joint pain, and degenerative joint diseases. Together with a history of patient complaint in a friendly environment, a thorough and functional total body examination, and a concomitant sensitive palpatory technique with specific joint mobility of the locomotor area involved, one can utilize certain criteria that help determine if and what manipulative or total body stabilization exercise-program treatment is recommended in that specific circumstance. Criteria used for the indication of orthopedic manual therapy include localized and referred pain, observation of soft-tissue abnormalities and the zone of irritation, pathologic motion barrier, characterized by motion restriction or hypomobility, or benign joint systemic hypermobility. Muscle imbalance always presents as regional, such as muscle weakening, shortening, or general myotendinous imbalance and/or enthesitis. The first effort or provisional treatment attempt is of great concern. After the expert opinion of treatment and elimination of possible contraindications, the manual therapist will be able to make the first diagnosis and prescribe an initial approach to treatment.

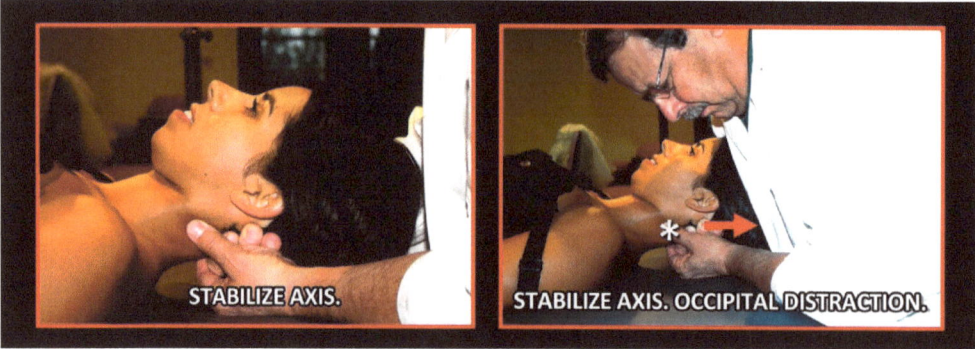

Figure 21. Initial orthopedic manual treatment. Source: Rocabado Institute, Chile. Long axis distraction of the cervical spine (C_0–C_1–C_2).

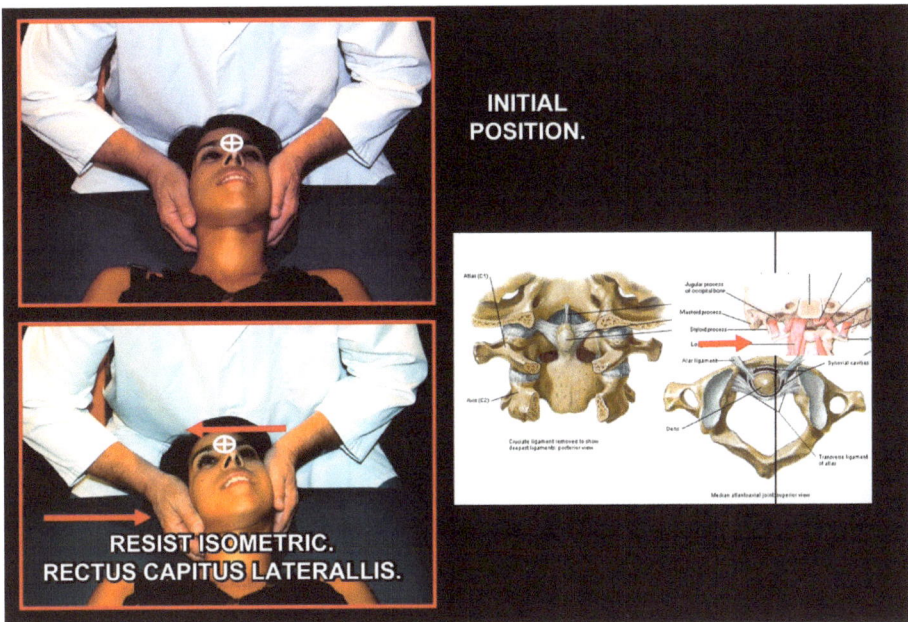

Figure 22. Normalization of C_2 left rotation. Source: Rocabado Institute, Chile. Employing alar ligament and rectus capitis laterallis using neuromuscular techniques.

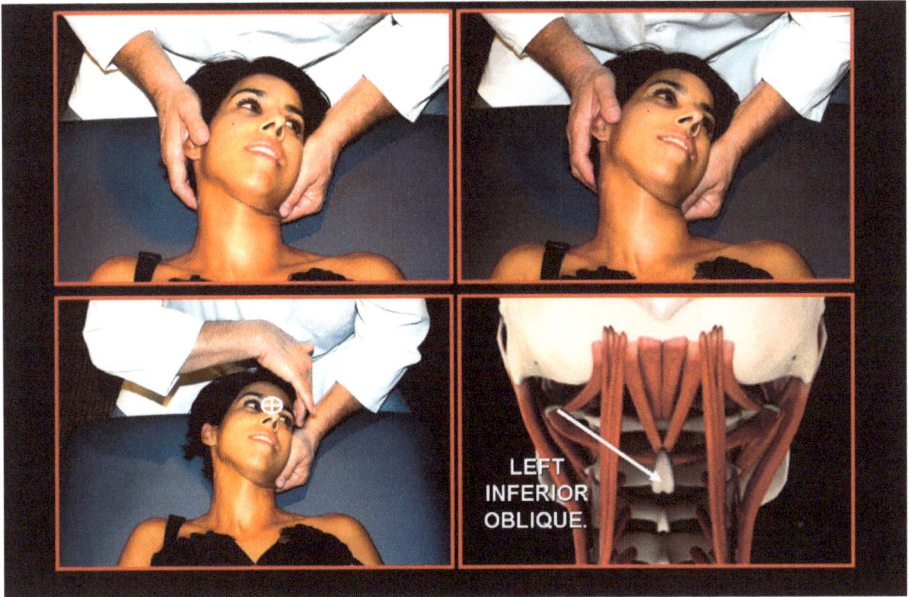

Figure 23. *Atlas* derotation, left direction. Source: Rocabado Institute, Chile. Employing left inferior oblique and right anterior rectus capitis muscles using neuromuscular techniques.

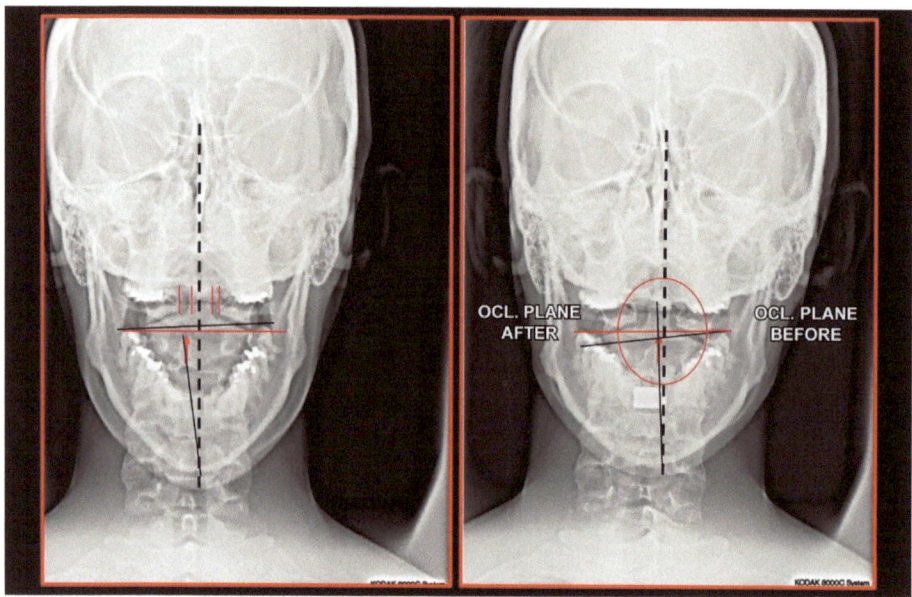

Figure 24. Radiographic situation before and after one session of orthopedic manual therapy.

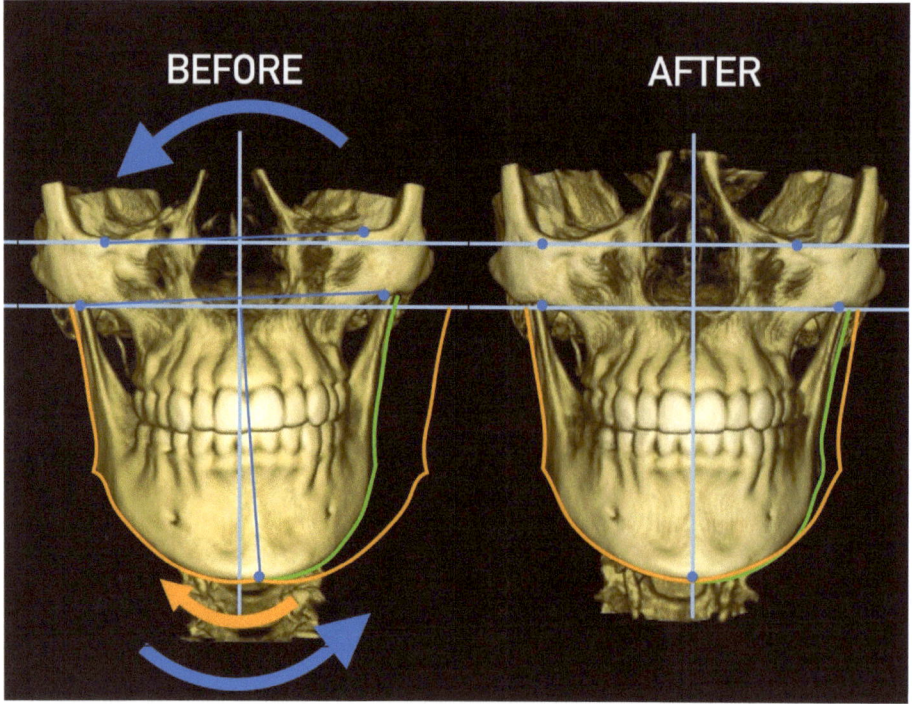

Figure 25. Effect of cervical vertebrae alignment. Anterior view.

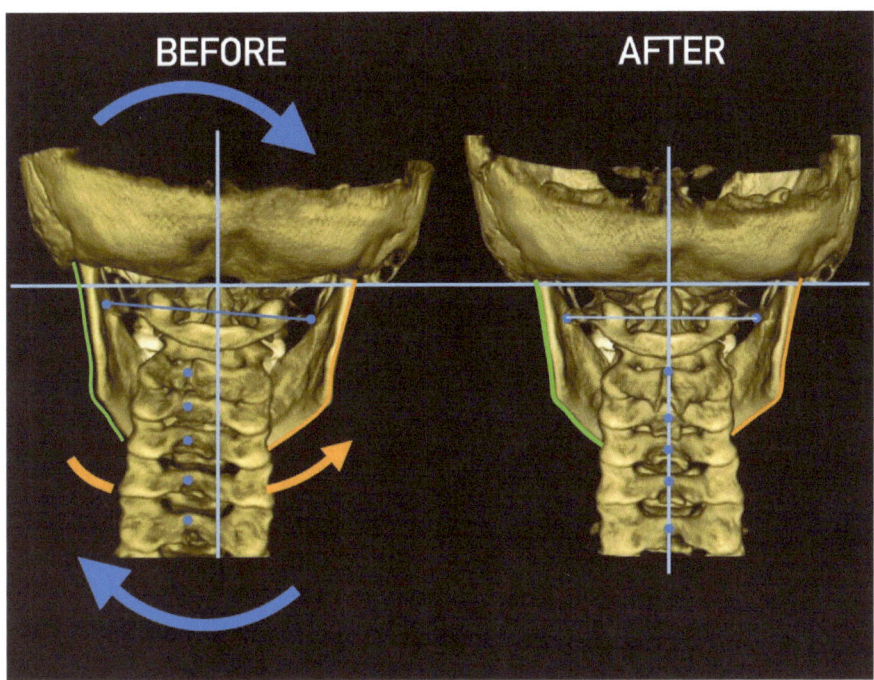

Figure 26. Effect of cervical vertebrae alignment. Posterior view.

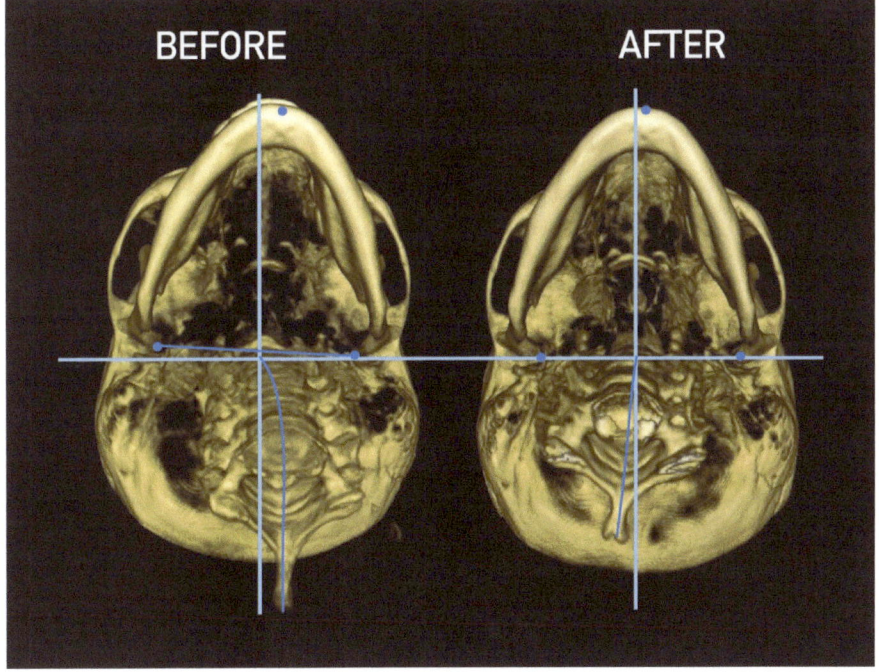

Figure 27. Effect of cervical vertebrae alignment. Inferior view.

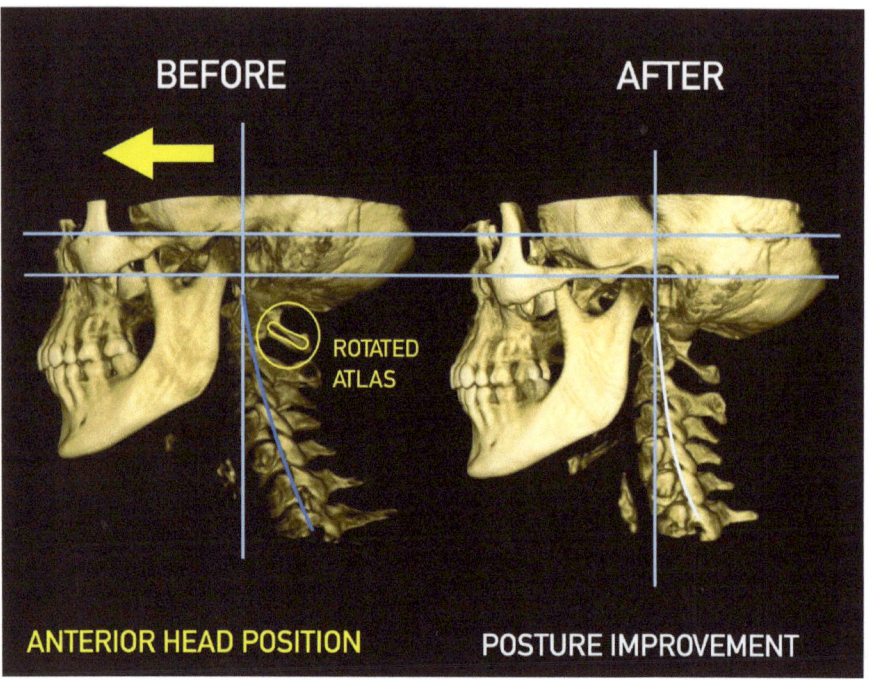

Figure 28. Effect of cervical vertebrae alignment. Lateral view.

11.3. Correction of Body Posture to Address TMJ Dysfunction

As early as the first half of the 20th century, Thompson and Brody described the influence of posture of the body on the position of the jaw [133]. Hansson et al. and Freesmeyer suggested that an alteration in the position of the hips may be an etiological cause for cranio-mandibular dysfunctions [134–136]. Gelb provided an important approach to the diagnosis and treatment of cranio-mandibular dysfunctions, pointing out that alterations in posture play an etiological role in cranio-mandibular dysfunctions, and proposes that dysfunctional treatment includes the correction of body posture [137] (Figure 29). Thus, Bergbreiter found a relationship between the alterations of the posture of the hips and TMJ, finding a prevalence of joint noise in TMJ on the side of the body with a lower hip [138]. Similarly, studies by Stute showed that TMJ alterations are more frequent on the same side of the body with the lowest hip [139]. Other authors report that in patients with postural alterations, the sensitivity to palpation of the masticatory muscles is increased [140,141].

Shup and Zernial propose that the anatomical relationships explain how the postural alterations of the hips influence the position of the head [142]. These would be the relationship between the sphenobasilar (sphenooccipital) synchondrosis and sacral bone, which is made through the dura and the muscle chains made up of the masticatory, hyoid, flexor, and extensor muscles of the neck and dorsal muscles with the muscles of the hips. This finding can be explained through kinematic chains, which in the human body represent circuits in the continuity of direction and planes through which the organizing forces propagate, generating adaptive compensations based on three principles: Balance, Economy and Comfort (no pain).

Under normal conditions, posture regulators are found in the support of the feet. These are mediated by two pairs of nerves, sensory afferents and motor efferents, and involve approximately 10% of the cerebral cortex. In conditions of dysfunction, posture mediation involves the stomatognathic system, through the information provided by TMJ structures [143] and occlusion, since the cranio-mandibular system joins the anterior and posterior kinematic chains, and, therefore, this system of complex control involves six cranial nerves and approximately 38% of the cerebral primary sensory and motor cortices.

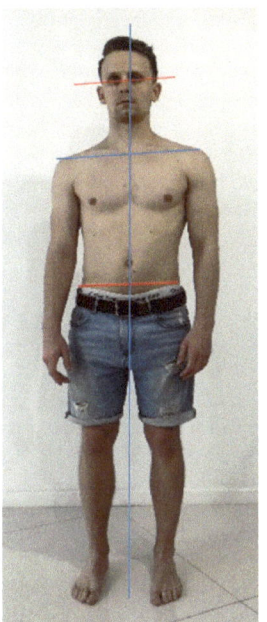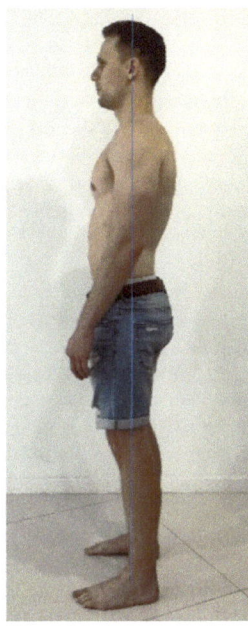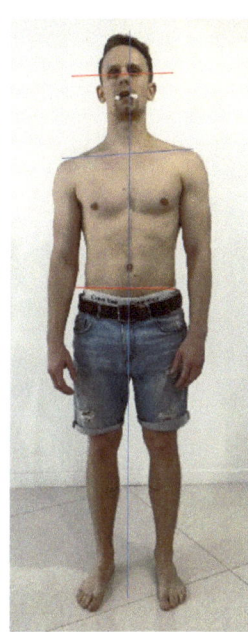

Figure 29. A 28-year-old patient with pain (5/10) and nonspecific muscle weakness in the right hip, evaluated by active hip flexion (pain) and unipodal balance (weakness). The informed consent from the patient was obtained for publication of photos. Source: Rocabado Institute, Chile. Note the misalignments at the shoulders (most evident), and the pelvis (less evident, however, the object of our intervention). The head is presented in the side bending/rotation to the right, and forwarded. The body posture is reassessed in both planes, this time avoiding occlusal contact with a soft disposable element. Although the shoulder misalignment is maintained, soft changes at the pelvic level can be seen: hip flexion's pain is 1-2/10 (lower), and unipodal stability improves subjectively, although weakness persists. There are no significant changes in the sagittal plane. Such clinical findings lead us to consider the management of local conditions that are not necessarily the cause, but rather the consequence of alterations in complex kinematic chains to be considered, to increase the effectiveness of interventions, combining dentistry and physiotherapy in such clinical situation's management.

In an adaptive scheme, the body will attempt to maintain balance, even if the system is not economical, but the priority will always be no pain. Thus, body posture affects balance in the activation of the kinematic chains. Following the premise that "Posture control is the result of a complex system that includes different sensor and motor components from visual, somatosensory and vestibular information", at the central level, there is a reciprocal influence between the trigeminal nerve and the vestibular nucleus, responsible for the masticatory function and balance control, respectively, and between the masticatory and cervical muscles. This influence would explain that dental malocclusions significantly impair posture control (and vice versa), even though research has not been conclusive.

Subcranial vertebral rotation conditions (Occiput-*atlas-axis*), generate three-dimensional positional changes at the temporomandibular articular (mandibular) fossa, as it forms an integrative part of the base of the skull, which directly affects the static and dynamic TMJ alignments, and can generate compressive and shear forces both at rest and during activity [45,143]. If we also consider the relationship between the vestibular system and balance, it is not surprising that the muscles involved in postural balance are in a condition of reflex inhibition, which may explain the changes in sensitivity and pain reported at the level of the masticatory musculature and iliac torsion phenomena ("lower hip"). It is, therefore, necessary that the study and diagnosis of cranio-mandibular dysfunctions/pathologies also consider the global analysis of the patient's posture.

11.4. Treatments Based of Concepts of Trigeminal-Cervical Convergence

Treating patients with headaches and facial pain with or without synovial temporomandibular disorders and dysfunctions based on the neurological aspect has significant advantages. Upper-cervical nociceptive neurons are the point of convergence between the cervical spine, mandibular, and upper jaw nociceptive neurons. This provides a neuroanatomic interrelation between synovial TMJ and cervical spine positional faults, with or without degeneration and/or pain. This suggests that synovial TMJ disorders can often overlap with cervical-spine disorders or pathology [144]. This is crucial when formulating a diagnosis or treatment plan with a broad perspective of a holistic well-being approach.

The convergence of cervical and trigeminal afferents on second-order neurons in the trigemino-cervical nucleus may refer to pain from the upper cervical spine into the head and face. Furthermore, "bi-directional interactions" between trigeminal and upper cervical afferents may also explain neck symptoms of trigeminal origin (e.g., migraine) [145].

In orthopedic manual therapy, the musculoskeletal concept is that the synovial joints, soft tissues that hold the joint together, and the muscles that move the joint have the same innervation; however, the nerves that supply the joint also supply the muscles that move the joint. This fundamental principle is also known as Hilton's law [20,146]. When the intra-joint terminals become irritated, the muscles that move the joint experience reflex muscle contraction. This increases the intra-joint tension and a vicious cycle is set up. Reinforcing this physiological concept is the fact that soft tissue damage precedes hard tissue injuries.

Details of the Rocabado principles of conservative temporomandibular joint dysfunction (TMD) treatment are beyond the scope of this article, but are described in detail in our previous studies [16,70,71,147]. Briefly, the TMD orthopedic manual therapy consists of the use of occlusal 24/7 splint, distraction of TMJ in order to increase the joint space and the vertical capsular/condylar dimension and wide range of myofascial techniques at the level of masticatory musculature, supra- and infrahyoid muscles, suboccipital, and paravertebral muscles [16,70,71]. Once the goal of cranio-cervico-mandibular and occlusion stability is achieved, the patient continues with a total general musculoskeletal stabilization program with a long-term approach and dental and physiotherapy control every six months [147]. Thus, the musculo-fascio-ligamento-capsular aspects of TMD, and not only the temporomandibular joint itself, is considered in both diagnosis and treatment. Importantly, both TMD and neck pain could cause facial pain, and are frequently associated with the development of craniofacial allodynia during painful exacerbation. The central sensitization that could be developed in these patients needs to be taken into account, as well [148,149].

11.5. Axis and Atlas Derotation

Considering these strong concepts in treating a facial pain or headache of cervical origin with or without concomitant synovial TMJ disorder, the position of the head in space in three dimensions, sagittal, coronal, and axial relation to the rest of the body, this concept becomes fundamental. It determines the functional position of the occipital bone with the *atlas* (first cervical vertebra) supporting through the condyles of the occiput, and the weight of the head. The *atlas* needs to be horizontal over the segment of C_2–C_3, with the *axis* (second cervical vertebra) in the skeletal midline to distribute the total weight of the head to the rest of the body (Figure 30). This is a stable, centric relation of the craniovertebral joints. The craniovertebral centric relation determines a horizontal transverse occlusal plane of the upper maxilla and mandible.

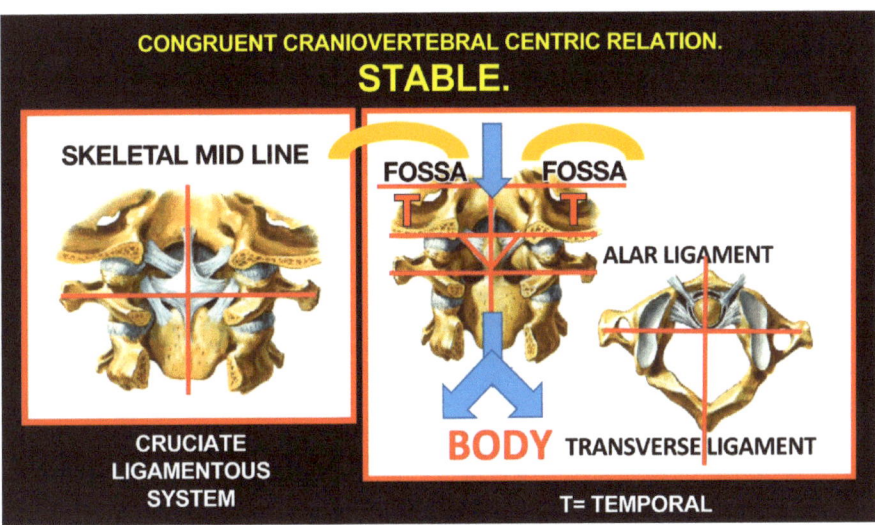

Figure 30. Stable, centric relation of the craniovertebral joints.

Importantly, the harmony of osseous structures remains the reflection of the dynamics of soft-tissue biomechanics. Moreover, soft-tissue damage proceeds in hard-tissue injury of the bone and joints. Cranial position and movement are controlled by more than 20 pairs of cervical muscles. This enormous dynamic condition controls not only the cranium, but determines the position of the mandibular fossa of the temporal bone in the three planes of space and undoubtfully the 3D position of the maxilla. Once we normalize the occipito-atlanto-axial relationship (not earlier!), we can begin determining the mandibulo-maxillary relations, or condyle-fossa congruent position with or without the disc interposed, or how mandibular occlusal contacts relate to maxillary occlusal contacts for rest position. These 40 muscles work simultaneously to stabilize and control the cranium as a stable foundation for mandibular proportional patterns of movement, which, consequently, can affect the intra-joint condyle-disc/disc-temporal arthrokinematics.

The cranium through the cervical spine in lordosis (physiological curvature of the cervical spine) needs to be stabilized over the horizontal shoulder girdle to permit the coordinated action of the masticatory, supra- and infra-mandibular, prevertebral, as well as middle and inferior pharyngeal-constrictor muscles with their antagonistic, deep craniovertebral and superficial paravertebral cervical muscles. Particular orthopedic manual therapy of the most common positional fault syndromes considers that these biomechanical conditions are illustrated, showing they are not problems associated with age, as often stated.

11.6. Treatments Focused on Temporomandibular Joint

Once the optimal craniovertebral position is acquired and stabilized and, thereby, the optimal position of mandibular condyle-fossa relationship is obtained, initial ("default") conditions for the treatment of the TMJ are obtained [45]. If the occlusion does not change significantly and the mandible can move freely in all directions without pain, an occlusal splint is not necessary. However, this happens in few cases. In most cases, an occlusal splint is necessary to provide free movement of the mandible in all directions, at the beginning of treatment in the anteroposterior direction (protrusion/retrusion of mandible) in particular. A plastic splint is most often fabricated on the upper jaw, so its bottom part is rigid and flat, with only slightly increased canine regions to obtain a basic, mutually protected occlusion [26,150,151]. In subsequent orthopedic manual therapy visits, the splint is grinded to obtain at least a 16-point contact with the lower teeth at rest, without right-left imbalance.

During these visits, the manual therapist works with TMJ using particular techniques, including long axis distraction of the joint, mobilization therapy, and a wide range of soft techniques affecting the masticatory (and other) muscles and craniomandibular ligaments. Further, help from a specialist in maxillofacial surgery may rarely be necessary; however, such treatment should be planned (its necessity diagnosed) and discussed with the patient prior to the start of the treatment.

11.7. Treatment of Occlusion

When the optimal occlusion is obtained, aligning the teeth to obtain an optimal maxillo-mandibular tooth relationship should follow, including proper contact of all upper and lower teeth according to the tripod concept and functional anterior guidance (separation of the lateral teeth when the mandible is protruded; sagittal Christensen's phenomenon), as well as lateral guidance (separation of the contralateral lateral teeth when the mandible is in laterotrusion; transversal Christensen's phenomenon), led by the upper canine (canine guidance) or more teeth (group function/group guidance). The most important factors in occlusion remain the absence of traumatic articulation, artificial mandibular guidance and/or occlusal interferences, in particular, mediotrusive molar interferences, thus avoiding muscular avoidance patterns towards these occlusal "hot spots" and other consequent problems [26] (for details, see Dawson, 2007; Greven et al., 2020 [152,153]). The occlusal alignment can be obtained by orthodontic, restorative, prosthetic dentistry, or their combination. Such alignment of the teeth allows the dental specialist to eliminate the splint and obtain optimal functional (including masticatory) ability of the dentition, without pain or disturbances.

11.8. Other Therapeutic Modalities

Apart from the principal approaches, there are several others, which may have adjuvant (not primarily curative) potential. Anesthetic nerve blocks generally play a dual role in both supporting diagnosis and pain relief. However, in the case of occipital neuralgia or COP, the response to anesthetic nerve blocks should not be considered pathognomonic, as its specificity is poor, and other primary and secondary headache disorders may also respond [10].

Transcutaneous electrical nerve stimulation therapy has been used in the conservative management of cervicogenic headaches, with reported benefits [154,155]. However, given the inherent difficulty of realistic placebo and blinding in TENS studies, the results should be interpreted cautiously [156].

Acupuncture or other alternative methods may be beneficial.

Psychotherapy, including meditation (e.g., mindfulness) and cognitive-behavioral therapy remains important supplemental therapies in a significant number of patients, due to the beneficial effect as they undergo this often long and demanding treatment process. Although most psychological problems are secondary, it still has an important therapeutic potential.

Pharmacological and surgical interventions should be reserved for selected patient populations in whom all other conservative and minimally invasive options have failed, to be weighed against the potential risk. They are not the primary focus of this article; thus, they are reviewed elsewhere [10].

12. Conclusions

The etiopathogenesis of COP is complex, but the data are available, understandable, and most importantly, clinically applicable. The key is the understanding of the mechanism of trigeminocervical functional convergence as well as the tricentric concept. Based on the understanding of neuroanatomical and neurophysical, neuromuscular relations, a precise diagnosis and a successful conservative treatment of these patients, based mainly on orthopedic manual therapy and occlusal treatment, is possible, reliable and reproducible.

Author Contributions: Conceptualization, J.Š. and M.R.; methodology, J.Š.; writing—original draft preparation, J.Š., R.Ž.; writing—review and editing, M.R., M.V., L.E.O., R.Ž.; visualization, R.Ž.; supervision, J.Š., M.R. All authors have read and agreed to the published version of the manuscript.

Funding: This research received no external funding.

Institutional Review Board Statement: Not applicable.

Informed Consent Statement: Informed consent of patient was obtained.

Data Availability Statement: Not applicable.

Acknowledgments: Authors thank to Jan Kucera from Boston University, Boston, MA, USA for valuable comments to the manuscript and to Jan Streblov and Martin Tomeček for their overall support of TMJ program at the 3DK clinic, Prague, Czech Republic.

Conflicts of Interest: The authors declare no conflict of interest.

References

1. Verma, S.; Tripathi, M.; Chandra, P.S. Cervicogenic Headache: Current Perspectives. *Neurol. India.* **2021**, *69*, 194–198.
2. Van Suijlekom, H.A.; Lamé, I.; Stomp-van den Berg, S.G.; Kessels, A.G.; Weber, W.E. Quality of Life of Patients with Cervicogenic Headache: A Comparison with Control Subjects and Patients With Migraine or Tension-Type Headache. *Headache* **2003**, *43*, 1034–1041. [CrossRef] [PubMed]
3. Fernandez, M.; Moore, C.; Tan, J.; Lian, D.; Nguyen, J.; Bacon, A.; Christie, B.; Shen, I.; Waldie, T.; Simonet, D.; et al. Spinal manipulation for the management of cervicogenic headache: A systematic review and meta-analysis. *Eur. J. Pain.* **2020**, *24*, 1687–1702. [CrossRef] [PubMed]
4. Bogduk, N. The anatomical basis for cervicogenic headache. *J. Manipulative Physiol. Ther.* **1992**, *15*, 67–70. [PubMed]
5. Bogduk, N.; Govind, J. Cervicogenic headache: An assessment of the evidence on clinical diagnosis, invasive tests, and treatment. *Lancet Neurol.* **2009**, *8*, 959–968. [CrossRef]
6. Bogduk, N. The neck and headaches. *Neurol. Clin.* **2014**, *32*, 471–487. [CrossRef]
7. Headache Classification Subcommittee of the International Headache Society. The International Classification of Headache Disorders: 2nd edition. *Cepthalagia* **2004**, *24*, 9–160.
8. Headache Classification Subcommittee of the International Headache Society. The International Classification of Headache Disorders 3rd edition (beta version). *Cephalgia* **2013**, *33*, 629–808. [CrossRef]
9. Sjaastad, O.; Fredriksen, T.A.; Pfaffenrath, V. Cervicogenic Headache: Diagnostic Criteria. Headache. *J. Head Face Pain* **1998**, *38*, 442–445. [CrossRef]
10. Barmherzig, R.; Kingston, W. Occipital Neuralgia and Cervicogenic Headache: Diagnosis and Management. *Curr. Neurol. Neurosci. Rep.* **2019**, *19*, 20. [CrossRef]
11. Fredriksen, T.A.; Antonaci, F.; Sjaastad, O. Cervicogenic headache: Too important to be left undiagnosed. *J. Headache Pain* **2015**, *16*, 6. [CrossRef] [PubMed]
12. Sjaastad, O.; Bakkteig, L.S. Prevalence of cervicogenic headache: Vaga study of headach epidemiology. *Acta Neurol. Scand.* **2008**, *38*, 442–445. [CrossRef] [PubMed]
13. Knackstedt, H.; Bansevicius, D.; Aaseth, K.; Grande, R.B.; Lundqvist, C.; Russel, M.B. Cervicogenic headache in the general population: The Akershus study of chronic headache. *Cephalalgia* **2010**, *30*, 1468–1476. [CrossRef] [PubMed]
14. Evers, S. Comparison of cervicogenic headache with migraine. *Cephalalgia* **2008**, *28*, 16–17. [CrossRef] [PubMed]
15. Lord, S.; Barnsley, L.; Wallis, B.; Bogduk, N. Third occipital headache: A prevalence study. *J. Neurol. Neurosurg. Psychiatr.* **1994**, *57*, 1187–1190. [CrossRef] [PubMed]
16. Rocabado, M.; Iglarsh, Z.A. *Musculoskeletal Approach to Maxillofacial Pain*; J. B. Lippincott Comp.: Philadelphia, PA, USA, 1991.
17. Dvorak, J.; Penning, L.; Hayek, J.; Panjabi, M.M.; Grob, D.; Zehnder, R. Functional diagnostics of the cervical spine using computer tomography. *Neuroradiology* **1988**, *30*, 132–137. [CrossRef]
18. Williams, P.L.; Bannister, H. *Gray's Anatomy*, 38th ed.; Churchill Livingstone: New York, NY, USA, 1995.
19. Kikuta, S.; Jenkins, S.; Kusukawa, J.; Iwanaga, J.; Loukas, M.; Tubbs, R.S. Ansa cervicalis: A comprehensive review of its anatomy, variations, pathology, and surgical applications. *Anat. Cell Biol.* **2019**, *52*, 221–225. [CrossRef]
20. Moore, K.L.; Dalley, A.F.; Agur, A.M.R. *Moore Clinically Oriented Anatomy*, 7th ed.; Lippincott Williams & Wilkins: Baltimore, MD, USA, 2014.
21. Renton, T.; Egbuniwe, O. Pain. Part 2A: Trigeminal Anatomy Related to Pain. *Dent. Update* **2015**, *42*, 238–240. [CrossRef]
22. Lazarov, N.E. Neurobiology of orofacial proprioception. *Brain Res. Rev.* **2007**, *56*, 362–383. [CrossRef]
23. Bogduk, N. Cervicogenic headache: Anatomic basis and pathophysiologic mechanisms. *Curr. Pain Head Rep.* **2001**, *5*, 382–386. [CrossRef]

24. Biondi, D.M. Cervicogenic headache: A review of diagnostic and treatment strategies. *J. Am. Osteopath. Assoc.* **2005**, *105*, 16–22.
25. Biondi, D.M. Noninvasive treatments for headache. *Expert. Rev. Neurother.* **2005**, *5*, 355–362. [CrossRef] [PubMed]
26. Okeson, J.P. *Management of Temporomandibular Disorders and Occlusion*, 8th ed.; Elsevier: New York, NY, USA, 2020.
27. Kerr, F.W. Facial, vagal and glossopharyngeal nerves in the cat. Afferent connections. *Arch. Neurol.* **1962**, *6*, 264–281. [CrossRef] [PubMed]
28. Kerr, F.W. The divisional organization of afferent fibres of the trigeminal nerve. *Brain* **1963**, *86*, 721–732. [CrossRef]
29. Cetas, J.S.; Saedi, T.; Burchiel, K.J. Destructive procedures for the treatment of nonmalignant pain: A structured literature review. *J. Neurosurg.* **2008**, *109*, 389–404. [CrossRef]
30. Giovanni, A.; Giorgia, A. The neurophysiological basis of bruxism. *Heliyon* **2021**, *7*, e07477. [CrossRef]
31. Louvi, A.; Yoshida, M.; Grove, E.A. The derivatives of the Wnt3a lineage in the central nervous system. *J. Comp. Neurol.* **2007**, *504*, 550–569. [CrossRef] [PubMed]
32. Lund, J.P. Mastication and its control by the brain stem. *Crit. Rev. Oral Biol. Med.* **1991**, *2*, 33–64. [CrossRef]
33. Cody, F.W.; Lee, R.W.; Taylor, A. A functional analysis of the components of the mesencephalic nucleus of the fifth nerve in the cat. *J. Physiol.* **1972**, *226*, 249–261. [CrossRef]
34. Daunicht, W.J.; Jaworski, E.; Eckmiller, R. Afferent innervation of extraocular muscles in the rat studied by retrograde and anterograde horseradish peroxidase transport. *Neurosci. Lett.* **1985**, *56*, 143–148. [CrossRef]
35. Porter, J.D.; Spencer, R.F. Localization of morphology of cat extraocular muscle afferent neurons identified by retrograde transport of horseradish peroxidase. *J. Comp. Neurol.* **1982**, *204*, 56–64. [CrossRef] [PubMed]
36. Dessem, D.; Luo, P. Jaw–muscle spindle afferent feedback to the cervical spinal cord in the rat. *Exp. Brain Res.* **1999**, *128*, 451–459. [CrossRef] [PubMed]
37. Goodwin, G.M.; Luschei, E.S. Effects of destroying spindle afferents from jaw muscles on mastication in monkeys. *J. Neurophysiol.* **1974**, *37*, 967–981. [CrossRef] [PubMed]
38. Ongerboer de Visser, B.W. Afferent limb of the human jaw reflex: Electrophysiologic and anatomic study. *Neurology* **1982**, *32*, 563–566. [CrossRef]
39. Luschei, E.S. Central projections of the mesencephalic nucleus of the fifth nerve: An autoradiographic study. *J. Comp. Neurol.* **1987**, *263*, 137–145. [CrossRef]
40. Daunton, N.G. Sensory components of bite–force response in the rat. *J. Comp. Physiol. Psychol.* **1977**, *91*, 203–220. [CrossRef]
41. Eichner, K. Über eine Gruppeneinteilung der Lückengebisse für die Prothetik. *Dtsch. Zahnärztl. Z.* **1955**, *10*, 1831–1834.
42. Malet, J. *Implant Dentistry at Glance*, 1st ed.; Wiley-Blackwell: London, UK, 2012.
43. Cheynet, F.; Guyot, L.; Richard, O.; Layoun, W.; Gola, R. Discomallear and malleomandibular ligaments: Anatomical study and clinical applications. *Surg. Radiol. Anat.* **2003**, *25*, 152–157. [CrossRef]
44. Connelly, S.T.; Tartaglia, G.M.; Silva, R.G. *Contemporary Management of Temporomandibular Disorders. Fundamentals and Pathways to Diagnosis*, 1st ed.; Springer: Zurich, Switzerland, 2019.
45. Olmos, S.R.; Kritz–Silverstein, D.; Halligan, W.; Silverstein, S.T. The effect of condyle fossa relationships on head posture. *J. Craniomand. Pract.* **2005**, *23*, 48–52. [CrossRef]
46. Von Piekartz, H.J.M.; Schouten, S.; Aufdemkampe, G. Neurodynamic responses in children with migraine or cervicogenic headache versus a control group. A comparative study. *Man. Ther.* **2007**, *12*, 153–160. [CrossRef]
47. Wei, W. Neural Mechanisms of Motion Processing in the Mammalian Retina. *Annu. Rev. Vis. Sci.* **2018**, *4*, 165–192. [CrossRef] [PubMed]
48. D'Attilio, M.; Filippi, M.R.; Femminella, B.; Festa, F.; Tecco, S. The influence of an experimentally–induced malocclusion on vertebral alignment in rats: A controlled pilot study. *Cranio* **2005**, *23*, 119–129. [CrossRef]
49. D'Attilio, M.; Scarano, A.; Quaranta, A.; Festa, F.; Caputi, S.; Piattelli, A. Modification of condyle anatomy following a monolateral bite rise: A histological study in rat. *Int. J. Immunopathol. Pharmacol.* **2007**, *20*, 43–47. [CrossRef] [PubMed]
50. Cardinal, L.; da Silva, T.R.; Andujar, A.L.F.; Gribel, B.F.; Dominguez, G.C.; Janakiraman, N. Evaluation of the three-dimensional (3D) position of cervical vertebrae in individuals with unilateral posterior crossbite. *Clin. Oral Investig.* **2022**, *26*, 463–469. [CrossRef] [PubMed]
51. Šedý, J. Response to: Cardinal L, da Silva TR, Andujar ALF, Gribel BF, Dominguez GC, Janakiraman N. Evaluation of the three-dimensional (3D) position of cervical vertebrae in individuals with unilateral posterior crossbite. *Clin. Oral Invest.* **2021**, *25*, 6961. [CrossRef]
52. Di Vece, L.; Faleri, G.; Picciotti, M.; Guido, L.; Giorgetti, R. Does a transverse maxillary deficit affect the cervical vertebrae? A pilot study. *Am. J. Orthod. Dentofacial. Orthop.* **2010**, *137*, 515–519. [CrossRef]
53. McGuinness, N.J.; McDonald, J.P. Changes in natural head position observed immediately and one year after rapid maxillary expansion. *Eur. J. Orthod.* **2006**, *28*, 126–134. [CrossRef]
54. Greenbaum, T.; Dvir, Z.; Reiter, S.; Winocur, E. Cervical flexion-rotation test and physiological range of motion—A comparative study of patients with myogenic temporomandibular disorder versus healthy subjects. *Musculoskelet. Sci. Pract.* **2017**, *27*, 7–13. [CrossRef]
55. Korbmacher, H.; Koch, L.; Eggers-Stroeder, G.; Kahl-Nieke, B. Associations between orthopaedic disturbances and unilateral crossbite in children with asymmetry of the upper cervical spine. *Eur. J. Orthod.* **2007**, *29*, 100–104. [CrossRef]

56. Milidonis, M.K.; Kraus, S.L.; Segal, R.L.; Widmer, C.G. Genioglossi muscle activity in response to changes in anterior/neutral head posture. *Am. J. Orthod. Dentofacial. Orthop.* **1993**, *103*, 39–44. [CrossRef]
57. Mohl, N. Head posture and its role in occlusion. *Int. J. Orthod.* **1977**, *15*, 6–14. [PubMed]
58. Ohmure, H.; Miyawaki, S.; Nagata, J.; Ikeda, K.; Yamasaki, K.; Al–Kalaly, A. Influence of forward head posture on condylar position. *J. Oral Rehabil.* **2008**, *35*, 795–800. [CrossRef] [PubMed]
59. Paco, M.; Duarte, J.A.; Pinho, T. Orthodontic Treatment and Craniocervical Posture in Patients with Temporomandibular Disorders: An Observational Study. *Int. J. Environ. Res. Public Health* **2021**, *18*, 3295. [CrossRef] [PubMed]
60. Sandoval, C.; Díaz, A.; Manríquez, G. Relationship between craniocervical posture and skeletal class: A statistical multivariate approach for studying Class II and Class III malocclusions. *Cranio* **2019**, *29*, 1–8. [CrossRef]
61. Proffit, W.R. *Contemporary Orthodontics*, 6th ed.; Elsevier: New York, NY, USA, 2019.
62. McNamara, J.A., Jr. Early intervention in the transverse dimension: Is it worth the effort? *Am. J. Orthod. Dentofacial. Orthop.* **2002**, *121*, 572–574. [CrossRef]
63. Michelotti, A.; Iodice, G.; Piergentili, M.; Farella, M.; Martina, R. Incidence of temporomandibular joint clicking in adolescents with and without unilateral posterior cross-bite: A 10-year follow-up study. *J. Oral Rehabil.* **2016**, *43*, 16–22. [CrossRef]
64. Fiorrilo, L. Spine and TMJ: A Pathophysiology report. *J. Funct. Morphol. Kinesiol.* **2020**, *5*, 24. [CrossRef]
65. Cruccu, G.; Ongerboer de Visser, B.W. The jaw reflexes. The International Federation of Clinical Neurophysiology. *Electroencephalogr. Clin. Neurophysiol.* **1999**, *52*, 243–247.
66. Morquette, P.; Lavoie, R.; Fhima, M.D.; Lamoureux, X.; Verdier, D.; Kolta, A. Generation of the masticatory central pattern and its modulation by sensory feedback. *Prog. Neurobiol.* **2012**, *96*, 340–355. [CrossRef]
67. Dellow, P.G.; Lund, J.P. Evidence for central timing of rhythmical mastication. *J. Physiol.* **1971**, *215*, 1–13. [CrossRef]
68. Sessle, B.J.; Yao, D.; Nishiura, H.; Yoshino, K.; Lee, J.C.; Martin, R.E.; Murray, G.M. Properties and plasticity of the primate somatosensory and motor cortex related to orofacial sensorimotor function. *Clin. Exp. Pharmacol. Physiol.* **2005**, *32*, 109–114. [CrossRef] [PubMed]
69. Hamm, T.M.; Trank, T.V.; Turkin, V.V. Correlations between neurograms and locomotor drive potentials in motoneurons during fictive locomotion: Implications for the organization of locomotor commands. *Prog. Brain Res.* **1999**, *123*, 331–339. [PubMed]
70. Rocabado, M. *Theoretical and Hans–on Master Class: Cervical and Craniomandibular Dysfunctions*, 1st ed.; SynergyOAcademy: Cluj-Napoca, Romania, 2018.
71. Rocabado, M. *Theoretical and Hans–on Master Class II: Cervical and Craniomandibular Dysfunctions*, 1st ed.; SynergyOAcademy: Cluj-Napoca, Romania, 2018.
72. Goadsby, P.J.; Ratsch, T. On the functional neuroanatomy of neck pain. *Cephalalgia* **2008**, *28*, 1–7. [CrossRef]
73. Campbell, D.G.; Parsons, C.M. Referred head pain and its concomitants. *J. Nerv. Ment. Dis.* **1944**, *99*, 544–551. [CrossRef]
74. Feinstein, B.; Langton, J.B.K.; Jameson, R.M.; Schiller, F. Experiments on referred pain from deep somatic tissues. *J. Bone Joint Surg.* **1954**, *36*, 981–997. [CrossRef]
75. Dreyfuss, P.; Michaelsen, M.; Fletcher, D. Atlanto-occipital and lateral atlanto-axial joint pain patterns. *Spine* **1994**, *19*, 1125–1131. [CrossRef]
76. Dwyer, A.; Aprill, C.; Bogduk, N. Cervical zygapophysial joint pain patterns I: A study in normal volunteers. *Spine* **1990**, *15*, 453–457.
77. Schellhas, K.P.; Smith, M.D.; Gundry, C.R.; Pollei, S.R. Cervical discogenic pain: Prospective correlation of magnetic resonance imaging and discography in asymptomatic subjects and pain suff erers. *Spine* **1996**, *21*, 300–312. [CrossRef]
78. Grubb, S.A.; Kelly, C.K. Cervical discography: Clinical implications from 12 years of experience. *Spine* **2000**, *25*, 1382–1389. [CrossRef]
79. Ashina, S.; Bendtsen, L.; Lyngberg, A.C.; Lipton, R.B.; Hajiyeva, N.; Jensen, R. Prevalence of neck pain in migraine and tension-type headache: A population study. *Cephalalgia* **2015**, *35*, 211–219. [CrossRef]
80. Johnston, M.M.; Jordan, S.E.; Charles, A.C. Pain referral patterns of the C1 to C3 nerves: Implications for headache disorders. *Ann. Neurol.* **2013**, *74*, 145–148. [CrossRef] [PubMed]
81. Shimohata, K.; Hasegawa, K.; Onodera, O.; Nishizawa, M.; Shimohata, T. The clinical features, risk factors, and surgical treatment of cervicogenic headache in patients with cervical spine disorders. *Headache* **2017**, *57*, 1109–1117. [CrossRef] [PubMed]
82. Amevo, B.; Aprill, C.; Bogduk, N. Abnormal instantaneous axes of rotation in patients with neck pain. *Spine* **1992**, *17*, 748–756. [CrossRef] [PubMed]
83. Watson, D.H.; Trott, P.H. Cervical headache: An investigation of natural head posture and upper cervical flexor muscle performance. *Cephalalgia* **1993**, *13*, 272–284. [CrossRef]
84. Okeson, J.P. *Orofacial Pain: Guidelines for Assessment, Diagnosis and Management*, 1st ed.; Quintessence: Chicago, IL, USA, 1996.
85. Paesani, D.A. *Bruxism: Theory and Practice*, 1st ed.; Quintessence Publishing: Berlin, Germany, 2010.
86. Harness, D.M.; Peltier, B. Comparison of MMPI scores with self-report of sleep disturbance and bruxism in the facial pain population. *Cranio* **1992**, *10*, 70–74. [CrossRef]
87. Pierce, C.J.; Chrisman, K.; Bennett, M.E.; Close, J.M. Stress, anticipatory stress, and psychologic measures related to sleep bruxism. *J. Orofac. Pain* **1995**, *9*, 51–56.
88. Rugh, J.D.; Harlan, J. Nocturnal bruxism and temporomandibular disorders. *Adv. Neurol.* **1988**, *49*, 329–341.

89. Bandodkar, S.; Tripathi, S.; Chand, P.; Singh, S.V.; Arya, D.; Kumar, L.; Singh, M.; Singhal, R.; Tripathi, A. A study to evaluate psychological and occlusal parameters in bruxism. *J. Oral Biol. Craniofac. Res.* **2022**, *12*, 38–41. [CrossRef]
90. Franks, A.S. Cervical spondylosis presenting as the facial pain of temporomandibular joint disorder. *Ann. Phys. Med.* **1968**, *9*, 193–196. [CrossRef]
91. Koopman, J.S.; Dieleman, J.P.; Huygen, F.J.; de Mos, M.; Martin, C.G.; Sturkenboom, M.C. Incidence of facial pain in the general population. *Pain* **2009**, *147*, 122–127. [CrossRef]
92. Choi, I.I.; Jeon, S.R. Neuralgias of the head: Occipital neuralgia. *J. Korean Med. Sci.* **2016**, *31*, 479–488. [CrossRef] [PubMed]
93. Khanfour, A.A.; El Sekily, N.M. Relation of the vertebral artery segment from C1 to C2 vertebrae: An anatomical study. *Alexandria J. Med.* **2015**, *51*, 143–151. [CrossRef]
94. Allen, W. The varieties of the atlas in the human subject, and the homologies of its transverse processes. *J. Anat. Physiol.* **1879**, *14*, 18–27. [PubMed]
95. Pekala, P.A.; Henry, B.M.; Pekala, J.R.; Hsieh, W.C.; Vikse, J.; Sanna, B.; Walocha, J.A.; Tubbs, R.S.; Tomaszewski, K.A. Prevalence of foramen arcuale and its clinical significance: A meta-analysis of 55,985 subjects. *J. Neurosurg. Spine* **2017**, *27*, 276–290. [CrossRef] [PubMed]
96. Friedrich, R.E. Ponticulus posticus is a frequent radiographic finding on lateral cephalograms in nevoid basal cell carcinoma syndrome (Gorlin-Goltz syndrome). *Anticancer Res.* **2014**, *34*, 7395–7399.
97. Limousin, C.A. Foramen arcuale and syndrome of Barre-Lieou. Its surgical treatment. *Int. Orthop.* **1980**, *4*, 19–23. [CrossRef]
98. Li, Y.; Peng, B. Pathogenesis, Diagnosis, and Treatment of Cervical Vertigo. *Pain Physician* **2015**, *18*, E583–E595.
99. Travell, J.G.; Simons, D. *Myofascial Pain and Dysfunction*, 1st ed.; Lippincott Williams & Wilkins: Philadelphia, PA, USA, 2013.
100. Zhuang, X.; Tan, S.; Huang, Q. Understanding of myofascial trigger points. *Chin. Med. J.* **2014**, *127*, 4271–4277.
101. Gerwin, R.D.; Dommerholt, J.; Shah, J.P. An expansion of Simons integrated hypothesis of trigger point formation. *Curr. Pain Headache Rep.* **2004**, *8*, 468–475. [CrossRef]
102. Sharav, Y.; Singer, E.; Schmidt, E.; Dionne, R.A.; Dubner, R. The analgesic effect of amitriptyline on chronic facial pain. *Pain* **1987**, *31*, 199–209. [CrossRef]
103. Clarkson, E.; Jung, E. Atypical Facial Pain. *Dent. Clin. North Am.* **2020**, *64*, 249–253. [CrossRef] [PubMed]
104. May, A.; Hoffmann, J. Facial pain beyond trigeminal neuralgia. *Curr. Opin. Neurol.* **2021**, *34*, 373–377. [CrossRef] [PubMed]
105. Marklund, M.; Braem, M.J.A.; Verbraecken, J. Update on oral appliance therapy. *Eur. Respir. Rev.* **2019**, *28*, 190083. [PubMed]
106. Antonaci, F.; Ghirmai, S.; Bono, S.; Sandrini, G.; Nappi, G. Cervicogenic headache: Evaluation of the original diagnostic criteria. *Cephalalgia* **2001**, *21*, 573–583. [CrossRef] [PubMed]
107. Van Suijlekom, J.A.; de Vet, H.C.W.; van den Berg, S.G.M.; Weber, W.E.J. Interobserver reliability of diagnostic criteria for cervicogenic headache. *Cephalalgia* **1999**, *19*, 817–823. [CrossRef] [PubMed]
108. van Suijlekom, H.A.; de Vet, H.C.W.; van den Berg, S.G.M.; Weber, W.E.J. Interobserver reliability in physical examination of the cervical spine in patients with headache. *Headache* **2000**, *40*, 581–586. [CrossRef]
109. Grzesiak, R.C. Psychologic considerations in temporomandibular dysfunction. A biopsychosocial view of symptom formation. *Dent. Clin. North Am.* **1991**, *35*, 209–226. [CrossRef]
110. Fillingim, R.B.; Ohrbach, R.; Greenspan, J.D.; Sanders, A.E.; Rathnayaka, N.; Maixner, W.; Slade, G.D. Associations of Psychologic Factors with Multiple Chronic Overlapping Pain Conditions. *J. Oral Facial Pain Headache* **2020**, *34*, 85–100. [CrossRef]
111. Van Suijlekom, H.; Van Zundert, J.; Narouze, S.; Van Kleef, M.; Mekhail, N. Cervicogenic headache. *Pain Pract.* **2010**, *10*, 124–130. [CrossRef]
112. Lampl, C.; Rudolph, M.; Deligianni, C.I.; Mitsikostas, D.D. Neck pain in episodic migraine: Premonitory symptom or part of the attack? *J. Headache Pain* **2015**, *16*, 566. [CrossRef]
113. Kuhn, W.F.; Kuhn, S.C.; Gilberstadt, H. Occipital neuralgias: Clinical recognition of a complicated headache. A case series and literature review. *J. Orofac. Pain* **1997**, *11*, 158–165.
114. de Sousa, J.E.; Halfon, M.J.; Bonardo, P.; Reisin, R.C.; Fernández Pardal, M.M. Different pain patterns in patients with vertebral artery dissections. *Neurology* **2005**, *64*, 925–926. [CrossRef] [PubMed]
115. Saeed, A.B.; Shuaib, A.; Al Sulaiti, G.; Emery, D. Vertebral artery dissection: Warning symptoms, clinical features and prognosis in 26 patients. *Can. J. Neurol. Sci.* **2000**, *27*, 292–296. [CrossRef] [PubMed]
116. Campos, C.R.; Calderaro, M.; Scaff, M.; Conforto, A.B. Primary headaches and painful spontaneous cervical artery dissection. *J. Headache Pain* **2007**, *8*, 180–184. [CrossRef] [PubMed]
117. Hack, G.D.; Koritzer, R.T.; Robinson, W.L.; Hallgren, R.C.; Greenman, P.E. Anatomic relation between the rectus capitis posterior minor muscle and the dura mater. *Spine* **1995**, *20*, 2484–2486. [CrossRef]
118. Hallgren, R.C.; Pierce, S.J.; Prokop, L.L.; Rowan, J.J.; Angela, L.S. Electromyographic activity of rectus capitis posterior minor muscles associated with voluntary retraction of the head. *Spine J.* **2014**, *14*, 104–112. [CrossRef]
119. Hallgren, R.C.; Pierce, S.J.; Sharma, D.B.; Rowan, J.J. Forward Head Posture and Activation of Rectus Capitis Posterior Muscles. *J. Am. Osteopath. Assoc.* **2017**, *117*, 24–31. [CrossRef]
120. Blumenfeld, A.; Siavoshi, S. The challenges of cervicogenic headache. *Curr. Pain Headache Rep.* **2008**, *22*, 47. [CrossRef]
121. Lance, J.W.; Anthony, M. Neck tongue syndrome on sudden turning of the head. *J. Neurol. Neurosurg. Psychiatr.* **1980**, *43*, 97–101. [CrossRef]

122. Bogduk, N. An anatomical basis for neck tongue syndrome. *J. Neurol. Neurosurg. Psychiatr.* **1981**, *44*, 202–208. [CrossRef]
123. Jansen, J.; Markakis, E.; Rama, B.; Hildebrandt, J. Hemicranial attacks or permanent hemicrania—A sequel of upper cervical root compression. *Cephalalgia* **1989**, *9*, 123–130. [PubMed]
124. Poletti, C.E.; Sweet, W.H. Entrapment of the C2 root and ganglion by the atlanto-epistrophic ligament: Clinical syndrome and surgical anatomy. *Neurosurgery* **1990**, *27*, 288–291. [CrossRef] [PubMed]
125. Jansen, J.; Bardosi, A.; Hildebrandt, J.; Lucke, A. Cervicogenic, hemicranial attacks associated with vascular irritation or compression of the cervical nerve root C2. Clinical manifestations and morphological findings. *Pain* **1989**, *39*, 203–212. [CrossRef]
126. Kuritzky, A. Cluster headache-like pain caused by an upper cervical meningioma. *Cephalalgia* **1984**, *4*, 185–186. [CrossRef] [PubMed]
127. Sharma, R.R.; Parekh, H.C.; Prabhu, S.; Gurusinghe, N.T.; Bertolis, G. Compression of the C-2 root by a rare anomalous ectatic vertebral artery. *J.Neurosurg.* **1993**, *78*, 669–672. [CrossRef] [PubMed]
128. Hildebrandt, J.; Jansen, J. Vascular compression of the C2 and C3 roots—Yet another cause of chronic intermittent hemicrania? *Cephalalgia* **1984**, *4*, 167–170. [CrossRef]
129. Hanzelka, T.; Dušek, J.; Ocásek, F.; Kučera, J.; Šedý, J.; Beneš, J.; Pavlíková, G.; Foltán, R. Movement of the patient and the cone beam computed tomography scanner: Objectives and possible solutions. *Oral Surg. Oral Med. Oral Pathol. Oral Radiol.* **2013**, *116*, 769–773. [CrossRef]
130. Minervini, G. Teledentistry in the management of patients with dental and temporomandibular disorders. *Biomed Res. Int.* **2022**, *2022*, 7091153. [CrossRef]
131. Haas, M.; Bronfort, G.; Evans, R.; Schulz, C.; Vavrek, D.; Takaki, L.; Hanson, L.; Leininger, B.; Neradilek, M.B. Dose-response and efficacy of spinal manipulation for care of cervicogenic headache: A dual-center randomized controlled trial. *Spine J.* **2018**, *18*, 1741–1754. [CrossRef]
132. Jull, G.; Trott, P.; Potter, H.; Zito, G.; Niere, K.; Shirley, D.; Emberson, J.; Marschner, I.; Richardson, C. A randomized controlled trial of exercise and manipulative therapy for cervicogenic headache. *Spine* **2002**, *27*, 1835–1843. [CrossRef]
133. Thompson, J.R.; Brody, A.G. Factors in the position of the mandible. *J. Am. Dent. Assoc.* **1942**, *29*, 925–941. [CrossRef]
134. Hansson, T.; Henée, W.; Hesse, J. *Funktionsstörungen im Kausystem*, 1st ed.; Hüthig Buch-Verlag: Heidelberg, Germany, 1990.
135. Hansson, T.L.; Christensen Minor, C.A.; Wagnon Taylor, D.L. *Physical Therapy in Craniomandibular Disorders*, 1st ed.; Quintessenz-Verlag: Berlin, Germany, 1992.
136. Freesmeyer, W.B. *Zahnärztliche Funktionstherapie*, 1st ed.; Hanser-Verlag: München, Germany, 1993.
137. Gelb, H. *New Concepts in Craniomandibular and Chronic Pain Management*, 1st ed.; Mosby-Wolfe: London, UK, 1994.
138. Bergbreiter, C. *Untersuchung über die Zusammenhänge Zwischen der Fehlstatik und den Funktionellen Befunden des Craniomandibulären Systems*; Inaug. Diss., Med. Fak.: Tübingen, Germany, 1993.
139. Stute, W. Sakrokraniomandibuläre Integrationsstörungen. In *Ganzheitliche Zahnheilkunde in der Praxis*; Becker, W., Ed.; Spitta-Verlag: Balingen, Germany, 1996.
140. Wallace, C.; Klineberg, I. Management of Craniomandibular Disorders. Part II: Assessment of Patients with Craniocervical Dysfunction. *J. Orofacial Pain* **1994**, *8*, 42–54. [PubMed]
141. Coy, R.E.; Flocken, J.E.; Adib, F. Musculoskeletal etiology and therapy of craniomandibular pain and dysfunction. *Cranio Clin. Int.* **1991**, *1*, 163–173. [PubMed]
142. Shup, W.; Zernial, P. *Zahnärztliche und kieferorthopädische Behandlungsmöglichkeiten bei Craniomandibulärer Dysfunktion*. Fachvereinigung deutscher Kieferorthopäden. (KFO-1G); W. Scupp: Köln, Germany, 1996.
143. Rocabado, M. *Atlas Clínico II, Congruencia Cráneo-cérvico-mandibular, Aplicación Clínica*, 1st ed.; Instituto Rocabado: Santiago de Chile, Chile, 2021.
144. Aniri, M.; Jull, G.; Bullock-Saxton, J.; Darnell, R.; Lander, C. Cervical musculoskeletal impairment in frequent intermittent headache. Part 2: Subjects with concurrent headache types. *Cephalgia* **2007**, *27*, 891–898. [CrossRef]
145. Dreyfuss, P.; Dreser, S.J.; Cole, A.; Mayo, K. Sacroiliac joint pain. *J. Am. Acad. Orthop. Surg.* **2004**, *12*, 255–265. [CrossRef]
146. Hilton, J. *On Rest and Pain: A Course of Lectures on the Influence of Mechanical and Physiological Rest in the Treatment of Accidents and Surgical Diseases, and the Diagnostic Value of Pain, delivered at the Royal College of Surgeons of England in the years 1860, 1861, and 1862*; William Wood & Company: West Chester, PA, USA, 1863.
147. Rocabado, M.; Gutierrez, R.; Gutierrez, M.F.; Gutierrez, M.J. Case report: Anterior open bite correction treatment by dental treatment and physical therapy through craniocervical mandibular and occlusal stabilization. *Cranio* **2021**, *10*, 1–6. [CrossRef]
148. Kang, J.H. Neck associated factors related to migraine in adolescents with painful temporomandibular disorders. *Acta Odontol Scand.* **2021**, *79*, 43–51. [CrossRef]
149. von Piekartz, H.; Lüdtke, K. Effect of treatment of temporomandibular disorders (TMD) in patients with cervicogenic headache: A single-blind, randomized controlled study. *Cranio* **2011**, *29*, 43–56. [CrossRef]
150. Williamson, E.H. Eugene, H. Williamson on occlusion and TMJ dysfunction. Interview by S. Brandt. *J. Clin. Orthod* **1981**, *15*, 333–350.
151. Williamson, E.H. Eugene, H. Williamson on occlusion and TMJ dysfunction (Part 2). *J. Clin. Orthod.* **1981**, *15*, 393–404+409–410.
152. Dawson, P.E. *Functional Occlusion: From TMJ to Smile Design*, 1st ed.; Elsevier: St. Louis, MO, USA, 2007.

153. Greven, G.; Piehslinger, E.; Haberl, T.; Betzl, C. Correlation between Internal Derangement of the Temporo-Mandibular Joint and Ipsi-Lateral Mediotrusive Molar Interferences-A Condylographic Study Using Virtual Articulation. *Int. J. Dent. Oral Health* **2020**, *6*, 1–6.
154. Gross, A.; Langevin, P.; Burnie, S.J.; Bédard-Brochu, M.S.; Empey, B.; Dugas, E.; Faber-Dobrescu, M.; Andres, C.; Graham, N.; Goldsmith, C.H.; et al. Manipulation and mobilisation for neck pain contrasted against an inactive control or another active treatment. *Cochrane Database Syst. Rev.* **2015**, *23*, 4249. [CrossRef] [PubMed]
155. Chen, L.; Zhang, X.L.; Ding, H.; Tao, Y.Q.; Zhan, H.S. Comparative study on effects of manipulation treatment and transcutaneous electrical nerve stimulation on patients with cervicogenic headache. *J. Chin. Integr. Med./Zhong. Xi. Yi.* **2007**, *5*, 403–406. [CrossRef] [PubMed]
156. Deyo, R.A.; Walsh, N.E.; Schoenfeld, L.S.; Ramamurthy, S. Can trials of physical treatments be blinded? The example of transcutaneous electrical nerve stimulation for chronic pain. *Am. J. Phys. Med. Rehabil.* **1990**, *69*, 6–10. [CrossRef]

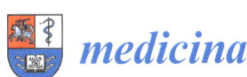

Review

Cranial and Odontological Methods for Sex Estimation—A Scoping Review

Laura Maria Beschiu [1], Lavinia Cosmina Ardelean [2,*], Codruta Victoria Tigmeanu [2] and Laura-Cristina Rusu [1]

[1] Department of Oral Pathology, Multidisciplinary Center for Research, Evaluation, Diagnosis and Therapies in Oral Medicine, "Victor Babes" University of Medicine and Pharmacy Timisoara, 2 Eftimie Murgu Sq., 300041 Timisoara, Romania

[2] Department of Technology of Materials and Devices in Dental Medicine, Multidisciplinary Center for Research, Evaluation, Diagnosis and Therapies in Oral Medicine, "Victor Babes" University of Medicine and Pharmacy Timisoara, 2 Eftimie Murgu Sq., 300041 Timisoara, Romania

* Correspondence: lavinia_ardelean@umft.ro

Abstract: The estimation of sex from osteological and dental records has long been an interdisciplinary field of dentistry, forensic medicine and anthropology alike, as it concerns all the above mentioned specialties. The aim of this article is to review the current literature regarding methods used for sex estimation based on the skull and the teeth, covering articles published between January 2015 and July 2022. New methods and new approaches to old methods are constantly emerging in this field, therefore resulting in the need to summarize the large amount of data available. Morphometric, morphologic and biochemical analysis were reviewed in living populations, autopsy cases and archaeological records. The cranial and odontological sex estimation methods are highly population-specific and there is a great need for these methods to be applied to and verified on more populations. Except for DNA analysis, which has a prediction accuracy of 100%, there is no other single method that can achieve such accuracy in predicting sex from cranial or odontological records.

Keywords: sex estimation; cranial methods; odontological methods; morphometric analysis; morphologic analysis; biochemical analysis

1. Introduction

The estimation of sex from osteological and dental records has long been an interdisciplinary field of dentistry, forensic medicine and anthropology alike, as it concerns all the above mentioned specialties.

In both forensic and archaeological cases, a reliable method to establish the sex of the deceased is paramount, as it is the first step towards a more detailed analysis of the human remains and helps in narrowing down the list of individuals and putting together a demographic pattern.

The estimation of sex from osteological remains can be achieved using three major types of methods: morphological assessment (non-metric) of teeth and bone traits that exhibit dimorphic features, morphometric assessment (by measuring specific quantifiable features of bones and teeth) and biochemical analysis, such as DNA analysis [1–4] or Barr bodies analysis [5] (Figure 1). DNA analysis is by far the most accurate method, but it is also the most expensive and may not be suited for large numbers of specimens [6,7].

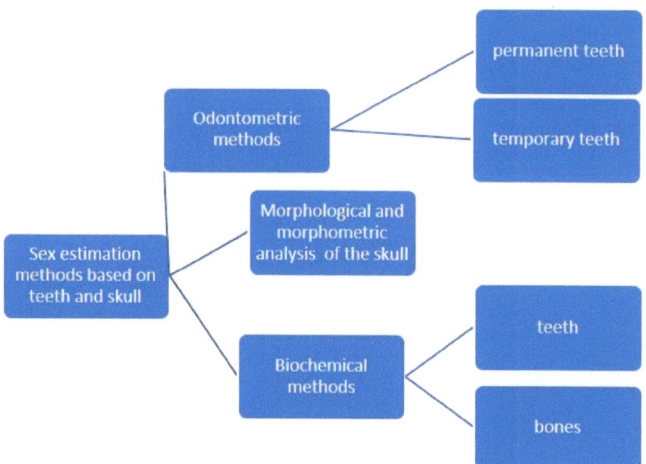

Figure 1. Odontological and cranial sex estimation methods (overview).

1.1. Morphological and Morphometric Methods

The morphological and morphometric assessment methods are both generally accepted techniques based on scientifically proven grounds, but they have limitations. For instance, morphological assessment (non-metric) is based on a certain subjective evaluation of the observer and also requires experience. Morphometric assessment (metric), on the other hand, is a laborious technique and depends on the exact determination of anatomical landmarks. Moreover, the population-specific variations in the skull make these methods almost impossible to generalize [8].

More recently, computer-aided techniques have facilitated the use of morphometric assessments, making them less subjective and time-consuming. Advances in three-dimensional image analysis have achieved rapid, automatic measurement of the entire outer surface of the craniofacial hard and soft tissue, as opposed to measurements of only limited distances and angles of the cranium. The digital analysis of the cranium and digital data storage have had a huge impact on sex estimation methods. The stored images, whether digital impressions or radiographic images, can be used time and time again for multiple analyses [9–11].

Almost all bones exhibit dimorphic features. Sex discrimination methods have proven successful in many bones, including the hyoid, ulna, sternal end of the rib, metacarpals and even metatarsals [12]. However, the pelvis shows the highest degree of dimorphism, followed by the skull [13], which has an accuracy for gender determination of up to 94% [14].

The anatomical structures of the skull used for the purpose of sex estimation are numerous: the frontal bone (position of squamous part, the appearance of the supraciliary arch, the sharpness and shape of the orbit, the frontal sinus—which remains stable and unchanged until old age and is, according to some studies, a unique structure, comparable to fingerprints) [15], the zygomatic bone (presence of marginal tubercle on the frontal process), the temporal bone (size and shape of the mastoid process, width of the zygomatic processes), the occipital bone (the nucal crest, the clivus), the mandible (angle between body and mandible ramus—angle of mandible, ramus height, base height), the shape of the nasal root, muscular insertions on bones, tooth size, face shape etc. [16] (Figure 2).

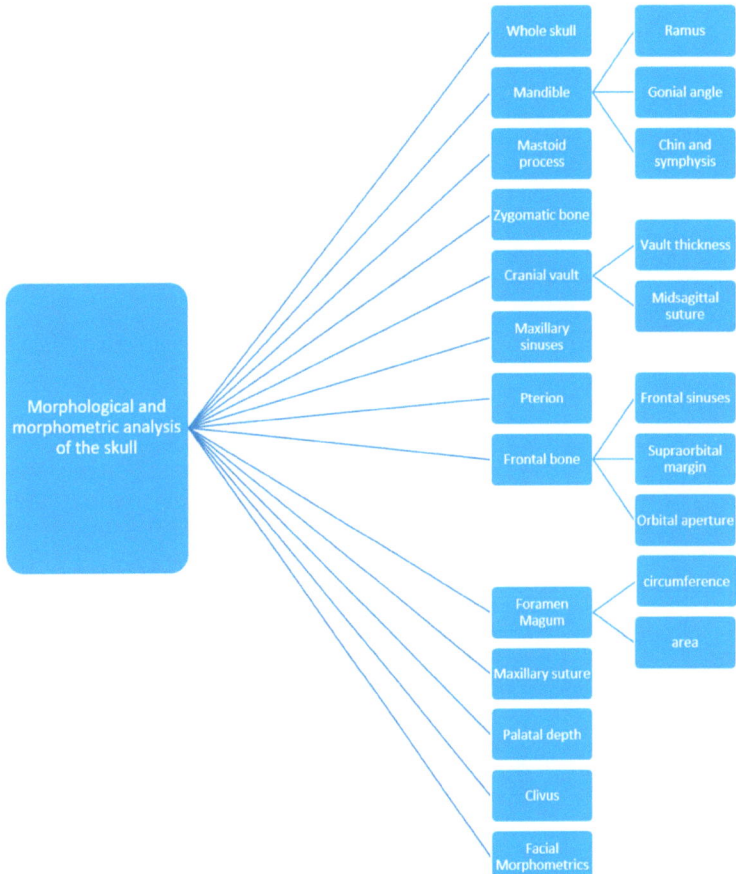

Figure 2. Parts of the skull used for sex estimation.

In many circumstances, whether in mass fatalities, explosions, mutilated bodies or poorly preserved archaeological records, the entire pelvis or skull cannot be retrieved and only fragmented parts of these bones are available for study. In these cases, the mandible plays a decisive role in sex estimation because it is the largest, strongest and one of the most dimorphic parts of the skull [17–19]. Dimorphism in the mandible is reflected in its shape and size; male bones are generally bigger and more robust than female bones. If only the mandible is available for assessment, gender determination has an accuracy of around 90% [16].

The mandible is usually one of the best preserved bones, along with the teeth, which are highly resistant to bacterial degradation, extreme heat and other types of aggressions and are therefore most likely to be preserved in fossil and archaeological records. Teeth can be heated to temperatures of 1600 °C without appreciable loss of microstructure [20] and, unlike skeletal bones, the human origin of teeth is rarely in doubt [21]. That is why the teeth form a highly valuable asset in estimating the sex of deceased individuals and are especially important in assessing children, where dimorphic aspects of the pelvis and other bones are not yet recognizable. In cases of fire or explosion, the thermal trauma causes major damage to the anatomical structures, leaving the teeth as the only way to establish the sex of the victims.

1.2. Biochemical Methods

Biochemical analyses for sex estimation purposes re based on DNA and Barr bodies from the dental pulp or from the hard tissue of the teeth. The DNA polymerase chain reaction (PCR) is more expensive and takes longer to obtain results, whereas the Barr bodies analysis is quicker and requires less equipment [5,22].

Due to their great tissue resistance, teeth can be considered as a reliable source of DNA, making them valuable in biochemical analysis methods as well. All structures of the tooth have proven value for extracting DNA material (enamel, cementum, dentine and pulp). The dental pulp contains fibroblasts, odontoblasts, endothelial cells, peripheral nerves, undifferentiated mesenchymal cells and nucleated components of blood, found in the coronal and radicular pulp, which are rich sources of DNA and free from contamination by external factors [23].

Amelogenin (AMEL) is the enamel-specific matrix formed during the first stages of tooth formation. It has been discovered that there are two types of AMEL genes, one found on the X chromosome and the other found on the Y chromosome. Hence, using PCR on the AMEL gene from DNA found in the dental pulp is a useful method to establish the sex of an individual [23]. PCR analyses that target regions of the amelogenin gene have become the method of choice for sex estimation of biological samples [24]. However, discrepancies have been noted with AMEL gene-based sex estimation, mostly due to X and Y deletion in the population and mutations in primer-binding sites. Some populations, such as Indians, appear to be affected by high frequencies of Y deletion. The presence of PCR inhibitors, degradation of the DNA samples and the presence of mixed DNA also contribute to inaccurate results obtained by amelogenin analysis and, therefore, other alternative techniques and markers have been suggested for sex estimation, such as STS, SRY, TSPY, DXYS156, SNPs, DYZ1 and next generation sequencing (NGS) [25].

Among the methods used to extract DNA from the dental pulp, the method using phenol chloroform appears to be quite cost-effective, but it is tedious and requires high precision. Newer extraction methods, such as Chelex 100^{TM} (Medox Biotech, Chennai, India) and QIA cube^{TM} (Qiagen, Hilden, Germany), could be substituted for the traditional method [23]. Recently, another method, termed the loop-mediated amplification method (LAMP reaction), which can give results within an approximately half an hour time limit, has been recommended as an alternative to conventional PCR techniques. Another advantage of the LAMP method is that it works under isothermal conditions, which stops further denaturation of the DNA [24].

Other biochemical analysis methods include the use of a fluorescent body test. It has been shown that, when chromosomes are stained with quinacrine mustard, they fluoresce differentially along their length when viewed under ultraviolet light, and the human Y chromosome fluoresces more brightly than the other chromosomes [20]. The reason for the bright fluorescence of the Y chromosome is not entirely clear. This technique has been used in forensic science for sex estimation from dried blood stains, saliva and hair since the 1970s [20]. The fluorescent Y body test has shown to be a reliable, simple and cost-effective technique for gender determination in the immediate postmortem period of up to one month after death. Therefore, its limitation is related to the post-mortem interval, making it only relevant for recently deceased individuals and, hence, impossible to use in archaeological findings [20].

The estimation of sex in ancient archaeological remains and fossils is also possible through DNA extraction techniques. The dawn of ancient DNA (aDNA) techniques was in 1983 at Berkeley, California, when Higuchi et al. extracted and sequenced ancient mitochondrial DNA (mtDNA) from a 150-year-old specimen of the quagga, a zebra-like species [26]. Then, in 1985, Svante Pääbo successfully investigated 23 Egyptian mummies for DNA content [27] and, in 1997, aDNA from Neanderthal specimens from the Feldhofer Cave in Germany was also successfully extracted [28].

Even today, the retrieval of mtDNA from ancient human specimens is not always successful owing to DNA deterioration and contamination. Usually, only short DNA fragments can be retrieved from ancient specimens. Degradation and contamination in long-term preserved specimens still make analysis very difficult. This is due to the technical difficulties with extraction, amplification and sequencing of ancient mtDNA. In recent years, NGS has mainly been applied to ancient samples. It seems that this technique is suitable for aDNA research [29]. According to the literature, short tandem repeat (STR) typing could represent a time-saving and cost-effective solution for sex estimation in archaeological sites [30].

The aim of this article is to review the current literature regarding methods used for sex estimation based on the skull and the teeth, covering articles published between January 2015–July 2022.

2. Materials and Methods

A digital search of PubMed/Medline and DOAJ was performed using the following criteria: "sex" AND ("determination" OR "estimation" OR "prediction") AND ("odontometric" OR "teeth"), "sex" AND ("determination" OR "estimation" OR "prediction") AND "human skull", "sex" AND "teeth" AND "ancient DNA". Filtering of the publication period was applied. The search retrieved 832,715 results. These results were then refined by their title and abstract so as to be in accordance with the inclusion criteria. The reference list of all identified articles was further manually searched for additional articles. This process of refining and excluding eventually left a total number of 97 articles. The set question was: *What methods are used for cranial and odontological sex estimation and which ones have the highest prediction accuracy?*

The PICO specialized framework was used to form the question and facilitate the literature search.

- Population: all ages, genders and ethnicities included;
- Intervention: cranial and odontological methods for sex estimation;
- Comparison: age range, sample size, method used, sex estimation accuracy;
- Outcome: to determine the methods and find out which ones have the highest sex estimation accuracy.

The inclusion criteria comprised the following:

- Population included: all ethnic groups;
- Patients, autopsy cases and skeletons from archaeological records;
- Original articles;
- With or without abstracts;
- Articles written in English;
- Methodologies based on both skull and teeth assessments;
- Both metric and non-metric methods;
- Both temporary and permanent teeth;
- Study focus relevant to our search question;
- No minimum number of individuals required.

The exclusion criteria comprised the following:

- Studies covering non-human subjects;
- Studies published before 2015;
- Abstracts without full reports;
- Review articles.

Titles and abstracts were scanned by two reviewers independently (L.M.B. and L.C.R.) for possible inclusion under the above mentioned criteria. Disagreements between authors were solved through discussions and consensus and mediated by a thirdg reviewer, L.C.A. The final decision was made based on the opinion of two out of the three reviewers. The PRISMA flow chart (Figure 3) was used and guidelines were followed [31]. Studies were assessed based on the reported data.

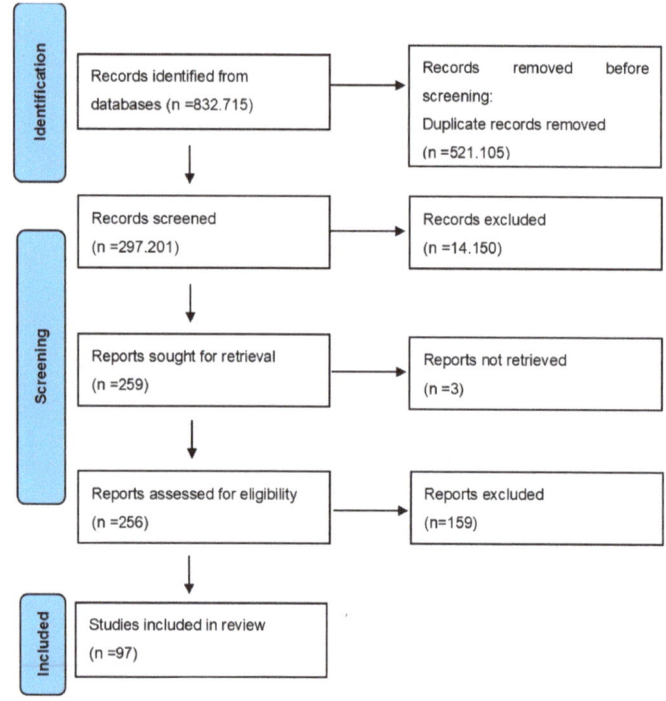

Figure 3. Prisma flow diagram.

The data extracted from each article comprised:
- Methodology used;
- Population /ethnicity;
- Sample size;
- Main conclusions;
- Accuracy of the method applied, where available.

All this information was analyzed and then tabulated in order to depict the results in a clearer manner, as the types of studies, the methodologies used and the conclusions drawn varied greatly.

3. Results

The studies were split into different categories and tabulated accordingly. The categories are as follows:
- Odontometric methods (Table 1);
- Radiographic methods (Table 2);
- Non-radiographic methods (Table 3);
- Ancient populations studies (Table 4);
- Biochemical methods (Table 5).

Table 1. Odontometric methods.

No.	Reference	Methodology	Population	No. of Cases/Age	Main Conclusions	Sex Estimation Accuracy
1	[32]	Linear and diagonal dimensions recorded at both crown and cementoenamel junction levels of extracted molars	Northwest Indian	73 males 57 females	The calculated index of sexual dimorphism was higher in lower molars than in the upper molars	Max 70%
2	[33]	Four odontometric parameters: ICW, IPW, AL and CW, measured directly with the subject	Indian	100 males 100 females	Maxillary parameters exhibited higher mean values in males compared to females	
3	[34]	MD and BL dimensions of all upper teeth	Indian	250 males 250 females	The MD and BL dimensions were statistically significant different between males and females	99.8% using stepwise discriminant functions
4	[35]	Lip prints; Mandibular Canine Index; Facial Index	Indian	50 males 50 females	Type II pattern in lips most common No significant difference in odontometric analysis	
5	[36]	Maxillary impressions; palatine rugae; MD canines; ICW; MD and BL of upper molars	Indian	60 males 60 females 20 families of 4 members	Females—more wavy rugaes Males—all measured indexes were higher than in females	
6	[37]	MD, BL measurements of 28 teeth	Indian	100 males 100 females 18–25 years old	Larger dimensions of teeth in males when compared to females	
7	[38]	Maxillary Canine Index and maxillary first molar dimensions	Indian	100 males 100 females 15–25 years old	BL dimension of maxillary first molar is a more reliable indicator for gender determination	
8	[39]	MD and BL dimensions of upper and lower *temporary teeth*	Indian	250 males 250 females 3–5 years old	Boys generally had larger crown diameters than girls	
9	[40]	Maximum ramus height, bigonion width and bicondylar breadth in OPG MD of upper central incisors, canines	Indian	100 males 100 females 18–30 years old	Ramus height—most dimorphic Permanent maxillary central incisor—more dimorphic than the maxillary canines	
10	[41]	MD—left mandibular canine	Indian	60 males 60 females 15–40 years old	Increased MD diameter in males	72.5%
11	[42]	CBCT and odontometrics of 28 teeth	Jordanian, Saudi, Egyptian	159 males 93 females 20–45 years old	Odontometric differences of 28 teeth between gender and among Saudi, Jordanian and Egyptian populations were insignificant ($p > 0.05$)	

Table 1. Cont.

No.	Reference	Methodology	Population	No. of Cases/Age	Main Conclusions	Sex Estimation Accuracy
12	[43]	MD and BL of permanent upper first molar	Indian	300 males 300 females 17–25 years old	The differences between males and females in MD and BL dimensions measured were statistically significant ($p < 0.05$)	
13	[44]	OPG—root length observed in all permanent teeth	Indian	500 males 500 females 21–60 years old	Sexual dimorphism in root length was observed in 13, 14, 15, 16, 23, 26, 33, 36, 43 and 46 (mesial) Most dimorphic teeth were canines	
14	[45]	MD of left and right canine, intercanine distance, MCI	Indian	100 males 100 females 18–25 years old	Significant sexual dimorphism of mandibular canines	73%
15	[46]	MD and BL of upper first molar	Indian	149 males 151 females 18–30 years old	BL crown dimension and the hypocone (distolingual) cusp showed the highest sexual dimorphism	64.3%
16	[47]	MCI and Pont Index	Indian	53 males 53 females 18–25 years old	MCI and Pont's Index showed significant sexual dimorphism	Standard right MCI could predict sex accurately at 75.4% Standard left MCI could predict sex accurately at 66.9%
17	[48]	MD diameter of permanent mandibular right and left canines, as well as mandibular intercanine distance	Indian	200 males 200 females 20–40 years old	The MD crown width of the permanent mandibular right and left canines, as well as the mandibular intercanine distance of the males, was found to be larger in size	78.8%
18	[49]	MD and BL diameter of mandibular canine and mandibular first molar—study casts	Indian	50 males 50 females 17–25 years old	Sexual dimorphism can be predicted by measuring mesiodistal dimension of mandibular canine and mandibular first molar	
19	[50]	Lip prints Finger prints MCI	Indian	25 males 25 females 18–25 years old	MCI was not found to be a significant indicator of gender Lip prints exhibited sexual dimorphism	

Table 1. Cont.

No.	Reference	Methodology	Population	No. of Cases/Age	Main Conclusions	Sex Estimation Accuracy
20	[51]	Dental measurements on upper right teeth	Brazilian	100 males 100 females 18–30 years old	Dental measurements are useful tools for sex determination, and the canine measurements showed a proportional correlation with stature	70.5%
21	[52]	Experimentally burned teeth at 400 °C, 700 °C and 900 °C	Portuguese		The perimeter at the CEJ and the combined measurements of the MD and BL diameters, at the same level, were quite promising in the post-burning analysis	>80%
22	[53]	MCI measured from dental casts	Portuguese	50 males 70 females 16–30 years old	MCI may not be particularly useful in sex prediction	64.2%
23	[54]	MD dimension of teeth from study castsPCA from the logarithm of the dental widths	Spanish	120 patients mean age: 14.48 ± 2.78 (males) mean age: 14.71 ± 2.69 (females)	Tooth dimension can be a considered a valuable complementary tool in sex determination for Spanish population	76.2%
24	[55]	MD widths of mandibular canines ICW From casts	Nepal	40 male 40 female	Sex predictability by using MCI showed poor sex predictability and should be used cautiously in Nepalese population	57.5–62.5%
25	[56]	Raman spectroscopy of teeth PCA of teeth from anthropological collection	Croatian	55 teeth 11–76 years old	The accuracy of classification models depends both on the tooth type (molar and premolar) and recording site (anatomical neck and apex) on the tooth	>90%
26	[57]	MD and BL dimensions of permanent teeth measured from dental casts and radiographs	Iranian	74 male 257 female 12–35 years old	Sex dimorphism is very strong in the dentition Ageing significantly reduces measurements Mandibular canines were the most dimorphic teethBolton ratio was not affected by sex	

ICW—intercanine width; IPW—interpremolar width; AL—arch length; CW—combined length of six maxillary anterior teeth; MD—mesiodistal; BL—buccolingual; OPG—ortopanthomography; CBCT—cone-beam computed tomography; MCI—Mandibular Canine Index; CEJ—cement–enamel junction; PCA—principal component analysis.

Table 2. Radiographic methods.

No.	Reference	Methodology	Population	No. of Cases/Age	Main Conclusions	Sex Estimation Accuracy
1	[42]	CBCT and odontometrics of 28 teeth	Jordanian, Saudi, Egyptian	159 males 93 females, 20–45 years old	Odontometric differences of 28 teeth between gender and among Saudi, Jordanian and Egyptian populations were insignificant ($p > 0.05$)	
2	[58]	A total of 99 cephalometric variables were compared, subjected to statistical analysis and tested for significance using the t-test	Dravidian	125 males 125 females 25–40 years old	Twenty-four variables showed statistical significance	52—78%
3	[59]	PA cephalometric analysis	Hispano-American Peruvians	1525 patients 5–44 years old	Significant differences between sexes Males, on average, are larger and have increased muscle attachment in their skeletons than females	63–75%
4	[60]	Mandible morphometry on CBCT scans	Korean	96 males 104 females 18–60 years old	Gender can be accurately predicted using this technique	67%
5	[61]	CT scans of FM	Indian	110 males 90 females	Shape and dimensions of FM should be taken into consideration during surgery involving the craniovertebral junction and in forensic and anthropological investigations	65%
6	[62]	Morphometric analysis of the mandible with OPG	Italian	50 males 20–68 years 50 females 21–62 years old	Mandible exhibits great sexual dimorphism	92.5%
7	[63]	Morphometric analysis with OPG	Indian	500 males 500 females 21–60 years old		69%
8	[64]	Submentovertex radiography	South Indian	75 males 75 females	Circumference in FM was the best sex indicator	67.3%
9	[65]	OPG measurements of the mandible	Chennai	150 OPGs 3–70 years old, divided into seven groups	Highly statistically significant differences between genders	
10	[66]	OPG measurements of the mandible	Indian	113 males 87 females 4–75 years old	Significant differences between all the parameters: gonial angle, height and width of the ramus of mandible	

Table 2. Cont.

No.	Reference	Methodology	Population	No. of Cases/Age	Main Conclusions	Sex Estimation Accuracy
11	[67]	Maxillary sinuses measured with OPG	Brazilian	32 males 32 females >20 years old	There were differences between the mean values of the maxillary sinus dimensions evaluated for both sexes However, when the values were between 27 mm and 31 mm for height, and 44 mm and 48 mm for width, it was impossible to determine the sex	
12	[68]	Maxillary sinus measurements with MRI scan	Indian	30 males 30 females 21–73 years old	Sexual dimorphism was shown by the volume of the maxillary sinuses on the left side	
13	[69]	CT scans of skulls	Malaysian	45 males 42 females 18–75 years old	Males showed higher values for all the parameters than females, except for the left orbital height	85.1%
14	[70]	Orbital aperture dimension with PA cephalogram	North Indian	250 males 250 females 20–50 years old	All the linear measurements, such as orbital height, orbital width and interorbital distance, were significantly greater in males than females	84.8%
15	[71]	Maxillary sinuses measured with CT scans	Indian	50 males 50 females >20 years old	Volume of left maxillary sinus of males is larger than that of females	84% in males 92% in females
16	[19]	Chin and mandibular symphysis measurements with CT scans	Caucasian	203 males 216 females >18 years old Age-matched samples	Chin width (the frontal view) was found to be a sexually selected trait; it can be considered as a parameter for sex determination The chin was found to be a more heterogeneous anatomical structure than symphysis and it was sexually more dismorphic	
17	[72]	Frontal sinus measured with PA cephalograms	Indian	100 males 100 females ≥14 years old	It was found that the left width and area are most suitable for gender determination	
18	[73]	CT scans of the gonial angle	Turkish	150 males 150 females Three age groups 20–80 years old	Males showed slightly smaller gonial angle values than those of females in all age groups Gonial angle is not a particularly good indicator to identify the sex from the cranium	

295

Table 2. Cont.

No.	Reference	Methodology	Population	No. of Cases/Age	Main Conclusions	Sex Estimation Accuracy
19	[74]	Mandibular CBCT scans	Brazilian	74 males 86 females 18–60 years old		95.1%
20	[75]	Bi-zygomatic distance and intervolt distance measured with"jug handle" radiograph	Indian	30 males 30 females 18–25 years old	Bizygomatic distance is a more reliable parameter to determine gender as compared to intervault distance	
21	[17]	Mandibular ramus and gonial angle measurements with OPG	North Indian	200 males 200 females 10–40 years old	The mandibular ramus showed a high sexual dimorphism, with condylar and coronoid ramus heights as the most significant predictor for age and sex estimation Gonial angle can only be used as an additional tool	
22	[18]	Mandibular rami measurements with OPG	South Indian	229 males 271 females 20–60 years old	Condylar height/maximum ramus height was found to be the best sex predictor	80.4%
23	[15]	CBCT measurements of the skull	Iranian	51 males 51 females 46.65 ± 12.72 years old		Highest accuracy related to mandible bone—89% Lowest accuracy related to FM—71%
24	[76]	Clivus measurements with CBCT scan	Indian	76 males 74 females 6–17 years old	The clivus length was statistically significant The clivus length was greater in male population	
25	[44]	OPG—root length observed in all permanent teeth	Indian	500 males 500 females 21–60 years old	Sexual dimorphism in root length was observed in 13, 14, 15, 16, 23, 26, 33, 36, 43 and 46 (mesial); The most dimorphic teeth are canines	
26	[77]	CT images used to measure the mediolateral, superoinferior and anteroposterior dimensions and the volume of the maxillary sinuses	Indian	15 males 15 females		83.3%

Table 2. Cont.

No.	Reference	Methodology	Population	No. of Cases/Age	Main Conclusions	Sex Estimation Accuracy
27	[78]	Lateral cephalograms—gonial angle	Indian	149 males 155 females 18–30 years old		56.3%
28	[79]	Morphometric evaluation of frontal sinus with PA radiographs	Saudi Arabian	200 males 200 females 14–70 years old	Right width and left width are most suited regressors for sex determination	67.70–95.90%
29	[80]	OPG—ten mandibular variables were measured	South Indian	192 males 192 females	Coronoid height was the single best parameter, providing an accuracy of 74.1%	Overall accuracy: 75.8%
30	[81]	Measurements of the mandibular ramus: maximum ramus breadth, maximum ramus height and coronoid height using Planmeca ProMax	Indian	80 OPGs	Greatest sexual dimorphism was noticed in the maximum ramus height	Prediction rate using all five variables: 83.8%
31	[82]	Linear tooth measurements with CBCT machine learning: naive Bayesian, random forest, support vector machine	Iranian	245 males 240 females	Naive Bayesian—highest accuracy for sex classification	Average accuracy: 92.31%
32	[83]	Roof, height and floor of pulp chamber Marginal enamel/dentine thickness Tooth width and crown length CBCT	Iranian	100 males 100 females Mean age: 21.28 ± 2.47	Maxillary first molars were more dimorphic than mandibular teeth Mesio-distal variables were more dimorphic than bucco-lingual ones	Highest accuracy: 84%
33	[84]	PCA with lateral cephalograms	Indian	54 males 51 females	Sex was clearly associated with occlusion	Over 96% variation between male and female
34	[85]	PCA of mandible surface CT scans	Japanese	23 males 22 females Mean age: 43.1 ± 14.6	Significant differences between male and female, the mandibular branch of males was larger than that of females, and the mandible angle was overhanging outside	

PA—postero-anterior; FM—foramen magnum; MRI—magnetic resonance imaging; CT—computed tomography; HBM—homologous body modeling.

Table 3. Non-radiographic methods (cranial morphometric studies on modern populations).

No.	Reference	Methodology	Population	No. of Cases/Age	Main Conclusions	Sex Estimation Accuracy
1	[9]	Morphological features from the 3D skull MKDSIF-FCM algorithm	Han Chinese		Accuracy improvements of nearly 8.6%, 3.5% and 2.2% compared to other algorithms	
2	[14]	Supraorbital margin and frontal bone quantified by wavelet transform and Fourier transform	Han Chinese	73 males 60 females 22–28 years old	Compared with the traditional methods, the correct rate is higher	90.9% for males 94.4% for females
3	[86]	Photographs of maxillary sutures—dry skulls	Thai	96 males 94 females	Maxillary suture length can be applied for sex estimation	79.47%
4	[87]	Cranial vault thickness—autopsy cases	Caucasion Negroid Mongoloid	1097 cases 103 <19 years old 994 >19 years old	Females appear to have a larger frontal cranial thickness Cranial vault thickness generally cannot be used as an indicator for sex	
5	[88]	Various craniometric measurements on dry skulls	Thai	100 males 36–96 years old 100 females 15–93 years old	Mastoid length (right and left), nasal height, FM length, cranial base length, bizygomatic breadth, FM breadth, biauricular breadth, upper facial breadth, basion-nasospinale length, maximum cranial length and biorbital breadth expressed significant sexual dimorphism	88–92.2%
6	[89]	Maxillary arch depth and palatal depth measured from dental casts	Indian	250 males 250 females 17–25 years	Only mean maxillary arch depth values were found to be statistically significantly different	
7	[90]	Anthropometric measurements of patients	Indian	50 males 50 females 30–40 years old	Significantly higher facial height, pronasale-to-menton distance and interzygomatic width in males as compared to females	
8	[91]	Measurements of FM in skulls	Indian	41 males 31 females >18 years old		Predictability of area was the highest: 70.3%
9	[92]	Palate measurements from dental casts	Jordanian	66 males 84 females 18–50 years old 75 males 75 females 6–12 years old	The palatal dimensions that reflect the palatal size were significantly higher in males than in females	

Table 3. Cont.

No.	Reference	Methodology	Population	No. of Cases/Age	Main Conclusions	Sex Estimation Accuracy
10	[11]	3D soft tissue craniofacial analysis	British and Irish white Europeans	102 British males 27 Irish males 132 British females 31 Irish females Below 13–over 50 years old	The magnitude of dimorphism in sex is revealed in facial, nasal and crania measurements Males are relatively larger than females, especially in the mouth and nasal regions	
11	[93]	Skull measurements	Greek	176 individuals		Multivariate combinations: >95%
12	[94]	Vault and midsagittal curve of the neurocranium measurements	Greek	94 males 82 females	In contrast to the midsagittal curve of the neurocranium, the shape of the cranial vault can be used as an indicator of sex in the modern Greek population	89.2%
13	[95]	Novel interlandmark distance measures across six regions of the cranium (dry skulls)	South Africans of European descent (white)	114 males 113 females		74–88.2%
14	[10]	3D geometric morphometric measurements of the cranium (dry skulls)	Greek	94 males 82 females	There are shape differences between the sexes in the upper-face and the orbits Size is significant for sexual dimorphism in the upper-face region	
15	[16]	Mastoid process measurements from dry skulls	Bosnian	50 males 47–71 year old 50 females 43–76 years old	There was a statistically significant difference between the genders on the basis of the mastoid process	
16	[96]	Mastoid measurements from dry skull	Indian	25 males 25 females >18 years old	The mastoid process is a good indicator for sex determination	83%
17	[12]	Mandible measurements from dry skulls	British	40 males 36 females	Mandibular metrics are good predictors for sex determination	77.3%
18	[8]	Computer vision cranial measurements	Malaysian	54 males 46 females 5–85 years old	CV methods are suitable for sex determination	78.2–86.2%
19	[97]	Virtual method—evaluating the exocranial surface	Czech	208 individuals	Highest accuracy for Czech population—96.2% Highest accuracy for inter-populational differences—92.8%	91.8%

Table 3. *Cont.*

No.	Reference	Methodology	Population	No. of Cases/Age	Main Conclusions	Sex Estimation Accuracy
20	[98]	Pterion surface evaluated by machine learning	Thai	100 skulls	PMP and PI distances were significantly longer in males	80.7%
21	[99]	Fully automated method with 3D models	CzechGreek	170 Czech 156 Greek	The method is efficient in estimating sex from cranial remains	Population-specific accuracy: 78.5–96.7% Population generic accuracy: 71.7–90.8%

PMP—distance from the center of the pterion to the mastoid process of the temporal bone; PI—distance from the center of the pterion to the mastoid process of the external occipital protuberance.

Table 4. Ancient population studies.

No.	Reference	Methodology	Population	No. of Cases/Age	Main Conclusions	Sex Estimation Accuracy
1	[4]	Various anthropological procedures of the skull and skeleton aDNA analysis	Croatian	84 adult medievalskeletons	For the mandible, the only measurement that showed sexual dimorphism was mandibular body height	Seven multivariate and five univariate discriminant functions for sex estimation with overall accuracy rates above 80%
2	[100]	Os coxae Skull Os coxae + skull		66 individuals 13–16th century	The preauricular sulcus, frontal bossing and arc compose should be reconsidered as appropriate traits for sex estimation	The combined estimate (97.7%) outperformed the os coxae-only estimate (95.7%), which outperformed the skull-only estimate (90.4%)

Table 5. Biochemical studies.

No.	Reference	Methodology	No. of Cases	Main Conclusions	Sex Estimation Accuracy
1	[23]	PCR analysis from dental pulp Amelogenin gene analysis Teeth subjected to different conditions	130 teeth	Teeth buried in soil yielded least amount of DNA over a period of time and no DNA could be obtained at high temperatures	
2	[101]	PCR analysis	Eight mesiodens teeth	Sex identification through DNA was possible in six out of eight cases	
3	[24]	DNA—amelogenin analysis	50 teeth subjected to different conditions, including extreme temperatures of 1050 °C	Pulpal tissue and degenerating odontoblastic processes provided enough DNA for sex identification	100% retrieval of DNA along with gender determination

Table 5. Cont.

No.	Reference	Methodology	No. of Cases	Main Conclusions	Sex Estimation Accuracy
4	[30]	DNA analysis of ancient petrous bone compared to femur and tooth	39 skeletal element from 13 individuals	Petrous bone is the best skeletal element with regard to DNA conservation in ancient remains	
5	[102]	Capillary electrophoresis (CE)-and massively parallel sequencing (MPS)-based analysis of petrous bone	Different sections of eight unknown cranial bones and additionally—where available—other skeletal elements	Short tandem repeat (STR) typing from the petrous bones leads to reportable profiles in all individuals	
6	[103]	DNA extraction from petrous bone and tooth	50 skeletal remains	More likely to obtain a complete STR profile from petrous bone material	
7	[104]	MS proteomics on 5000 year old teeth	11 Neolitic human teeth	The method represents an alternative for sex estimation when DNA is not exploaitable	The targeted proteomics assay allowed the confirmation of the sex in all the samples
8	[105]	Enamel peptide analysis by liquid chromatography and mass spectrometry without destruction of analyzed teeth	8 permanent, 15 deciduous teeth from fossil remains	Analysis of teeth enamel peptidome is sutable for sex determination of human fossil remains	
9	[106]	Enamel peptides	43 teeth from 29 nonadult individuals 40 gestational weeks to 19 years old from archaeological sites in England	The method enables forensic identification of nonadult human remains, including perinates	28 out of 29 individuals were identified

The most frequently employed parameters were MCI, MD diameter of the lower canines and ICW. Out of the total of 26 studies, 18 were performed on an Indian population. Girish et al. reported the highest accuracy of sex estimation (99.8%) by measuring the BL and MD dimensions of all upper teeth [34].

The most frequently used radiographic method was OPG, followed by CT and CBCT. The highest accuracy of sex estimation was reported by Gamba et al. (95.1%), using CBCT scans for mandibular sexual dimorphism analysis [74].

To our knowledge, so far, Gowland et al.'s study is the only one addressing the sex determination from the teeth of pre-birth individuals [106].

4. Discussion

In the period between January 2015 and July 2022, a large number of studies have dealt with the issue of sex estimation of individuals from measurements or analyses of the teeth and cranium, which shows the importance of the subject.

4.1. Populations

The most studies by far were undertaken by Indian researchers on contemporary populations, as shown in Tables 1–3 [17,18,24,33,44,61,63,66,68,70–72,75–78,80,81,84,89–91,96].

With regard to European populations, Greek studies seem to be more frequent [10,93,94,99], but there are also British [11,12], Portuguese [52,53], Spanish [54], Croatian [4,56], Bosnian [16], Italian [62] and Czech [97,99] studies, a study concerning Caucasians in general [19] and one concerning South Africans of European descent [95]. A number of articles concerned Saudi Arabian, Egyptian, Malaysian, Chinese, Korean, Jordanian, Nepalese, Iranian, Japanese, Thai, Turkish, Brazilian, Peruvian and Australian populations [4,8,9,14,43,55,57,59,60,67, 69,73,74,82,83,85,86,88,92,98]. One study described 1097 autopsy cases of Caucasian, Mongoloid and Negroid individuals [87]. The type of population on which morphometric studies have been conducted is important, as the results are largely population-related and not applicable to other ethnicities. This does not apply to biochemical studies, however, where the conclusions are unrelated to the ethnicity of the individuals involved.

4.2. Sample Size

A few articles stand out, due the large samples involved, having over 500 cases and, in some, as many as 1296 [34,44,59,87]. Girish et al.'s odontometric study comprised 500 cast measurements—half male, half female—and their ability to differentiate gender in the population using stepwise discriminant functions was found to be very high, with 99.8% accuracy [34]. Govindaram et al.'s study is the only study reviewed that involved the measurement of roots of permanent teeth in order to find sexual dimorphism. It also had a large sample of 1000 cases, with only patients with the past three generations living in Tamil Nadu and Tamil mother tongue accepted for study. The study found a number of roots displaying sexual dimorphism, while the upper and lower canines were the most dimorphic [44]. De Boer et al. used a sample of 1097 autopsy cases with multiple ancestral origins belonging to Caucasian, Negroid and Mongoloid races, for which cranial vault thickness was measured. Differences were found between males and females, with females apparently having larger frontal cranial thickness, but the conclusion drawn was that cranial vault thickness "cannot be used as a proxy for configuring the anthropological biological profile" [87].

4.3. Sex Estimation in Children

Perez et al.'s article was the first study attempting to use Rickett's PA cephalometric analysis to establish the sex of an individual of a Peruvian population. Apart from being the first study to use this type of PA analysis, its strength resides in the fact that the sample size was large (1296 cases) and also involved children (5–44 year old), which is rare in this type of study (Tables 1–3). However, their accuracy rate was between 63–75% and they concluded that Rickett's PA cephalometric analysis is not adequate for sex determination [59].

Other studies that included children or children's skulls include those of Singh et al., Rajkumari et al., Poongodi et al., Noble et al. and Mustafa et al. [39,65,66,92,107]. Singh's research was performed on 500 dental casts belonging to 250 boys and 250 girls aged 3 to 5 and found significant differences between the dimensions of temporary teeth in girls and boys, with boys having larger tooth dimensions than girls [39]. This was the single odontometric study on temporary teeth that met our search criteria. Another study involving children is that of Rajkumari et al., which aimed to find sexual dimorphism by analyzing mandibular dimensions with OPG. It included the OPGs of 150 patients aged 3 to 70 years and the measurements performed were: maximum ramus width (MaxRW), minimum ramus width (MinRW), condylar height (ConH), coronoid height (CorH), projective ramus height (PH) and gonial angle (GA), recorded bilaterally. They found that MaxRW (R/L), ConH (R/L), CorH (R/L), PH (R/L) and GA (R/L) showed highly statistically significant differences between the genders [65]. Poongodi et al. also included OPGs of both children and adults (ages 4–75) in their research and the results showed significant variables in the GA and the height of the ramus [66]. Mustafa et al. searched for sexual dimorphism in the palatal arch and in the size of the incisive papillae measured from 150 dental casts of Jordanian children and reported significant size differences both in the palatal arch and the incisive papillae in children [92].

Noble et al.'s research used multidetector computed tomography (MDCT) to scan 152 juvenile crania of a Western Australian population. They acquired fifty-two 3D landmarks that were analyzed using Procrustean geometric morphometrics and found little quantifiable sexual dimorphism in individuals younger than 12 years of age, whereas, in older individuals, at 18 years of age, the prediction accuracy rates are as high as 94%, and the authors concluded that simple, linear interlandmark distances of crania could be an option for preliminary classification of skeletal remains [107].

Ziganshin et al. used liquid chromatography and mass spectrometry to analyze tooth enamel peptides from 15 deciduous teeth from fossil remains. A specific peptide containing phosphorylated Ser66 residue was found only in the enamel from deciduous teeth, suggesting its role in the enamel formation of deciduous teeth [105].

Gowland et al.'s study addressed sex determination from the teeth of nonadult human remains, including pre-birth individuals, using dimorphic enamel peptide analysis [106].

4.4. Odontometric Studies

Odontometric studies searched for sexual dimorphism in teeth dimensions, whether measuring upper or lower teeth, all teeth or only specific teeth. The measurements were performed intraorally [37,40,43]; from dental casts [36,38,54,55,57] or, in some cases, radiographs [40,41,57]; or using Raman spectroscopy [56], and their conclusions vary greatly in terms of the accuracy rate found (Figure 4).

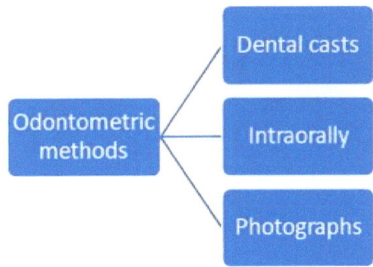

Figure 4. Types of odontometric methods.

The canines, maxillary central incisors and first molars (both upper and lower) [43,46] were the teeth most frequently measured and, among them, the mandibular canines seem to come up the most [40,41,45,55]. The mesiodistal and buccolingual diameters of the teeth were also frequently assessed parameters, as was the Mandibular Canine Index (MCI) [35,36,48,54,55,57].

4.4.1. Mandibular Canine Index

Regarding the MCI, the results reported are very different. While Priyadharshini et al., Krishnan et al. and Silva et al. found that the MCI was not particularly useful in sex determination (Silva et al. found an accuracy rate of 64.2%) [35,50,53], other studies seem to disagree and show quite high accuracy rates, between 66.98% and 78.8%, in determining the sex by MCI [45,47,48].

4.4.2. Other Teeth Measurements

Studies conducted on 28 teeth have also come up with different results. Alam et al.'s cross-sectional CBCT study performed on 159 males and 93 females of Saudi, Jordanian and Egyptian origin found that the odontometrics of the second maxillary and mandibular molars were insignificant in terms of sex estimation [42]. However, the study conducted by Girish et al. on 250 males and 250 females of Indian ancestry concluded that the ability to differentiate gender in the population using stepwise discriminant functions was very high, with 99.8% accuracy, with males showing statistically larger teeth than females [34].

Larger dimensions of teeth in males were found in Dash et al.'s study as well. They measured the MD and BL dimensions of all teeth, excluding the third molars, in an Indian population [37]. Similar to Priyadharshini et al., Krishnan et al. and Silva et al., they also concluded that canines and premolars showed no statistical difference between sexes [35,50,53].

Gouveia et al.'s research stands out from the odontometric studies through their methods. They employed experimentally burned teeth (at 400 °C, 700 °C and 900 °C) to perform measurements and test the sexual dimorphism. However, they conclude that most of the standard measurements, although presenting significant sex differences, were "not reliable enough to allow for correct sex classifications close to 100% both before and after the burning", but they managed to achieve correct sex classification above 80% [52].

4.5. Morphometrics of the Skull

Articles using morphometrics of the skull in various forms, whether through direct measurements of the skull, through radiological scans or using 3D facial computed applications, are quite difficult to compare because the methods vary greatly (Figure 5) and their conclusions are also very different.

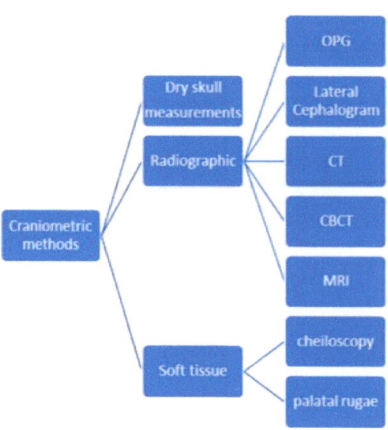

Figure 5. Types of craniometric methods.

Among the parts of the cranium most frequently assessed, studies concerning the mandible are the most frequent. Eight articles using OPG scans of the mandible, two articles using mandibular CBCT measurements, two articles using lateral cephalogram to measure mandibular parameters [78,84] and two articles employing CT (one to assess the chin and the mandibular symphysis [19] and one the mandible surface [85]) were reviewed. The most frequently measured parameters were GA and ramus height (RH).

4.5.1. Dimorphism of the Gonial Angle

With regard to GA, Sambhana et al., in an OPG based study on a South Indian population, concluded that the GA did not show significant sexual dimorphism [80]. This was similar to the study by Bulut et al. [73], which examined 150 male and 150 female CT scans of the mandible of a Turkish population between the ages of 20 and 80 years old, divided into three groups for more accuracy, and concluded that the GA is not a particularly good indicator for sex identification and should not be used as a sole criterion [73]. Belaldavar et al. also found a low accuracy rate for the GA (56.3%) in their research on lateral cephalometric radiographs of 155 males and 149 females of Indian origin, aged 18–30 [78]. In contrast, Rajkumari et al., in their research on 150 OPGs, concluded that the GA, along with other mandibular parameters, such as MaxRW, ConH, CorH, and PH, showed highly statistically significant differences between the genders [65]. Similar results were found by Poongodi et al. in their OPG study, concluding that the GA and the RH are significant variables in determining the sex [66]. The study of Suzuki et al., using CT, found significant differences between Japanese males and females, the gonial angle overhanging outside in male cases [85].

4.5.2. Dimorphism of the Ramus Height

RH is also often employed in morphometrics of the crania in studies performed with OPG and CBCT, with a high accuracy of prediction rates, between 69% and 83.8% [40,58,60,62,63,80,81]. With regards to this parameter, studies seem to agree more than for other parameters. Except for one study, that of Bašić et al., which only found sexual dimorphism in the mandible in its body height, the others reported high sexual dimorphism in the mandibular ramus [4]. The main difference between the study by Bašić et al. compared to all others that involved mandibular ramus measurements is that Bašić's study was based on measurements of medieval Croatian skeletons, whereas the others were radiographic studies conducted on modern populations, most of them Indian [40,58,63,80,81] and one Saudi Arabian [60] and one Italian [62]. A particularly large sample of cases was analyzed by More et al. (500 male and 500 female digital OPGs), and the conclusion drawn was that the overall accuracy for diagnosing sex from the mandibular ramus was 69.0% [63]. Damera et al., in their study, reported that the greatest sexual dimorphism of the mandible was expressed in the maximum RH, giving an accuracy in the prediction rate of 83.8% [81]. Missier et al., in their study on 250 lateral cephalograms, reported that the RH, along with the ramus length and Conylion to Gnathion measurements, showed the highest sex-determining dependability (78%) in the mandible [58]. Similar findings were presented by Sambhana et al. in their study conducted on 384 OPGs, which resulted in an overall accuracy of 75.8%, with the CorH being the single best parameter, providing an accuracy of 74.1% [80]. The CT-based study by Suzuki et al. found significant differences regarding the size of the mandibular branch between Japanese males and females, the mandibular branch of males being larger [85].

4.5.3. Dimorphism of the Chin and Mandibular Symphysis

Tunis et al.'s study regarding the chin and mandibular symphysis had a large (419) adult, age-matched sample of Caucasian origin. They concluded that males had a significantly wider and taller chin than females and, with regard to the symphysis, their study showed the existence of sexual dimorphism in the observed symphysis metric characteristics; i.e., males exhibited higher, thicker and larger symphyses that were more lingually oriented compared with those of females [19]. This was the only study reviewed concerning the chin and the mandibular symphysis.

4.5.4. Dimorphism of the Foramen Magnum

Regarding the FM as a tool for sex determination, there were two types of measurements performed: area and circumference. Raikar et al. found circumference to be the best predictor of sex, achieving an accuracy rate of 67.3% [64], whereas Kamath et al.'s study found the area of the FM to be the best sex predictor [91]. Both studies were based on Indian populations, Raikar's study being performed on 150 submentovertex radiographies while Kamath's study was undertaken with measurements from 72 skulls.

Vinutha et al., in their research, measured the anteroposterior and transverse diameters of the FM, as well as the circumference, and 65% of cranial CT scans overall were sexed correctly based on these measurements [61].

Nourbashkh et al. performed research based on measurements of the skulls of 102 people. The frontal sinus, maxillary sinus, mandible and FM were assessed. They concluded that the highest accuracy was related to the mandible bone, with 89% (the RH had the highest value), and the lowest accuracy was related to the FM, with 71% [15].

Mahakkanukrauh et al. also measured the FM in their research, along with other measurements of dried skulls of Thai origin, and found significant differences between the genders [88].

4.5.5. Dimorphism of the Maxillary Sinuses

The maxillary sinuses have also served as a tool for sex identification, but the results reported vary greatly. De Queiroz et al. measured the height and width of the maxillary sinuses and found a limited applicability for sex estimation because, when the individuals' maxillary sinus dimensions were between certain values, it was impossible to determine the sex [67]. Rani et al.'s study was based on MRI scans of the maxillary sinuses, which was found to be an adequate method for sex estimation, with the highest sexual dimorphism being found in the volume of the left side maxillary sinus [68]. Similar results were presented by Bangi et al. in their CT study on maxillary sinuses, showing that the volume of the left maxillary sinus of males is larger than that of females [71]. Another CT-based study on maxillary sinuses was undertaken by Prabhat et al., who reported a high gender prediction accuracy of 83.3%; however, their sample size was relatively low (30 patients) [77]. In fact, except for Bangi's research (100 cases) [71], the other reviewed studies regarding maxillary sinuses had relatively small samples: 64 cases in de Queiroz et al.'s study [67] and 60 subjects in Rani et al.'s study [68].

4.5.6. Dimorphism of the Left Side versus the Right Side of the Skull

With respect to the left side of the cranium being more sexually dimorphic than the right side, Rani et al. found in their studies that the highest percentage of sexual dimorphism was shown in the left maxillary sinus [68], and similar results were reported by Bangi et al. [71]. Soman et al. also reported that the left width and area of the frontal sinus are more suitable for gender estimation [72].

4.5.7. Dimorphism of the Mastoid

Regarding the mastoid, two articles were reviewed, one performed on 100 adult modern Bosnian skulls [16] and the other also performed on skulls, this time of Indian origin, all 50 adults [96]. They both concluded that the mastoid process is a good indicator for sex estimation, and the latter gave an accuracy rate for prediction of 83%. The limitation of using the mastoid process as sex estimation in forensic or anthropological investigations is related to the fact that the mastoid region is considered as one of the slowest and later-growing regions of the cranium, showing a higher degree of sexual dimorphism in adulthood, so it can only be used in adults [96].

4.5.8. Dimorphism of the Palate, the Pterion and the Orbital Aperture of the Frontal Bone

Significant differences between sexes were also found in other parts of the cranium, such as the palate, pterion and orbital aperture of the frontal bone.

Two articles regarding the palate were reviewed: one performed by Mankapure et al. on 500 dental casts of adult Indian patients by measuring the arch depth and the palatal depth, which concluded that only the mean maxillary arch depth values are statistically significantly different between sexes [89]. The other study regarding the palate was undertaken by Mustafa et al. [92] on 300 dental casts, among which 150 were children. They measured the palatal arch dimensions and the size of the incisive papillae in both the adult and children groups and the shape of the incisive papillae in the adult group only. They found that the size of the palatal arch was significantly higher in adult males than females, and there were also significant differences between the size and the shape of the incisive papillae in adults. In the children group, the palatal width and length significantly predicted the sex, while the size of the incisive papillae was also significantly different between the two genders. Their conclusions strongly suggest that the palatal dimensions and their overall size are sexually dimorphic [92].

Regarding the orbital aperture, only the research done by Kanjani et al. met our search criteria. This was performed with PA cephalograms of 250 adult males and 250 adult females of North Indian origin, and the parameters measured were the maximum height and width of the right and left orbits, along with the interorbital distance. The study reported 84.8% accuracy after subjecting the obtained values to discriminant function analysis [70].

The study by Uabundit et al., carried out on 124 dried skulls, aimed to classify and examine the prevalence of all types of pterion variations using morphometric measurements and machine learning models to estimate sex and age. The main conclusion was that the random forest algorithm could predict sex with 80.7% accuracy [98].

4.6. High Sex Prediction Accuracy

Among the articles reviewed, few of them report a very high sex prediction accuracy based on morphometric or odontometric methods. Mahakkanukrauh et al.'s study, which performed various cranial measurements of the skull of 200 Thai individuals, reported that, according to discriminant analysis, percentage accuracies obtained from both direct and stepwise methods were distinctly high (88.0–92.2%) [88].

Yang et al. investigated the superior orbital margin and frontal bone of the skull in a Chinese population and proposed a technology of objective sex estimation for the skull using wavelet transforms and Fourier transforms. Their results showed that the accuracy rate for male and female sex discrimination was between 90.9% and 94.4% [14].

A very high accuracy rate was also reported by Shireen et al. in their study regarding the sexual dimorphism of the frontal sinus in a Saudi Arabian population. Their reported accuracy rates were between 67.70% and 95.90% [79]. Nuzzolese et al., in their OPG-based study on the mandible, also reported that the efficacy of cross-validated discriminant analysis indicated a high level of robust and significant classification based on their 25 chosen landmarks, with 92.5% correct overall classifications [62].

The odontometric study with the highest accuracy rate reported was that of Girish et al., performed on cast models of all upper teeth except the third molars. They measured the MD and BL dimensions of these teeth and found that the ability to differentiate gender in the population using stepwise discriminant functions had a 99.8% accuracy [34].

4.7. Machine Learning

Machine learning and virtual methods to assess dimorphism are, most likely, the way forward in this field. Not only are they becoming more and more accurate, but they are also less time consuming, less invasive and more cost-efficient compared to other methods [9,97–99]. Parts of the skull or the skull as a whole are more frequently assessed through these methods, as in the studies undertaken by Gao et al. [9], Chovalpoulou et al. [94,99], Arigbabu et al. [8], Musilova et al. [97], Uabundit et al. [98] and Bertsatos et al. [99]. However, soft tissue can also serve to determine the dimorphic features of the face, as in Agbolade et al.'s study [11]. Noble et al.'s study on juvenile crania also employed machine learning methods [107].

4.8. Biochemical Analysis

The biochemical methods used for sex estimation were performed either on teeth alone [23,24,101], on teeth and bone [30,103] or on bone alone [102].

Both Chowdhury et al., and Dutta et al. [23,24] performed their research on teeth subjected to different conditions mimicking environmental conditions, such as teeth buried in soil or under extreme heat, and attempted to amplify the Amel gene from dental pulp or dentin using the PCR reaction. Chowdhury et al. found that the amount of DNA extracted decreases as the period of time in which teeth were exposed increases, that teeth buried in soil yielded the least amount of DNA over a period of time and that no DNA could be obtained at high temperatures (350 °C) [23]. Dutta et al.'s research was performed on 50 teeth samples also exposed to different conditions, such as sea water, room temperature, soil and incineration (500–1050 °C) [24]. They achieved 100% retrieval of DNA along with gender determination, even under extreme environmental conditions (1050 °C), which was not reported elsewhere in the literature and gives the study particular strength. Their reported limitation lies in the high number of PCR cycles needed and in the fact that it was time-consuming in cases of salt-water exposure and incineration [24].

Both Pilli et al.'s and Gonzalez et al.'s studies compared the quality of DNA extracted from teeth to that extracted from petrous bone and their results were similar, in that both studies found that the petrous bone was the best skeletal element with regard to skeletal conservation [30,103]. Pilli et al.'s research was conducted on ancient skeletal remains from the 6th to 7th century CE and found that it was also possible to obtain a complete STR profile when analyzing ancient bones [30]. Gonzalez et al. also performed a histological analysis as well to compare the microscopic structure of a petrous bone to that of a tooth and the microscopic structure of fresh petrous bone to that of an archaeological or forensic sample, trying to understand why the petrous bone is an advantageous substrate in ancient DNA studies. They found a "peculiar microstructural characteristic, unique to the petrous bone, that might explain the good preservation of DNA in that substrate" [103].

Kulstein et al. based their research on comparing the petrous bone to other parts of cranial bones in trying to retrieve DNA. They showed that STR typing from the petrous bones led to reportable profiles in all individuals. They also compared the efficacy of two techniques—namely, CE typing and MPS analysis—and showed that "MPS has the potential to analyze degraded human remains and is even capable to provide additional information about phenotype and ancestry of unknown individuals" [102].

The study by Froment et al. emphasized the high potential of MS-based proteomics as an alternative for sex estimation of ancient remains when DNA is not exploitable [104].

The studies by Ziganshin et al. [105] and Gowland et al. [106] investigated the role of enamel peptides in the sex determination of human remains, with promising results.

5. Conclusions

Except for biochemical analysis, there is no single morphometric or morphological method reporting 100% accurate results regarding sex estimation. However, the multitude of methods tested and the continuous development of new techniques, especially computer-aided technologies and high-quality radiological images, and advances in the dental and forensic research fields have improved gender determination methods over the last years and will probably continue to do so in the future. The high volume of articles and the high number of researchers, with various backgrounds, concerned about this topic show the importance of this subject for scientists, dentists, forensic investigators and anthropologists alike.

Author Contributions: Conceptualization, L.M.B.; methodology, L.M.B. and L.-C.R.; software, C.V.T.; writing—original draft preparation, L.M.B., L.-C.R., C.V.T. and L.C.A.; writing—review and editing, L.C.A. and L.-C.R.; supervision, L.C.A.; project administration, L.-C.R. All authors have read and agreed to the published version of the manuscript.

Funding: This research received no external funding.

Institutional Review Board Statement: Not applicable.

Informed Consent Statement: Not applicable.

Data Availability Statement: Not applicable.

Conflicts of Interest: The authors declare no conflict of interest.

References

1. Krishan, K.; Chatterjee, P.M.; Kanchan, T.; Kaur, S.; Baryah, N.; Singh, R.K. A review of sex estimation techniques during examination of skeletal remains in forensic anthropology casework. *Forensic Sci. Int.* **2016**, *261*, e1–e165. [CrossRef] [PubMed]
2. Bedalov, A.; Bašić, Ž.; Marelja, I.; Dolić, K.; Bukarica, K.; Missoni, S.; Šlaus, M.; Primorac, D.; Andjelinović, Š.; Kružić, I. Sex estimation of the sternum by automatic image processing of multi-slice computed tomography images in a Croatian population sample: A retrospective study. *Croat. Med. J.* **2019**, *60*, 237–245. [CrossRef]
3. Bubalo, P.; Baković, M.; Tkalčić, M.; Petrovečki, V.; Mayer, D. Acetabular osteometrie standards for sex estimation in contemporary Croatian population. *Croat. Med. J.* **2019**, *60*, 221–226. [CrossRef]
4. Bašić, Ž.; Kružić, I.; Jerković, I.; Andelinovic, D.; Andelinovic, Š. Sex estimation standards for medieval and contemporary Croats. *Croat. Med. J.* **2017**, *58*, 222–230. [CrossRef] [PubMed]
5. Gupta, M.; Mishra, P.; Shrivastava, K.; Singh, N. An Overview of age, sex and race determination from teeth and skull. *Adv. Hum. Biol.* **2015**, *5*, 20–31.
6. Buonasera, T.; Eerkens, J.; de Flamingh, A.; Engbring, L.; Yip, J.; Li, H.; Haas, R.; DiGiuseppe, D.; Grant, D.; Salemi, M.; et al. A comparison of proteomic, genomic, and osteological methods of archaeological sex estimation. *Sci. Rep.* **2020**, *10*, 11897. [CrossRef] [PubMed]
7. Loreille, O.; Ratnayake, S.; Bazinet, A.L.; Stockwell, T.B.; Sommer, D.D.; Rohland, N.; Mallick, S.; Johnson, P.L.F.; Skoglund, P.; Onorato, A.J.; et al. Biological sexing of a 4000-year-old egyptian mummy head to assess the potential of nuclear DNA recovery from the most damaged and limited forensic specimens. *Genes* **2018**, *9*, 135. [CrossRef]
8. Arigbabu, O.A.; Liao, I.Y.; Abdullah, N.; Mohamad Noor, M.H. Computer vision methods for cranial sex estimation. *IPSJ Trans. Comput. Vis. Appl.* **2017**, *9*, 19. [CrossRef]
9. Gao, H.; Geng, G.; Yang, W. Sex Determination of 3D skull based on a novel unsupervised learning method. *Comput. Math. Methods Med.* **2018**, *2018*, 4567267. [CrossRef]
10. Chovalopoulou, M.E.; Valakos, E.D.; Manolis, S.K. Sex determination by three-dimensional geometric morphometrics of craniofacial form. *Anthropol. Anzeiger.* **2016**, *73*, 195–206. [CrossRef]
11. Agbolade, O.; Nazri, A.; Yaakob, R.; Ghani, A.A.; Cheah, Y.K. Morphometric approach to 3D soft-tissue craniofacial analysis and classification of ethnicity, sex, and age. *PLoS ONE* **2020**, *15*, e0228402. [CrossRef] [PubMed]
12. Cole, C.; Eliopoulos, C.; Zorba, E.; Borrini, M. An anthropometric method for sex determination from the mandible: Test on British medieval skeletal collections. *J. Biol. Res.* **2017**, *90*, 30–35. [CrossRef]
13. Tise, M.L.; Spradley, M.K.; Anderson, B.E. Postcranial sex estimation of individuals considered Hispanic. *J. Forensic Sci.* **2013**, *58*, S9–S14. [CrossRef] [PubMed]
14. Yang, W.; Zhou, M.; Zhang, P.; Geng, G.; Liu, X.; Zhang, H. skull sex estimation based on wavelet transform and Fourier transform. *Biomed. Res. Int.* **2020**, *2020*, 8608209. [CrossRef] [PubMed]
15. Nourbakhsh, R.; Razi, S.; Razi, T. Evaluation of relation of dimensional measurement of different anatomic skull structures to determine sexual dimorphism in cone beam CT images of an Iranian population. *J. Res. Med. Dent. Sci.* **2018**, *6*, 33–38. [CrossRef]
16. Sarač-Hadžihalilović, A.; Hojkurić, E.; Musić, M.; Hasanbegović, I.; Ajanović, Z.; Dervišević, L.; Brkić, S. Model "P" in gender prediction based on the mastoid process. *Med. Glas.* **2020**, *17*, 279–6284. [CrossRef]
17. Behl, A.; Grewal, S.; Bajaj, K.; Baweja, P.; Kaur, G.; Kataria, P. Mandibular ramus and gonial angle—Identification tool in age estimation and sex determination: A digital panoramic radiographic study in north indian population. *J. Indian Acad. Oral. Med. Radiol.* **2020**, *32*, 31–36. [CrossRef]
18. Kartheeki, B.; Nayyar, A.S.; Sindhu, Y.U.; Lakshmana, N. Accuracy of mandibular rami measurements in prediction of sex. *Arch. Med. Health Sci.* **2017**, *5*, 50–54. [CrossRef]
19. Sella Tunis, T.; Hershkovitz, I.; May, H.; Vardimon, A.D.; Sarig, R.; Shpack, N. Variation in chin and mandibular symphysis size and shape in males and females: A CT-Based study. *Int. J. Environ. Res. Public Health* **2020**, *17*, 4249. [CrossRef]
20. Veeraraghavan, G.; Lingappa, A.; Shankara, S.P.; Mamatha, G.P.; Sebastian, B.T.; Mujib, A. Determination of sex from tooth pulp tissue. *Libyan J. Med.* **2010**, *5*, 5084. [CrossRef]
21. Zagga, A.; Ahmed, H.; Ismail, S.; Tadros, A. Molecular sex identification of dry human teeth specimens from Sokoto, Northwestern Nigeria. *J. Forensic Dent. Sci.* **2014**, *6*, 132–138. [CrossRef] [PubMed]
22. Capitaneanu, C.; Willems, G.; Thevissen, P. A systematic review of odontological sex estimation methods. *J. Forensic Odontostomatol.* **2017**, *35*, 1–19.
23. Chowdhury, R.; Singhvi, A.; Bagul, N.; Bhatia, S.; Singh, G.; Goswami, S. Sex determination by amplification of amelogenin gene from dental pulp tissue by polymerase chain reaction. *Indian J. Dent. Res.* **2018**, *29*, 470–476. [CrossRef] [PubMed]
24. Dutta, P.; Bhosale, S.; Singh, R.; Gubrellay, P.; Patil, J.; Sehdev, B.; Bhagat, S.; Bansal, T. Amelogenin gene—The pioneer in gender determination from forensic dental samples. *J. Clin. Diagn. Res.* **2017**, *11*, ZC56–ZC59. [CrossRef] [PubMed]
25. Dash, H.R.; Rawat, N.; Das, S. Alternatives to amelogenin markers for sex determination in humans and their forensic relevance. *Mol. Biol. Rep.* **2020**, *47*, 2347–2360. [CrossRef]
26. Higuchi, R.; Bowman, B.; Freiberger, M.; Ryder, O.A.; Wilson, A.C. DNA sequences from the quagga, an extinct member of the horse family. *Nature* **1984**, *312*, 282–284. [CrossRef]
27. Pääbo, S. Molecular cloning of ancient Egyptian mummy DNA. *Nature* **1985**, *314*, 644–645. [CrossRef]

28. Krings, M.; Stone, A.; Schmitz, R.W.; Krainitzki, H.; Stoneking, M.; Pääbo, S. Neandertal DNA sequences and the origin of modern humans. *Cell* **1997**, *90*, 19–30. [CrossRef]
29. Nesheva, D.V. Aspects of ancient mitochondrial dna analysis in different populations for understanding human evolution. *Balk. J. Med. Genet.* **2014**, *17*, 5–14. [CrossRef]
30. Pilli, E.; Vai, S.; Caruso, M.G.; D'Errico, G.; Berti, A.; Caramelli, D. Neither femur nor tooth: Petrous bone for identifying archaeological bone samples via forensic approach. *Forensic Sci. Int.* **2018**, *283*, 144–149. [CrossRef]
31. Page, M.J.; McKenzie, J.E.; Bossuyt, P.M.; Boutron, I.; Hoffmann, T.C.; Mulrow, C.D.; Shamseer, L.; Tetzlaff, J.M.; Aki, E.A.; Brennan, S.E.; et al. The PRISMA 2020 statement: An updated guideline for reporting systematic reviews. *BMJ* **2021**, *372*, n71. [CrossRef] [PubMed]
32. Tabasum, Q.; Sehrawat, J.S.; Talwar, M.K.; Pathak, R.K. Odontometric sex estimation from clinically extracted molar teeth in a North Indian population sample. *J. Forensic Dent. Sci.* **2017**, *9*, 176. [CrossRef] [PubMed]
33. Grewal, D.S.; Khangura, R.K.; Sircar, K.; Tyagi, K.K.; Kaur, G.; David, S. Morphometric analysis of odontometric parameters for gender determination. *J. Clin. Diagn. Res.* **2017**, *11*, ZC09–ZC13. [CrossRef] [PubMed]
34. Girish, H.C.; Murgod, S.; Savita, J.K. Gender determination by odontometric method. *J. Forensic Dent. Sci.* **2017**, *9*, 44. [CrossRef]
35. Priyadharshini, K.; Ambika, M.; Sekar, B.; Mohanbabu, V.; Sabarinath, B.; Pavithra, I. Comparison of cheiloscopy, odontometric, and facial index for sex determination in forensic dentistry. *J. Forensic Dent. Sci.* **2018**, *10*, 88–91. [CrossRef]
36. Pereira, T.; Shetty, S.; Surve, R.; Gotmare, S.; Kamath, P.; Kumar, S. Palatoscopy and odontometrics for sex identification and hereditary pattern analysis in a Navi Mumbai population: A cross-sectional study. *J. Oral. Maxillofac. Pathol.* **2018**, *22*, 271–278. [CrossRef]
37. Dash, K.; Panda, A.; Behura, S.; Ramachandra, S.; Bhuyan, L.; Bandopadhyay, A. Employing dimensional disparity of teeth to establish the gender in Odisha population: A dimorphic study. *J. Int. Soc. Prev. Community Dent.* **2018**, *8*, 174–178. [CrossRef]
38. Phulari, R.S.; Rathore, R.; Talegaon, T.; Jariwala, P. Comparative assessment of maxillary canine index and maxillary first molar dimensions for sex determination in forensic odontology. *J. Forensic Dent. Sci.* **2017**, *9*, 110. [CrossRef]
39. Singh, A.; Bhatia, H.P.; Sood, S.; Sharma, N. Demystifying the mysteries: Sexual dimorphism in primary teeth. *J. Clin. Diagn. Res.* **2017**, *11*, ZC110–ZC114. [CrossRef]
40. Satish, B.N.V.S.; Moolrajani, C.; Basnaker, M.; Kumar, P. Dental sex dimorphism: Using odontometrics and digital jaw radiography. *J. Forensic Dent. Sci.* **2017**, *9*, 43. [CrossRef]
41. Chennoju, S.K.; Ramaswamy, P.; Swathi, E.; Smitha, B.; Sankaran, S. Discriminant canine index—A novel approach in sex determination. *Ann. Stomatol.* **2015**, *6*, 43–46. [CrossRef]
42. Alam, M.K.; Alzarea, B.K.; Ganji, K.K.; Kundi, I.; Patil, S. 3D CBCT human adult odontometrics: Comparative assessment in Saudi, Jordan and Egypt population. *Saudi Dent. J.* **2019**, *31*, 336–342. [CrossRef] [PubMed]
43. Shireen, A.; Ara, S. Odontometric analysis of permanent maxillary first molar in gender determination. *J. Forensic Dent. Sci.* **2016**, *8*, 145–149. [CrossRef]
44. Govindaram, D.; Bharanidharan, R.; Ramya, R.; Rameshkumar, A.; Priyadharsini, N.; Rajkumar, K. Root Length: As a determinant tool of sexual dimorphism in an ethnic Tamil population. *J. Forensic Dent. Sci.* **2018**, *10*, 96–100. [CrossRef] [PubMed]
45. Rajarathnam, B.; David, M.; Indira, A. Mandibular canine dimensions as an aid in gender estimation. *J. Forensic Dent. Sci.* **2016**, *8*, 83–89. [CrossRef]
46. Yadav, A.B.; Angadi, P.V.; Yadav, S.K. Sex assessment efficacy of permanent maxillary first molar cusp dimensions in Indians. *Contemp. Clin. Dent.* **2015**, *6*, 489–495. [CrossRef]
47. Gupta, J.; Daniel, M.J. Crown size and arch width dimension as an indicator in gender determination for a Puducherry population. *J. Forensic Dent. Sci.* **2016**, *8*, 120–125. [CrossRef]
48. Patel, R.A.; Chaudhary, A.R.; Dudhia, B.B.; Macwan, Z.S.; Patel, P.S.; Jani, Y.V. Mandibular canine index: A study for gender determination in Gandhinagar population. *J. Forensic Dent. Sci.* **2017**, *9*, 135–143. [CrossRef]
49. Agrawal, A.; Manjunatha, B.; Dholia, B.; Althomali, Y. Comparison of sexual dimorphism of permanent mandibular canine with mandibular first molar by odontometrics. *J. Forensic Dent. Sci.* **2015**, *7*, 238–243. [CrossRef]
50. Krishnan, R.P.; Thangavelu, R.; Rathnavelu, V.; Narasimhan, M. Gender determination: Role of lip prints, finger prints and mandibular canine index. *Exp. Ther. Med.* **2016**, *11*, 2329–2332. [CrossRef]
51. Couto, D.M.S.E.; Gallassi, N.C.D.; Gomes, S.L.; Ulbricht, V.; Pereira Neto, J.S.; Daruge, E., Jr.; Francesquini, L., Jr. Brazilian's dental anthropometry: Human identification. *J. Forensic Dent. Sci.* **2019**, *11*, 73–77. [CrossRef] [PubMed]
52. Gouveia, M.F.; Oliveira Santos, I.; Santos, A.L.; Gonçalves, D. Sample-specific odontometric sex estimation: A method with potential application to burned remains. *Sci. Justice* **2017**, *57*, 262–269. [CrossRef] [PubMed]
53. Silva, A.M.; Pereira, M.L.; Gouveia, S.; Tavares, J.N.; Azevedo, Á.; Caldas, I.M. A new approach to sex estimation using the mandibular canine index. *Med. Sci. Law.* **2016**, *56*, 7–12. [CrossRef] [PubMed]
54. Daniele, G.; Matilde, S.S.A.; María, M.; Rafael, R.V.; Milagros, A.M. Sex estimation by tooth dimension in a contemporary Spanish population. *Forensic Sci. Int.* **2020**, *317*, 110549. [CrossRef] [PubMed]
55. Atreya, A.; Shrestha, A.; Tuladhar, L.R.; Nepal, S.; Shrestha, R.; Sah, S.K. Sex Predictability by using mandibular canine index. *J. Nepal Health Res. Counc.* **2020**, *17*, 501–505. [CrossRef]
56. Gamulin, O.; Škrabić, M.; Serec, K.; Par, M.; Baković, M.; Krajačić, M.; Babić, S.D.; Šegedin, N.; Osmani, A.; Vodanović, M. Possibility of human gender recognition using Raman spectra of teeth. *Molecules* **2021**, *26*, 3983. [CrossRef]

57. Rakhshan, V.; Ghorbanyjavadpour, F.; Ashoori, N. Buccolingual and mesiodistal dimensions of the permanent teeth, their diagnostic value for sex identification, and Bolton indices. *Biomed. Res. Int.* **2022**, *2022*, 8381436. [CrossRef]
58. Missier, M.; Samuel, S.; George, A. Facial indices in lateral cephalogram for sex prediction in Chennai population—A semi-novel study. *J. Forensic Dent. Sci.* **2018**, *10*, 151–157. [CrossRef]
59. Perez, I.; Chavez, A.; Ponce, D. Applicability of the Ricketts' posteroanterior cephalometry for sex determination using logistic regression analysis in Hispano American Peruvians. *J. Forensic Dent. Sci.* **2016**, *8*, 111. [CrossRef]
60. Albalawi, A.; Alam, M.; Vundavalli, S.; Ganji, K.; Patil, S. Mandible: An indicator for sex determination—A three-dimensional cone-beam computed tomography study. *Contemp. Clin. Dent.* **2019**, *10*, 69–73. [CrossRef]
61. Vinutha, S.P.; Suresh, V.; Shubha, R. Discriminant function analysis of Foramen Magnum variables in South Indian population: A study of computerised tomographic images. *Anat. Res. Int.* **2018**, *2018*, 2056291. [CrossRef] [PubMed]
62. Nuzzolese, E.; Randolph-Quinney, P.; Randolph-Quinney, J.; Di Vella, G. Geometric morphometric analysis of sexual dimorphism in the mandible from panoramic x-ray images. *J. Forensic Odontostomatol.* **2019**, *37*, 35–44. [PubMed]
63. More, C.B.; Vijayvargiya, R.; Saha, N. Morphometric analysis of mandibular ramus for sex determination on digital orthopantomogram. *J. Forensic Dent. Sci.* **2017**, *9*, 1–5. [CrossRef]
64. Raikar, N.; Meundi, M.; David, C.; Rao, M.; Jogigowda, S. Sexual dimorphism in Foramen Magnum dimensions in the South Indian population: A digital submentovertex radiographic study. *J. Forensic Dent. Sci.* **2016**, *8*, 180. [CrossRef] [PubMed]
65. Rajkumari, S.; Nikitha, K.; Monisha, S.; Nishagrade, S.; Thayumanavan, B.; Murali, B. Role of orthopantamograph in forensic identification: A retrospective study among Chennai Population. *J. Pharm. Bioallied. Sci.* **2019**, *11*, S393–S396. [CrossRef]
66. Poongodi, V.; Kanmani, R.; Anandi, M.S.; Krithika, C.L.; Kannan, A.; Raghuram, P.H. Prediction of age and gender using digital radiographic method: A retrospective study. *J. Pharm. Bioallied. Sci.* **2015**, *7*, S504–S508. [CrossRef]
67. de Queiroz, C.L.; Terada, A.S.S.D.; Dezem, T.U.; Gomes de Araújo, L.; Galo, R.; Oliveira-Santos, C.; Alves da Silva, R.H. Sex determination of adult human maxillary sinuses on panoramic radiographs. *Acta Stomatol. Croat.* **2016**, *50*, 215–221. [CrossRef]
68. Rani, S.U.; Rao, G.V.; Kumar, D.R.; Sravya, T.; Sivaranjani, Y.; Kumar, M.P. Age and gender assessment through three-dimensional morphometric analysis of maxillary sinus using magnetic resonance imaging. *J. Forensic Dent. Sci.* **2017**, *9*, 46. [CrossRef]
69. Ibrahim, A.; Alias, A.; Nor, F.M.; Swarhib, M.; Abu Bakar, S.N.; Das, S.; Abdullah, N.; Noor, M.H.M. Study of sexual dimorphism of Malaysian crania: An important step in identification of the skeletal remains. *Anat. Cell Biol.* **2017**, *50*, 86–92. [CrossRef]
70. Kanjani, V.; Rani, A.; Kanjani, D. Morphometric analysis of the orbital aperture in North Indian Population: A retrospective digital forensic study. *Int. J. Appl. Basic Med. Res.* **2019**, *9*, 85–88. [CrossRef]
71. Bangi, B.B.; Ginjupally, U.; Nadendla, L.K.; Vadla, B. 3D evaluation of maxillary sinus using computed tomography: A sexual dimorphic study. *Int. J. Dent.* **2017**, *2017*, 9017078. [CrossRef] [PubMed]
72. Soman, B.; Sujatha, G.; Lingappa, A. Morphometric evaluation of the frontal sinus in relation to age and gender in subjects residing in Davangere, Karnataka. *J. Forensic Dent. Sci.* **2016**, *8*, 57. [CrossRef] [PubMed]
73. Bulut, O.; Freudenstein, N.; Hekimoglu, B.; Gurcan, S. Dilemma of gonial angle in sex determination: Sexually dimorphic or not? *Am. J. Forensic Med. Pathol.* **2019**, *40*, 361–365. [CrossRef] [PubMed]
74. Gamba, T.D.O.; Alves, M.C.; Haiter-Neto, F. Mandibular sexual dimorphism analysis in CBCT scans. *J. Forensic Leg. Med.* **2016**, *38*, 106–110. [CrossRef]
75. Chandra, S.; Chaturvedi, N.; Sah, K.; Sinha, S.; Hamza, A. Craniometric measurement by jug handle view: An aid for gender determination. *J. Indian Acad. Oral. Med. Radiol.* **2018**, *30*, 398–401. [CrossRef]
76. Chaurasia, A.; Patil, R.; Katheriya, G. Radiomorphometeric evaluation of clivus in indian paediatric population visiting a tertiary dental hospital-a cone beam computed tomography study. *J. Clin. Diagn. Res.* **2018**, *12*, ZC05–ZC08. [CrossRef]
77. Prabhat, M.; Rai, S.; Kaur, M.; Prabhat, K.; Bhatnagar, P.; Panjwani, S. Computed tomography based forensic gender determination by measuring the size and volume of the maxillary sinuses. *J. Forensic Dent. Sci.* **2016**, *8*, 40–46. [CrossRef]
78. Belaldavar, C.; Acharya, A.B.; Angadi, P. Sex estimation in Indians by digital analysis of the gonial angle on lateral cephalographs. *J. Forensic Odontostomatol.* **2019**, *37*, 45–50.
79. Shireen, A.; Goel, S.; Ahmed, I.; Sabeh, A.; Mahmoud, W. Radiomorphometric evaluation of the frontal sinus in relation to age and gender in Saudi population. *J. Int. Soc. Prev. Community Dent.* **2019**, *9*, 584–596. [CrossRef]
80. Sambhana, S.; Sanghvi, P.; Mohammed, R.; Shanta, P.; Thetay, A.R.; Chaudhary, V. Assessment of sexual dimorphism using digital orthopantomographs in South Indians. *J. Forensic Dent. Sci.* **2016**, *8*, 180. [CrossRef]
81. Damera, A.; Mohanalakhsmi, J.; Yellarthi, P.; Rezwana, B. Radiographic evaluation of mandibular ramus for gender estimation: Retrospective study. *J. Forensic Dent. Sci.* **2016**, *8*, 74. [CrossRef] [PubMed]
82. Esmaeilyfard, R.; Paknahad, M.; Dokohaki, S. Sex classification of first molar teeth in cone beam computed tomography images using data mining. *Forensic Sci. Int.* **2021**, *318*, 110633. [CrossRef] [PubMed]
83. Paknahad, M.; Dokohaki, S.; Khojastepour, L.; Shahidi, S.; Haghnegahdar, A. A Radio-Odontometric analysis of sexual dimorphism in first molars using cone-beam computed tomography. *Am. J. Forensic Med. Pathol.* **2022**, *43*, 46–51. [CrossRef] [PubMed]
84. Johnson, A.; Singh, S.; Thomas, A.; Chauhan, N. Geometric morphometric analysis for sex determination using lateral cephalograms in Indian population: A preliminary study. *J. Oral Maxillofac. Pathol.* **2021**, *25*, 364. [CrossRef]

85. Suzuki, K.; Nakano, H.; Inoue, K.; Nakajima, Y.; Mizobuchi, S.; Omori, M.; Kato-Kogoe, N.; Mishima, K.; Ueno, T. Examination of new parameters for sex determination of mandible using Japanese computer tomography data. *Dentomaxillofac. Radiol.* **2020**, *49*, 20190282. [CrossRef]
86. Sinthubua, A.; Ruengdit, S.; Das, S.; Mahakkanukrauh, P. A new method for sex estimation from maxillary suture length in a Thai population. *Anat. Cell Biol.* **2017**, *50*, 261–264. [CrossRef]
87. De Boer, H.H.; Van der Merwe, A.E.; Soerdjbalie-Maikoe, V.V. Human cranial vault thickness in a contemporary sample of 1097 autopsy cases: Relation to body weight, stature, age, sex and ancestry. *Int. J. Legal Med.* **2016**, *130*, 1371–1377. [CrossRef]
88. Mahakkanukrauh, P.; Sinthubua, A.; Prasitwattanaseree, S.; Ruengdit, S.; Singsuwan, P.; Praneatpolgrang, S.; Duangto, P. Craniometric study for sex determination in a Thai population. *Anat. Cell Biol.* **2015**, *48*, 275–283. [CrossRef]
89. Mankapure, P.K.; Barpande, S.R.; Bhavthankar, J.D. Evaluation of sexual dimorphism in arch depth and palatal depth in 500 young adults of Marathwada region, India. *J. Forensic Dent. Sci.* **2017**, *9*, 153–156. [CrossRef]
90. Singh, A.; Sreedhar, G.; George, J.; Shukla, V.; Vashishta, V.; Negi, M.P.S. Anthropometric study using craniofacial features to determine gender in Lucknow population. *J. Forensic Dent. Sci.* **2017**, *9*, 120–124. [CrossRef]
91. Kamath, V.G.; Asif, M.; Shetty, R.; Avadhani, R. Binary logistic regression analysis of Foramen Magnum dimensions for sex determination. *Anat. Res. Int.* **2015**, *2015*, 459428. [CrossRef] [PubMed]
92. Mustafa, A.G.; Tashtoush, A.A.; Alshboul, O.A.; Allouh, M.Z.; Altarifi, A.A. Morphometric study of the hard palate and its relevance to dental and forensic sciences. *Int. J. Dent.* **2019**, *2019*, 1687345. [CrossRef] [PubMed]
93. Bertsatos, A.; Papageorgopoulou, C.; Valakos, E.; Chovalopoulou, M.E. Investigating the sex-related geometric variation of the human cranium. *Int. J. Legal Med.* **2018**, *132*, 1505–1514. [CrossRef]
94. Chovalopoulou, M.E.; Valakos, E.D.; Manolis, S.K. Sex determination by three-dimensional geometric morphometrics of the vault and midsagittal curve of the neurocranium in a modern Greek population sample. *HOMO—J. Comp. Hum. Biol.* **2016**, *67*, 173–187. [CrossRef] [PubMed]
95. Small, C.; Schepartz, L.; Hemingway, J.; Brits, D. Three-dimensionally derived interlandmark distances for sex estimation in intact and fragmentary crania. *Forensic Sci. Int.* **2018**, *287*, 127–135. [CrossRef]
96. Bhayya, H.; Avinash Tejasvi, M.; Jayalakshmi, B.; Reddy, M.M. Craniometric assessment of gender using mastoid process. *J. Indian Acad. Oral Med. Radiol.* **2018**, *30*, 52–57. [CrossRef]
97. Musilová, B.; Dupej, J.; Brůžek, Š.; Velemínská, J. Sex and ancestry related differences between two Central European populations determined using exocranial meshes. *Forensic Sci. Int.* **2019**, *297*, 364–369. [CrossRef]
98. Uabundit, N.; Chaiyamoon, A.; Iamsaard, S.; Yurasakpong, L.; Nantasenamat, C.; Suwannakhan, A.; Phunchago, N. Classification and morphometric features of pterion in Thai population with potential sex prediction. *Medicina* **2021**, *57*, 1282. [CrossRef]
99. Bertsatos, A.; Chovalopoulou, M.E.; Brůžek, J.; Bejdová, Š. Advanced procedures for skull sex estimation using sexually dimorphic morphometric features. *Int. J. Legal Med.* **2020**, *134*, 1927–1937. [CrossRef]
100. Inskip, S.; Scheib, C.L.; Wohns, A.W.; Ge, X.; Kivisild, T.; Robb, J. Evaluating macroscopic sex estimation methods using genetically sexed archaeological material: The medieval skeletal collection from St John's Divinity School, Cambridge. *Am. J. Phys. Anthropol.* **2019**, *168*, 340–351. [CrossRef]
101. Srivastava, M.; Tripathi, S.; Astekar, M.; Singal, D.; Srivastava, A.; Vashisth, P. Sex determination from mesiodens of Indian children by amelogenin gene. *J. Forensic Dent. Sci.* **2017**, *9*, 125–129. [CrossRef] [PubMed]
102. Kulstein, G.; Hadrys, T.; Wiegand, P. As solid as a rock—Comparison of CE- and MPS-based analyses of the petrosal bone as a source of DNA for forensic identification of challenging cranial bones. *Int. J. Legal Med.* **2018**, *132*, 13–24. [CrossRef] [PubMed]
103. Gonzalez, A.; Cannet, C.; Zvénigorosky, V.; Geraut, A.; Koch, G.; Delabarde, T.; Ludes, B.; Raul, J.S.; Keyser, C. The petrous bone: Ideal substrate in legal medicine? *Forensic Sci. Int. Genet.* **2020**, *47*, 102305. [CrossRef] [PubMed]
104. Froment, C.; Hourset, M.; Sáenz-Oyhéréguy, N.; Mouton-Barbosa, E.; Willmann, C.; Zanolli, C.; Esclassan, R.; Donat, R.; Thèves, C.; Burlet-Schiltz, O.; et al. Analysis of 5000 year-old human teeth using optimized large-scale and targeted proteomics approaches for detection of sex-specific peptides. *J. Proteom.* **2020**, *211*, 103548. [CrossRef] [PubMed]
105. Ziganshin, R.H.; Berezina, N.Y.; Alexandrov, P.L.; Ryabinin, V.V.; Buzhilova, A.P. Optimization of method for human sex determination by peptidome analysis of teeth enamel from teeth of different biological generation, archeological age, and degrees of taphonomic preservation. *Biochemistry* **2020**, *85*, 614–622. [CrossRef]
106. Gowland, R.; Stewart, N.A.; Crowder, K.D.; Hodson, C.; Shaw, H.; Gron, K.J.; Montgomery, J. Sex estimation of teeth at different developmental stages using dimorphic enamel peptide analysis. *Am. J. Phys. Anthropol.* **2021**, *174*, 859–869. [CrossRef]
107. Noble, J.; Cardini, A.; Flavel, A.; Franklin, D. Geometric morphometrics on juvenile crania: Exploring age and sex variation in an Australian population. *Forensic Sci. Int.* **2019**, *294*, 57–68. [CrossRef]

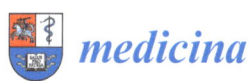

Article

A Comparative Analysis of Dental Measurements in Physical and Digital Orthodontic Case Study Models

Elena-Raluca Baciu [1], Dana Gabriela Budală [1,*], Roxana-Ionela Vasluianu [1,*], Costin Iulian Lupu [1], Alice Murariu [2], Gabriela Luminița Gelețu [2], Irina Nicoleta Zetu [2], Diana Diaconu-Popa [1], Monica Tatarciuc [1], Giorgio Nichitean [3] and Ionuț Luchian [4]

[1] Department of Implantology, Removable Dentures, Dental Technology, Faculty of Dental Medicine, University of Medicine and Pharmacy "Grigore T. Popa", 700115 Iasi, Romania
[2] Department of Surgery, Faculty of Dental Medicine, University of Medicine and Pharmacy "Grigore T. Popa", 700115 Iasi, Romania
[3] Faculty of Dental Medicine, University of Medicine and Pharmacy "Grigore T. Popa", 700115 Iasi, Romania
[4] Department of Periodontology, Faculty of Dental Medicine, University of Medicine and Pharmacy "Grigore T. Popa", 700115 Iasi, Romania
* Correspondence: dana-gabriela.bosinceanu@umfiasi.ro (D.G.B.); roxana.vasluianu@umfiasi.ro (R.-I.V.)

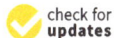

Citation: Baciu, E.-R.; Budală, D.G.; Vasluianu, R.-I.; Lupu, C.I.; Murariu, A.; Gelețu, G.L.; Zetu, I.N.; Diaconu-Popa, D.; Tatarciuc, M.; Nichitean, G.; et al. A Comparative Analysis of Dental Measurements in Physical and Digital Orthodontic Case Study Models. *Medicina* 2022, 58, 1230. https://doi.org/10.3390/medicina58091230

Academic Editors: Giuseppe Minervini and Stefania Moccia

Received: 9 August 2022
Accepted: 2 September 2022
Published: 6 September 2022

Publisher's Note: MDPI stays neutral with regard to jurisdictional claims in published maps and institutional affiliations.

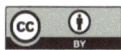

Copyright: © 2022 by the authors. Licensee MDPI, Basel, Switzerland. This article is an open access article distributed under the terms and conditions of the Creative Commons Attribution (CC BY) license (https://creativecommons.org/licenses/by/4.0/).

Abstract: *Background and Objectives:* Study models are essential tools used in the dental teaching process. The aim of the present study was to compare the values obtained by manual and digital orthodontic measurements on physical and digital case study models. *Materials and Methods:* The physical experimental models were obtained by traditional pouring (improved stone-type IV gypsum products) and by additive manufacturing (resins). The digital experimental models were created by scanning the physical ones, using a white light-emitting diode (LED) source and an L-shaped dental scanner—Swing DOF (DOF, Seoul, Korea). The physical study models were first measured using a digital caliper, and then, they were scanned and evaluated using the DentalCad 3.0 Galway software (exocad GmbH, Darmstadt, Germany). The Pont, Linder–Harth, and Bolton indices, which are used in orthodontics for training students, were derived using the available data. *Results:* When comparing the linear measurement mean ranks taken on physical study models to those of digital models, no statistically significant differences ($p > 0.05$) were found. A similar result was also shown when the dentoalveolar growth indicators were analyzed. *Conclusions:* It can be concluded that dental study models made by direct light processing (DLP) and pouring type IV class gypsum are both acceptable for orthodontic teaching purposes.

Keywords: dental study model; additive manufacturing; direct light processing; arch measurements

1. Introduction

Dental models are an indispensable diagnostic and legal tool for all dental disciplines regarding the processes for training future dentists. They may also be used as a documentary tool, working well as a duplicate model. Furthermore, plaster models are valued by the academic community for their use in evaluating patient progress and documenting research [1,2].

Traditionally, dental models are made in the laboratory using gypsum products with different levels of hardness, depending on the model's purpose. These are obtained from dental arch impressions—which are recorded using elastic materials or intraoral scanners—producing positive images of a patient's teeth and the surrounding tissue, which must be reproduced as accurately as possible. Intraoral scanners are becoming more and more common, but little is known about their accuracy for full-arch scans, despite their increasing use in daily life [3,4]. The accuracy of a scan is affected by intraoral conditions, such as the optical digitalization unit's restricted area, possible fogging of the digitalization unit, the patient's and dentist's movements, intraoral light, the presence of humidity (saliva or blood), the soft tissue, or the optical scanning equipment used (scanning wands) [5].

Traditional stone dental models have notable advantages, including their affordability, simplicity of use, accuracy in details impression reproduction, compatibility with impression materials, dimensional stability, and great mechanical properties. The disadvantages of using them include the need for additional storage space and the risk of fracture and deterioration [6].

In contrast, digital models have a number of advantages, such as low cost, less time consumed, the ability to share online images with other practitioners and patients, the fact that they are durable and not prone to degradation, lower laboratory and chairside expenses, computerized storage, enhanced patient instruction, and better professional productivity and efficiency [7–9]. In cases of periodontal patients, digital dental models are recommended, as they reduce the trauma caused by the impression procedure [10].

Despite these benefits, digital models are not yet routinely used in daily practice because of some disadvantages in their application, including data loss in cases of degradation in electronic storage, dependence on third parties, time-consuming software support, the need to learn the operating system, and high equipment costs.

The additive rapid prototyping/three-dimensional (3D) printing methods most often used in dentistry are stereolithography (SLA), digital light processing (DLP), selective laser sintering (SLS), selective laser melting (SLM), electron beam processing (EBM), PolyJet photopolymer printing, and fused deposition modeling (FDM) [11–13].

Both DLP and SLA printing techniques employ similar printing principles (layer-by-layer solidification of a light-polymerizable liquid polymer under laser illumination) but require different devices [14]. To build extremely accurate models with fine-grained geometries, SLA makes use of a moving ultraviolet (UV) laser beam, whereas DLP makes use of fixed UV light from a projector [15,16]. The polymerization of each multilayer resin deposit occurs far more quickly (in a matter of seconds) than with SLA, making DLP a preferable process for dental laboratories with an industrial character. It also has a lower cost than SLA by saving material (photopolymers and ceramic-filled resins) [17]. The digital light-processing indications are as follows: dental models, cast coping, resin patterns, wax pattern splints, temporary restorations, surgical guides, aligners, retainers, and castable crowns and bridges [18–21].

The accuracy of printed models may vary greatly due to the materials (aging process), equipment, and procedures used in the technical fabrication processes [22].

The degree of dental arch development may be assessed by looking at the size and space of the teeth in relation to one another [23]. Many variables, both hereditary and environmental, can lead to dental anomalies and occlusal problems [24]. Malocclusions can be induced by volume anomalies, which are one of the contributing factors. Incidence of different dental defects are explored in several studies; however, few focused on malocclusions in relation to the teeth [25].

During the educational orthodontic evaluation of the study models, the Linder–Harth and Pont indices and the Bolton analysis are frequently used. The Linder–Harth approach, which was developed from Pont's index, is useful for estimating the width of the dental arch. These methods employ both measured and calculated values based on formulas [26,27]. When establishing the difference between these values, it is possible to determine whether or not there is a dental arch abnormally present in transversal planes. However, the transverse sizes of dental arches are not governed by the size of the teeth but by the gnathic type of the arch [27].

Bolton's analysis was developed in 1958 and assesses whether there is a volume difference between the maxillary and mandibular permanent teeth. Bolton [28] also discovered a relationship between the total mesiodistal widths of the teeth and suggested that an anterior ratio value of 77.2% and overall ratio value of 91.3% are needed for ideal occlusion. The frontal ratio is the only one that can be determined in cases in which there are edentulous spaces in the lateral area.

A difference of more than 1.5 mm in the size of mandibular and maxillary teeth is clinically important, with involvement in the future treatment plan [29].

The purpose of the present study is to compare the values obtained by traditional and digital orthodontic measurements on physical and digital case study models.

In order to achieve the proposed objective, we formulated two null hypotheses:
- the linear measurement values are not influenced by the method, the material, or the obtainment technique used in the case study models;
- the lack of space is undisturbed by the obtained values using various measurement techniques and dental study models.

2. Materials and Methods

2.1. Patient Selection and Impression Recording

The study protocol (Figure 1) was approved by the Ethics Committee of "Grigore T. Popa" University of Medicine and Pharmacy of Iasi (No. 196/03.06.2022), and the included participants consented to the procedures.

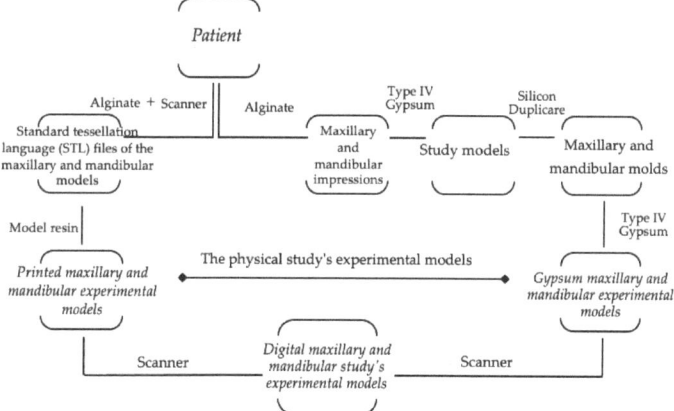

Figure 1. The study protocol's design: from patient to digital case study models.

To perform the experimental models, alginate maxillary and mandibular impressions were taken from patients.

Patients had to meet the following criteria in order to be included in the study: over 18 years of age; cooperative; no general diseases; no previous experience of anaphylactic reactions; completely erupted permanent dentition from the first molar; no interproximal caries or fillings, prosthetic crowns, or bridges; no teeth anomalies, edentation, orthopedic, or orthodontic treatments in their history; and diagnosed with Class I malocclusion.

The impressions were registered at the Faculty of Dentistry, Iasi, Romania. To achieve this stage, medium-sized plastic–steel impression trays (Guangzhou Aurora Health Products Company, Hunan, China), perforated for a better retention of the impression material, together with Orthoprint (Zhermack SpA, Badia Polesine, Italy) alginate material, were used. After the appropriate amount of powder with water was measured out and prepared in accordance with the manufacturer's recommendations, the final impressions were transported to the dental laboratory, in a 100% humidity medium, within 30 min, and then poured [30].

2.2. The Methods of Producing the Case Study Models

2.2.1. The Physical Models

Traditional pouring and additive manufacturing/digital light processing were used to create 4 sets of experimental models. Each set (using same material and method) included 4 study models—2 maxillary and 2 mandibular; therefore, a total of 16 models were obtained (Figure 2).

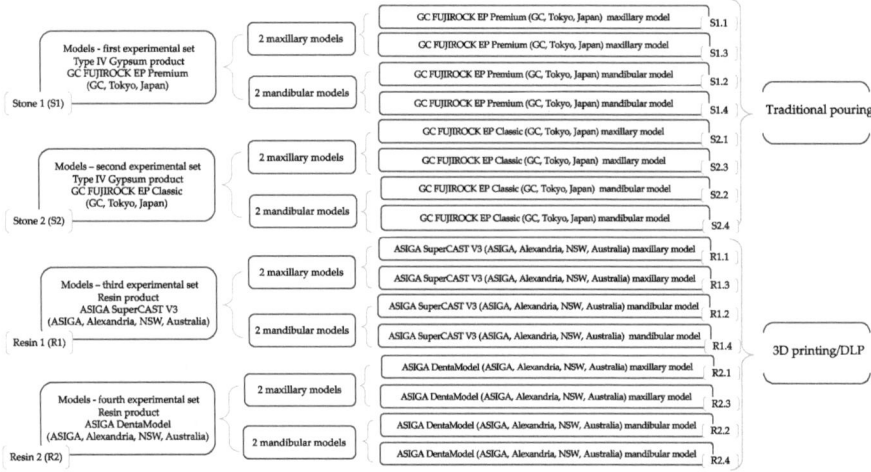

Figure 2. Experimental case study models.

Dental Stone Models

Silicon Duplicate Elite Double 22 (Zhermack SpA, Badia Polesine, Italy) was used to duplicate the models. When using Type IV gypsum powder, the manufacturer's recommended dosage of water was followed. For 30 s, the gypsum paste was molded under a vacuum to produce a homogenous paste with a semi-fluid consistency, free of air inclusions, after it was spatulated. The gypsum material was gradually poured in the mold placed on the vibration table. After 60 min, the models were removed from the molds and stored for 48 h at room temperature [31]. All models were poured by the same dental technician.

Three-Dimensionally Printed Models

The scanned images (Swing DOF Scanner—DOF, Seoul, Korea) of the recorded impressions were automatically converted to standard tessellation language (STL) format by the dedicated scanner software. The files were then imported using the Asiga Composer software, version 1.2 (ASIGA, Alexandria, NSW, Australia) to be manufactured on a digital light processing printer, 3D MAX UV Asiga (ASIGA, Alexandria, NSW, Australia).

The following settings were used:
- Support scripts: contact with the model—0.5 mm; height leveling—2 mm; support spacing—2 mm; material strength—40×; and torsion tolerance—0.
- Thickness layer—0.05 mm.
- "Fast print" mode with separation detection and anti-aliasing.

At each printing cycle, two models in a series were printed in a horizontal position (Figure 3). Each cycle lasted for approximately one hour. The printed models were stored for 24 h at room temperature [22].

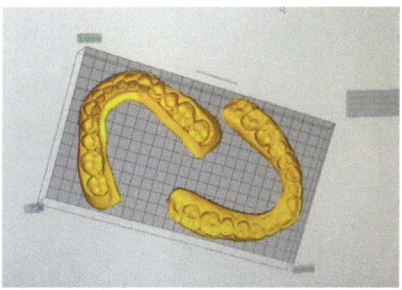 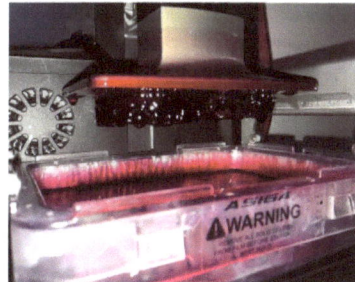

Figure 3. The 3D-printed models: from STL files to printed models.

2.2.2. The Digital Models

The digital models were created by scanning the physical ones, using a white light LED source and an L-shaped dental scanner—swing DOF (DOF, Seoul, Korea). The data were saved in an STL-format file.

2.3. Dental Measurement

We evaluated the reproducibility of dental arch characteristics, such as mesiodistal widths of incisors, canines, premolars, and first molars, as well as interpremolar and molar widths, using manual and digital linear measurements as follows:

- The upper arch interpremolar width was measured between central grooves on the occlusal surface of the first premolars.
- The superior intermolar distance was measured between mesial pits on the occlusal surface of first molars.
- The distance between the contact points of the lower premolars was assessed for the lower premolar diameter.
- The distance between the tips of the distobuccal cusps of the first lower molar was used as the point of measurement for the lower molar diameter [26–28].

2.3.1. Traditional Dental Measurement

The measurements were taken with a portable digital caliper Gedore No. 711 (GEDORE Austria GmbH, Österreich, Austria) with 0.01 mm accuracy, which was previously calibrated. Each measurement was performed twice, at one-day intervals, by the same operator. The operator was instructed to measure a maximum of 8 dental study models in a single day so that fatigue related to errors may be reduced. The procedure was repeated in order to include all of the models, and a Microsoft Excel spreadsheet was used to record the results of the measurements that were taken in millimeters. A total of 448 manual measurements were performed.

2.3.2. Modern Dental Measurement

The digital measurements made on the scanned experimental dental models followed the same guidelines. The digital models were analyzed using DentalCAD 3.0 Galway (exocad GmbH, Darmstadt, Germany). The three-dimensional images were rotated and enlarged on screen to facilitate measurements (Figure 4).

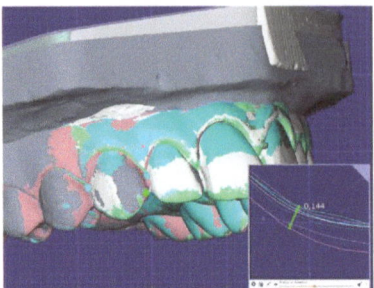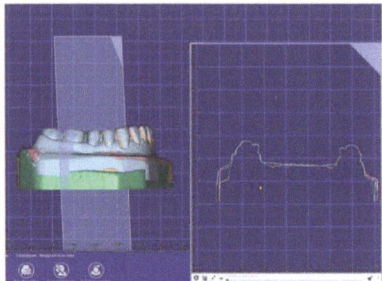

Figure 4. DentalCAD 3.0 Galway (exocad GmbH, Darmstadt, Germany) measurements on the digital study models.

A total of 14 measurements were made on each dental digital model by the same operator.

2.4. Orthodontic Model Analysis

Using these measured values for the orthodontic model analysis [26–28], the Pont and Linder–Harth indices, Bolton's anterior, and the overall ratio were calculated (Table 1).

Table 1. The formulas used to calculate the development of the arches.

Methods	Equations	
Pont index	Sum of incisors (SI) = sum of mesio-distal width of the maxillary incisors	
	Interpremolar arch widths =	$\dfrac{\text{sum of the widths of the maxillary incisors} \times 100}{80}$
	Intermolar arch widths =	$\dfrac{\text{sum of the widths of the maxillary incisors} \times 100}{64}$
Linder–Harth index	Interpremolar arch widths =	$\dfrac{\text{sum of the widths of the maxillary incisors} \times 100}{85}$
	Intermolar arch widths =	$\dfrac{\text{sum of the widths of the maxillary incisors} \times 100}{65}$
Bolton's analysis	Anterior ratio =	$\dfrac{\text{sum of the widths of the 6 mandibular anterior teeth}}{\text{sum of the widths of the 6 maxillary anterior teeth}} \times 100$
	Overall ratio =	$\dfrac{\text{sum of the widths of the 12 mandibular teeth}}{\text{sum of the widths of the 12 maxillary teeth}} \times 100$

2.5. Statistical Analysis

Statistical analysis was performed using SPSS, version 20 (SPSS Inc., Chicago, IL, USA). The obtained data were subjected to multiple Mann–Whitney U tests for pairwise comparisons among groups represented by manual and digital measurements on physical and digital models. The statistical analysis was conducted at a significance level of $p < 0.05$.

3. Results

3.1. Evaluation of the First Hypothesis

The following data were compared in order to test the first study hypothesis:

- The average values obtained by manual measurements of the mesiodistal widths of the incisors, canines, premolars, and first permanent molars, as well as the interpremolar and molar widths at the level of the traditionally models (type IV gypsum) versus 3D-printed models (resins).
- The average values acquired by digital measurements of the mesiodistal widths of the incisors, canines, premolars, and first permanent molars, as well as the interpremolar and molar widths at the level of scanned models: type IV gypsum digital model versus resin (3D printing) digital model.

- The average values produced by manual measures as opposed to digital measurements of the mesiodistal widths of the incisors, canines, premolars, and first permanent molars, as well as the interpremolar and molar widths at the level of the traditional models (type IV gypsum).
- The average values obtained by manual measurements, as opposed to digital measurements, of the mesiodistal widths of the incisors, canines, premolars, and first permanent molars, as well as of the interpremolar and molar widths at the level of the additive processing models (resins).

The findings from the statistical analysis for the maxillary and mandibular arches are shown in Tables 2 and 3.

Table 2. Maxillary pairwise comparison of the 14 studied diameters using the Mann–Whitney U test.

Pairwise Comparison		Mean Rank	p-Value [a]
Type IV gypsum versus resin DigitalCalliper	S1.1 + S1.3 + S2.1 + S2.3 DigitalCalliper	28.45	0.980
	R1.1 + R1.3 + R2.1 + R2.3 DigitalCalliper	28.55	
Type IV gypsum versus resin Exocad	S1.1 + S1.3 + S2.1 + S2.3 Exocad	28.75	0.909
	R1.1 + R1.3 + R2.1 + R2.3 Exocad	28.25	
DigitalCalliper versus Exocad Type IV gypsum products	S1.1 + S1.3 + S2.1 + S2.3 DigitalCalliper	28.50	1.000
	S1.1 + S1.3 + S2.1 + S2.3 Exocad	28.50	
DigitalCalliper versus exocad Resins	R1.1 + R1.3 + R2.1 + R2.3 DigitalCalliper	28.70	0.928
	R1.1 + R1.3 + R2.1 + R2.3 Exocad	28.30	

[a] The Mann–Whitney U test was used. The significance level was set at 0.05; S1.1—maxillary stone (GC FUJIROCK EP Premium—GC, Tokyo, Japan) model, no.1; S1.3—maxillary stone (GC FUJIROCK EP Premium—GC, Tokyo, Japan) model, no.3; S2.1—maxillary stone (GC FUJIROCK EP Classic—GC, Tokyo, Japan) model, no.1; S2.3—maxillary stone (GC FUJIROCK EP Classic—GC, Tokyo, Japan) model, no.3; R1.1—maxillary resin (ASIGA SuperCAST V3—ASIGA, Alexandria, NSW, Australia) model no.1; R1.3—maxillary resin (ASIGA SuperCAST V3—ASIGA, Alexandria, NSW, Australia) model no.3; R2.1—maxillary resin (ASIGA DentaModel—ASIGA, Alexandria, NSW, Australia) model no.1; and R2.3—maxillary resin (ASIGA DentaModel—ASIGA, Alexandria, NSW, Australia) model no.3.

Table 3. Mandibular pairwise comparison of the 14 studied diameters using the Mann–Whitney U test.

Pairwise Comparison		Mean Rank	p-Value [a]
Type IV gypsum versus resin DigitalCalliper	S1.2 + S1.4 + S2.2 + S2.4 DigitalCalliper	28.71	0.922
	R1.2 + R1.4 + R2.2 + R2.4 DigitalCalliper	28.29	
Type IV gypsum versus resin Exocad	S1.2 + S1.4 + S2.2 + S2.4 Exocad	29.09	0.787
	R1.2 + R1.4 + R2.2 + R2.4 Exocad	27.91	
DigitalCalliper versus Exocad Type IV gypsum products	S1.2 + S1.4 + S2.2 + S2.4 DigitalCalliper	27.95	0.799
	S1.2 + S1.4 + S2.2 + S2.4 Exocad	29.05	
DigitalCalliper versus Exocad Resins	R1.2 + R1.4 + R2.2 + R2.4 DigitalCalliper	28.23	0.902
	R1.2 + R1.4 + R2.2 + R2.4 Exocad	28.77	

[a] The Mann–Whitney U test was used. The significance level was set at 0.05; S1.2—mandibular stone (GC FUJIROCK EP Premium—GC, Tokyo, Japan) model no.2; S1.4—mandibular stone (GC FUJIROCK EP Premium—GC, Tokyo, Japan) model no.4; S2.2—mandibular stone (GC FUJIROCK EP Classic—GC, Tokyo, Japan) model no.2; S2.4—mandibular stone (GC FUJIROCK EP Classic—GC, Tokyo, Japan) model no.4; R1.2—mandibular resin (ASIGA SuperCAST V3—ASIGA, Alexandria, NSW, Australia) model no.2; R1.4—mandibular resin (ASIGA SuperCAST V3—ASIGA, Alexandria, NSW, Australia) model no.4; R2.2—mandibular resin (ASIGA DentaModel—ASIGA, Alexandria, NSW, Australia) model no.2; and R2.4—mandibular resin (ASIGA DentaModel—ASIGA, Alexandria, NSW, Australia) model no.4.

Even if there were differences in the mean ranks of the obtained results (with greater values recorded in digital measurements), they were not statistically significant ($p > 0.05$).

3.2. Evaluation of the Second Hypothesis

In order to evaluate the second hypothesis, the following values were compared:
- The values obtained by manual and digital measurements of the Pont index, the Linder–Harth index, and Bolton's analysis on traditionally poured versus 3D-printed models.
- The values obtained by manual versus digital measurements of the Pont index, the Linder–Harth index, and Bolton's analysis on physical and digital models.

A similar result for excessive mesiodistal mandibular teeth (Bolton's overall ratio > 91.3%) was noticed from a comparative examination of the average values obtained in the case of the investigated indices (Figures 5 and 6).

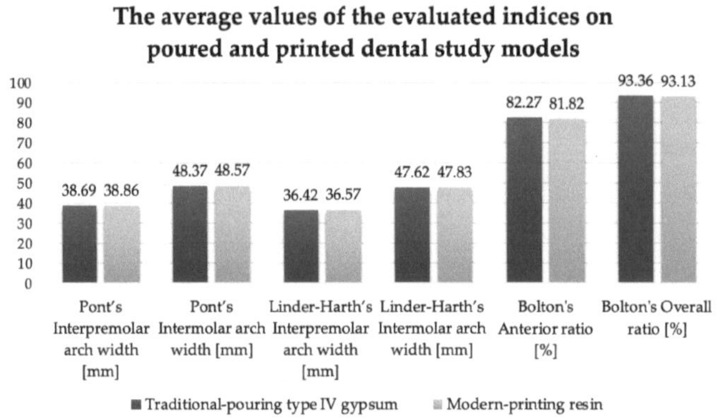

The average values of the evaluated indices on poured and printed dental study models

Index	Traditional-pouring type IV gypsum	Modern-printing resin
Pont's Interpremolar arch width [mm]	38.69	38.86
Pont's Intermolar arch width [mm]	48.37	48.57
Linder-Harth's Interpremolar arch width [mm]	36.42	36.57
Linder-Harth's Intermolar arch width [mm]	47.62	47.83
Bolton's Anterior ratio [%]	82.27	81.82
Bolton's Overall ratio [%]	93.36	93.13

Figure 5. The average values of the evaluated indices on the experimental case study models.

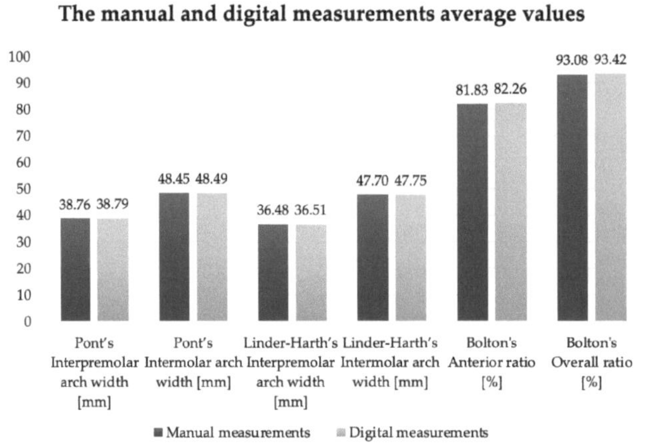

The manual and digital measurements average values

Index	Manual measurements	Digital measurements
Pont's Interpremolar arch width [mm]	38.76	38.79
Pont's Intermolar arch width [mm]	48.45	48.49
Linder-Harth's Interpremolar arch width [mm]	36.48	36.51
Linder-Harth's Intermolar arch width [mm]	47.70	47.75
Bolton's Anterior ratio [%]	81.83	82.26
Bolton's Overall ratio [%]	93.08	93.42

Figure 6. The average values of the evaluated indices by manual and digital measurements.

Table 4 shows statistically significant values for the measured indices: Pont interpremolar and intermolar arch widths ($p < 0.05$) and Linder–Harth interpremolar and intermolar arch widths ($p < 0.05$) at the level of printed models versus traditional ones. When the difference between the calculated and the measured values was evaluated, a statistically insignificant result ($p = 0.83$—Pont's and Linder–Harth's interpremolar arch widths; $p = 0.59$—Pont's and Linder–Harth's intermolar arch widths) was obtained.

Table 4. Traditional pouring versus 3D printing comparison of the analyzed indices using the Mann–Whitney U test.

Orthodontic Analysis		Traditional Pouring Versus 3D Printing	Mean Rank	p-Value [a]
Pont index	Interpremolar arch widths	Traditional pouring	2.50	0.020 *
		3D printing	6.50	
	Intermolar arch widths	Traditional pouring	2.50	0.020 *
		3D printing	6.50	
	The difference between the calculated and the measured interpremolar arch widths values	Traditional pouring	6.00	0.083
		3D printing	3.00	
	The difference between the calculated and the measured intermolar arch widths values	Traditional pouring	6.00	0.059
		3D printing	3.00	
Linder–Harth index	Interpremolar arch widths	Traditional pouring	2.50	0.021 *
		3D printing	6.50	
	Intermolar arch widths	Traditional pouring	2.50	0.020 *
		3D printing	6.50	
	The difference between the calculated and the measured interpremolar arch widths values	Traditional pouring	6.00	0.083
		3D printing	3.00	
	The difference between the calculated and the measured intermolar arch widths values	Traditional pouring	6.13	0.059
		3D printing	2.88	
Bolton's analysis	Anterior ratio	Traditional pouring	5.75	0.149
		3D printing	3.25	
	Overall ratio	Traditional pouring	5.63	0.189
		3D printing	3.38	

[a] The Mann–Whitney U test was used. * The significance level was set at 0.05.

In the case of the overall ratio (Bolton's analysis, $p < 0.05$), a statistical significance between the mean ranks of manual versus digital measurements (Table 5) was established. However, the difference between the average values was 0.34 mm, which is considered to have no clinical significance.

Table 5. Manual versus digital measurement comparison of the analyzed indices using the Mann–Whitney U test.

Orthodontic Analysis		Manual Versus Digital Measurements	Mean Rank	p-Value [a]
Pont index	Interpremolar arch widths	Manual measurements	4.50	1.000
		Digital measurements	4.50	
	Intermolar arch widths	Manual measurements	4.50	1.000
		Digital measurements	4.50	
	The difference between the calculated and the measured interpremolar arch widths values	Manual measurements	5.75	0.149
		Digital measurements	3.25	
	The difference between the calculated and the measured intermolar arch widths values	Manual measurements	4.63	0.885
		Digital measurements	4.38	

Table 5. Cont.

Orthodontic Analysis		Manual Versus Digital Measurements	Mean Rank	p-Value [a]
Linder–Harth index	Interpremolar arch widths	Manual measurements	4.50	0.885
		Digital measurements	4.50	
	Intermolar arch widths	Manual measurements	4.50	1.000
		Digital measurements	4.50	
	The difference between the calculated and the measured interpremolar arch widths values	Manual measurements	5.75	0.149
		Digital measurements	3.25	
	The difference between the calculated and the measured intermolar arch widths values	Manual measurements	4.63	0.885
		Digital measurements	4.38	
Bolton's analysis	Anterior ratio	Manual measurements	3.00	0.083
		Digital measurements	6.00	
	Overall ratio	Manual measurements	2.63	0.028 *
		Digital measurements	6.38	

[a] The Mann–Whitney U test was used. * The significance level was set at 0.05.

4. Discussion

Numerous authors highlighted dental digital models as beneficial. Some of these advantages include simpler data transmission, reduced treatment planning, and shorter diagnostic time when compared with traditional model setups and reconstruction [32–34]. However, when considering the usefulness of digital models, the following question arises: are they reliable?

Two previous systematic reviews, by Fleming et al. [35] and Luu et al. [36], respectively, compared the validity of digital model measurements with those from plaster models. According to the authors' findings, the digital model evaluations were correct.

The study results show that there were no statistically significant differences in the mean rank of the obtained linear measurement values on the physical and digital case study models, which means that the first null hypothesis was verified.

Similar findings were obtained by Sousa et al. [37], who evaluated the reliability of measurements made on 3D digital models obtained by scanning plaster models with laboratory scanners. The authors emphasized the increased ability to enlarge and rotate the pictures of the digital model image, as well as the software's simplicity of use in detecting landmarks.

Abizadeh et al. [6] found a statistically significant difference between model analysis on plaster models and digital models created by model scanning. Measurements of plaster models were more accurate than measurements of digital models due to the fact that the digital model scans were not a true 1:1 replica of the plaster ones.

The current investigation included study models obtained by full dental arch impressions with alginate material. The results indicate that printed and traditional models both properly reproduce dental arch details. In contrast, a recent study conducted by Sayed et al. [38] concluded that stone casts generated using polyvinyl siloxane and alginate impression and pouring type IV die stone have a higher linear dimensional accuracy than 3D-printed casts.

According to Nestler et al. [39], both extrusion-based and photopolymerization-based printers were precise, although Asiga MAX UV (ASIGA, Alexandria, NSW, Australia) had the highest accuracy. In contrast, Sayed et al. [38] found that the greatest number of distortions above 0.5% were produced by the digital model with full-arch-prepared abutment teeth obtained using the same printer.

Choi et al. [40] and Jin et al. [41] found no statistically significant differences between measurements taken from the physical plaster and printed models using the stereolithography method.

In a systematic review of the literature, Etemad-Shahidi et al. [42] evaluated the accuracy of full-arch dental models manufactured using different 3D-printing technologies and concluded that other factors, such as the layer thickness, base design, postprocessing, and storage can equally influence the accuracy of the resultant 3D-printed models.

It is well documented in the literature that tooth size differences (TSD) play an important role in orthodontic finalization, particularly in the front area. Knowing about TSD and other variables provides the practitioner an advantage when making a final treatment selection to achieve great results.

The existing studies on TSD used traditional measuring compasses or digital calipers to estimate mesiodistal tooth widths using plaster or digital models [43,44].

Furthermore, it is demonstrated that measurements taken from 3D digital models are a viable alternative to those taken from physical models, since storing records is faster, more reliable, and easier to complete. Accuracy is measured using digital calipers, which are widely regarded to be the gold standard [44–49].

According to the "clinically acceptable" term [48,50–52], the results of the present study reveal that the values had differences of less than 0.5 mm between traditional and 3D-printed models, as well as between manual and digital measurement methods. On the other hand, for prosthodontic applications, the accuracy requirements for dental models are often greater, and a measurement discrepancy of less than 0.2 mm was shown to be clinically acceptable in [53].

Despite minor differences in the measurements of mesiodistal tooth width and arch length on digital models, Leifert et al. [54] found that digital models were clinically acceptable and repeatable when compared to traditional models.

Wan Hassan et al. [50] questioned the accuracy of dental measurements in various degrees of crowded dentitions when measuring stone casts and reconstructed rapid prototyping models.

The findings of the current study show greater mesiodistal teeth width values recorded in digital rather than manual measurements. Similar results were also obtained by Cuperus et al.'s [55] research using an intraoral scanner to create the digital models.

The difference between manual and digital recordings, according to Naidu et al. [48], is explained by the absence of a physical barrier when placing measurement points on virtual models; the difficulty in scanning the contact points, which results in small amounts of missing data that must be interpolated by a computer algorithm; and the operator's training and proficiency, which can cause minor variations in contact point locations between the stone and digital models.

Even if—as in the case of Pont and Linder–Harth interpremolar and intermolar arch widths ($p < 0.05$) and Bolton's overall ratio ($p < 0.05$)—a statistically significant difference between the manual and digital measurements was observed, the discrepancies were deemed to have no clinical implications. In this context, the second null hypothesis must also be accepted.

The reasons for the significant differences between physical and digital study models could be a highlighted correction of tooth position, the increased accuracy of the virtual setup compared with the manual one, and the superimposition of moving objects that may affect the geometry of digital models [48,56].

Similar to other in vitro studies, this research had several limitations. One limitation was that only one laboratory scanner, one type of 3D printer, and one software for digital measurements were employed. Another limitation was the difficulty of measuring tooth widths with a digital caliper on physical mandibular models due to access and the difficulty of resting at the exact mesial and distal landmarks in crowded areas.

Digital technology limitations were represented by the scanning procedure (the accuracy of physical models may be affected when imaging powder is applied to them before scanning), the "shape assumption" problem, which occurs when the software uses a computer algorithm to fill the interproximal inaccurate or uncaptured data, and the process of printing, which can produce its own errors [57,58].

Additional research is needed to evaluate the accuracy of dental case study models obtained using various scanners (intraoral and laboratory), printers, and production parameters, with measurements made using dedicated applications.

5. Conclusions

Within the limitations of the current study, it can be concluded that the precision of digital measurements of teeth widths, using DentalCAD 3.0 Galway (exocad GmbH, Darmstadt, Germany) on digital models, was comparable to direct measurements with a portable digital caliper Gedore No. 711 (GEDORE Austria GmbH, Österreich, Austria) on physical dental models.

Digital measurements of mesiodistal teeth width showed higher values compared with manual ones; therefore, the difference between the average values recorded had no clinical significance.

For orthodontic teaching purposes, dental study models manufactured by direct light processing (DLP) and traditional pouring are both acceptable.

Author Contributions: Conceptualization, E.-R.B., C.I.L., A.M., G.L.G., I.N.Z., D.D.-P. and M.T.; methodology, E.-R.B., C.I.L., A.M., G.L.G., I.N.Z., D.D.-P. and M.T.; software, G.N., D.G.B. and R.-I.V.; validation, I.L., D.G.B. and R.-I.V.; investigation, E.-R.B., C.I.L., A.M., G.L.G., I.N.Z., D.D.-P. and M.T.; resources, E.-R.B., C.I.L., A.M., G.L.G., I.N.Z., D.D.-P. and M.T.; writing—original draft preparation, E.-R.B., C.I.L., A.M., G.L.G., I.N.Z., D.D.-P. and M.T.; writing—review and editing, D.G.B. and R.-I.V.; visualization, D.G.B. and R.-I.V.; supervision, I.L.; project administration, I.L. All authors have read and agreed to the published version of the manuscript.

Funding: This research received no external funding.

Institutional Review Board Statement: The study was carried out in accordance with the latest version of the Declaration of Helsinki and was approved by the Research Ethic Committee of the University of Medicine and Pharmacy, Iasi, Romania (Number: 196/03.06.2022).

Informed Consent Statement: Informed consent was obtained from the subject involved in the study.

Data Availability Statement: The data that support the findings of this study are available on request from the corresponding author.

Acknowledgments: We would like to thank Drăghici Dental, Iași, Romania, for providing us all the experimental models and for the technical assistance regarding digital measurements.

Conflicts of Interest: The authors declare no conflict of interest.

References

1. Pachêco-Pereira, C.; De Luca Canto, G.; Major, P.W.; Flores-Mir, C. Variation of orthodontic treatment decision-making based on dental model type: A systematic review. *Angle Orthod.* **2015**, *85*, 501–509. [CrossRef]
2. Marty, M.; Broutin, A.; Vergnes, J.N.; Vaysse, F. Comparison of student's perceptions between 3D printed models versus series models in paediatric dentistry hands-on session. *Eur. J. Dent. Educ.* **2019**, *23*, 68–72. [CrossRef] [PubMed]
3. Pozzi, A.; Arcuri, L.; Lio, F.; Papa, A.; Nardi, A.; Londono, J. Accuracy of complete-arch digital implant impression with or without scanbody splinting: An in vitro study. *J. Dent.* **2022**, *119*, 104072. [CrossRef] [PubMed]
4. De Francesco, M.; Stellini, E.; Granata, S.; Mazzoleni, S.; Ludovichetti, F.S.; Monaco, C.; Di Fiore, A. Assessment of Fit on Ten Screw-Retained Frameworks Realized through Digital Full-Arch Implant Impression. *Appl. Sci.* **2021**, *11*, 5617. [CrossRef]
5. Amin, S.; Weber, H.P.; Finkelman, M.; El Rafie, K.; Kudara, Y.; Papaspyridakos, P. Digital vs. conventional full-arch implant impressions: A comparative study. *Clin. Oral Implant. Res.* **2017**, *28*, 1360–1367. [CrossRef]
6. Abizadeh, N.; Moles, D.R.; O'Neill, J.; Noar, J.H. Digital versus plaster study models: How accurate and reproducible are they? *J. Orthod.* **2012**, *39*, 151–159. [CrossRef] [PubMed]
7. Akdeniz, B.S.; Aykaç, V.; Turgut, M.; Çetin, S. Digital dental models in orthodontics: A review. *J. Exp. Clin. Med.* **2022**, *39*, 250–255.
8. Gül Amuk, N.; Karsli, E.; Kurt, G. Comparison of dental measurements between conventional plaster models, digital models obtained by impression scanning and plaster model scanning. *Int. Orthod.* **2019**, *17*, 151–158. [CrossRef] [PubMed]
9. Horton, H.M.; Miller, J.R.; Gaillard, P.R.; Larson, B.E. Technique comparison for efficient orthodontic tooth measurements using digital models. *Angle Orthod.* **2010**, *80*, 254–261. [CrossRef]
10. Goriuc, A.; Jităreanu, A.; Mârțu, I.; Dascălu, C.G.; Kappenberg-Nițescu, D.C.; Solomon, S.M.; Mârțu, A.; Foia, L.; Țapu, I.; Istrate, B.; et al. Experimental EDX analysis of different periodontal splinting systems. *Exp. Ther. Med.* **2021**, *22*, 1384. [CrossRef]

11. Baciu, E.R.; Cimpoeșu, R.; Vițalariu, A.; Baciu, C.; Cimpoeșu, N.; Sodor, A.; Zegan, G.; Murariu, A. Surface Analysis of 3D (SLM) Co–Cr–W Dental Metallic Materials. *Appl. Sci.* **2021**, *11*, 255. [CrossRef]
12. Mârțu, I.; Murariu, A.; Baciu, E.R.; Savin, C.N.; Foia, I.; Tatarciuc, M.; Diaconu-Popa, D. An Interdisciplinary Study Regarding the Characteristics of Dental Resins Used for Temporary Bridges. *Medicina* **2022**, *58*, 811. [CrossRef] [PubMed]
13. Tancu, A.M.; Pantea, M.; Totan, A.; Tanase, M.; Imre, A. 3D Printed Dental Models-A comparative analysis, Rev. *Mater. Plast.* **2019**, *56*, 51–54. [CrossRef]
14. Alharbi, N.; Wismeijer, D.; Osman, R.B. Additive manufacturing techniques in prosthodontics: Where do we currently stand? a critical review. *Int. J. Prosthodont.* **2017**, *30*, 474–484. [CrossRef] [PubMed]
15. Hussein, M.O.; Hussein, L.A. Optimization of Digital Light Processing Three-Dimensional Printing of the Removable Partial Denture Frameworks; The Role of Build Angle and Support Structure Diameter. *Materials* **2022**, *15*, 2316. [CrossRef] [PubMed]
16. Unkovskiy, A.; Schmidt, F.; Beuer, F.; Li, P.; Spintzyk, S.; Kraemer Fernandez, P. Stereolithography vs. Direct Light Processing for Rapid Manufacturing of Complete Denture Bases: An In Vitro Accuracy Analysis. *J. Clin. Med.* **2021**, *10*, 1070. [CrossRef] [PubMed]
17. Tzivelekis, C.; Sgardelis, P.; Waldron, K.; Whalley, R.; Huo, D.; Dalgarno, K. Fabrication routes via projection stereolithography for 3D-printing of microfluidic geometries for nucleic acid amplification. *PLoS ONE* **2020**, *15*, e0240237. [CrossRef]
18. Shaikh, S.; Nahar, P.; Ali, H.M. Current perspectives of 3d printing in dental applications. *Braz. Dent. Sci.* **2021**, *24*, 1–9. [CrossRef]
19. Iliescu, A.A.; Perlea, P.; Iliescu, M.G.; Gorea, V.; Nicolau, G. Printarea 3D în tehnologia dentara-statusul actual. *Med. Stomatol.* **2017**, *45*, 9–13.
20. Ender, A.; Mehl, A. Accuracy of complete-arch dental impressions: A new method of measuring trueness and precision. *J. Prosthet. Dent.* **2013**, *109*, 121–128. [CrossRef]
21. Pantea, M.; Ciocoiu, R.; Tancu, A.M.C.; Nină, D.M.; Petre, A.; Antoniac, I.V.; Melescanu-Imre, M. Comparative Study on Two Methods Used in Obtaining 3D Printed Dental Models. *Mater. Plast.* **2019**, *56*, 812. [CrossRef]
22. Joda, T.; Matthisson, L.; Zitzmann, N.U. Impact of Aging on the Accuracy of 3D-Printed Dental Models: An In Vitro Investigation. *J. Clin. Med.* **2020**, *9*, 1436. [CrossRef]
23. Fernandez, C.C.A.; Pereira, C.V.C.A.; Luiz, R.R.; Vieira, A.R.; De Castro Costa, M. Dental anomalies in different growth and skeletal malocclusion patterns. *Angle Orthod.* **2018**, *88*, 195–201. [CrossRef] [PubMed]
24. Devi, L.B.; Keisam, A.; Singh, H.P. Malocclusion and occlusal traits among dental and nursing students of Seven North-East states of India. *J. Oral Biol. Craniofac. Res.* **2022**, *12*, 86–89. [CrossRef] [PubMed]
25. Uslu, O.; Akcam, M.O.; Evirgen, S.; Cebeci, I. Prevalence of dental anomalies in various malocclusions. *Am. J. Orthod. Dentofac. Orthop.* **2009**, *135*, 328–335. [CrossRef]
26. Rykman, A.; Smailiene, D. Application of Pont's Index to Lithuanian Individuals: A Pilot Study. *J. Oral Maxillofac. Res.* **2015**, *6*, e4. [CrossRef]
27. Domenyuk, D.A.; Vedeshina, E.G.; Dmitrienko, S.V. Mistakes in Pont (Linder-Harth) method used for diagnosing abnormal dental arches in transversal plane. *Arch. Euromed.* **2016**, *6*, 23–26.
28. Bolton, W. The clinical application of a tooth-size analysis. *Am. J. Orthod.* **1962**, *48*, 504–529. [CrossRef]
29. Mollabashi, V.; Soltani, M.K.; Moslemian, N.; Akhlaghian, M.; Akbarzadeh, M.; Samavat, H.; Abolvardi, M. Comparison of Bolton ratio in normal occlusion and different malocclusion groups in Iranian population. *Int. Orthod.* **2019**, *17*, 143–150. [CrossRef]
30. Wadhwa, S.S.; Mehta, R.; Duggal, N.; Vasudeva, K. The effect of pouring time on the dimensional accuracy of casts made from different irreversible hydrocolloid impression materials. *Contemp. Clin. Dent.* **2013**, *3*, 313–318. [CrossRef]
31. Millstein, P.L. Determining the accuracy of gypsum casts made from type IV dental stone. *J. Oral Rehabil.* **1992**, *19*, 239–243. [CrossRef]
32. Shastry, S.; Park, J.H. Evaluation of the use of digital study models in postgraduate orthodontic programs in the United States and Canada. *Angle Orthod.* **2014**, *84*, 62–67. [CrossRef]
33. Palmer, N.G.; Yacyshyn, J.R.; Northcott, H.C.; Nebbe, B.; Major, P.W. Perceptions and attitudes of Canadian orthodontists regarding digital and electronic technology. *Am. J. Orthod. Dentofac. Orthop.* **2005**, *128*, 163–167. [CrossRef] [PubMed]
34. Kuroda, T.; Motohashi, N.; Tominaga, R.; Iwata, K. Three-dimensional dental cast analyzing system using laser scanning. *Am. J. Orthod. Dentofac. Orthop.* **1996**, *110*, 365–369. [CrossRef]
35. Fleming, P.S.; Marinho, V.; Johal, A. Orthodontic measurements on digital study models compared with plaster models: A systematic review. *Orthod. Craniofac. Res.* **2011**, *14*, 1–16. [CrossRef]
36. Luu, N.S.; Nikolcheva, L.G.; Retrouvey, J.M.; Flores-Mir, C.; El-Bialy, T.; Carey, J.P.; Major, P.W. Linear measurements using virtual study models. *Angle Orthod.* **2012**, *82*, 1098–1106. [CrossRef]
37. Sousa, M.V.; Vasconcelos, E.C.; Janson, G.; Garib, D.; Pinzan, A. Accuracy and reproducibility of 3-dimensional digital model measurements. *Am. J. Orthod. Dentofac. Orthop.* **2012**, *142*, 269–273. [CrossRef] [PubMed]
38. Sayed, M.E.; Al-Mansour, H.; Alshehri, A.H.; Al-Sanabani, F.; Al-Makramani, B.M.A.; Mugri, M.H.; Ahmed, W.M.; Alqahtani, N.M.; Bukhary, D.M.; Alsurayyie, F.H.; et al. Accuracy of Master Casts Generated Using Conventional and Digital Impression Modalities: Part 2—The Full Arch Dimension. *Appl. Sci.* **2022**, *12*, 2148. [CrossRef]
39. Nestler, N.; Wesemann, C.; Spies, B.C.; Beuer, F.; Bumann, A. Dimensional accuracy of extrusion- and photopolymerization-based 3D printers: In vitro study comparing printed casts. *J. Prosthet. Dent.* **2021**, *125*, 103–110. [CrossRef]

40. Choi, W.J.; Lee, S.J.; Moon, C.H. Evaluation of accuracy of 3-dimensional printed dental models in reproducing intermaxillary relational measurements: Based on inter-operator differences. *Korean J. Orthod.* **2022**, *52*, 20–28. [CrossRef]
41. Jin, S.J.; Kim, D.Y.; Kim, J.H.; Kim, W.C. Accuracy of Dental Replica Models Using Photopolymer Materials in Additive Manufacturing: In Vitro Three-Dimensional Evaluation. *J. Prosthodont.* **2019**, *28*, e557–e562. [CrossRef] [PubMed]
42. Etemad-Shahidi, Y.; Qallandar, O.B.; Evenden, J.; Alifui-Segbaya, F.; Ahmed, K.E. Accuracy of 3-Dimensionally Printed Full-Arch Dental Models: A Systematic Review. *J. Clin. Med.* **2020**, *9*, 3357. [CrossRef] [PubMed]
43. Tomassetti, J.J.; Taloumis, L.J.; Denny, J.M.; Fischer, M.S., Jr. A comparison of 3 computerized Bolton tooth-size analyses with a commonly used method. *Angle Orthod.* **2001**, *71*, 351–357. [PubMed]
44. Zilberman, O.; Huggare, J.A.; Parikakis, K.A. Evaluation of the validity of tooth size and arch width measurements using conventional and three-dimensional virtual orthodontic models. *Angle Orthod.* **2003**, *73*, 301–306.
45. O'Mahony, G.; Millett, D.T.; Barry, M.K.; McIntyre, G.T.; Cronin, M.S. Tooth size discrepancies in Irish orthodontic patients among different malocclusion group. *Angle Orthod.* **2011**, *81*, 130–133. [CrossRef]
46. Zerouaoui, M.F.; Bahije, L.; Zaoui, F.; Regragui, S. Study of variations of the Bolton index in the Moroccan population depending on Angle malocclusion class. *Int. Orthod.* **2014**, *12*, 213–221. [CrossRef]
47. Stevens, D.R.; Flores-Mir, C.; Nebbe, B.; Raboud, D.W.; Heo, G.; Major, P.W. Validity, reliability, and reproducibility of plaster vs. digital study models: Comparison of peer assessment rating and Bolton analysis and their constituent measurements. *Am. J. Orthod. Dentofac. Orthop.* **2006**, *129*, 794–803. [CrossRef]
48. Naidu, D.; Freer, T.J. Validity, reliability, and reproducibility of the iOC intraoral scanner: A comparison of tooth widths and Bolton ratios. *Am. J. Orthod. Dentofac. Orthop.* **2013**, *144*, 304–410. [CrossRef]
49. Bowes, M.; Dear, W.; Close, E.; Freer, T.J. Tooth width measurement using the Lythos digital scanner. *Aust. Orthod. J.* **2017**, *33*, 73–81. [CrossRef]
50. Wan Hassan, W.N.; Yusoff, Y.; Mardi, N.A. Comparison of reconstructed rapid prototyping models produced by 3-dimensional printing and conventional stone models with different degrees of crowding. *Am. J. Orthod. Dentofac. Orthop.* **2017**, *151*, 209–218. [CrossRef]
51. Hirogaki, Y.; Sohmura, T.; Satoh, H.; Takahashi, J.; Takada, K. Complete 3-D reconstruction of dental cast shape using perceptual grouping. *IEEE Trans. Med. Imaging* **2001**, *20*, 1093–1101. [CrossRef]
52. Bell, A.; Ayoub, A.F.; Siebert, P. Assessment of the accuracy of a three-dimensional imaging system for archiving dental study models. *J. Orthod.* **2003**, *30*, 219–223. [CrossRef] [PubMed]
53. Papaspyridakos, P.; Chen, Y.-W.; AlShawaf, B.; Kang, K.; Finkelman, M.; Chronopoulos, V.; Weber, H.-P. Digital workflow: In vitro accuracy of 3D printed casts generated from complete-arch digital implant scans. *J. Prosthet. Dent.* **2020**, *124*, 589–593. [CrossRef] [PubMed]
54. Leifert, M.F.; Leifert, M.M.; Efstratiadis, S.S.; Cangialosi, T.J. Comparison of space analysis evaluations with digital models and plaster dental casts. *Am. J. Orthod. Dentofac. Orthop.* **2009**, *136*, 16.e1–16.e4. [CrossRef]
55. Cuperus, A.M.; Harms, M.C.; Rangel, F.A.; Bronkhorst, E.M.; Schols, J.G.; Breuning, K.H. Dental models made with an intraoral scanner: A validation study. *Am. J. Orthod. Dentofac. Orthop.* **2012**, *142*, 308–313. [CrossRef]
56. Rossini, G.; Parrini, S.; Castroflorio, T.; Deregibus, A.; Debernardi, C.L. Diagnostic accuracy and measurement sensitivity of digital models for orthodontic purposes: A systematic review. *Am. J. Orthod. Dentofac. Orthop.* **2016**, *149*, 161–170. [CrossRef]
57. Alrasheed, W.A.; Owayda, A.M.; Hajeer, M.Y.; Khattab, T.Z.; Almahdi, W.H. Validity and Reliability of Intraoral and Plaster Models' Photographs in the Assessment of Little's Irregularity Index, Tooth Size-Arch Length Discrepancy, and Bolton's Analysis. *Cureus* **2022**, *14*, e23067. [CrossRef]
58. Morton, J.; Derakhshan, M.; Kaza, S.; Li, C. Design of the Invisalign system performance. *Semin. Orthod.* **2017**, *23*, 3–11. [CrossRef]

MDPI AG
Grosspeteranlage 5
4052 Basel
Switzerland
Tel.: +41 61 683 77 34

Medicina Editorial Office
E-mail: medicina@mdpi.com
www.mdpi.com/journal/medicina

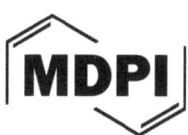

Disclaimer/Publisher's Note: The statements, opinions and data contained in all publications are solely those of the individual author(s) and contributor(s) and not of MDPI and/or the editor(s). MDPI and/or the editor(s) disclaim responsibility for any injury to people or property resulting from any ideas, methods, instructions or products referred to in the content.

www.ingramcontent.com/pod-product-compliance
Lightning Source LLC
LaVergne TN
LVHW072316090526
838202LV00019B/2298